S0-AUZ-170

BARRON'S

GUIDE TO MEDICAL AND DENTAL SCHOOLS

EIGHTH EDITION

by
Dr. Saul Wischnitzer
with Edith Wischnitzer

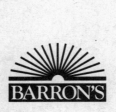

BARRON'S

© Copyright 1997 by Barron's Educational Series, Inc.
Prior editions © 1995, 1993, 1991, 1989, 1987, 1985, 1982 by
Barron's Educational Series, Inc.

Portions adapted from *Barron's Guide to Medical, Dental, and
Allied Health Science Careers* by Saul Wischnitzer.

All rights reserved.
No part of this book may be reproduced in any form, by
photostat, microfilm, xerography, or any other means, or
incorporated into any information retrieval system,
electronic or mechanical, without the written permission
of the copyright owner.

All inquiries should be addressed to:
Barron's Educational Series, Inc.
250 Wireless Boulevard
Hauppauge, NY 11788

Library of Congress Catalog Card No. 96-47470

International Standard Book No. 0-8120-9788-2

Library of Congress Cataloging-in-Publication Data

Wischnitzer, Saul.
    Barron's guide to medical & dental schools / Saul
Wischnitzer, with Edith Wischnitzer.—8th ed.
        p.   cm.
    "Portions adapted from Barron's guide to medical,
dental, and allied health science careers by Saul
Wischnitzer"—T.p. verso.
    Includes bibliographical references and index.
    ISBN 0-8120-9788-2
    1. Medicine—Vocational guidance. 2. Dentistry—
Vocational guidance. 3. Osteopathic medicine—
Vocational guidance. I. Wischnitzer, Edith.
II. Wischnitzer, Saul. Barron's guide to medical,
dental, and allied health science careers. III. Title.
R690.W558   1997
610'.71'173—dc21   96-47470
                                       CIP

PRINTED IN THE UNITED STATES OF AMERICA
98765432

CONTENTS

LIST OF TABLES

LIST OF SAMPLE DOCUMENTS

ACKNOWLEDGMENTS

Acknowledgment is made to the following organizations for allowing us to reprint copyrighted or previously published material in this book.

The American Association of Colleges of Osteopathic Medicine for permitting us to reprint the current AACOMAS application form.

The American Dental Association Survey Center for allowing us to use data in Tables 17.1, 17.2, and 19.1 from its Annual Supplemental Reports on Dental Education 1994–95, as well as for the sample DAT material used in Chapter 18.

New York University School of Medicine for permitting us to reprint its current application form.

Hugo R. Seibel and Kenneth E. Guyer for permission to reprint a Model MCAT exam from their book *Barron's How to Prepare for the Medical College Admission Test*, 8th edition. © copyright 1997 by Barron's Educational Series, Inc.

The efforts and cooperation of Ms. Max Reed, Senior Editor for this book at Barron's, is very much appreciated.

DEDICATION

This book is dedicated to our children, Judah and Rachel, whose help, cooperation, and encouragement made its publication possible. We are especially grateful to our son who applied his computer skills in preparing the format for the data capsules for all the professional schools. His contribution has significantly enhanced both the appearance and value of this book.

PREFACE

Of the many decisions facing you, the choice of a career is among the most important and it obviously requires very careful consideration. The competitive nature of our contemporary society has created marked pressures for an early choice, but the selection of a career is best determined after evaluation of your interests, abilities, and life goals. If you are considering medicine or dentistry, you will need the most current information about schools, admissions policies, and educational programs, as well as up-to-date data, to make the most realistic decision to overcome the barriers to success.

This book has been written to help you arrive at a decision and to provide you with both facts and advice on planning a career in medicine or dentistry, starting with high school and continuing through college and into professional school. The author has attempted to answer the most basic questions and to provide you with sources for more detailed information. Sound advice and current information are not only essential because of the strong competition that exists today, but also necessary because of the rapidly changing nature of medical education.

While your ultimate success naturally will depend on your abilities, the advice presented in this book can help you make the decisions that must be made during high school and college, which can be so crucial to achieving your goals.

In 1974 *Barron's Guide to Medical, Dental, and Allied Health Science Careers* was published. The favorable reception it was given resulted in the publication of new editions of the book in 1975 and 1977. With the very rapid increase in interest in health science careers, an expanded fourth edition of the book would have resulted in a volume that would be too cumbersome to be readily useful as a handbook for prospective students. Thus, it was decided to publish the book as two separate volumes: one dealing with medicine and dentistry, and the other, *Futures in Health,* with the allied health sciences. This volume is the eighth edition of the former.

Medicine and dentistry have been combined into a single volume because they are closely related. Among the considerations that they have in common are the facts that: (1) at the outset of one's study of the biological sciences in high school, a choice between the two careers need not be made; (2) a definitive career decision can, if necessary, be deferred until the junior year of college because of their common educational pathway; (3) in some special cases applying to both medical and dental school may be desirable; (4) at some institutions medical and dental students take courses in the basic sciences together; (5) dental clinics are often located in hospitals that are centers for postgraduate medical as well as dental training; (6) medicine and dentistry sometimes overlap, especially in surgical specialties relating to the mouth and neck. As a result of the interrelationship of these two sciences some dental schools award the Doctor of Dental Medicine (DMD) degree rather than the traditional Doctor of Dental Surgery (DDS) degree.

In preparing this eighth edition, the book has been completely redesigned in format and thus its appearance has radically changed. For the first seven editions this manual was published in double column format. This has been altered (except for school profiles) to a single column, which, along with a larger and more attractive type size, significantly enhances the book's readability. In addition, data summaries have been inserted at the beginning of each school's profile. Supplementing these dramatic changes are 18 others of major significance, enumerated below.

In preparing this new edition, the facts and statistics have been updated so the book is optimally current. The following major changes or additions have been introduced: (1) All medical and dental school profiles have been reviewed and, where required, updated. (2) The comprehensive data in Tables 5.1, 7.1, 10.1, and 21.3 have been made current. (3) A discussion of enhancing memorization is presented. (4) How to succeed as a premedical student is analyzed. (5) The admission of disabled students is discussed. (4) The meaning of rejection is evaluated. (5) A detailed explanation for using Table 5.1,

Basic Data on the Medical Schools, has been added. (6) The in-depth medical school profiles have been placed in a separate chapter (Chapter 6) along with an explanation of their use. (7) The chapter on opportunities for women (Chapter 7) has been greatly expanded and significantly revised. (8) The listing of summer programs for minority groups has been updated. (9) A section on successfully managing educational indebtness has been added to Chapter 9, Financing Your Medical Education. (10) Evolving new medical curricula are discussed. (11) A new chapter on postgraduate education and training (Chapter 11) has been added. (12) The discussion of family practice (primary care) has been expanded. (13) A presentation of the curriculum of each osteopathic school has been added. (14) Practice options for physicians beginning their careers are presented and detailed. (15) A new chapter, Physicians and Medicine in the Twenty-First Century, has been introduced (Chapter 15). (16) The number of sample DAT questions has been expanded, and more sample essays for the AMCAS application have been added. (17) Appendix F, providing Tracking Tables that organize the application process, has been added. (18) Information on the World Wide Web as related to medical and dental applications is included in Appendix H.

The new material has, in part, been added because prospective physicians should become aware of the changing climate in medicine, which will undoubtedly have a significant impact on their professional lives. Medical practice has been revolutionized by dramatic improvements in the diagnosis and treatment of diseases. This has resulted in changing medical practitioners from generalists to specialists. These improvements have also resulted in increasing the expectations of the public as to what can be delivered in the way of patient care. The failure to meet these expectations has resulted in increasing numbers of malpractice suits.

There has also been a profound increase in patient service needs as a result of the fact that Medicare and Medicaid subsidize a large part of health care costs, which have been increased dramatically. Governmental financing of such programs has given the government significant power in the regulation of many phases of medical practice (such as the length of a patient's stay in a hospital and the level of reimbursement for services).

Some material in this edition stems in large measure from the author's experience as a private, professional advisor of premedical and predental students. This has added a broader dimension to the book's perspective, as a result of exposure to a large pool of individuals with a variety of pre- and postcollegiate backgrounds at many different schools.

Finally, the reader should know that this manual is designed to do more than assist you in a very comprehensive way, in your quest to gain admission to professional school. It serves, especially for those seeking careers in medicine, as a guide into and through your postgraduate training on both the residency and fellowship levels. It also gives you an insight into the options available when you consider entering medical practice. Thus, depending at what point in your education you begin to make use of this book, it can be of service for many years and thus should be kept readily available as a permanent part of your personal library.

The author welcomes comments from readers. Please send them to the publisher at the address on the copyright page.

Saul Wischnitzer, PhD
Queens, New York
February 1997

ABBREVIATIONS

AACOMAS	American Association of Colleges of Osteopathic Medicine Application Service
AADS	American Association of Dental Schools
AADSAS	American Association of Dental Schools Application Service
AAMC	Association of American Medical Colleges
AMA	American Medical Association
AMCAS	American Medical College Application Service
AMSA	American Medical Student Association
AOA	American Osteopathic Association
CACMS	Committee on Accreditation of Canadian Medical Schools
CDA	Commission on Dental Accreditation
COTRANS	Coordinated Transfer Application System
DAT	Dental Admission Test
FLEX	Federation Licensing Examinations
GPA	grade point average
HMO	Health Maintenance Organization
IMG	International Medical Graduate
IPA	Independent Practitioners' Association
LCME	Liaison Committee on Medical Education
MCAT	Medical College Admission Test
Med-MAR	Medical Minority Applicant Registry
MSKP	Medical Sciences Knowledge Profile
MSTP	Medical Scientist Training Program
NBME	National Board of Medical Examiners
NIH	National Institute of Health
NIRMP	National Intern and Resident Matching Program
OMSAS	Ontario Medical School Application Service
PPA	Private Practitioners' Association
USMLE	United States Medical Licensing Examination
WAMI	Wyoming, Alaska, Montana, Idaho
WHO	World Health Organization
WICHE	Western Interstate Commission for Higher Education

PART ONE

MEDICINE

---

1 Medicine as a Career

On being a physician
Why study medicine?
Historical overview
The need for physicians
Physician surplus: current debate
Desirable attributes for a medical career
The challenge to becoming a physician

ON BEING A PHYSICIAN

Physicians are acknowledged practitioners of the art of medicine. They are expected to be people of high ethical standards since they are entrusted with the intimate details of life and death. They are expected to have the capacity and enthusiasm for difficult work extended over long hours, and they must be able to perform efficiently under a chronic load of heavy responsibility.

Physicians are expected to be able to reason quickly and accurately and to have life-long desires to continually add to their accumulated body of medical knowledge by learning about new developments in their profession. They are expected to be able to communicate with their patients in order to teach them hygienic measures and to adequately explain the nature and significance of a disease. They are also expected to be willing to serve the community in a capacity beyond that of their professional training. Physicians are people who have ordinary physical and emotional needs, yet who have a great purpose in life. Their practice can be the source of enrichment of their own life as well as the lives of others.

When setting your sights toward a medical career, your goal should be to become a *good* physician. Ideally, this means becoming a doctor who will (1) blend book knowledge with common sense; (2) provide compassion with candor; (3) strive to maintain perspective by focusing on the whole patient rather than solely on the disease; (4) allow time to listen to those seeking help; (5) perceive the real meaning of the patient's words; (6) communicate with patients in a way they can easily understand; (7) think independently; (8) rely on your own mind and clinical judgment; (9) utilize tests and consultants to verify hypotheses; (10) be aware of limitations of lab procedures; (11) be cognizant of your own fallibility; and (12) not be afraid to admit when you don't know something.

WHY STUDY MEDICINE?

The medical profession offers much to a young person. It provides an avenue for attaining satisfaction of many of the most fundamental human desires. Medicine can satisfy your intellectual curiosity; it permits you to successfully apply the enormous body of information that has been accumulated in recent decades to reduce pain and suffering and extend the average life span. At the same time, it presents the challenge of the many unsolved problems that await solution through laboratory or hospital work.

Medicine can satisfy your desire for human service by enabling you to bring help and comfort to others. Medicine can satisfy your desire to work in a profession that has prestige. While prestige is no longer granted automatically, it does come with the faithful discharge of responsibilities and obligations. Medicine can also satisfy your desire for a substantial income. This income, which is superior to that of most other professions, is earned by the long and difficult hours demanded of the physician. Medicine is a profession that can, to a significant extent, satisfy your desire for independent and individual achievement in a society that is becoming increasingly overstructured.

An MD degree and the completion of all three components of the United States Medical Licensing Examination (USMLE) enables you to practice medicine anywhere in the United States. With this degree, you can care for people at all stages: you can bring them into the world, treat their childhood and young adult illnesses, help them deal with their middle-age crises, and assist them in coping with the increasingly frequent and troublesome illnesses of advancing years.

If teaching appeals to you, you can enjoy guiding the next generation of physicians. Educating medical students, residents, and postdoctoral fellows will enhance your own creative abilities and stimulate your own thought processes.

If you have a flair for writing, there is a vast potential to use literary expression in writing lucid scientific papers, analytic essays, or even nonscientific works. Just remember the background of Arthur Conan Doyle, W. Somerset Maugham, or Lewis Thomas, to mention a few prominent physician-writers.

Should laboratory work be more to your liking, with suitable postdoctoral training (or an MD-PhD degree), you may want to become involved in valuable research that can lead to finding cures for diseases and possible disease prevention. Much work is being done today in the field of genetic engineering, which impacts greatly on congenital disorders and various metabolic abnormalities.

Medicine therefore represents the broadest spectrum of opportunities for an individual to render service to others while at the same time attaining his or her own goals in life in a satisfying manner. Medicine provides the widest range of career options in a variety of roles, such as small-town doctor, family practitioner, specialist, superspecialist, clinical investigator, academician, public health officer, administrator, and varying combinations of these positions. Making the choice, rather than having the choice, is the issue medical students and residents face at some point in their training.

HISTORICAL OVERVIEW

In seeking to become a physician, you are planning to join a fraternity of professional men and women who have a profound influence, both physically and emotionally, on the lives of many millions of people. The roots of medicine penetrate deeply into the history of humankind. Cave paintings reveal the existence of "healers" as far back as the Ice Age. The medical practitioners of ancient China developed acupuncture and a smallpox vaccination method. Western medicine is indebted to the "scientific" approach developed in ancient Greece and Rome by men such as Hippocrates and Galen. These advances were preserved through the Dark Ages by the Arab world. In medieval Europe medical science stagnated until the rebirth of learning and experimentation in the Renaissance.

In the United States during the colonial era, medicine was largely a hit-or-miss affair. The pushing of the frontiers westward developed a pioneer type of doctor. A step forward was achieved in the last half of the eighteenth century when medical schools in the United States began conferring the MD degree and it was no longer necessary to journey abroad to obtain one. In 1910 the Flexner report, Medical Education in the United States and Canada, brought about a revolution in medical education and placed it on a sound basis by establishing standardized requirements of medical education. Flexner's basic recommendations included the following:

1. Medical education should be conducted in the context of a university. This would help ensure that students would gain a scientifically oriented foundation for the practice of medicine.

2. Schools should be changed from a "diploma mill" or trade school status to that of providing a professional school education.

3. The upgraded medical schools should be provided with a full-time faculty, because practicing physicians lacked time to devote themselves adequately to teaching.

Flexner's report resulted in a drastic reduction in the number of then-existing medical schools.

The impact of the Flexner report extended far beyond improving the quality of medical education. Ultimately it was responsible for the preeminence in biomedical research and the development of specialty medicine in this country.

Well before the turn of this century, Americans made major contributions to medical science, especially in the battle against infectious diseases. In the last half of the twentieth century, American medicine has become a world leader. Thus, to become a physician means entering a fellowship with a healing tradition that extends back to the beginnings of civilization.

Highlights in American medical education are summarized below:

1765—University of Pennsylvania opens the nation's first medical school.
1848—Elizabeth Blackwell is the first American woman to receive a medical degree.
1870—An estimated 15,000 Americans travel to Germany and Austria over the course of the next four decades for modern medical education.
1893—Johns Hopkins University Medical School opens and is the first to require a baccalaureate degree for admission and four years of study for a medical degree.
1910—The Flexner report recommends closing half of American medical schools.
1952—Case Western University introduces an organ system-based curriculum.
1956—Federal Health Facilities Research Act enhances research efforts in medical schools.
1968—McMaster University of Canada introduces problem-based learning.
1992—About 18% of U.S. physicians and 42% of medical students are women.
   —Number of students applying to medical schools reaches an all-time high.
1993–1995/6—The record number of medical school applicants continues.

THE NEED FOR PHYSICIANS

Until about 1980, the increasing need for additional manpower in the health professions, and particularly medical manpower, was shown in governmental studies of both urban and rural areas. Thus medical educators strongly urged that efforts be made to increase the number of physicians and other health science personnel. As a result, increased financial support, especially from the federal government, resulted in expanding first-year enrollment by both enlarging existing medical school class size and by establishing new colleges of medicine. Thus, for example, the number of first-year students increased from about 8,000 in 1960–1961 to more than 11,000 in 1970–1971 and then to about 16,500 first-year places in the early 1980s. All of the six two-year basic science schools were converted to four-year MD-granting institutions. Also, in the 1980s nine new schools became operational, thereby ultimately providing about 750 to 1,000 additional places.

The increase in the number of medical schools and their class size has resulted in a significant narrowing of the gap between physician supply and demand. The number of active physicians increased roughly 12% from 285,000 to 318,000 in the 1965 to 1970 period as against a population growth of only 5%. A similar rate of increase also occurred between 1970 and 1980 as well as in the following decade. The current projection is for about a 17% increase in the number of physicians during the 1990s. The total number of active physicians is projected to be 666,000 by the year 2000. This would result in a physician-to-population ratio of 241 per 100,000 by the year 2000, which is higher than the 1988 ratio of 223 per 100,000. Thus, on a numerical basis, the gap between physician supply and demand apparently will be closed. A major study of future physician manpower needs, known as the GEMENAC report, which projected an oversupply of physicians, has given rise (not surprisingly) to anxiety among some pre-medical and medical students, as well as to residents, regarding the need for their services in the twenty-first century.

There are a number of factors to consider when evaluating the conclusion of this report. First, as with all projections based on statistical analysis, they need not be self-fulfilling. Second, a major and unknown impact on the validity of the report's conclusions is the very significant (and long overdue) increase in the enrollment of women in medical schools; women now constitute more than 35% of the student population and their number may rise to 45% or more. An unknown, but perhaps significant, number of these women may initially opt for a specialty of their primary interest but later, to meet personal and/or family needs, gravitate to fields that demand less time. This may leave a void in the supply of physicians specializing in internal medicine, surgery, and other time-intensive fields. Third, the number of American graduates of foreign medical schools may diminish, in view of the drastic change in the "atmosphere" with regard to this option. Fourth, with the size of the applicant pool subject to cyclical fluctuation, there could at some point possibly be a sharp decline (as took place in the mid-1980s). There would then be a tendency for some schools to reduce the size of their entering class, and thus the total number of medical school graduates may, under these conditions, diminish. All the while the population will undoubtedly continue to grow, increasing the demand for medical services (already being fueled by public health education programs).

The aforementioned considerations may have contributed to the significant downward revision in the size of the projected physician surplus that was made by the Department of Health and Human Services over that originally contained in the 1980 GEMENAC report. The overall question of whether there will be a physician surplus, and how big the surplus will be, cannot be resolved with any degree of certainty. The situation is more complex than simply the ratio of the number of physicians to the total population. There is an important issue of an unequal distribution of physicians with rural and inner city areas remaining underserved even when the overall number of physicians has significantly increased. In addition, there is an increasing pressure to deemphasize specialization and strongly encourage the expansion of the number of primary care or family practice physicians. In view of these considerations, the increased number of physicians will definitely have its impact. *It will require that prospective practitioners be more flexible in the choice of a specialty and in the location of their practice, and above all be very dedicated to their chosen profession.*

PHYSICIAN SURPLUS: CURRENT DEBATE

A new major debate is developing over the issue of physician surplus. It was fueled by a report by a commission of health care policy experts funded by the Pew Foundation. The commission recommended that 20% of the nation's medical schools be closed by the year 2005. It warned of a surplus of 100,000 to 150,000 physicians in the next century, and urged closing some schools as the best way to solve the problem, although it did not identify which schools should be shut down.

The conclusion by the Pew commission that there will be a surplus of physicians is consistent with the earlier findings of other organizations and the GEMENAC report discussed above. Not surprisingly, there has been a cool reaction by those in academic medicine to the recommendation that schools be closed. They advocate two other courses of possible action, namely downsizing schools and limiting access to graduate training by foreign graduates. Currently, U.S. schools graduate about 17,000 physicians a year, but there are 24,000 first-year graduate positions available. The 7,000 extra spaces are filled by foreign medical graduates. The commission did recommend that graduate medical training be capped at 110% of U.S. medical graduates. Some educators believe that solving the foreign graduate problem by itself will resolve the issue and downsizing will be unnecessary. This is because they feel that once this number is down, the marketplace will in a natural way readjust the specialist-to-generalist ratio and uneven geographic distribution of physicians, thus eliminating surplus physicians.

One major element strongly impacts upon the issue of physician surplus, namely managed care. Since the number of specialists will be reduced under managed care, more physicians will enter primary care, altering our health care system's infrastructure more rapidly than expected.

It is clear that the present decade is a time of change and uncertainty; it will take time till this situation becomes clarified. The current debate reinforces the conclusion noted above that prospective physicians must be strongly committed, need to show flexibility and openmindedness, and above all stay informed.

DESIRABLE ATTRIBUTES FOR A MEDICAL CAREER

The changing environment for medical practice that is gradually taking place, which is discussed later in this chapter, will fully impact on those who will practice in the twenty-first century. Thus, while ten specific desirable attributes are noted below, one major personal quality should be emphasized at this point, namely, the need for a strong commitment to medicine. Having such a commitment will serve to overcome the inevitable obstacles, which include a less attractive environment in which to practice, high tuition costs, a long education and training period, and lower income expectations. An intense commitment will permit one to meet the inevitable challenges and overcome any setbacks that may be encountered. It will also serve to avoid incurring the disappointment that withdrawal from a career goal for nonacademic reasons would generate.

There are ten basic qualities that are desirable for prospective physicians to have.

1. *Intelligence.* Medical studies and practice require an ability to learn, retain, and integrate a vast amount of scientific data through study, experimentation, and experience.

2. *Scientific interest.* Medicine, while an applied science, rests upon an understanding of the fundamental biological and chemical activities that we define as life. An understanding of its dynamic processes requires a solid grounding in chemical, physical, and biological principles. What is especially desirable is a mastery of the scientific mode of inquiry and the attainment of good manipulative skills.

3. *Favorable personality.* A successful practice involves an ability to establish and maintain a good rapport with people at all levels. Thus, you must realize that you will have to treat people coming from different walks of life and associate with colleagues who have different backgrounds. It is very desirable to have warmth and empathy and, thus, be able to reflect a positive response to the needs, suffering, and fears of others in a manner that can provide both reassurance and respect. Another desirable personality characteristic is broadmindedness. This is reflected by a wide breadth of interests, the desire for a wide range of experiences, the habit of forming value judgments independently, the ability to establish close friendships, an open-mindedness to nonconforming ideas, and the capacity of putting issues in their proper perspective.

4. *Physical and emotional strength.* Those who plan a career in medicine must possess the capability of enduring the rigorous physical and emotional demands of many years of study and training. You must be able to maintain the self-discipline required during such a prolonged preparatory period. Medical school and

specialty training require a disposition capable of expending an enormous amount of energy. This innate characteristic is reflected in the records of those achieving a high degree of academic success while being simultaneously involved in a variety of extracurricular activities. This suggests that as busy practitioners such individuals will also be able to participate in a variety of non-professional activities.

5. *Ability to tolerate uncertainty and frustration.* The practice of medicine is based on the fact that every patient is unique, that frequently one must intervene thera-peutically before all the facts are available, and that even after securing all rele-vant data it may be necessary to select from several courses of action that are quite different and possibly contradictory. Thus you must have a personality that enables you to function in an atmosphere of ambiguity where clear-cut and pre-cisely defined treatment modalities are lacking. Moreover, since the response to even the most appropriate therapeutic regime may prove disappointing, you also must be able to withstand the frustrations of clinical failure in spite of excellent medical treatment.

6. *Well-organized work habits.* It is crucial to professional success that prospective medical students maximize their expenditure of time and effort. This will ensure that opportunities will not be lost and information will not go to waste.

7. *Capacity for self-education.* Willingness to learn a great deal about a topic with-out the prospect of gaining external reward for doing so is essential. The reason is that much of what will be learned in medical school will either be forgotten and/or become obsolete. Inherent in self-education is the necessity to hone one's critical faculties. This will permit clear thinking and independent formulation of judgments. Self-education also includes an ability to assimilate and sustain by continual learning a large knowledge base, as well as the ability to define and solve problems by interpreting data, reasoning critically, and applying learned information.

8. *Social awareness.* A gradual change is taking place in health care delivery, in which the focus is not exclusively on the individual patient out of the context of the many psychological and social factors that affect health and produce illness. It is thus incumbent to have an awareness of the current climate relative to the sociomedical issues involved in providing health care to the varying population groups.

9. *Achievement.* Evidence of some special achievement, in any one of a variety of fields, is an asset for a prospective medical school applicant. Thus an applicant may have climbed a well-known mountain, organized a band, or learned how to captain a small fishing boat. Achievements that demonstrate initiative, leader-ship potential, and/or the ability to establish satisfactory interpersonal relation-ships are indicative of the potential for achievement in the challenging field of medicine.

10. *Creativity.* The ability to marshall one's intellectual resources to meet chal-lenges is an especially valuable asset. This capability for creativity may be reflected in self-confidence and by an ability to detect and define problems, to think originally, to question established scientific dogmas, and to demonstrate intellectual courage.

The four years of high school and first three years of college provide the opportu-nity to determine to what extent you possess these basic attributes. The grades you receive, especially in your science courses, will provide a basis for judging your intel-lectual ability. Your response to various science courses, as well as other contacts with experimentation and scientific inquiry in class or possibly in summer work, will enable you to evaluate your natural response to this area of studies. Your ability to get along with your fellow students and friends should provide a basis for judging your personality. Finally, how you stand up to the demands of your school work and personal problems will provide some basis for evaluating your inner tenacity and determination.

Objective self-analysis at the end of high school and at the end of each college year will help to ensure that your choice of a medical career is realistic and will provide a stimulus for greater performance. Such analysis may, on the other hand, call for reconsideration and a possible change in your career goal. If this is the case, the change should be made promptly after consultation with your guidance counselor and parents, in order to avoid loss of time and almost certain disappointment at a later date.

The aim of the self-evaluation should not be to determine if you are outstanding in all the basic attributes necessary for a successful medical career; rather you should ascertain if you are above average in the sum total, at least average in each, and do not have very serious deficiencies in any. What is to be sought is a determination of how close one actually comes to a hypothetical standard, realizing that there is a broad spectrum of acceptability determined by a balancing of all factors.

THE CHALLENGE TO BECOMING A PHYSICIAN

The first step to becoming a physician is to decide that at all times you will be realistic and honest with yourself. Before you reach the stage of applying to a medical school, you should periodically reevaluate your abilities and the sincerity of your conviction to become a physician. You should determine if you possess the intelligence, scientific aptitude, personality, and inner strength—that are essential for success as a physician.

Each prospective medical school applicant must in time face the reality that he or she will be but one out of more than 45,000 applicants competing for a place in freshman medical school classes. The competition is very intense and more than 50% of the applicants fail to attain their goal (at least on the first try). You should also be aware that since each applicant applies to about ten medical schools, there are more than 300,000 applications to be processed. This means screening 500 to 7,500 applicants to fill 50 to 250 places. The initial screening process rejects some individuals outright and ranks others for further action, determining if they merit a prompt interview or should be put on hold for an interview at a later date. It is, therefore, important to realize at the outset that in addition to your intellectual achievements and potential, the mechanics of the admission process itself is critical. Knowing which schools and how many schools to apply to, presenting your qualifications, writing your essay, and handling yourself well at interviews are all vital elements in achieving your goal. The admission process is the culmination of your efforts to become a physician. It involves marketing your personal assets to the maximum extent possible. It is therefore important for you to get to know your strengths and weaknesses in order to make sure that you accentuate the strengths and minimize or, if possible, even eliminate the weaknesses. The image that you indirectly project by means of the transcripts, recommendations, and MCAT scores submitted in your behalf, and that you directly project in your interview, will determine the success of your attempt to secure a place in a medical school. Once you have been accepted for admission, it is almost a certainty (because of the negligible failure rate) that in due course you will be awarded your medical degree.

Future Challenges

After completing their studies and training, the challenge of the practitioners of the twenty-first century will be (1) to maintain the traditional commitment to service as the central theme of their work in spite of increasing regulation; (2) to remain committed to life-long learning as medical knowledge has an increasingly shorter half-life of validity; (3) to seek to resolve the social and ethical problems that arise as technological capabilities increase within a humanistic framework. For further discussion of these challenges, see Chapter 15, Physicians and Medicine in the Twenty-First Century.

2 Preparing for Medical School

High school
College
Postbaccalaureate programs
Humanistic aspects of premedical education

HIGH SCHOOL

High school is a period of social adjustment and a time when the student becomes increasingly aware of what adult responsibilities are. Thus, while high school is a transitional era, it is a critical one in that it is usually the time when your career goals become tentatively formulated. Career ambitions may change as you become exposed to new areas of knowledge and as old ones are explored more deeply, but it is advantageous to have some general educational goals rather than to drift aimlessly.

A *final* decision to choose medicine as a career need not be made in high school and probably should be deferred until the end of the sophomore year of college. Two questions, however, need to be answered in high school: Do you intend to go to college? Do you have a genuine interest in science? It is essential to plan an educational program of high school studies that will make it feasible to gain admission to a suitable college as well as to test the validity of your preliminary career decision.

Program of Studies

Having decided to attend college and possibly become a premedical student, you should select your high school program to include courses that meet at least the minimum requirements for admission to a liberal arts college. The program should therefore include:

English: 4 years

Laboratory science: 2 years

Modern foreign or classical language: 2 years

Mathematics: 2½ years

Social studies: 2 years

You should enlarge upon these requirements as much as is feasible by taking electives to obtain a well-rounded academic background. Concentrate in a science with the aim of making your other college courses less demanding, and thereby enhance your chances of securing higher grades in all your courses. This approach can help strengthen your science course average, which is one of the factors in the medical school selection process.

Mastering good study habits and computer literacy are essential elements that should be achieved in high school, since they will have a significant impact on your success in college. Set up regular hours for study, learn how to read quickly and effectively, and learn how to take lecture notes and develop test-taking skills. Good achievement in your academic studies, especially in science, should be a major challenge of your high school education.

During high school you should participate in a variety of extracurricular activities, including athletics and science clubs, especially premedical groups such as the Future Physician Club or Medical Explorer Post of the Boy Scouts of America. While in high school you should acquire a good ability to communicate—both orally and in writing. Seek help if there is a serious problem in these areas. Your summers should be spent profitably and should involve activities that bring you into active contact with people. Working in a hospital or laboratory may also provide some useful experience, but such activities are probably best deferred until the college years.

Take the appropriate college entrance examination required by the colleges you plan to apply to—either SAT I or the ACT (American College Testing program). If your scores are in the upper percentiles, you should feel encouraged about your potential success.

COLLEGE

The Selection of a College

There is a wide choice of colleges open to the high school graduate whose ultimate goal is medical school. Students should make their choice from one of the liberal arts colleges or universities accredited by one of the six regional accrediting agencies. This helps ensure that the school has met at least the minimum educational standards for institutions of higher learning. You should determine your personal preference either for a small school, with its opportunities for more personalized instruction and closer interaction with faculty and fellow students, or for a larger university, with its wider curricular and extracurricular opportunities. Factors such as cost should also be carefully considered. Take into account also the size of the library, the student-faculty ratio, the local environment, and the academic pressures. In addition, evaluate each college keeping in mind the following points:

1. Does the college offer the premedical courses that are prerequisites for admission to medical school? Examine the school's catalog to determine this.

2. Does the college have dynamic and modern science departments and adequate laboratory facilities?

3. Does the list of faculty members in the catalog indicate a competent staff? (Note, for example, the number of faculty with doctorate degrees.)

4. When you visit the school, do students speak well of the science and mathematics departments?

5. Does the school have good library facilities? A visit to the library will give you an insight into its quality.

6. Does the college have a high academic reputation? Examination of the freshman class profile, which should be available from high school counselors, will shed light on this point.

7. Does the college consistently send a significant portion of its premedical graduates to medical school? This information is very helpful in assessing the school's reputation and the quality of its premedical students. Discuss this question with the college's seniors, its premedical advisor, and its science professors.

8. Does the college have a premedical advisory program? A knowledgeable and dedicated premedical advisor will help ensure academic guidance, current information, and assistance at the time the student is planning to apply to medical and/or dental school.

A comparative evaluation of these and other issues involves reading the schools' catalogs and visiting each of the campuses under consideration. A visit offers the opportunity of meeting students, admissions and guidance personnel, and professors, and of discussing the aspects of the schools with those who are most familiar with them.

It is very important to give careful consideration to the college you select, for it will undoubtedly have a major impact upon your career. The undergraduate school at which you matriculate can affect your performance. In addition, it is one of the factors in the selection of medical students. Because of this, it is very desirable to secure a quality education at a well-established or prestigious college or university. A private school may give you an edge. To secure admission to a college that will improve your career potential requires competitive grades, attractive SAT I or ACT scores, impressive recommendations, and personal achievement(s).

Program of Studies

You should realize at the outset of your college career that every medical school admissions committee will initially screen your application by viewing your grades as a whole. This is expressed by your grade point average (GPA), which simply represents the total of your average for each academic year divided by the number of years you have attended college (usually three at the time you apply, plus any summer school work completed). Then your science course average, your achievement in your major and in the more challenging premedical requirements (such as organic chemistry and physics), and honors work or independent study are all scrutinized. This means that it is imperative that you apply all your talents (and remedy any deficiencies) at the time you begin college studies. It is risky to wait until you are faced with serious academic problems to decide to buckle down to the demands of your courses. It is difficult, although certainly not impossible, to rectify the results of one unimpressive semester, let alone an entire year. Thus, for example, a B or 3.0 for your first freshman semester will give you a maximum B+ or 3.5 average for the year only if your second semester is straight A or 4.0. Similarly, a 3.0 for the entire freshman year would demand a perfect sophomore year to bring you up to a B+ level. In addition, a mediocre semester or a mediocre year can seriously undermine your self-confidence and raise doubts about the wisdom of your career decision. This type of situation is undoubtedly one of the underlying factors in the significantly high incidents of changes in majors among freshman premeds.

Your Major

Historically, premedicine has changed to keep pace with advancements in medical education. In colonial America, premedical education as such was nonexistent. However, as medical education became more sophisticated, so by necessity did premedical education come into existence. During this century there have been varying trends in premedical programming. The older school of thought was that a specialized preprofessional program was mandatory. As a result, a formal "premedical major" with a prescribed program of study was established. A strong movement away from this approach began in the mid-1950s. Students were encouraged to select any major that was of interest, but if it was in one of the sciences (as was frequently the case) they were also urged to obtain broad exposure to the humanities and social sciences as well. Currently the pressure, due to diminished time allotted to the basic sciences in medical school, has given impetus to encouraging students to complete more science courses in college, so that the pendulum has swung somewhat in the direction of a science major. While completing a science major, students automatically take the required premedical courses.

The specific choice of which science to major in is yours alone. You should, before making a decision, evaluate your school's science departments in terms of their requirements, quality of teaching, and grading attitudes. To do so, you should read the school catalog and talk to faculty members and senior-level students. The choice should be the one in which you will be academically most successful and in which you stand a good chance of developing a good relationship with members of the department staff. A correct decision as to your major will help ensure that your GPA, science cumulative average, and the quality of your recommendations—three critical medical school selection factors—will be strong.

Most premedical students major in biology (zoology) or chemistry, but some major in biochemistry, physics, or even computer science, all of which have a relevance to medicine. However, choosing to major in a science unrelated to the art of healing, such as geology or engineering, will certainly not impede an applicant from gaining admission.

It should be strongly emphasized that being a nonscience major is not a liability so far as medical school admission is concerned, but may even be an asset. Humanities majors, although representing the smaller segment of the applicant pool, have as good an admissions track record as science majors. Thus, should your current interest lie in the classics, foreign languages, history, or philosophy, and your career goal is medicine, you should pursue a humanities major and seek to develop an attractive set of credentials supported by solid achievement in the premedical science prerequisites. This approach is especially valid now that medical educators are stressing the importance of developing and retaining the humanistic attributes as medical and postgraduate students. Thus what is critical is not your major, but the nature of your achievement and development as a college student.

These remarks should alleviate the concerns of those who fear that being a liberal arts major would impede their chances for admission into medical school. Another factor influencing prospective medical students against becoming liberal arts majors is the concern that they would then be less competitive in facing the demands of a science-oriented curriculum. A comparative study of science and nonscience majors from three medical schools has shown, however, that this is not the case. This conclusion was based on performance on both parts of the National Board Examination (now USMLE) and on clinical-year grade point averages. There is no reason not to assume that the same is applicable to medical students as a whole. This finding should further encourage college freshmen to feel free in their choice of a major.

Premedical Requirements

Regardless of your choice of a major, you should arrange to include the basic premedical science courses plus lab requirements, namely, two years of chemistry and one each of biology and physics, in your first three years of college study. The purpose of premedical science course requirements is twofold: (1) to determine the compatibility between the student and science, since medicine academically is the science of the human body, and (2) to provide the premedical student with a background on which to launch future studies in the basic medical sciences.

The required premedical science courses you take should not be those designed for the nonscience major. If possible, stagger your laboratory courses so that you don't take too many at one time. These courses require additional time both in the laboratory and outside of the classroom. However, none of these courses should be deferred to the senior year. They are all needed in preparation for the MCAT. One or more of these courses may be in progress when taking the spring MCAT.

The course requirements are purposely limited in order to allow broad latitude for the planning of individualized programs. Table 2.1 lists the courses required by medical schools. The symbol on the right indicates how many schools require that course for admission.

It should be noted that some advanced science courses, as well as some nonscience courses, while not officially required for admission by some schools, may nevertheless be listed in their catalogs as "recommended" or "desirable."

In summary, while the premedical core studies in the sciences will usually absorb the greatest portion of one's time and energy, one must place these in the proper perspective of the entire program of undergraduate education. For just as the patient should be viewed as a whole rather than as merely a collection of organ systems, so too should the person be educated as a whole in order to face both the academic as well as the nonacademic challenges that lie ahead. In essence this means that the student should attempt to secure a meaningful balance between the physical and biological sciences, and the humanities and social sciences. In this way, not only will the college experience be more pleasurable, but also one's sense of purpose and ethical values will be developed, and a more humanistic physician can evolve in a mechanistically oriented society.

Table 2.1
SUMMARY OF REQUIRED COURSES
+ required by more than 100 schools
− required by fewer than 20 schools

Course	
Chemistry	
Inorganic (or General) Chemistry	+
Organic Chemistry	+
Qualitative Analysis	−
Quantitative Analysis	−
Physical Chemistry/Quantitative Analysis	−
Biochemistry	−
Other	−
Biology	
General Biology (or Zoology)	+
Embryology	−
Genetics	−
Comparative Anatomy	−
Cell Biology	−
Molecular Biology	−
Other	−
Physics	
General Physics	+
Other	−
Mathematics	
College Mathematics	−
College Algebra	−
Analytical Geometry	−
Trigonometry	−
Calculus	−
Other	−
Humanities	
English	+
Language	−
Other	−
Social and Behavioral Sciences	
Sociology	−
Psychology	−
Behavioral Science	−
Social Science	−
Other	−

Special Educational Opportunities

Most liberal arts colleges offer special educational opportunities that can enhance the character of your program of study. These programs not only improve the quality of your college educational experience but also increase the strength of your medical school application and thereby improve your admission chances. You should not arbitrarily utilize any of these programs but should incorporate them into your program only if you are sure that they will definitely help you attain your career goal. The six special programs discussed below are advanced placement credit, honors courses, independent study, graduate-level courses, pass/fail courses, and summer school courses.

Advanced Placement Credit

When a student has acquired advanced placement credit for excelling in a science on the high school level, one or more required premedical courses will be waived. As a result, there will be a gap in grade information in this area. It is frequently desirable in such cases to substitute a suitable number of elective courses for the waived courses. You should select substitute elective courses carefully, determining that your high school background is adequate, and discussing the course requirements with the instructor. You should also consider auditing the basic science course from which you have been excused in advance of taking the elective; this would not only provide a useful background but would also enable you to develop a set of lecture notes that could prove helpful for review when you are studying for the MCAT. For example, if your general biology requirement has been waived, you should review the principles of biology by yourself or audit a course if possible. This preparation is essential, even if you do not major in biology. In this case, your elective course grades will serve to indicate to the admissions committee your academic potential in this important area. If you do major in biology, a good grounding in its principles will serve you well for a variety of electives you choose during the course of your studies.

Honors Courses

There is no question that completing an honors section of a course can strengthen your admission potential. This, however, is true only if you get an A in such a course. Receiving a B grade may serve to depress your GPA (and, where applicable, your science average) even though in reality a B in an honors section may be equivalent to an A in a standard section. In some cases, however, grades for honors courses may be weighted, in order to provide an equivalency factor. Thus, before enrolling in an honors section, you should determine, by talking to the instructor and students involved in the course, just how much additional work it requires and how the grade is evaluated. If you have the time and are confident of your ability to master the requirements, then enrolling in an honors section is reasonable. In any case, the honors credit should be noted in your application documents. The course can be educationally rewarding and provide a good source for securing an impressive letter of recommendation.

Independent Study

Another approach that can add significantly to the attractiveness of your credentials is satisfactory completion of an independent study program. Such an undertaking can demonstrate that you are willing and able to accept the responsibility of a special educational challenge. Your motives must, however, be sincere so that you will apply yourself maximally in order to ensure that your research is impressive and is completed on schedule. As a result of such an activity you will undoubtedly develop a special favorable relationship with your mentor, who will then be able to strongly support your candidacy for admission to medical school at the appropriate time.

Independent study should be undertaken only if you are sure that it will not have a negative impact on your educational responsibilities as a whole. You need to be especially careful in selecting a project that can be realistically completed by the date you set. It is best if you can complete any independent study project before you apply to medical school so that recommendations resulting from this work can be submitted when they can be most effective. A good time to carry out such a project may be the summer after you complete your junior-year studies. By then you should have completed all your premedical science course requirements and satisfactorily taken your MCAT. Your only remaining commitment will be preparing your application(s) to medical school. There is no objection, if time is available, to undertake independent study during the regular academic year.

Graduate Courses

Occasionally, the option of taking a graduate-level course is available to undergraduates. You should not assume, unless specifically told, that you will be graded differently from the graduate students taking the course with you. Thus the note of caution regarding the impact of the grade applicable here. Graduate courses can be demanding, and successful completion of such a challenge can demonstrate impressively your ability to respond effectively to the academic challenge of medical school. If you do successfully complete graduate courses, make sure to bring it to the attention of the medical school by noting it on your essay or in your interview.

Pass/fail Courses

These are courses that your school permits you to take for credit without getting a grade. It is not advisable to take any courses in biology or chemistry on this basis since the implication would be that your level of performance was not satisfactory. Thus while the absence of a grade would preclude any negative impact on your GPA and science average, your image could suffer. On the other hand, taking a medically unrelated science (such as geology) or a nonscience course of special interest on a pass/fail basis is quite legitimate. It shows evidence of your desire to secure a broad education, which certainly is desirable.

Summer Courses

There is no inherent objection to the completion of courses during the summer. Moreover, it may prove useful or even desirable to do so in order to get some required nonscience courses out of the way and thereby lighten your course load during the regular academic year. Thus some students take one or two nonscience courses at the end of their sophomore year so they can lighten their course load during their junior year when they have to take organic chemistry or physics and also study for the MCAT.

It may even prove advantageous to take one or more science electives during the summer, if they are not offered at your school during the regular academic year, or if you cannot fit them into your schedule. In addition, summer electives can help improve your science average. Thus if your BCPM (biology, chemistry, physics, and math) average comes close to a critical level, taking summer courses can bring these figures up. It is worthwhile to consider attending summer school to do so. Again, it is important to realize that it can take an A or two A's to do this, and that special care needs to be taken before utilizing this double-edged option.

Succeeding in College

Four factors are involved in doing well in college: academic ability, determination, good study skills, and proper time management. There are, however, a good number of pitfalls that should and can be avoided to enhance your chances for success. The following are ten tips that may prove helpful:

TIP 1   Prepare for lectures
Being acquainted with the general subject material in advance of a lecture will permit you to understand it better as well as to integrate the new information with the knowledge you already have.

TIP 2   Guard your time
The social demands of college life can be very time consuming. You need to determine your obligations and priorities. Study time needs will inherently vary. Thus, you should not feel pressured by classmates to give up needed study time for social activities.

TIP 3   Avoid test cramming
The proven method of successful studying involves repetition. Thus, earlier review of material covered and keeping up with class assignments will serve to reduce the need for cramming prior to examinations.

TIP 4   Seek assistance
Failure to comprehend a topic should not be a source of embarrassment. Instead, you should be motivated to secure help from teachers, upperclass students, or other classmates.

TIP 5   Utilize free time

Free time between classes can be an occasion for extra study. This time can be useful because you may not be as tired then as in the evening hours. Also, use the free time for class preparation or review purposes.

TIP 6   Listening is an art

When sitting in on a lecture, avoid being distracted by a classmate or even by the instructor's mannerisms. Rather, focus your attention on the content of the talk.

TIP 7   Proper note taking

Students vary in their ability to take accurate lecture notes, which can be sketchy or disorganized. It is well worth the effort to review and, if necessary, rewrite lecture notes so that they will be legible, complete, and accurate.

TIP 8   Review

Daily brief review and regular periodic review of the material being studied will serve to enhance your knowledge of the subject matter and reduce the time needed for study for examinations.

TIP 9   Proper reading

If you read an assigned chapter in its entirety for the first time, you may be overwhelmed by its detail. To get the most out of your reading, skim the subject titles and subheadings, opening and concluding sentences, in order to get a knowledge of the main ideas and to be better prepared to absorb the details.

TIP 10   Underlining with purpose

If reading material is first "screened," as noted above, and then read, you are in a better position to judge what to underline. You will then be able to underscore with discrimination and to highlight passages that will prove more meaningful when you review them at a later date.

The following discussion covers (1) organizing oneself, (2) writing term papers, and (3) taking examinations.

Organizing for College Life

It is important to be aware of the fact that during high school, competition may not necessarily be very intense, because not all students are considering college or postgraduate careers. Under these circumstances, students may not be motivated to acquire good study habits in order to succeed. This is especially true if they find that, with a modest amount of work, they can attain adequate grades to be admitted to a college, even the one of their choice. Upon entering college, where competition is usually much more intense, knowing how to study is obligatory if the student is to have a good enough academic record to get into a professional school.

College life is very time consuming; it preempts the largest block of one's daily activities. It has built-in time commitments, such as: (1) the need to attend lecture and recitation classes, as well as laboratory sessions; (2) library research and term paper writing; and (3) study in preparation for periodic midterm and final examinations. In addition to these educational time demands, there are those of a personal nature, such as eating, relaxation, social life, and participation in extracurricular activities. Leading a balanced college life that meets both your personal and educational needs is the most desirable formula for achieving academic success. It also ensures enjoying your stay in college, which is a unique time in one's life.

The key to adequately meeting both your school and personal obligations is the proper allocation of your time. This can be done either in a disorganized or in an orderly manner (without the need for extreme regimentation). Thus, if you establish a seven-day grid (Fig. 2.1, page 19), with a time plan schedule from 8:00 A.M. to 10:00 P.M., you can readily see: (1) if you have allotted the needed time to meet all your responsibilities, and

(2) how much spare time you have available and where it is in order to meet unforeseen demands and unexpected challenges.

Having formulated your semester's course of study, you should initially fill in the time where you have scheduled lectures, recitations, and laboratory sessions. Next, you should factor into your schedule that one hour of class time on average requires two hours of study time. Thus, a typical 16-hour semester course load requires 32 hours of study time, resulting in a basic total weekly educational time commitment of 48 hours (exclusive of special test study time). Place any other regular commitments into the time grid, such as travel to and from school, attendance at religious services, social obligations, etc. With these items placed in their proper time frame, your actual available free time becomes readily evident and can then be allotted to meet your personal needs.

You should recognize that allocation of study time also needs to be flexible, since: (1) the same course may demand a varying amount of study time at different intervals during the course of a semester, depending on such variables as complexity of topics and frequency of examinations; and (2) different courses vary significantly in their overall study time requirements, depending on their inherent difficulty, quality of the instruction, and ability of the student. With this in mind, you should be prepared to make appropriate adjustments in your initial study time schedule to accommodate changing circumstances. It is obviously also essential that you prioritize your study time so that you place appropriate emphasis not only on time allotment, but also in the sequence in which you study your subjects in the context of their importance and difficulty. Successfully completing the highest priority assignments should be satisfying enough to motivate you to proceed with other, perhaps less appealing, projects. It is vital for your health and the success of your study efforts that you allot adequate time for meals, recreation, relaxation, and sleep.

Failure to provide time for any of these four vital areas can diminish the efficiency of your study efforts. A consistent fulfillment of your study plans will allow you more freedom to enjoy your rest periods without feeling any sense of guilt for having taken time off.

It is also important that you put to good use the time breaks between classes for relaxation, makeup reading, or review of material, prior to a lecture or lab. This will allow you to get the most out of these learning opportunities.

Time-demanding projects, such as term papers or laboratory reports, should be placed into your study time schedule as soon as it is practical. You can then work on them in a timely fashion, rather than hastily completing them in order to meet a competing assignment.

Genuine study involves intense concentration that can usually be done more efficiently in short time intervals. Thus, you should try to utilize study time blocks of 30 to 60 minutes to avoid mental fatigue. Also, try to avoid studying closely related subjects in sequence, so as to minimize the confusion between them.

Another major benefit that comes from having and adhering to a study schedule is that it reduces the possibility of your work piling up. Such a situation can produce stress that may impede your academic progress. It is obvious that studying under pressure is not as effective as studying under favorable conditions.

With an appropriate study plan—one that has periodically been reviewed and adjusted—potential problems with exams can be avoided. You will find that, under these circumstances, you will not need to cram for tests, but, rather, you will be able to review intensively. Moreover, you will likely retain the basic information longer and be able to build upon it, as you absorb more advanced material.

Physical Setting

After establishing an appropriate study schedule, it is essential to secure a suitable and conducive atmosphere, where your study plan can be carried out. The first place to consider is your home or dorm room. This location is a good choice if you are its sole occupant and can enjoy the privacy and solitude that is necessary for successful study. However, the presence of siblings in the home or roommates in the dorm may make this location impractical, unless you can control entry or gain the cooperation of the occupant(s).

Learning in the Classroom

Benefiting from Lectures

Lectures provide an excellent way of securing ideas, facts, and viewpoints. To get the most out of lectures, it is important to improve your listening skills. To accomplish this, the following should be taken into consideration:

TIP 1   Your lecture seat

Your position in the classroom can influence your level of concentration. If you find your attention wandering, try to move to a place that is preferably near the front and, if possible, near the center. Try to avoid sitting in a crowded area.

TIP 2   Preparation

Orient yourself before the lecture as quickly as possible. This may take the form of a brief review of the previous lecture and/or highlights of a reading assignment.

TIP 3   Note taking

Take notes with discrimination. You need to use judgment as to the extent of note taking that a course requires. Speaking to students who took the course with the same instructor, and did well, will give you some general guidelines as to the extent of note taking that is desirable.

When presented with new information, fresh ideas, complex or condensed information during the course of a lecture, detailed note taking is mandatory. Similarly, concepts or facts that may be inconsistent with those known or held by you should be recorded because this type of information tends to be easily disregarded or dismissed because of the inherent conflict between what you hear and what you believe to be true.

TIP 4   Identifying main ideas

The central themes of a lecture should be determined. Their significance should be enhanced by "fleshing them out" with illustrations, diagrams, or supporting numerical data. Major ideas become genuinely meaningful when one associates some details with them.

TIP 5   Accuracy

Lecture notes are a condensation of the teacher's presentation. If you use the note-taking approach, as is commonly done, rather than taping the lecture, an accurate representation of the information is needed. This should be done with the aim of using as condensed a written record as possible, while concentrating on making sure that you secure all of the principles and facts. To achieve this goal, you may find it helpful to develop a personalized shorthand system. This requires consistently using abbreviations and symbols and not being concerned with the presence of incomplete sentence flow.

TIP 6   Reworking notes

At the first available opportunity, your rough notes should be rewritten so that their meaning is clear and the notes can be used at a future date for review and to prepare for exams. In rewriting your notes, you should rework them by filling in gaps and adding any relevant details that you recall. The process of reworking your notes can be valuable because it helps you better understand and absorb the material and it enhances your note-taking skills—an essential part of the learning process.

TIP 7   Rethinking concepts

After the lecture, discuss the principles presented with your classmates to be sure that you understood them properly. Only when your notes are intelligible should you raise any counter-arguments to the issues discussed.

Fig. 2.1.
TIME PLAN

		Monday	Tuesday	Wednesday	Thursday	Friday	Saturday
A.M.	8:00						
	9:00						
	10:00						
	11:00						
	12:00						
P.M.	1:00						
	2:00						
	3:00						
	4:00						
	5:00						
	6:00						
	7:00						
	8:00						
	9:00						
	10:00						

Recitation Classes

Many courses consist of two (or three) lectures per week and one recitation or discussion hour. This arrangement is especially desirable where lecture classes are large and the only opportunity available to discuss the course material is during a recitation hour. The following is suggested in order to get the most from the recitation interval:

TIP 1   Complete assignments

The need to finish assignments and be prepared is especially important in recitation classes. Being knowledgeable about the issues, both in terms of general principles and specific facts, facilitates participation in recitation classes. Thus, reading the assigned material is essential to feeling comfortable in and getting the most out of these classes.

TIP 2   Supplemental reading

The lecturer may provide a list of or refer to supplemental reading material. Becoming familiar with at least some of this material can enhance your ability to participate in discussions. Therefore, you should have notes available that contain highlights from any of the supplementary material you have read so that you can use that material appropriately and efficiently. You may wish to bring copies of relevant articles with you to class.

TIP 3   Prepare questions

During the lecture sessions, especially where large groups are involved, questions may arise that invariably remain unanswered. These should be noted and the list of questions should be brought to the recitation session, where they can be raised as topics for discussion. Getting a clear definition of terms is especially desirable. In addition, you may also wish to identify any discrepancies or apparent contradictions between the lecture and reading material that deserves resolution. Questions that arise in the course of reading should also be noted.

TIP 4 Clarify lectures

Rewriting your lecture notes may bring to your attention areas where further clarification is desirable. The recitation hour provides an opportunity to eliminate any confusion.

TIP 5 Test preparation exercise

Listen to the questions being asked and note your answers in order to compare them with those of your instructor. This will provide you with an estimate of your level of knowledge and you can see where there are gaps in your pool of information.

Writing Term Papers

Term papers are traditional college assignments. In general, they are usually not favored by students because they challenge the individual much more than study assignments. However, the preparation of term papers provides a useful vehicle to learn how to properly and clearly express yourself. This is a vital communication skill that is invaluable in the world you will work in.

Our educational system in large measure is a structured one, requiring that you simply recall information that has been presented. Preparing term papers requires independent thought, since it necessitates your evaluating and synthesizing information from multiple sources. As a result, you can formulate conclusions that you support with facts, thereby reflecting your ability to reason along logical lines.

Writing an attractive and effective term paper requires proper topic selection (assuming you have a choice), ability to obtain appropriate information (research skills), talent at organization, and clearly expressing your thoughts.

Instructors usually provide submission deadlines for the term paper. Once you know the deadline, you should set up a work schedule so that you can meet it. This should consist of the following interim deadlines:

topic selection date

rough draft date

semifinal draft date

final draft date

Obviously, you will need adequate and appropriate spacing between these four stages. By getting right to work, you can proceed in a systematic manner. You will also find yourself under less pressure. Concentrate on the quality of your work rather than only progressing toward its completion. If you delay working on your term paper, you will eventually need a crash program to catch up. This could impair the quality of your end product as well as your other educational obligations, which may then have to be neglected to meet this commitment. The above schedule should allow about one week between each of the drafts so that you can have a fresh look at the material before you move on to the next stage. These time intervals should be included in your overall work schedule.

Selecting a Topic

Your instructor will usually provide you with general guidelines on dealing with the term paper, including the general topic. The choice of a specific topic may well be left to you. The idea is to find a topic that will be of strong interest. This is especially important because it will serve to motivate you to face up to the challenging task in a forceful and positive manner.

If the instructor does not assign a specific topic nor offer a list of topics from which to choose, your initial approach should be to look at your text and determine relevant issues that fall into the general topic category. The bibliography dealing with the topic may provide some clues that are worth pursuing. Some additional research involving encyclopedias and/or current periodicals may shed light on possible appropriate topics that deserve consideration.

In selecting a topic, it is critical that you avoid choosing one that is too broad and thus cannot be readily covered, or, on the other hand, selecting a topic that is too narrow for you to find adequate source material to meet the needs of the topic. Even after making a topic decision, you need to be prepared to be flexible in determining its ultimate scope. As you proceed with organizing and writing your first draft, you may decide to enlarge or shorten the original desired coverage. Your initial clue as to the possible need to make any adjustment will come from the review of the library index and periodical index, which will provide insight as to the amount of information that is available. You must bear in mind the approximate length of the term paper as prescribed by the course instructor. Excessive length or brevity relative to the guidelines set should be avoided.

Before you invest extensive effort, but after you have formulated your term paper topic, you should check its appropriateness with your instructor. If you have selected more than one topic, present them all to your instructor, but indicate your preference. If you have difficulty choosing a topic, but have ideas that merit further discussion, arrange to do so with your instructor. Your discussions should be prearranged, by appointment, so that you can receive the time and attention you need. Avoid a spur-of-the moment inquiry. Also avoid any arranged meeting that you attend without any ideas to discuss. Offering some ideas of your own will demonstrate that you have given serious consideration to selecting a topic. This may lead to an exchange of ideas with your instructor that can produce possible subjects for further consideration. If you have no ideas to offer, you will convey a negative impression that is obviously not in your best interest.

Researching a Term Paper

Prepare an outline to serve as an organizational guide. This guide will enhance the presentation of your thoughts in a clear, organized, and concise manner.

There are two types of outlines that are used—topic and sentence outlines. Topic outlines are used in short essays and consist of a few words or phrases that highlight the major topics or subtopics that the essay will cover. Sentence outlines are used in longer writing projects and consist of one-sentence summaries for each of the topics or subtopics. This is used in term papers and will force you to determine exactly what you want to say. Such a sentence outline can serve to help determine the overall validity of the organizational scheme you have formulated for the project.

A suitable starting point for your research is an encyclopedia. Consult both general and specialized types. Try to have the reference librarian help you in your search for source material.

One of the keys to successful research is taking adequate notes. A useful way to do this is to record information on 5 × 7 cards, writing on one side only so that the cards can later be spread out. You should fully identify your reference source for sorting. For books, you should indicate title, author(s), publisher, year of publication, page where information is found, and total number of pages. For articles, you need to identify the name of the periodical, title of article, author(s), volume, issue number, date, and inclusive page numbers.

Material in books that contain important information or tables and/or charts should be photocopied, using the library's (coin operated) copy machine.

In cases where you copy text verbatim, you must use quotation marks, or you should paraphrase the text, using your own words to summarize the author's views. If you do not do this you will be guilty of plagiarism—a serious academic offense.

If your topic involves an issue that has more than one view, seek material that presents the alternative viewpoints, using the various reference sources noted earlier. You may need to broaden your reference heading if you are unable to adequately secure information under the headings you are currently using. If the standard sources are inadequate, you may want to make use of *The New York Times Index* and/or *Readers' Guide to Periodical Literature* (starting with the most recent edition). You probably will need to look through back issues as well as microfilm in your search for source material. You also may have to utilize the resources of other libraries to acquire all of the material you need.

These include public, central municipal, and college libraries. Universities frequently have specialized departmental libraries that can prove to be invaluable in your research.

To facilitate your effort, avoid repeating the information you have already recorded. Merely note the additional source for inclusion in your bibliography. Any work done by the instructor should obviously be noted in the body of the text, if appropriate, and certainly in the bibliography. (The reason for this should be obvious.) Avoid working on a project with someone else, even if you have the instructor's approval, because collaboration has inherent difficulties and an especially superior product is usually expected.

When you find that you have obtained the information you seek and sources provide only confirmatory data, you can begin preparing the rough draft of your term paper. Using a computer is strongly recommended.

The Rough Draft

Before starting your rough draft, review your outline and amend it as necessary. Then arrange your research index cards according to your outline. Number your cards in sequence.

Make a special effort to draft the initial paragraph so that it contains the premise of your paper and so that it comes across in a forceful manner. Next, you should clarify how you intend to achieve the goal of establishing the proposed premise.

Having defined your goals, you can now proceed to outline your research data, using the information from your cards to present your ideas. When presenting an author's ideas or providing support from one of your sources for a statement you are making, note with a superscript the card number containing the reference source. At this writing phase, place your emphasis on quality of the ideas, rather than on the flow of the language. At the next stage you can concentrate on improving the paper by elaborating on the details of your presentation. This rough draft should be clear and concise and should accurately present the information you secured in the course of your research. If it is appropriate to use a chart or table to support your argument, note the place in the text where it belongs.

After presenting the facts and viewpoints based on your research and evaluating them, you need to arrive at a concluding paragraph that can be supported by what you have established.

At the conclusion of this phase of the project, it is essential to pause for several days, so that you will have an opportunity to gain a fresh overview of what you have written in your rough draft. After the appropriate interlude, reread the draft to see if it is properly organized and if there is continuity between the paragraphs. If not, amend it by relocating paragraphs or merely adding appropriate connecting phrases. While making any of these necessary changes, make notes about any other alterations you wish to incorporate in the text and proceed to work on the next stage of the term paper.

Semifinal Draft

Examine each paragraph carefully to see that the opening sentence serves to introduce the theme of the paragraph. The balance of the paragraph should provide the supporting detail. Evaluate the paragraph for clarity and elaborate where necessary to be sure that you have fully expressed your thoughts. However, try to avoid excessively lengthy paragraphs.

The effort that you put into preparing the semifinal draft will determine how much work will be needed for the final draft. You should use a word processor or computer to prepare your paper. This makes correcting much easier and should obviously facilitate carrying out any alterations due to grammatical errors.

At this point, you should once again set your paper aside for a few days before you tackle the final draft. During this interlude, it would serve you well if you were able to arrange for an outsider to review your draft, especially a person who is qualified to check for spelling, grammar, and punctuation, as well as for clarity and continuity. With potentially useful comments in hand, you are now in a position to review your semifinal draft and get the paper ready for submission.

Final Draft

Your term paper will need a title page. If a format has not been assigned by the instructor, prepare a title page on your own. It should contain the title of your paper, the course name, number, and section, the name of the instructor, and your own name. The title you select should be informative and attention-grabbing.

Your final draft should incorporate the comments that you feel are appropriate from an outside reader. In rereading it, try to avoid radical alterations that may introduce new difficulties in continuity and exposition. This stage is designed to put the final touches on your paper, rather than make major revisions of it.

The final copy should have a two-inch border along the left margin (for comments) and should be double-spaced (except for lengthy quotations, which can be single-spaced).

All text pages should be numbered, preferably using the format page 1 of 10, page 2 of 10, etc. Place your name at the top of each page to ensure that it will not be lost. If a table of contents is needed, prepare one.

References should be numbered sequentially in Arabic and placed as close to the relevant material as possible. They should be identified, preferably on separate pages at the end of the paper. Your instructor may provide references and a style manual or sheet showing how these should be presented. If none is provided, your librarian can show you a source for this information.

Find a suitable presentation binder for your term paper, one that will make a positive impression without being flashy or costly. Make sure the pages are in the proper order before you insert them in your binder.

Taking Examinations

An integral part of our educational system is taking examinations. While it is acknowledged that they are imperfect measures of an individual's knowledge or ability, they are an accepted means of determining academic progress and thus help to establish a basis for advancement.

In addition to being a grading tool, exams can have a positive value in that they can encourage or motivate the student to achieve. Doing well on exams can improve one's self-esteem.

Students sometimes tend to fear exams, being concerned that they will not perform well. This can become a self-fulfilling prophecy, because it can lead to anxiety and this, in turn, can interfere with one's performance on the exam. Intense pre-examination anxiety must be avoided (realizing, of course, that some degree of nervousness is reasonable).

Knowing that you have done everything necessary to prepare for an exam should provide you with a sense of self-confidence that is strong enough to achieve a potentially good performance. Relaxing before an exam is therefore very desirable.

Reducing anxiety

A major prerequisite for reducing anxiety is to get a good night's sleep just prior to the exam. This should be obtained, if at all possible, without the use of any sleep-inducing aids so as to avoid any chance of a hangover that could interfere with your performance the next day.

A more active approach that may prove helpful is to employ one of the common tension-reducing methods. A common exercise is to sit down (in a comfortable chair, when possible), close your eyes, and take deep breaths. Hold each breath for about five seconds before exhaling. You should find your tension diminishing as you proceed with counting your breaths (approximately 20). Practicing this exercise will improve the results.

When possible, avoid mingling with other anxious students just prior to the exam, since this can have a negative effect on your state of mind. Waiting just outside the door of the exam room for the instructor to arrive is not recommended, nor is trying to get information from others at the last minute. You should, however, avoid being too far from the exam room at the appointed time, since being there on time is essential to remaining calm. If the exam room was or is one of your classrooms, try to sit in your usual seat, if possible. Remember that once the exam starts, and you focus attention on it, your nervousness should be gone.

General Exam Advice

Here are some important tips:

TIP 1   Readiness

Be prepared with several pens, pencils, and erasers; wear a watch, if possible.

TIP 2   Record data early

If you are afraid you will forget some vital memorized information, put it down in an appropriate place in your exam booklet for possible future reference (if your test proctor permits it).

TIP 3   Read instructions

Before beginning the exam, read all the instructions carefully. Underline key words (such as compare, differentiate, causes, reasons, etc.) in the instructions. The same advice applies to any essay questions. Note whether you are given a choice of parts of the exam or questions within a part and if there are any extra credit questions.

TIP 4   Record clues

If, while reading the essay question, highlights of answers come to mind, put them down so they can be referred to at a later time.

TIP 5   Balance your time

If you know how the exam is weighted pointwise, allot your time in answering the questions in a proportional manner.

Nature of Exams

Your exam can have three formats: objective, subjective, or a combination of both types of questions. Objective questions appear in the form of true-false, multiple-choice, matching, or completion. Science and mathematics exams are usually presented using an objective format. This is also true in other areas, where a large class size is involved, since it facilitates rapid grading. Objective exams are thought by some to entail less bias. Subjective examinations, on the other hand, consist of essay questions, with reasoning, analysis, and opinion rendering. This is the preferred type for humanities and social science courses. Subjective exams are viewed favorably because they are thought to measure the depth of knowledge and understanding.

Taking Objective Exams

Objective exams are recognition tests; you should not read into the question any elements that are not self-evident. The most straightforward, rather than obscure, meaning should be considered. Your answer should be based on the lectures and reading assignments for the course.

Questions have equal value, so avoid spending too much time on any one in particular. Answering all the questions that you know at the outset will provide you with time to consider and act on those you do not know. This includes guessing.

Accept questions at face value; do not add, change, or delete words to make the meaning more acceptable to you.

On multiple-choice completion questions, try to answer the question in your own words first, then find the answer that most closely approximates it. This is likely to be the correct one. In alloting time, expect multiple-choice questions to take twice as long per question as true-false questions. Also, when entering answers on an IBM card, one solid black stroke is enough; multiple strokes are superfluous and avoiding them will save some time.

True-false Questions

1. Beware of mandatory words: "never," "always," "must." They presuppose that, if any exceptions exist, the answer must be false. If guessing an answer to a question that has a mandatory word, then the answer chosen should also be false.

2. Similarly, you have to beware when such mandatory words as "generally," "normally," and "seldom" are used, since they clearly imply exceptions to the question and these would make the statement false. When guessing in this context, it is best to choose true.

Multiple-choice Questions

If you are uncertain about any of these questions and you have to guess, use the following guidelines:

1. If two answers contain similar sounding words, pick one of these.

2. If two answers are almost identical, choose one of these.

3. If among the choices an answer is unusually short or long, select one of these.

4. Eliminate extreme answers from consideration and choose from among the others.

5. If you are unable to make any choice, select the third answer. It has the highest probability of being correct.

Taking Subjective Exams

Subjective exams, in addition to recall, require organization and, frequently, conclusions. The following suggestions can prove helpful:

1. Read all the questions carefully and then select the easiest question to answer first.

2. After selecting the question, do not begin writing your response immediately. Rather, organize your answer in a longer order by noting down headings and subheadings, and then proceed.

3. The essay should be structured so that you initially present your position, follow it up with relevant data or arguments, and then draw the appropriate conclusions (offering other options when desirable).

4. Allot an appropriate amount of time for each question. When the time is up, wrap up your conclusions and move on.

5. At the outset, merely identify the question without repeating it. This will save time.

6. Try to have a strong lead sentence in each paragraph, with the following sentences supporting or flowing from this opening one.

7. When possible, use the technical vocabulary of the course.

8. Try to make your sentences short and as uncomplicated as possible. The sentences should not be mere definition statements, but should be supported by facts or arguments when possible. These should, preferably, be arranged in order.

9. If providing a definition, try to give it a broad meaning and use the instructor's wording when possible.

10. If you have answered in what you consider a satisfactory manner, do not seek to "flesh it out" with irrelevant information.

11. If you do not know an answer to an essay question and have left it to the end and still have no recall, write on a closely related issue in the hope that you will get partial credit.

12. Leave some space after each essay question in the case you recall some additional information later and time permits you to come back.

13. Neatness is very desirable; if it is difficult to read your writing, the instructor may be negatively biased. Write your essay in ink to enhance neatness.

14. Write your essay on one side of the page, leaving the other side for use, if necessary, later.

Upon Exam Completion

When you finish the exam, you will have a natural impulse to want to leave the room. You should make use of any remaining time to review your answers. Answers to objective questions should be altered if you feel that they were misinterpreted or answered wrong. Do not do so merely on impulse.

Review of your answers may also bring to your attention any questions that have inadvertently gone unanswered or may have been answered in the wrong place (a not uncommon situation that can prove disastrous). In a situation where you were forced to guess, rereading a question may bring the correct answer to mind. For essays, rereading can bring to light a point or issue that was overlooked, probably because we think faster than we write. Computations should be rechecked, especially the position of decimal points.

After leaving the classroom, make notes pertaining to the questions asked so that you have an idea of the type of exams the instructor gives, a useful reference for future exam preparation.

Memorization Techniques

Over the past several decades medical educators have been carefully scrutinizing the curriculum in order to update it and keep it relevant to the demands of a modern medical practice. One of the unstated goals is to reduce the extent of memorization needed and concentrate on the reasoning processes involved in problem solving. While some progress has been made, there is and will always remain a mass of essential information that has to be memorized, in college, medical school, and postgraduate training, in order to successfully complete these programs.

Below are some memorization techniques that may prove beneficial during your education. They can be divided into three categories:

A. Organize

TIP 1 Remove distractions

If you are not distracted by some outside elements, such as conversation, radio, or television, you obviously will be able to concentrate more effectively on the task at hand.

TIP 2 Get a good night's sleep

After a good night's sleep, one is usually mentally more alert in the morning than later in the day. Take advantage of this fact and try to grasp the major concepts early in the day, before you start to memorize the details.

TIP 3 Relax

When you are relaxed, new data can be absorbed more readily and you will likely retain it with a greater degree of accuracy. Being tense will prove mentally distracting and counterproductive.

TIP 4   Stand while studying

Some people find it helpful to try memorizing while standing up. You should determine if this works for you.

TIP 5   Create associations

Store information that you already know in some way that you can recall. When you want to add new data, it is desirable to link the "new" with similar data that you already know.

TIP 6   Generate images

Draw sketches and/or diagrams and use them to link together facts and illustrate relationships.

TIP 7   Scan over the material

Before beginning a reading assignment, skim over it in order to recognize the main ideas the writer seeks to convey.

TIP 8   Recite and repeat

When you recite material out loud, you double the effect by first reading the item and then hearing it, thereby involving two different senses. The effect will be further reinforced by repeating the information.

TIP 9   Write it

When an important fact comes spontaneously to mind, promptly write it down. Even if you do not refer to it later, the act of recording it will serve to place it in your mind's memory bank.

B. Think

TIP 10   Overstudy

Study somewhat more than you feel is necessary to ensure a feeling of self-confidence. This will also reinforce your prior memorization efforts.

TIP 11   Spread out learning

Make use of the valuable intervals between required assignments and commit information to memory that you expect to need later.

TIP 12   Look for connections

Interesting things are remembered more readily; if you have a subject that is not especially appealing, try to find something that is more interesting to relate it to. By establishing a connection, you will elevate your interest in the subject and be more likely to remember it.

TIP 13   Be selective

In committing material to memory, choose what is necessary or essential. Do not fill your mind with trivia or data that does not need to be memorized and can be easily retrieved.

TIP 14   Combine memory techniques

To secure maximal effect, memory techniques should be combined, with one technique reinforcing another.

C. Recall

TIP 15   Unblocking

You can possibly unlock your memory by stimulating the recall of related information; therefore, if you cannot recall an answer, try jotting down answers to related questions. This may cause the sought-after answer to come to mind.

TIP 16   Determine your memory style

Determine from experience what techniques work best for you. Also, ascertain what memory vehicle leaves the most lasting impression: reading, hearing, or seeing. Try wherever possible to use the one approach that works best for you.

TIP 17   Use your information

Repeated use will help you retain data. This is best exemplified by one's recall of telephone, social security, or bank account numbers.

TIP 18   Be positive

Develop the conviction that you do not really forget but that you simply misplace information and all you need to do is to find where in your memory file you stored that needed information.

Succeeding as a Premedical Student

In the preceding section detailed advice is outlined on various important aspects affecting your potential success as a college student in general. This section focuses on ways to enhance your career prospects, specifically as a college premedical student.

It is essential that throughout your college career, you evaluate your progress at regular intervals, certainly at the end of each semester. While doing this, it is important that you keep abreast of the admissions criteria and standards at medical schools that traditionally accept students from your school. To secure this information, you may have to tap several sources; tips on potential sources for useful information are outlined below:

TIP 1   Make connections

Establish early contact with other premed students, especially those on academic levels above you. This may most easily be done at premed club meetings. Discuss with others their plans and application experiences, where appropriate. Remember, however, that such students, while able to relate personal insights, may not have authoritative opinions. If what they say doesn't sound correct, seek clarification from your premed advisor.

TIP 2   Get information

Seek to obtain additional data (beyond that provided in Table 5.1), regarding current admissions criteria relative to grade point average, science cumulative average, and MCAT scores. This information will allow you to put your own performance in perspective as you progress through college. If such a self-evaluation raises concerns on your part, discuss them with your advisor as early as possible so as to not be negatively impacted psychologically and filled with self-doubt.

TIP 3   Obtain publications

Determine if your premed society or advisory office has prepared a student handbook or has a file with current admissions information, charts, and tables. This will add to your knowledge base.

TIP 4   Attend meetings

Many premedical groups organize "career nights," where speakers, frequently alumni, discuss different career options in the health professions. This may be supplemented by field trips that may involve visits to local medical schools. Additional information can be obtained by attending meetings where medical school representatives report on their admissions policies and procedures.

TIP 5   Seek advice

Arrange to meet with your advisor periodically so that he or she can assess your progress and get to know you. Your meetings can be both formal and informal, as an individual and as part of a group. It is important, especially at a large school, that you lose anonymity and become known to your advisor, who, in due course, will be writing recommendations on your behalf.

Another set of factors associated with your success as a premed student involves academic components (such as GPA and science cum). The following additional tips are relevant to this important area:

TIP 1   Plan well

Work out for yourself a basic four-year curriculum that fulfills the college's general prerequisites as well as those in your major (and minor) and premed course for graduation requirements. Discuss your plan with students who may have followed a similar program as well as with your advisor, to see if it is realistic.

TIP 2   Schedule appropriately

Once your overall college program is in place, structure your semesters' schedules so that there is a suitable balance of time blocks allotted to lectures, laboratory sessions, study, and relaxation intervals, as well as extracurricular activities.

TIP 3   Select carefully

In choosing the course section, bear in mind that more demanding courses such as chemistry or physics might best be taken earlier in the day, when you are more alert and receptive. In addition, ask other students about the different faculty members offering the same course, to determine their teaching characteristics. Are they devoted to educating their students? Do they mark their exams excessively hard? Are their exams aimed at eliciting what you really know? Are they reasonable to deal with? Avoid being influenced by students who may be biased because they feel that they were unfairly treated by a professor, unless there is a consistent pattern to this teacher's actions. In other words, you are seeking to obtain information to ensure that your chances for succeeding in your coursework are good.

TIP 4   Improve your average

To meet the credit requirement for graduation, you usually have to take electives. These should be carefully selected in terms of your general interest, rounding out your educational background, how the course fits in your schedule, time demands of the course, and the projected grade for the course. By selecting wisely, you can help boost your grade point average, since the computer does not distinguish between elective and required courses in automatically computing your GPA.

TIP 5   Elect a summer session

As the term proceeds you may find your schedule to be too demanding and that it is jeopardizing your overall performance. You should then consider dropping a course to lighten your load, perhaps making up the course during the following summer. Consult an appropriate school advisor before doing so.

Extracurricular and Summer Activities

Your nonacademic activities usually will not be decisive elements in your admission to medical school but they can be helpful. You would be well advised to participate in your college premedical society, as well as other organizations that may be related to medicine less directly. Participation in community, political, or sports activities helps in presenting the image of a well-rounded and adjusted individual to admissions officers.

If possible, plan your summer activities so that they can be useful for your career goals. Such activities include hospital work, research, or other activities involving interpersonal contacts. For example, at the end of the freshman year, try to find activities that involve working with people, such as youth camp work or community projects. During the summer following the sophomore year, try to gain some hospital experience. Though summer positions in hospitals are not readily available, try for employment as an orderly, operating or emergency room assistant, or nurse's aide. Also consider a position as a clinical laboratory assistant or a position in a mental hospital or nursing home.

The summer between the junior and senior year could also be spent in hospital work. Students with an interest in research might try obtaining a position at a medical school or in a government laboratory. In addition, a summer spent participating in a research project can provide an understanding of the scientific method in action. It will afford experiences in designing experiments and in collecting and evaluating data.

When working on a summer project, make a definite effort to ensure that your supervisor becomes acquainted with both you and your work. It may prove useful later when you begin securing letters of recommendation to be sent to the medical schools.

As a prospective professional, you should take a job in a hospital, not just to be able to list this activity on your application, but to be able to look at yourself and your reactions to the sick patient, to understand that medical practice is not all heroics and glory, but many hours of hard work. You should try to familiarize yourself with the roles of the various members of the health care team so that you recognize that each has a crucial function in the entire process. In this way you can see if it is the physician's role that is most compatible with your life goals.

Several excellent summer job opportunities exist in a few states at the following institutions:

California
Personnel Department
University of California
Lawrence Livermore Laboratory
P.O. Box 808-N
Livermore, CA 94550

Connecticut
Summer Student Research Fellowship
Department of Medical Education
Hartford Hospital
80 Seymour Street
Hartford, CT 06102-5037

Illinois
Summer Student Research Fellowship Program
Office of Research Administration
Michael Reese Medical Center
29th Street and Ellis Avenue
Chicago, IL 60616

Maine
Research Training Office
The Jackson Laboratory
Bar Harbor, ME 04609

New York
Research Participation Program in Molecular Biology
Roswell Park Cancer Institute
Elm and Carlton Streets
Buffalo, NY 14263

Summer Scientific Work Program
Franklin Hospital Medical Center
900 Franklin Avenue
Valley Stream, NY 11582

Brookhaven National Laboratory
Science Education Center
Building 438
P.O. Box 5000
Upton, NY 11973-5000

Pennsylvania
Mellon Research Summer Program in Psychiatry for Undergraduates
Western Psychiatric Institute and Clinic
3811 O'Hara Street
Pittsburgh, PA 15213

Texas
Surgical Laboratory Program
Baylor College of Medicine
Texas Medical Center
Houston, TX 77030

The Premedical Advisor and/or Committee

The premedical advisor can help you in planning the sequence of courses needed to meet the requirements at most medical schools. He or she will also offer suggestions as to which schools to apply to, when to take the MCAT, and how to interpret the scores. The advisor is usually assisted by a committee of faculty members who evaluate your academic performance and potential as well as your overall fitness to study medicine. The premedical committee maintains a file of your records and evaluations by individual members.

It is the obligation of the advisor or committee to provide the medical schools with supporting information in your behalf (see pages 42 and 43). Some medical schools will utilize their own recommendation forms that they send out to be completed. Most rely on the college's forms and even accept them in lieu of their own. Undergraduate schools vary in the format they use to provide their evaluation. Many use a letter of recommendation drafted by the advisor or a member of the committee who knows the student. It may include written comments about the applicant submitted by faculty members, and it will reveal the committee's consensus of the student's abilities and potential and may rate the applicant in comparison to others applying during the year from the same school. Some schools provide a letter of recommendation and a separate sheet of faculty comments. Others may provide a letter and a quantitative rating sheet (see page 44) and possibly also a comment sheet.

Attributes listed on rating sheets, and the ratings used, vary from school to school. However, in general they refer to the applicant's personal as well as academic attributes and attempt to portray them in a quantitative and objective manner.

In view of the generally high caliber of applicants to medical school, recommendations (and interviews) have assumed major importance in the application process. Thus, students should make themselves and their abilities well known to faculty members. Their knowledge of you should be as thorough as possible so that they can rate you not only quantitatively but also qualitatively. Recommendations by science professors, whether they know you from coursework or as an individual, are of special value. Of particular usefulness are evaluations from honors work or independent study supervisors who can comment on such qualities as initiative, determination, and reliability.

To facilitate preparation of letters of recommendation in your behalf, some college premedical committees require that prospective applicants complete a standard form that may be several pages long (see pages 38 to 41). This mechanism provides the committee with data relative to your personal life, family background, outside jobs, extracurricular activities (both school or non-school related), and special interests. They may also request that you submit a tentative list of the schools you wish to apply to as well as an essay relevant to your application to medical school. By this means, not only is a database available to the committee to formulate your letter of recommendation, but you will also be able to secure advice on where to apply and how many schools to apply to (see also page 57). In addition, your premedical committee essay can serve as a prototype for your AMCAS essay. If your school does not use such a form, you may, nevertheless, wish to use the sample format shown to provide information to your premedical advisor and/or committee. In addition, you may wish to solicit your advisor's (or an English composition instructor's) reaction to your essay as to content, style, and effectiveness in "marketing" your candidacy for admission.

Finally, a word of caution about advisors. It is essential that you are courteous and respectful at all times in your dealings with members of your college faculty and especially with your preprofessional advisor. Your advisor will be responsible for transmitting the qualitative impression of the faculty to the medical schools. Thus, your advisor's good will is most desirable and can be developed, not by ingratiating yourself, but by establishing a genuine relationship.

On the other hand, it is not necessary to accept your advisor's recommendations as the only truth if you have valid reasons to question it. As with physicians, there are both good and mediocre advisors. Moreover, there are no licensing or certification processes for accrediting advisors as there are for MDs or DDSs. The institution usually selects a member of its science faculty who may be interested in doing advisory work and assigns the responsibility to this individual, in turn relieving that person of some teaching responsibilities. The quality of the advice you will receive will depend upon the advisor's innate ability, experience, conscientiousness, other academic responsibilities, and number of other advisees. Thus, the extent of personal attention students receive varies greatly. All too frequently, student counseling is provided on a "clinic"-type basis. Students frequently turn to upperclass-level premeds (especially seniors) for advice; their advice can be misleading since their experience is limited, even if they have been successful in getting into medical school. In the event that you have reservations about some important issue, you can seek to validate your advisor's recommendations by discreetly discussing them with another faculty member on a confidential basis, by asking a friend at another school to pose the same question or problem there, or by contacting a medical school admission office or a private counseling service.

POSTBACCALAUREATE PROGRAMS

While the vast majority of medical school applicants are college seniors, a small, yet increasingly significant, number consists of those with a postbaccalaureate premedical education. This group is made up of individuals who: (1) seek to change their present career, (2) have been uncommitted as to a career choice and now have decided on medicine as a profession, or (3) sought but failed to secure admission to medical school and are now trying to improve their chances upon reapplying.

The following schools offer postbaccalaureate educational programs that provide a wide range of academic and nonacademic support. Programs extend for one or two years. Some are geared toward non-science majors, while others assist in preparation for the MCAT.

California
Postbaccalaureate Program
Educational and Community Programs
College of Medicine (125 Medical Surge I)
University of California, Irvine
Irvine, CA 92717
(714) 856-4603

Reapplicant Summer Course (RSC)
Special Admissions Support Program
School of Medicine
University of California, San Diego
Data Building, Room 102
9500 Gillman Drive
La Jolla, CA 92093
(619) 734-4170

Postbaccalaureate Premedical Program
Mills College
Office of Graduate Studies
Oakland, CA 94613
(510) 430-3309; fax: (510) 430-3314

Health Professions Postbaccalaureate Advancement Program
Health Profession Office
California State University, Fullerton
800 West State College Boulevard
Fullerton, CA 92634
(714) 773-3980

Postbaccalaureate Reapplicant Program
Office of Minority Affairs
School of Medicine
University of California, Davis
Davis, CA 95616
(916) 752-1852

Connecticut
Postbaccalaureate Programs
U. Conn. Post-Bac Program
School of Medicine
University of Connecticut
263 Farmington Avenue
Farmington, CT 06030
(203) 679-3874; fax: 679-1282

Florida
Postbaccalaureate Program
College of Arts and Sciences
University of Miami, Coral Gables
P.O. Box 248004
Coral Gables, FL 33124
(305) 284-5176

Illinois
Medical-Dental Education Preparation Program
Admissions Coordinator
MEDPREP, Wheeler Hall
School of Medicine
Southern Illinois University
Carbondale, IL 62901
(618) 536-6674

Maryland
Postbaccalaureate Premedical Program
Goucher College
1021 Dulaney Valley Road
Baltimore, MD 21204
(800) 697-4646

Postbaccalaureate Premedical-Predental Program
Department of Biological Sciences
Towson State University
Towson, MD 21204
(301) 830-3042

Massachusetts
Health Careers Program
Harvard University Extension School
51 Brattle Street
Cambridge, MA 02138
(617) 495-2926

Postbaccalaureate Prehealth Program
Program Administrator
Office of Professional and Continuing Studies
Tufts University
112 Packard Avenue
Medford, MA 02155
(617) 627-3562

Michigan
Advanced Baccalaureate Learning Experience (ABLE) Program
A254 Life Sciences Building
College of Human Medicine
Michigan State University
East Lansing, MI 44824
(517) 355-2405

Postbaccalaureate Premedical Program
Office of Student and Minority Affairs
University of Michigan Medical School
1301 Catherine Road
5109C Medical Science I Building
Ann Arbor, MI 48109
(313) 764-8185

Nebraska
Postbaccalaureate Program
Department of Pharmacology
School of Medicine
Creighton University
Omaha, NE 68178
(402) 280-3185

New York
Postbaccalaureate Premedical Program
Office of Preprofessional Programs
405 Lewisohn Hall
Columbia University
New York, NY 10027
(212) 305-3595

Postbaccalaureate Program
Prehealth Advising Office
Rm. 904 Main Building
College of Arts and Sciences
New York University
100 Washington Square East, Room 904
New York, NY 10003
(212) 998-8160

Postbaccalaureate Program
Coordinator, Post-Bac Program
School of Medicine and Biomedical Sciences
3435 Main Street, 40 CFS Building
Buffalo, NY 14214
(716) 829-2811

North Carolina
Postbaccalaureate Development Program
Office of Minority Affairs
Bowman Gray School of Medicine
Medical Center Boulevard
Winston-Salem, NC 27157
(910) 716-4201

Ohio
Postbaccalaureate Program
MEDPATH Office
1072 Graves Hall
College of Medicine
Ohio State University
333 West 10th Avenue
Columbus, OH 43210
(614) 292-3161; fax: (614) 698-4041

Postbaccalaureate Program
Director, Center for Excellence
College of Osteopathic Medicine
Ohio University
Grosvenor Hall
Athens, OH 45701
(614) 593-2365; fax: (614) 593-0892

Pennsylvania
Postbaccalaureate Program
Division of Special Studies
Bryn Mawr College
Bryn Mawr, PA 19010
(215) 526-7350

Postbaccalaureate Premedical Linkage and Non-linkage Programs
Postbac Premedical Programs
241 Mellon Hall
Duquesne University
Pittsburgh, PA 15282
(412) 396-6445; fax: (412) 396-5587

Postbaccalaureate Prehealth Program
Coordinator, Prehealth Programs
University of Pennsylvania College of General Studies
Philadelphia, PA 19104
(215) 898-4847

Texas
Postbaccalaureate Program
Director, Medical Student Recruitment
University of Texas Medical Branch
Ashbel Smith G120
Galveston, TX 77555
(409) 772-5256

Vermont
Postbaccalaureate Premedical and Allied Health Sciences Program
Chief Health Science Advisor
Bennington College
Bennington, VT 05201
(802) 442-5401

Virginia
Medical Academic Advancement Program
Office of Student Academic Support
School of Medicine
Health Sciences Center, Box 446
University of Virginia
Charlottsville, VA 22908
(804) 924-2189

HUMANISTIC ASPECTS OF PREMEDICAL EDUCATION _____

Aside from the intellectual and technical challenges that medical education presents, there are a variety of other considerations that must be faced by professional school students. Among these are the realizations that:

1. There is a great diversity in the patients that one sees. One is not surrounded by a homogeneous population, but by all types of people—rich and poor, young and old, educated and illiterate.

2. There are emotional as well as physical factors to be dealt with in patient care, including crises in the lives of patients.

3. The issues of pain and suffering, of dying and death are aspects of life that are distant from the young, healthy student who must learn to cope with them in a sympathetic, although somewhat detached, manner.

4. There are ethical issues to consider that cannot be defined scientifically, such as who shall be born, who shall live, who shall die.

Medical school does not adequately prepare one for the aforementioned problems and thus it is the premedical experiences and training that tend to mold one's values on these subjective issues. Only by an in-depth exposure to the human condition through literature, religion, and philosophy can the student develop the capacity to face the nonacademic aspects of the medical professions.

The inexperienced medical student is usually unable to assess the issues that defy scientific definition—the issues of human diversity, suffering, life and death. These questions are peripheral to mastering the mass of scientific information and technical skills during the preclinical years. It is during the premedical years that the opportunity exists to acquire the exposure that molds values relative to nonquantifiable moral issues. If these ethical guidelines can be acquired by formal and/or informal education in the course of one's college years as a premedical student, then a solid foundation will have been laid for the medical training that will follow, and ultimately a well-rounded physician will emerge to practice in the twenty-first century.

Request Form for Letter of Recommendation

_____ UNIVERSITY

Prehealth Professions Committee

Re: Request for Preparation of a Letter of Recommendation

Please prepare supporting material on the applicant's behalf for (check one or more):

medical _____, dental _____, osteopathy _____, podiatry _____,

optometry _____, other (specify) _____

Application for class entering: _____   Today's date _____

Name:_____   Date of birth: ____/_____/____
    (last)   (first)   (middle)

Local address: _____
        (number and street)   (city)   (state)   (zip)

Permanent address: _____
            (number and street)   (city)   (state)   (zip)

Telephone number: _____
            (area code)   (number)

Citizenship: U.S. _____   Other: (specify) _____

Father's occupation: _____   Mother's occupation: _____

Credits transferred (if any): _____, Completed: _____, In progress: _____

The data below should refer only to the applicant's performance at _____ University.

Current Grade Point Average: _____ Science cum (including math): _____

Major: _____ Major average: _____ Minor: _____ Minor average: _____

Has the applicant's education to date been continuous other than for vacations?

Yes: _____ No: _____

If the answer to the previous question is in the negative, indicate what the applicant has done while out of attendance or since graduation.

_____

_____

_____

Has the applicant ever been placed on probation (academic or disciplinary)?

Yes: _____ No: _____

If the answer to the previous question is yes, clarify the circumstances involved.

_____

_____

_____

Employment history: Complete as fully as possible.

	Position	Place of employment	Dates of employment	Hours worked/week
Summer prior to beginning college				
Freshman year				
Summer between freshman and sophomore years				
Sophomore year				
Summer between sophomore and junior years				
Junior year				
Summer between junior and senior years				
Senior year				

Furnish, in detail, the following information:

Extracurricular (school-related) activities (clubs, projects, positions in student government, student organizations, college or university committees, etc.)

_____

_____

_____

_____

Non-school-related activities (social, fraternal, religious, community, political, etc.)

_____

_____

_____

Hobbies: _____
_____
_____

Special interests (not previously covered):_____
_____
_____

Provide a TENTATIVE list of those schools to which the applicant plans to apply:

_____   _____   _____

_____   _____   _____

_____   _____   _____

_____   _____   _____

_____   _____   _____

_____   _____   _____

Is the applicant interested in a professional degree (DDS, MD, OD, DO, DPM, DVM) only?
(Check one.) Yes: _____ No: _____

Is the applicant interested in a combined MD/PhD degree? Yes: _____ No: _____

TYPE an essay (limited to two pages), in which the applicant considers the following topics, as
they personally relate:

1. How did your interest in the sciences begin and how did it develop?

2. What circumstances and considerations have motivated you to consider undertaking a career
   in the health sciences?

3. From where does your knowledge of the health sciences and of health care delivery stem (is it
   based on family exposure, work, reading, talking with practitioners, volunteer work, etc.)?

4. Why do you seek to enter the health professions? What do you hope to contribute? What do
   you feel you have to offer? What do you hope to derive from working in this area?

5. What are your plans in the event that you are not accepted (aside from reapplication)?

Type the essay, double-spaced, on this page. If you need more space, you may use additional pages.

AMCAS or AADSAS applications should be single-spaced. The suggestion for double spacing here is to permit emendation by your advisor.

Letter of Recommendation in Support of a Superior Candidate

_____ University
Premedical Advisory Committee

September 30, 1995

Chairperson
Admissions Committee

Re: Steven B. _____

Dear Doctor:

In the course of several extended interviews with Steven B. _____, I have gotten to know him academically and personally. I found that he is an attractive individual from both perspectives and therefore I am writing this recommendation.

Steve has been a solid achiever his entire life. After a superior (94) performance at Stuyvesant High School, one of New York City's top three, he enrolled at _____ College. He selected this school because of its modest size and the quality liberal arts education it offers. After adjusting to college life during his first semester, his record over the past three years has gone from about B+ to above A–. His science performance has been consistently superior in both the required premedical courses and in all his electives. He has a special aptitude for mathematics and has even tutored in this area.

What I found especially interesting in Steven's background is that he is one of the rare breed of premeds who is a genuine liberal arts student, having majored in East Asian studies. One of his professors cultivated his interest in this area, which blends well with his innate interest in people. This quality is also reflected by his involvement in a hospice program, which prospective medical students rarely get exposed to. Steve's perspective of medicine is well rounded, from having become an EMT, and also because he worked in the emergency and operating rooms at several local hospitals.

Steve is very affable, outgoing, open, and has a ready sense of humor. It is easy to establish a good rapport with him, which his future patients will surely come to appreciate. He has impressed me with his perceptive analysis of people and tolerant attitude toward them. Steve is a hard worker whose unusual physical strength permits him to be employed in his free time for very extended periods (a quality that should serve him well during his residency). He is also self-disciplined, having to resist a predisposition to becoming overweight. Being on the rugby team at _____, and now its captain, has been an asset in this regard. Steven is a young man of high integrity, with a genuine service orientation and a keen sense of observation.

In summary, Steven B. _____ stands out not merely on a quantitative paper profile, but rather as a total person. His warm personality, open-mindedness, and motivation make him attractive even among a large pool of qualified applicants.

Sincerely,

Chief Premedical Advisor

Letter of Recommendation to Enhance a Candidate's Status

_____ University

September 30, 1995
Chairperson
Admissions Committee   Re: Daniel H. _____

Dear Doctor:

I am writing on behalf of Daniel H. _____, whom I have gotten to know very well during the course of his extended visits to my office.

I am especially stimulated to write on behalf of Daniel in the light of what I foresee as the special qualities that I think physicians planning to practice in the next century should have. It is my feeling that there is a need for prospective physicians to feel that their sense of satisfaction will be the major fulfillment factor in their future medical practice. Daniel _____, to my mind, is an individual with such an outlook.

Daniel was born and raised on Long Island, where he attended private elementary and high schools. His parents both have a higher education. He enrolled at _____ University for his undergraduate studies because he desired the advantages that a smaller institution affords. _____ University premedical curriculum is rather unusual in that organic chemistry precedes inorganic chemistry. Daniel was academically unprepared for this regimen; nevertheless, by intensively applying himself he received a satisfactory grade in this course. This situation, however, impacted negatively on his freshman GPA (approximately 3.0). Subsequently, his performance steadily improved to the point where his GPA for junior year was 3.85. Clearly, his ability to face up to challenges and his determination to achieve his goal are most evident from his overall performance during the past three years. His science GPA (excluding freshman year) is superior and is reflected and confirmed in his strong showing on both of the science subtests of the spring, 1994 MCAT. His low quantitative score is probably an aberration. I believe it is to be of no significance in terms of a reflection on his ability. Nevertheless, he is retaking the exam because of his determination to rectify this situation.

What is especially striking about Daniel is that he comes from a family that has passed on a very successful business (wholesale fruit and vegetables) through several generations. His father, not surprisingly, would be quite amenable to his becoming active in the business upon graduating college and eventually attaining financial success. However, Daniel is seeking a service-oriented career.

Daniel has impressed me with the genuineness of his motivation and the sincerity of his conviction. He clearly realizes that the component of personal satisfaction is one of the most important aspects of a career in medicine. His considerable exposure to medicine has not only reinforced his interest in this field, but has provided him with evidence that such service can provide a unique means of personal gratification.

In summary, Daniel possesses solid academic and personal credentials and, in my mind, has the innate attributes that a prospective physician should possess. I strongly recommend him to your next freshman class.

Sincerely,

Chair, Premedical Advisory Committee

_____UNIVERSITY
_____
_____

CONFIDENTIAL REPORT ON CANDIDATE FOR ADMISSION TO PROFESSIONAL SCHOOL

Date _____

The following evaluation is submitted for your guidance by the Health Sciences Advisory Office of _____ (the college of arts and sciences for men of _____ University). This evaluation is based on a careful study of written evaluations by, and consultation with, those members of the faculty who have had personal knowledge of the candidate and his work in both lecture and laboratory courses.

NAME OF CANDIDATE _____ I.D. No._____
This student has completed _____ years of college. His cumulative average to date is _____ (A = 4).
Candidate for School of ( ) Medicine   ( ) Denistry   ( ) Podiatry   ( ) Optometry   ( ) Other _____

	OUTSTANDING	VERY GOOD	GOOD	AVERAGE	POOR
PERSONAL ATTRIBUTES					
1. Appearance and Social Manner					
2. Maturity and Emotional Stability					
3. Communication Skills					
4. Interpersonal Relations					
5. Cooperation and Reliability					
6. Self-Confidence					
ACADEMIC ATTRIBUTES					
7. Industry and Perseverance					
8. Originality and Resourcefulness					
9. Laboratory Skills					
10. Native Intelligence and Judgment					
11. Scientific Aptitude					

Summary evaluation of the applicant's
fitness for professional study and practice.*

*Determined by averaging the student's ratings of items 7 through 11 together with his cumulative academic average, according to a mathematical formula under which 4.0 is the highest possible rating. Students whose combined index falls between:

3.7 and 4.0 are rated "outstanding"
3.4 and 3.6 are rated "very good"
2.9 and 3.3 are rated "good"
2.3 and 2.8 are rated "average"
2.0 and 2.2 are rated "poor"

_____
Health Sciences Advisor

REMARKS_____
_____

NOTE: The above student has waived his right to inspect and review this recommendation under the Family Education Rights and Privacy Act of 1974. Therefore please keep this document confidential.

3 Applying to Medical School

GENERAL CONSIDERATIONS

There are two basic factors that determine admission to medical school independently of the personal qualifications of each candidate. These factors are the total number of first-year places available and the total number of applicants for admission. Now fewer than half of those that apply are accepted to American medical schools; about half of those that are rejected are considered qualified to attend medical school.

In the decade between the Great Depression and World War II, the number of medical schools remained substantially unchanged and the number of first-year students actually decreased slightly. In the next two decades (1940–60), nine new schools were established and, as a result, first-year enrollment increased by about 50%. In the 15-year period 1960–75, 27 new schools came into being, bringing with them nearly another 65% increase in enrollment. Over the next decade (1976–86), only seven new schools became operational. Currently, only one is being considered for development on the mainland. All of this points to the end of the era of medical school expansion, at least for this century.

During the long period of expansion (1940–86), the total number of freshman places changed as a result of the opening of new institutions or the enlarging of class size at existing schools. The data indicates that two-thirds of the increase in enrollment was due to the latter and one-third to the former. This is understandable because new schools usually start with small enrollments and then expand.

Prospects for the Future

The era of new medical school development and expansion has ended. The goal of 15,000 first-year enrollments, set by medical educators to meet national health care needs, has not only been met but even surpassed. For quite a number of years approximately 16,000 freshman medical students have enrolled each year. All indications are that the available number of freshman places has peaked, since no new schools are likely to open and significant expansion of first-year class size will not take place.

During the mid-1980s there was a continuous and marked decline in the number of medical school applicants, which reached an all-time low in 1988, with a 1.6:1 applicant/acceptee ratio. Since then, the decline has not only bottomed out, but the applicant pool has consistently increased since 1989. By 1993 the number of applicants surpassed the previous peak year of 1974, and has reached new heights over each of the past three years (see graph).

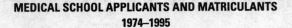

MEDICAL SCHOOL APPLICANTS AND MATRICULANTS
1974–1995

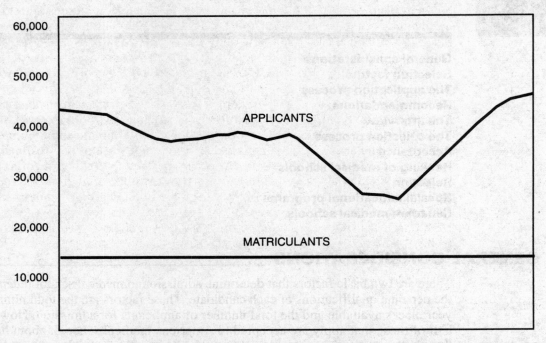

Educators link the increase in the applicant pool to the prolonged economic recession, with many professions no longer providing assured job opportunities. Medicine has retained its attractiveness as a means of providing a secure economic future. Consequently, students with a variety of majors are applying to medical school. Moreover, the surge in applicants has also been fueled by women, who now make up 40% of all medical students, and by Asian Americans. (Representation by other groups such as African-Americans and Hispanic Americans has not been growing.)

In the light of the exceptional circumstances associated with the change in the size of the applicant pool, it is very difficult to predict at this time what the admission prospects will be during the balance of this decade. Clearly, economic conditions over the next few years will impact strongly on this issue. During the interval a sustained large applicant pool is very likely.

First-year Applicants

During the decade from 1950 to 1960, the number of applicants significantly decreased (from 22,000 to 14,000 per year) and there was a corresponding decrease in the applicant/acceptee ratio (from 3.1:1 to 1.7:1). From the early 1960s to its peak in 1974, there was a continual increase in the number of applicants (from 14,000 to 43,000 per year). Since then the number of applicants has markedly declined (to 28,000 in 1987). Therefore, the applicant/acceptee ratio decreased from 2.8:1 to 1.7:1. The decreased applicant pool may have been due, in part, to the fact that academically weak students declined to apply, and thus in reality competition for a place in a freshman class was still intense.

From what has been noted above, it is obvious that there was a significant increase in the odds of gaining admission by those who applied during the 1975–88 period, when on average, the applicant/acceptee ratio was about 2:1, over applicants of the preceding 10 years when the ratio was closer to 3:1. In the years 1987–92, the competition turned out to be less than it had been since 1975. This was due to the significant gradual decline in the total number of applicants, which was estimated to have been about 1,000 per year. From 1989 to 1995 there was a strong and steady increase in the number of applicants, rising dramatically from 26,900 to 46,500, while the number of available places has remained about the same (approximately 16,000). This suggests that, for the balance of this decade, a near 3:1 applicant/acceptee ratio is likely.

While a near 3:1 ratio presents a formidable challenge, it need not be taken as reflecting any particular individual's chance for admission. Rather, it should be taken as a general reflection of the level of competition. The reason for this is that the applicant pool no longer consists almost entirely of white males as it did for well over the first half of this century. The pool now contains a sizable female segment and a smaller minority segment, which together make up more than 50% of the freshman class each year. This situation makes it more difficult to define the exact odds for any particular individual to gain admission solely on the basis of the applicant/acceptee ratio. The problem of mathematically defining the intensity of competition is compounded by the fact that about one-fourth of the total applicant pool may be repeaters, whose chances for admission usually are significantly less than are those of new applicants. Thus, in trying to assess your own overall chances, many factors come into play. These include sex, race, residency, age, and financial status in addition to intellectual achievement and potential.

Impact of Applicant Pool Size

Over the eight-year span (1988–96), the most dramatic fluctuation in the size of the applicant pool in a half century took place, from a very depressed number (about 27,000), to a remarkable record high (about 46,000). Such an enormous change in so short a time is unlikely to recur in the foreseeable future. It does, however, serve to impressively demonstrate how the size of the applicant pool significantly influences one's chances of getting into medical school as well as a variety of factors associated with the admissions process. Even under more normal circumstances, there are cyclical phases in the size of the pool of applicants and the impact of an above or below average number of applicants (about 35,000) will also be felt, although to a lesser degree, in a variety of ways. Therefore, consideration of the multifaceted influence of the impact of the applicant pool size is very important.

During interludes when the applicant pool is very large (such as the mid-1970s and mid-1990s), competition to secure a place is naturally extremely high. Under these circumstances, the following also takes place:

1. The chances for applicants with average credentials to gain admission is markedly diminished.

2. For the more attractive applicant the number of multiple acceptances received will likely be reduced.

3. The number of schools to which an applicant should apply will probably increase; consequently, the overall cost to applicants of the entire admissions process (such as application fees and interview expenses) will be higher.

4. The response from medical schools may be slower due to the large volume of applications that need to be processed when the pool is large.

5. Less attractive financial aid packages may be offered to applicants.

6. Competition will also be intense in the selection of women and minority group applicants who make up a sizable segment of most freshman classes.

7. Marked deficiencies in an applicant's record will carry more weight than usual, to the applicant's disadvantage; therefore, chances of the applicant securing an interview, which would allow the opportunity to explain a possible weakness in that applicant's record, are unfortunately diminished.

8. Tuition will more likely remain high when the applicant pool is large.

During a period when the applicant pool is low (as in 1984–87), the reverse of the above considerations come into play, to a degree dependent on the extent of the depression in the number of applicants.

In light of these considerations, it is important for all applicants to be alert to the status of the current size and direction of movement of the applicant pool for the few years prior to the time they plan to apply. They could then anticipate the general impact that the existing applicant pool situation will have upon them.

Early Admission

Most applicants to medical school plan to have their baccalaureate degree before beginning medical study. For a typical entering class, less than 5% of the first-year students lacked their bachelor's degree. (For details, see Table 5.1.)

There is considerable variation in policy regarding the admission of students after only three years of college study. The percentage of early admissions varies between none and 25%. In any case, only the exceptional student should consider applying for early admission, since only such an applicant will have a good chance of being accepted and the best chance of successfully completing his/her study. Applying early and not being accepted, however, does not prejudice your chances for admission the following year.

If you are interested in the early admission program, compare the colleges that offer such programs, using the information included in Table 5.1.

SELECTION FACTORS

The admissions process is theoretically geared to recognize applicants who measure up to a hypothetical image of the person who, in the consensus of the medical school's admissions committee, will prove to be a successful medical student and in time a qualified and dedicated practitioner. Those who are accepted may not have all the qualities that a committee seeks. There may even be some areas of weakness in a candidate's profile. The weaknesses, however, can be offset by strengths in other areas so that on balance the applicant's overall picture is one that meets the standards that each school sets. In other words, one need not be the ideal candidate in order to achieve success.

It should also be realized, as was implied earlier, that some applicants may, at first glance, possess an impressive array of qualifications but nevertheless do not succeed in gaining admission. These candidates unfortunately proved unable to effectively project to the committee, either indirectly through their application or directly at their interviews, all the strengths they possess. Having solid credentials and being able to market yourself as a prospective good physician make up the winning combination that will open the door to a place in a freshman medical school class.

Some selection factors, such as GPA or MCAT scores, can readily be put into quantitative terms, while others, such as personality or motivation, cannot. Nevertheless, both types of factors are important and have a strong bearing on the outcome of the admissions process. Specifically, they determine if you qualify to be placed at some point into the applicant interview pool and at a later time into the applicant acceptance pool.

Academic Achievement

Academic achievement is measured in terms of your grade point average, science course performance, and college(s) attended.

Grade Point Average (GPA)

The application that each medical school receives on behalf of an individual applicant will contain a facsimile of the candidate's college transcript and, where applicable, any postgraduate record. It will show the courses taken and grades received during the regular academic year as well as during any summer. (Those high school courses and grades for which advanced placement credit were given are also listed.) Courses that the applicant is taking or is planning to take are also frequently requested. This self-designed record is checked for accuracy against official transcripts sent by your school and will form the basis of your GPA.

Recently, with the competition for places in entering classes intense because of the large number of applicants, the GPA for the *average* matriculant was 3.5. This can be interpreted to mean that a significant number of the approximately 16,000 students accepted—which represents only 35% of the applicant pool—had an average below 3.5. On the other hand, the entire pool average was 3.3. This indicates that some applicants with 3.5 or higher failed to gain admission, thus emphasizing that a high GPA by itself does not guarantee acceptance into medical school. The corollary is also true, namely, that having an average below 3.3 also does not mean you will not be accepted. As a matter of fact, 8% of those accepted had averages of 2.5 or less. All this suggests that your chances will be markedly diminished if your average goes below 3.3. The lower the GPA, the greater the need to compensate for this weakness by high MCAT scores and recommendations. Also, achieving improved grades in the later years of college, especially in the sciences, will contribute to a more favorable reception of your application. All this emphasizes the fact that you should not view the GPA as an entity in itself; rather, it has to be taken along with all other considerations, and a low GPA by itself should not discourage you from applying. Therefore, the quantitative factors will remain a very vital, and for most applicants, a critical element of the selection process. You should strive to attain as high a level of achievement as possible. This is essential because passing the initial admissions screening is usually dependent on your academic achievement.

While the GPA is one of the major factors examined as part of the initial screening process, it is usually viewed in the context of the applicant's overall educational data. The reasons are that the GPA is subject to grade inflation, is relative to the college attended and the course of studies pursued, and only represents an overall level of performance rather than the direction of the performance.

Medical school admissions officers know that grade inflation—namely, artificially high grades that do not accurately reflect the level of academic achievement—is a common phenomenon of undergraduate education. Thus, while they do not minimize the value of a high GPA, they do not necessarily take it at face value. Admissions officers seek to establish how authentic the GPA is by checking to see at which college the grades were earned. Therefore, an applicant with a good GPA attending a college with low admission selection standards will not be much better off than another applicant with somewhat lower grades who is enrolled at a more selective school. Also, the GPA is viewed in the context of the applicant's course of study. An applicant who met the premedical course requirements by completing bona fide courses designed for science majors will obviously be favored over one whose courses were intended for nonscience majors. Similarly, an applicant who is successfully completing a science major will tend to be more credible than one who is not doing so.

The breakdown of an applicant's GPA frequently provides a more significant insight into an applicant's achievement than does the numerical value of the GPA. Thus, a consistent level of performance would tend to imply that this is the applicant's optimal achievement level. On the other hand, an erratic performance pattern, either upward or downward, may well reflect a person's response to the academic challenge being faced. An upward pattern suggests an ability to adjust to college, overcome an initial disappointing performance level, and then proceed to attain a high level of achievement even when the educational demands are increasing. A downward pattern would tend to indicate the reverse—namely, the inability to maintain a sustained high level of achievement in the face of increased educational pressures. In other words, when the values of GPAs are the same, a GPA with a consistently good achievement level and an upward pattern will have a greater impact on the screening and selection process than a similar GPA with a downward achievement trend.

Science Course Grades

The science course grades on your record are another factor considered in the admissions process. This is reasonable since medicine is the application of scientific principles that are intensively studied during the first two years of professional school. While a straight A science average is certainly not mandatory for admission to medical school, a solid level of consistently good performance (3.5 or better) will serve to demonstrate the potential to cope with the intellectual demands of the basic medical sciences.

Your science grades and the effort it took to achieve them will also help you evaluate your own abilities and the wisdom of your career choice. Incidentally, it is not essential to enjoy all your premedical science courses, but a genuine interest in science is essential.

It should be emphasized that just as the GPA's impact is relative to the college attended, so too is the science coursework judged. Similarly, the grade pattern for work completed over a three-year period can be of special value. Consistently good grades and an upward trend clearly present a positive image of your science potential.

College Attended

It has already been noted that the college attended affects the evaluation of an applicant's GPA and science coursework by the admissions committee. It also has an overall impact on admission chances in general, for three reasons. First, attendance at a university that has an affiliated medical school offers a degree of priority for acceptance into the university's own medical college, because medical schools traditionally accept a significant number of freshman from their own college. Second, it appears, at least statistically speaking, that an applicant from a private undergraduate institution has a greater chance of acceptance at a private medical school. Third, coming from a college that has established a good medical school admission track record is a decided advantage. There is an initial favorable bias because of the positive image that such an institution's name generates.

Intellectual Potential

Your academic performance, usually after a three-year period of undergraduate studies, provides a reasonable measure of your intellectual potential. Its usefulness, however, is tempered by the status of the school you attend, by the possibility of grade inflation, and possibly by the impact of pass/fail grades. For these reasons there are two additional factors considered in obtaining a comprehensive and reliable determination of the future performance of a medical student: MCAT scores and recommendations.

MCAT Scores

The Medical College Admission Test (MCAT) is a lengthy, standardized, multiple-choice examination that is given twice each year. It is designed to determine your skills in problem solving in the natural and biological sciences, your verbal reasoning ability, and your written expository aptitude. The MCAT is an indicator of your academic potential. The test is designed in such a manner that the value of memorization is deemphasized, while analysis and synthetic intellectual capabilities are tested. This clearly implies that one of the major goals in college should be to develop "thinking" skills in exactly these areas. This can best be done over an extended period of time rather than by cramming for a few weeks or even months, and/or depending on commercial MCAT preparation programs.

The MCAT score is particularly important because it provides a quantitative measurement that easily lends itself, together with your GPA (and science average), to a screening formula. Because of the large volume of applications, such formulas are used by *some* medical schools as a rapid preliminary evaluation technique. The formula baseline figure, which can be adjusted during the admission season, can determine if your application deserves more careful examination. This may involve reviewing your recommendations, essay, and extracurricular activities to determine the possibility of an invitation for an interview. The MCAT score by itself will also be used to assess the validity of your academic record. This is especially true when the problem of grade inflation exists and when the academic caliber of a school is unknown or uncertain.

The MCAT is therefore an admission obstacle that must be overcome by all premedical students because almost all schools require this examination (for exceptions, see for example, the University of Rochester or Johns Hopkins profile, Chapter 6). This examination should not be looked upon as a major admission barrier, but rather, from a positive perspective, as a potential asset that can enhance your admission potential. Therefore, if you have a high GPA, good MCAT scores will confirm your status as an attractive applicant and thus speed processing your application toward the interview stage. On the other hand, if you are a borderline or weak applicant, impressive MCAT scores can significantly strengthen the chance of having your application reviewed more thoroughly. It is at this point that your letters of recommendation will have a special influence in determining your true intellectual potential.

Letters of Recommendation

Letters of recommendation supplement the quantitative data provided by transcripts and MCAT scores. They add a positive or negative tone to the overall impression that your college work and aptitude test have established. All medical schools expect recommendations, preferably from your Health Professions Advisory Committee or from several natural science and other faculty members at your school.

Personal Attributes

Aside from your academic achievements and intellectual potential, a number of personal attributes can have an impact of varying degree on your admission chances. These attributes can be placed into categories, which will be discussed below.

Extracurricular and Summer Activities

See discussion in Chapter 2, page 30.

Exposure to Medicine

This factor was, in part, discussed in Chapter 2, "Extracurricular and Summer Activities." It should be noted that in addition to unstructured observation and service opportunities as a hospital volunteer, some institutions offer formal premedical observation programs on a group basis. In the course of such a program, premedical students, like medical interns, rotate through various departments and may even be given lectures by attending physicians on the staff. Some programs provide a small stipend. These types of programs can provide an invaluable opportunity for prospective medical students, by permitting them a direct personal view of the actual world of medicine and the realities of medical training. To learn about such exceptionally meaningful opportunities, make inquiries at the volunteer office of local hospitals; also ask your premedical advisor or senior premedical students who may have already participated in such a program.

Special Achievements

Medical schools usually look for applicants who, for one reason or another, stand out among the large pool of qualified individuals seeking admission. Therefore, gaining acceptance into honor societies or receiving awards for scholastic achievement or service will strengthen your admission potential. Demonstrated leadership capacity will also enhance your appeal. Achievements such as serving as a student senator at your college, gaining election to an important student office, organizing a band, forming a volunteer group of students to visit the sick at your school infirmary or the elderly and handicapped in the neighborhood, or tutoring underprivileged youngsters would all be a strong plus on your credentials. These kinds of accomplishments demonstrate that you have initiative, concern for others, an ability to interact constructively as part of a team effort (a requirement for modern patient care), and the determination to succeed. All these qualities are desirable in applicants seeking to enter such professions as medicine.

Individual Status

Your individual status can have a significant bearing on your chances for admission. Five factors are involved: citizenship, state of residence, age, sex, and minority status. Each of these factors is discussed separately, below.

Citizenship

U.S. medical schools have more qualified applicants than places available to train them. Moreover, the tuition paid by medical students covers only part of the actual training costs, with the balance made up by the school, state, and federal funding. Consequently, medical schools naturally have as their primary obligation the training of U.S. citizens and thus only rarely accept noncitizens into their freshman classes. Applicants not holding citizenship status, including Canadians, are clearly at a great disadvantage when applying for admission to U.S. schools. This handicap can be somewhat diminished if the applicant can secure a green card and establish permanent residency status, as well as initiate the first formal steps toward citizenship.

State of Residence

The state where you reside is another major factor in determining your chances for success. Many state schools have significantly lower tuition levels for their residents and exclude nonresidents from admission as well. They have this policy because they are funded by state taxes and thus believe that their primary obligation is to train professionals who not only live in the state but who are likely to set up practice there. The state of your residence should be carefully considered when the time comes to make up the list of schools to which you plan to apply.

If your state has only a few medical schools, you need not consider this an insurmountable obstacle because there are quite a few private schools that do not discriminate against out-of-state residents, although they may demonstrate geographical preferences to applicants from a general section of the country.

To be classified as a legal or bona fide resident of a state, you usually must maintain domicile in that state for at least 12 months preceding the date of first enrollment in an institution of higher education in that state. Student status at an institution of higher education (for example, as an undergraduate) does not constitute eligibility for residence status with regard to graduate-level work in the same state. You must maintain residence in a non-student capacity for the prescribed time in order to gain residence status. The student's eligibility to establish residence is also determined by his or her status as an adult or a minor. (A minor is any person who has not reached the age of 21, 18 in some states.) For minors, the legal residence is that of his or her parents, surviving parent, or legal guardian. As a result of Supreme Court rulings, the right of state schools to charge higher fees for out-of-state students has been upheld, but it may now be easier for such nonresident students who are 18 or older to establish legal residence and thus take advantage of the lower rate.

Two groups of states generally offer prospective applicants a statistically better chance of admission: those with many freshman places and relatively few in-state applicants (such as Illinois and Texas) and those with no in-state medical school but with special admission arrangements with other state schools (such as Maine and Wyoming).

Age

Medical schools prefer applicants who are in the 20–25 age group. Exceptions are made for select individuals, but the upper acceptance limit is usually about 35. The most favored applicants of the older group are those whose postcollege careers have been associated with medicine: research assistants, physician assistants, graduate students in one of the biomedical sciences, or holders of advanced degrees in one of these areas. Less attractive are applicants who would like to give up established careers as dentists, podiatrists, engineers, lawyers, accountants, or physicists, and who now seek to become physicians because of personal disillusionment with present activities. The latter group, seeking a career change instead of personal advancement, represent a higher risk than the former, because of concern that the pattern of giving up one's existing career might be repeated at a later time when this same individual is in medical school, training, or practice.

In the light of the aforementioned, an applicant whose age is above 25 (and preferably under 35) should present solid credentials in science course requirements, acceptable MCAT scores, good evidence of familiarity with the demands and responsibilities of a medical career, and above all, very convincing reasons for giving up a current career and seeking one as a physician (see Appendix A).

That there exists a significant pool of postbaccalaureate students who become premeds is evident from the fact that there are many schools (see list in Chapter 2) that offer special programs designed so these students can meet the premedical science course requirements. In addition, the University of Miami may offer advanced placement for those having a science PhD. Thus, it is possible that highly motivated and well-qualified career changers can succeed in spite of inherent difficulties, if they can establish a strong case for themselves and present it effectively.

Sex

The applicant's sex can influence the admission process. All medical schools accept both males and females as applicants and most encourage strongly motivated and well-qualified women to seek admission. Women currently make up at least 40% of the national freshman class admitted. Some schools are more liberal in admitting women than others (see Table 7.1). A detailed discussion of women in medicine is found in Chapter 7.

Minority Status

If you can claim minority status—namely, if you are African-American, Native American/Alaskan native, Mexican American, Puerto Rican, Asian or Pacific Islander, or other Hispanic—you will be given special consideration, because most schools actively seek to enroll minority group members in their freshman classes. As a result, minority students currently make up about 10% of the national freshman class. A more detailed discussion of minority opportunities can be found in Chapter 8.

Disability

Reliable surveys indicate that there are over 100 medical students with disabilities and upwards of 1,000 physicians-in-training with physical or learning disabilities. In 1970 Temple University Medical School in Philadelphia accepted a blind student who is currently a practicing child psychiatrist. The goal of disabled students is to gain admission on their own merit, and to secure reasonable accommodations from the school in order to be able to attend it. However, what constitutes "reasonable" accommodations and whether severely impaired students can be adequately trained has been a subject of considerable debate. The Americans with Disabilities Act (ADA) has greatly enhanced educational opportunities for disabled students; however, the law's loophole of allowing tests to measure skills provides a legal basis for a medical school to reject disabled applicants, claiming that they are lacking critical faculties and abilities that are fundamentally essential to practice medicine. Therefore, deficiencies in sensory skills could prevent them from observing patients or taking a history, deficiencies in motor skills could prohibit performing diagnostic procedures, and problems in communication skills may inhibit contact with patients or fellow physicians. Such limitations may serve as a basis to disqualify a disabled individual from gaining admission to any medical school. Not everyone shares this view, and a small, active group of disabled physicians is seeking to educate the medical community about the compensatory technology available for the handicapped medical student or physician.

Disabled students who feel that they have been rejected because of their disability can sue on grounds of discrimination as this is a violation of the ADA legislation. A blind Ohio premed student did so and won (but only after years of court battles). More recently, profoundly deaf and quadriplegic premedical students were admitted to medical school.

The current effort toward encouraging production of more primary care physicians, a physically demanding practice area, is not favorable to potential disabled applicants. Nevertheless, no generalization can be made regarding the chances of disabled premeds to gain admission. All individuals seeking a medical career have to judge for themselves their chances for gaining admission, satisfactorily completing their studies and training, and establishing a successful practice. Indeed, while there are major obstacles in the path of the disabled, they do not need to be insurmountable in the face of solid ability and intense determination.

Personal Characteristics

These include a wide variety of factors, such as personality, maturity, appearance, and ability to communicate, many of which become evident at the interview. They can have a decisive impact on your admission chances at that time.

In summary, there are more than ten factors that, to varying degrees, play a role in the admission process. An honest assessment of yourself in terms of each of these factors will give you an insight into your own chances for admission.

THE APPLICATION PROCESS

How to Apply

Traditional Application

There are currently two means of applying—directly to the school and indirectly through the American Medical College Application Service (AMCAS).

Non-AMCAS Schools

The direct approach involves submitting a separate application to any school that is *not* a member of AMCAS. The application for each of these schools should be returned with a check covering the fee, which varies in amount from school to school. Table 5.1 in Chapter 5 gives the application fees for each of the non-AMCAS schools. Appendix B has a sample application from a non-AMCAS school. The non-AMCAS schools requiring separate application are:

Baylor
Brown
Columbia
Harvard
Johns Hopkins
New York University
Texas A & M
Texas Tech.
University of Missouri, Kansas City
University of North Dakota
University of Rochester
University of Texas (Dallas, Galveston, Houston, San Antonio)
Yale

AMCAS Schools

If the schools to which you wish to apply are members of AMCAS, you must obtain an AMCAS Application Request Card from your Premedical Advisory Office or from AMCAS, Section for Student Services, Association of American Medical Colleges, 2450 N Street NW, Suite 201, Washington, D.C. 20037. Telephone: (202) 828-0600. The AMCAS Application Booklet will be sent to you and this booklet will serve as your application to all AMCAS schools to which you are applying. The cost will be determined by the number of AMCAS schools selected. AMCAS reproduces your application as well as your transcript and all your MCAT scores (but not your recommendations) for distribution to the schools. AMCAS will send you a Transmittal Notification (see sample on page 56), confirming that the schools you selected were sent the biographic and academic information shown on the form, which is based on the contents of your application. The decision regarding admission continues to rest with the individual medical schools. Schools presently subscribing to AMCAS are indicated in Table 5.1. It should be noted, however, that after viewing your AMCAS application, some schools may require a final application and charge an additional fee of $10 to $60.

When applying, whether it be directly to the schools or through AMCAS, be sure to consider the following points:

1. All application forms should be filled out neatly; preferably use a typewriter.

2. All questions should be answered carefully, fully, and accurately.

3. Where free space is provided for any comments, such as on the AMCAS application, use the space judiciously. Thus, where some clarification of your academic record is desirable (such as a prolonged illness that was responsible for poor grades during a certain semester, or where a transfer to another school occurred), advantage should be taken of the opportunity to do so. An impressive essay on your motivation to become a physician is also appropriate (see pages 59–60 and Appendix C).

4. The photograph submitted should be of good quality and should provide a favorable likeness.

5. Arrangements should be made for a transcript and the necessary recommendations to go to each non-AMCAS school. Only one copy of the transcript is needed for AMCAS, but copies of your recommendations should be sent directly to all AMCAS schools.

AMCAS-E Application

This is the electronic medical school application to AMCAS that is an alternative to the traditional one that needs to be filled out manually (see comparable sample, Appendix B). The electronic application is available in a Windows version from AMCAS's Web site (see below). AMCAS-E diskette packets will also be shipped to preprofessional health advisors, medical schools, and individuals. Those with access to the Web may place their orders for individual copies of the software or they may download the software directly from the AMCAS's Web site at: http://www.aamc.org/stuapps/admiss/amcasreq/download.htm

For technical support, e-mail *AMCAS @ aamc.org.,* typing AMCASETECH in the subject line. All other inquiries should be submitted to *AMCAS @ aamc.org,* typing A51500 in the subject line.

When to Apply

The earliest date when medical schools begin accepting applications varies; the exact dates for each school are indicated in Table 5.1. As a rule, your application should be submitted in July or August of the year preceding your planned enrollment. Naturally, the earlier your application is received, the earlier you will receive consideration. Thus, in the case of superior students, it may ensure an early acceptance that would reduce

ASSOCIATION OF AMERICAN MEDICAL COLLEGES

Section for Student Services
2450 N Street, N.W., Suite 201
Washington, D.C. 20037-1131
Telephone (202) 828-0600

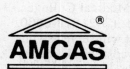

Your AMCAS Application has been forwarded to the schools listed below, with the biographic and academic information and MCAT scores which appear on this Transmittal Notification (TN). Please check all items carefully and notify AMCAS in writing immediately of any discrepancies. In all correspondence with AMCAS or medical schools, be sure to indicate your complete name, cycle/file number, Social Security Number and telephone number.

11/04/96   Cycle: 096-NEW

To: Alice Smith
           70 Poss St.
           Brooklyn, N.Y. 11211

Soc Sec #: 105-47-5167
Cycle/File #: 096-25130
Entering Class: 1997

Phone: 718-768-6325
Leg Res:
        KINGS   NY

Citizenship: UNIDENTIFIED
Visa Type: PERMANENT RESIDENT
Birthplace: WARSAW
       POLAND
Birthdate: 05/07/74   Age: 22   Sex: FEMALE
Num of Dep: 02

Self Desc: WHITE
Minority/Consider/Ethnic: NO
                Financial: YES
Fee Waiver: NO
Military Service: NO
Previous Med School: YES

Early Decision: NO
Advisor Information Release: YES

Colleges Attended	Major	Program	Degree	Degree Dates	Attended
NY UNIVERSITY	NEURO SCI	UNDERGR	BS	06/97	92-93
LONG IS U BROOKLYN CAMPUS	PHYS THERAPY	UNDERGR	ND		90-92
FOREIGN COLLEGE NOT CODED	PREV MED SCH	GRADUAT	ND		88-89

	BCPM		AO		Total		MCAT Scores
	GPA	HOURS	GPA	HOURS	GPA	HOURS	Test Date(s) Oct.
FR	3.00	19.0	3.70	15.0	3.31	34.0	Series Number
SO	3.68	11.0	3.50	15.0	3.58	26.0	Verbal Reasoning 9
JR	3.58	16.0	2.70	4.0	3.40	20.0	Physical Sciences 9
SR							Writing Sample N
PBU							Biological Sciences 10
CUG	3.38	46.0	3.48	34.0	3.42	80.0	
GRD							

Supplementary Hours: 13.0
Pass/Fail-Pass   0.0
Pass/Fail-Fail   0.0
Advanced Placement   0.0
CLEP   0.0

Number of MCAT(S) Taken: 0
MCAT Date: 09/96

Your application was Transmitted to:	Date of Application	Yr(s) Prev Applied

Code	School		
115	CORNELL	100196	
120	ALBERT EINSTEIN	100196	
136	SUNY-BROOKLYN	100196	
151	NEW YORK MED	100196	
801	MOUNT SINAI	100196	
805	SUNY-STONYBROOK	100196	

anxiety and make it unnecessary to apply to additional schools. Moreover, prolonged delay in applying means that you will be competing for a smaller number of openings since part of the class may be filled by the time your application is received. Deadlines for receipt of applications at each college are also listed in Table 5.1.

Early Decision Program (EDP)

From the students' point of view, applying to medical school is both an expensive and an emotionally trying experience. From the medical schools' point of view, selection is both a time-consuming and laborious process. To reduce the burden somewhat for both parties, the procedures of early decision have been introduced and adopted by some schools. Thus, if you are anxious to attend a particular school and you feel that you have a good chance of gaining admission, you should submit your application before the early decision deadline (usually August 1) to the selected school (but to none other at this time). Once your supporting data have been received, an interview will be scheduled if desirable and a prompt decision will be sent to you (usually about October 1). If this decision is in the affirmative you are obligated to accept the offer and refrain from seeking admission elsewhere. If you are rejected, you can then go ahead and apply to as many schools as you wish. Only if you have a sincere interest in attending a particular school and only if you have a good chance of being accepted should you use the early decision approach.

Medical schools participating in the early decision plan are indicated in Table 5.1. It should be realized that schools offering this option will fill only a part of their freshman class by this means. The remainder of the places, which will probably be the bulk of the class, will be filled by students applying under the standard procedure.

Where to Apply

The decision as to which schools to apply to is in part determined by the total number of applications you plan to file. The estimated national average for the past 20 years has remained 9–10 per applicant. The actual number you should send out is best determined by your financial means and a realistic evaluation of your chances for gaining acceptance. One of the financial considerations that should be taken into account is the cost for out-of-town interviews.

Table 3.1 offers a generalization regarding the number of applications that should be submitted in accordance with your academic record. The exact number of applications within each range should be determined by financial considerations, test scores, and possibilities for favorable interviews. A large volume of applications may be less important than selectivity as to which schools you should apply to since, in many cases, applications to some schools for some students are a waste of time, money, and effort.

Table 3.1
RELATIONSHIP OF ACADEMIC RECORD TO SUGGESTED NUMBER OF APPLICATIONS

Academic Record	Number of Applications
A– to A+	5–10
B+ to A–	10–15
B to B+	15–20
C to B	20–30

Consider the following criteria when determining to which schools you will apply:

1. At which medical schools will you find students of your caliber?
2. Where have students from your undergraduate college gained acceptance in recent years?

3. Which schools can you afford to attend? Determine what your financial means are and exactly how much you can pay for tuition and room and board without overextending yourself.

4. Which schools are located in areas that meet your personal needs? Do you prefer a large metropolitan area or a smaller town environment?

5. If you are planning to apply to an out-of-state school, does the school accept a significant number of nonresident students? Consider the possibility of schools located farther from home, even though these may not be the choices of your fellow students.

6. What schools offer curricula that are amenable to your style of intellectual endeavor? Carefully compare the curricula for differing schools to find the type which you find most appealing (see Chapter 6).

The Essay (See also Appendix C)

The AMCAS application is four pages long and the questions asked are straightforward. Detailed instructions are included.

Page two of the application is entitled "For Personal Comments" and is completely blank. It enables you to communicate directly with the admissions personnel who screen the applications and with those who evaluate the candidates. Your essay can thus be considered your brief or appeal for a place in the next freshman class. It affords you the opportunity to express yourself and to present your attributes in the most appealing manner possible, so the reader will want to get to know you personally by means of an interview.

One approach to drafting your essay can be to itemize all the information you wish to convey: biographical highlights, motivational factors behind your career choice, significant life experiences, and information about yourself or your past performance that needs elaboration or clarification. Having identified the key elements, you can next proceed to preparing a preliminary draft. The lead and concluding paragraphs probably deserve special attention since they will more likely be read during an initial scan of your essay. Once the draft is prepared, put it aside for a few days and then reread it and revise it as much as you feel is required. You may want to repeat this once again before your rough draft is completed.

You should next seek one or more outside reviewers to read and frankly criticize your essay. This may come from an able senior premed student, an English professor at your school, a young physician, or your premedical advisor. Since the essay is yours, you have the final decision of how much to revise your draft essay. You should realize that the more people you ask, the more pressure for revision there will be. Thus, a reasonable cutoff point is desirable; that is, when you are satisfied that your essay presents an honest image of you in the best possible light. When you reach that point, have your essay typed neatly and accurately and make sure it stays within the allotted one page.

There is no "ideal" essay; the samples of conventional and unconventional essays shown on page 59 and 60 are designed only to give you an insight into what other premeds have written. If your essay "sells" you as a potential attractive candidate, you have done your job.

RECOMMENDATIONS

Letters of recommendation can have a significant impact if they describe you in realistic, qualitative terms (and when they rank you with respect to others applying from your class). When the letter writers discuss not your quantitative achievements (midterm and final or course grades), but you as a person (in terms of your innate potential, motivation, personality, reliability), the communication will be effective. If your recommendation profile makes you stand out as a potential quality medical student and physician,

Sample Conventional Essay

During my freshman and sophomore years at University A, I worked as a physical therapy assistant on a voluntary, part-time basis at Medical Center B in Hometown. In the course of this experience, the most important conversation I had relevant to my career goal was with a nurse. I had observed that she was exceptionally intelligent, knowledgeable, and competent and I asked her why she had elected to become a nurse rather than a doctor. "A physician has to make a lifetime commitment to medicine; his profession must be his first priority. I am not prepared to have my profession dominate my life." Her response did not surprise me, it only served to reinforce my commitment to a profession in which I had become actively involved.

For the summer of 19-, while I could have continued my work in physical therapy, I chose to seek a position which I felt would provide a new perspective from which to view medicine. Upon returning to Bigtown, I began working at the Department of Radiology of Medical Center C. My activities were concentrated in the Special Procedures Division where one of my duties involved assisting the nurses to prepare the patient and the room for the scheduled test. I observed the procedures which usually were angiograms, venograms, or percutaneous nephrostomies. I was usually provided with a detailed explanation in the course of the procedure which was informative and educational. At the conclusion of the procedure, I listened to the radiologist read the X-rays and learned about the patient's problems and the appropriate treatments mandated. The staff, after getting to know me, encouraged my spending time with many of the apprehensive patients to try to alleviate some of their anxieties and to be generally supportive. In addition, for one hour each day, I attended classes with the interns where I learned basic human anatomy, how to interpret some of the nuances of complicated X-rays and listened to a discussion of some of the interesting cases that occurred each week. My experiences at Medical Center C were so stimulating that I immediately applied for placement for the following summer and was accepted.

In June 19-, I began to work as a research assistant for Dr. Teicher, a surgeon at Medical Center C. The research concerns the reliability of the criteria for the diagnosis of appendicitis. The justification for the research is the problematic nature of diagnoses as evidenced by the significant negative laparotomy rate. The aim of this study is to assess the feasibility of increasing the diagnostic accuracy. A large part of my activities involves using the hospital computer to retrieve, study, and evaluate appropriate patient charts in order to enlarge the statistical sample. My activities have not only made me more appreciative of the importance of medical research, but also it has shown me how some physicians combine their practice with clinical research.

After reading the article "The Ordeal: Life As a Medical Resident" in *The New York Times Magazine*, my understanding of the strong commitment a physician must make was strengthened. Unlike the nurse in Hometown, I have been impressed by the many doctors who lead rich and rewarding home lives as well as being totally dedicated to their profession.

Besides a sense of dedication, I am aware that appropriate academic ability is needed to meet the demands of medical school and postgraduate training. I elected to attend University A because it is an excellent institution of high education and I wanted to be on my own so as to develop the self-confidence necessary to manage my life. My high academic performance and my science MCAT scores confirm my ability to handle the anticipated demands of the basic medical sciences. In the light of both my clinical exposure and educational preparation, I feel confident that I will be prepared for the demands of medical education, training, and practice. I look forward to beginning this exciting and challenging adventure.

*Note: Names and places in this and the following essay have been changed.

Sample Unconventional Essay

Raindrops pelted my body as I absently stared at the small concentric circles formed from the fusion of a raindrop and a puddle. I loosely gripped the 14-foot fiberglass pole with my perspiring hands, and though: the pole vault—decathlon—third event—second day—the bar set at a logically impossible height, as Mr. Spock would say. Pressure. Whatever the outcome, I would not deny myself the challenge. So I strode down the slick runway, planted the pole, and launched myself up and over the bar—and subsequently into the giant sponge of a pit that sucked me into its depths. Of course, a requirement after a successful vault is back flip in the pit, which I immediately performed to the delight of the roaring crowd—all 23 of them. Thus ends another chapter in THE LIFE AND TIMES OF JOE WHITE.

Now let us turn to a later chapter, Joe White: The Road to Becoming a Physician.

My ambition to become a physician arose from my desire to help people. But not to help people like a waiter or a mechanic helps people. I want to help people who truly require my services. The first thing that anyone must do in order to help another is to care. I believe this to be the most important quality of a physician. And I believe that I possess this quality. I do, however, realize that it is not always easy to care about someone—especially if he does not seem to care about himself. My experiences with many different types of people will be valuable when caring for patients. However, my motives are not all so unselfish. I have always been fascinated with the structure and functions of the body. My high school and college educations have given me a broad background from which to build. By becoming a physician I will be able to further pursue my inquiry into the functioning of the body.

The road to becoming a physician may be full of potholes, detours, and do not enters. The way is not easy. But, I do not know the meaning of the word "quit" and do not intend to look it up.

Now that I have explained my motivation, let me explain my commitment. When I arrived at Chatham College, I obtained employment in the Health Center as an assistant laboratory technician/phlebotomist, where I have been working ever since. This job has provided me the important experience of interacting with patients. Then the director of the Health Center requested that I join his Student Health Advisory Committee, which functions to inform the student body of various health issues.

To obtain more knowledge about physicians and the practice of medicine, I served as a volunteer in a cardiology department. From this experience I learned much (relatively speaking) about cardiology and realized that the life of the physician was not all roses.

My academic life has not been limited to books. I worked with Dr. Jim Pike of Chatham College on epilepsy research. I enjoyed this very much and found it to an interesting and informative experience.

There was much more to my life than scholastics. I spent many a night with the love of my life—hockey. My club team was able to successfully compete against Division II and III teams. I also spent a good deal of time playing the gentleman's game of rugby.

Through my various activities I have encountered many different types of people. This fall I will be exposed to an entirely new environment. I will be taking a break from my regular science courses in order to study in Paris, where I hope to expand my cultural and intellectual horizons.

I hope that these excerpts from the book of my life have given you a little insight into me as a person. The next chapter is still in the planning stages, but after it is written I will be sure to send you a copy of Joe White: The Physician.

your admission chances will be significantly enhanced and the possibility of your being invited for an interview will be strengthened. If, on the other hand, your letters of recommendation are bland or noncommittal, your chances of getting an interview will not be helped.

It is *your* responsibility to see that recommendations in your behalf are sent to the medical schools. You can strengthen the quality of your recommendations by making sure that your health professions advisor gets to know you and has a favorable impression of you. In addition, you will be called upon to submit faculty evaluations to the health professions committee or to send out separate letters of recommendation. It is clearly advantageous to ensure that these individuals really know you. This can best be achieved by asking appropriate questions during recitation periods, at personal conferences, or better still, in the course of doing a research or independent study project. All this requires appropriate initiative on your part, which can pay rewarding dividends at the time you apply to medical school.

Letters from prestigious professors, as reflected by their academic rank, are obviously more impressive and effective than those from teaching assistants or faculty instructors. It is not advisable to ask for a recommendation unless you are fairly confident that the individual knows you well enough and is known to follow through on such requests. Otherwise you may end up with a perfunctory recommendation and such a letter may even be late in coming. Therefore, you should tactfully ask the people from whom you are requesting letters if they feel that they are in a position to write about you in a manner that will help your admission chances.

It is also appropriate to arrange to have letters of recommendation sent in your behalf (to your school committee or directly to the medical schools) by a hospital staff member where you have worked (in a volunteer or paid capacity), or other employers, or by faculty members who have known you well as the result of working for them on a special project; these letters can supplement your committee's recommendation. Letters from clergy, family physicians, relatives, friends, or alumni (unless the latter know you exceedingly well) are not only ineffective but may be self-defeating. Such letters leave the clear impression that you have weak credentials that need such unsolicited outside support to merit attention.

In order to arrange that a committee recommendation be sent out in your behalf, your advisory office may require that you complete forms comparable to an AMCAS application and be interviewed by your premedical advisor and/or advisory committee. These proceedings can serve as a "trial run" in preparation for the actual application process. It is therefore advantageous for you to prepare, early in your upper junior semester, a short statement incorporating autobiographical highlights, an outline of your personal attributes, relevant information about your exposure to medicine, and a brief discussion of your motives for selecting a medical career. This statement should be given to professors from whom you have requested recommendations at the time you request them, in order to facilitate their task; it can also be used in completing forms requested by your committee and later by AMCAS.

THE INTERVIEW

At the outset, it should be realized that the interview is not just a brief exchange between yourself and one or more representatives of the school that has requested your appearance. The interview should not be looked upon as a one-sided affair, but rather as an opportunity for a dialogue that has advantages for both the school and you.

The school uses the interview to determine

1. if your personal attributes are as appealing as your academic record (this goes, of course, for a student who is already academically acceptable), and if your personal attributes will enable you to overcome any deficiency that may appear.

2. if your personal attributes will place you in the overall acceptable range (if you are considered academically borderline).

3. if you are considered to have some obvious academic or physical deficiency, whether you have the personal attributes to overcome the deficiency.

The interview will permit you to

1. have an opportunity to sell yourself by projecting as favorable an image as possible, and thus overcoming any deficiencies in your record.

2. familiarize yourself with the campus and with its facilities, as well as with members of its student body.

3. obtain firsthand answers to questions about the school that may not yet have been answered.

Significance of the Interview

The receipt of the letter requesting that you come for an interview clearly indicates that the medical school is seriously interested in you. The large volume of applications has meant that admissions officers have to be highly selective in granting interviews. Admissions officers have at their disposal only a limited number of interviewers, who are usually faculty members and whose time is obviously very valuable. Thus, obtaining an invitation to come for an interview means either that they wish to confirm a tentative decision that you are acceptable or they think that you deserve a chance to prove that you merit admission in spite of some possible weakness. The interviewer will endeavor to appraise such personal qualifications as responsiveness, a warmth of personality, poise, ability to communicate ideas clearly and concisely, and soundness of motivation.

In the interviewer's written report, these criteria will usually be touched upon.

1. *Physical appearance:* Grooming, bearing, and self-confident manner.

2. *Personality:* Friendliness, ability to establish rapport and charm, sense of humor.

3. *Communication skills:* Ability to express ideas clearly, fluently, and intelligently.

4. *Motivation:* Soundness of career choice, conviction of interests.

5. *Maturity:* Ability to undertake responsibility that the career entails.

6. *Interests:* What educational, social, and cultural interests do you have?

7. *Level of concern:* Do you have a genuine interest in people, their problems, and helping them solve them—empathy?

8. *Emotional stability:* Composure while under pressure.

9. *Intellectual potential:* Have you truly demonstrated superior intellectual abilities?

10. Overall subjective reaction of the interviewer to the applicant.

Evaluate yourself in terms of items 1 to 9 as honestly as possible and work to improve your weaknesses. By subjecting yourself to mock interviews by your peers, you can determine where your weaknesses are, and how well you are doing to overcome them. Allow your mock interviewers to be honest and candid (even if it hurts your feelings).

Preparation for the Interview

There are a number of steps that you can take that will help to prepare you for your interview.

1. Read the catalog of the school and become familiar with any special facilities or programs it has to offer.

2. Discuss with fellow applicants from your college the nature of their experiences at interviews at various schools.

3. Dress neatly and be properly groomed.

4. Arrive for the interview early, so that you locate the interview site with time to spare for an adjustment to your surroundings.

5. If your interviewer is late, do not indicate annoyance for being kept waiting. (He or she probably was delayed by something important.)

6. Act naturally and avoid looking nervous.

7. Answer the questions raised without trying to anticipate what you think the interviewer may wish to hear.

8. Avoid controversial subjects and don't raise sensitive issues.

9. Be prepared to explain your specific interest in the school you are visiting.

10. If you inadvertently flub a question, don't let it upset you for the rest of your interview.

11. Be well rested, alert, and honest. Do not exaggerate your scholastic achievements or extracurricular activities.

12. If you worked on a research (or other) project, be prepared to discuss it fluently and concisely.

13. If you have had exposure to medicine by working at a hospital, be prepared to discuss it if asked, or work it into the conversation in an appropriate manner.

14. If you can, find out the departmental affiliation of your interviewer in advance from an admissions office secretary, or by checking his or her name in the school catalog. You may then be able to raise a topic of special mutual interest (if being interviewed by a surgeon, you may wish to mention that you observed an appendectomy).

15. Do not hesitate to ask questions about the school and its program—or about the interviewer's activities (such as how much time does he or she have for research).

16. Talk to a classmate who has had an interview at the school. Get his or her impressions of the school and interview. Remember that it is unlikely that you will get the same interviewer—but it is possible.

17. If the school is of special interest to you, you may wish to contact an alumnus in attendance or a recent graduate.

18. Bear in mind that the school is trying to get a sense of you as a person—to see what motivates you—to understand why you want to enter the health sciences, and to become convinced that you are a worthy, potential colleague.

The following steps will be of additional help in preparing for the interview:

19. Prepare rehearsed answers to the typical questions that may be asked at an interview. You can tape record your responses and hear how you sound.

20. See if you can appropriately fit or slip your rehearsed answers in during the interview in a manner that is casual and doesn't sound canned. The latter can be accomplished by pausing for a moment before answering a question that you are prepared for, acting as if you are preparing your answers.

21. Try to sell your favorable assets by fitting them into the interview (hospital work, research experience, community activities, research articles published, etc.). Know your strengths thoroughly.

22. Try to establish a rapport with the interviewer from the very outset. Walk in with a greeting, a smile on your face, and a firm handshake. On leaving, express your appreciation for the time the interviewer gave you.

23. Try to avoid, where possible, "yes" or "no" answers. Rather, give the pros and cons of the issue and your views in a brief and concise manner. Show that you can be analytical while at the same time avoid being overly talkative.

24. If you don't understand the question, ask the interviewer to clarify it.

25. Look directly at your interviewer; act relaxed; avoid squirming in your seat.

26. If you don't know an answer, admit it rather than guess wildly. If pressed for a reply, qualify it as being an "on the spur of the moment" judgment, that is open to change on further reflection.

27. Don't open up discussions on your own, such as on politics or religion. If asked, don't be defensive. Interviewers seek a sense of confidence even on controversial issues.

28. Avoid disparaging your school or specific instructors or students. It will not help make you look better.

29. If you have a video camera and VCR, tape yourself during a practice interview and see how you look and sound. Note if your body language conveys a positive or negative impression. Try to improve your performance in a second taping at a later session.

30. If you have serious problems handling interviews (such as being very shy or having a speech defect), seek professional help by taking a course that teaches interview skills.

Typical Interview Questions

Be prepared to answer some typical questions that frequently come up, some of which follow.

1. Why did you attend _____ College?
2. What are your extracurricular activities?
3. Why do you want to become a physician?
4. What books and newspapers do you read?
5. What do you do during the summer?
6. How will you finance your education?
7. What other schools have you applied to?
8. What do you plan to specialize in?
9. Why did you get a poor grade in _____?
10. Do you have any questions?
11. Which medical school is your first choice?
12. What kind of social life do you have?
13. Describe your schedule at _____ .
14. What were your favorite courses taken?
15. Did you participate in any special science projects in high school or college?
16. Will your religious convictions interfere with your studies or practice?
17. How did you arrive at your decision to become a physician?
18. What area of medicine do you wish to enter?
19. Describe a typical day in your life.
20. Do you feel you should have gone to a different college?

21. What do you do in your spare time?
22. Tell me about yourself and your family.
23. What do you think are the most pressing social problems?
24. Describe your study habits.
25. What are your hobbies?
26. What experiences led you to your career choice?
27. What are your plans for marriage and a family?
28. Why isn't _____ your first choice?
29. What are the characteristics of a good physician (or dentist)?
30. Why do you think you are better suited for admission than your classmates?
31. What is the status of the medical doctor in modern society?
32. What has been your most significant accomplishment to date?
33. If you had great willpower, how would you change yourself?
34. What are the characteristics of a mature person?
35. What can be determined about an applicant at an interview?
36. What books have you read recently?
37. Describe your research at _____ .
38. What is your opinion on _____ (major current event issues)?
39. What newspaper do you read and which columnist do you like the best?
40. How do you cope with frustrating situations?
41. What will you do if you are not accepted?
42. How do you rank among the preprofessional students at your school?
43. Have you ever worked with people, and if so in what capacity?
44. Who has had the greatest influence on your life?
45. What made you apply to our school?
46. What are your weaknesses?
47. Describe your exposure to medicine at _____ .
48. If you are accepted to more than one school, how will you decide which to attend?
49. How do you see yourself ten years from now?
50. Why did your grades go down in your _____ semester?
51. Why do you want to work with people who are ill?
52. How will you finance your education and yourself while you are a medical student?
53. At what point in your life did you decide to become a physician?
54. How do you know you will be happy if you become a physician?
55. Will the level of income affect your choice of a specialty, and do you think physicians are overpaid?
56. How do you feel about treating HIV positive or AIDS patients?
57. What do you think about legalizing medically sanctioned euthanasia?
58. What is an HMO? Would you want to be employed by one as a physician?

59. Will the question of the likelihood of malpractice suits affect your choice of a specialty?

60. What makes you think you will be prepared for medical school by the time you graduate from college?

Atypical Interview Questions

1. What is your favorite piece of music?

2. Do you know enough about hockey to compare the _____ and the _____ _____ teams?

3. What would you do to improve the quality of life in large cities?

4. Describe the difference between lactose and glucose.

5. What movies did you see recently?

6. If you were to have a year off, what would you do with it?

7. What is your favorite form of entertainment?

8. What is your opinion of socialized medicine?

9. What do you feel are physicians' obligations to their patients?

10. How would you respond to a patient who you learn is terminally ill?

11. How do your parents feel about your career goals?

12. What are the characteristics of aromatic compounds?

13. Why do you think that life was based on the carbon atom?

14. What do you think about and how did you prepare for the MCAT?

15. Can you explain why your MCAT scores went up (down) when you took the test a second time?

16. Would you be willing to serve in an area where there is a physician shortage?

17. What subspecialty are you considering?

18. What message would you like me to convey to the admissions committee in your behalf?

19. What were your most favorite and least favorite courses in college?

20. What demands do you think medicine will make upon you?

21. How will marriage and having a family fit in with your career plans?

22. Have you been interviewed or accepted at any other school?

23. What are your thoughts about the expected physician surplus?

24. What are your views on abortion, gay rights, capital punishment, and animal experimentation?

25. What are your thoughts about the use of animals for medical research?

26. What do you feel should be the physician's role as far as abortion is concerned?

27. What are your opinions about the issue of universal health care?

28. How do you feel about the level of compensation of interns and residents (house staff)?

29. Do you feel an obligation to treat the indigent or uninsured patients?

30. What three words describe you best?

31. What do you do for recreation?

32. What do you think of the idea of closing some medical schools to limit the output of physicians and thus avoid a physician surplus?

33. Do you have a physician role model? If so, who and why do you perceive that person as a role model?

34. If you were an interviewer, what one question would you always ask an applicant?

You can improve your performance by preparing for it (as indicated in the preceding sections) and by learning from the mistakes you may have made at the interviews you have had. Thus, after each interview, evaluate your performance along the following lines.

1. Did I come across effectively?

2. Where did I flounder and become excessively talkative?

3. Did I keep my cool after a blunder?

4. Was there some basic information I should have known, but didn't?

5. Were my prepared responses effective?

6. Did I sell myself, especially my assets, adequately and effectively?

7. Did I establish a good rapport and behave in a well-mannered way?

8. Did I seem to show the appropriate interest in the school at which I was being interviewed?

9. Was I able to slip in information that I wanted the interviewer to know about me?

10. What would I have done differently?

With honest answers, you can then go on and prepare more effectively for the next interview. The results should be better. The first interview is usually the toughest. Try to schedule it with a school that is not your first choice, if this is at all possible.

THE SELECTION PROCESS

Medical school admissions committees have a complicated and difficult task. Selecting future medical students requires assessing diverse information about each applicant in order to make decisions that affect the lives and careers of applicants, the attainment of their schools' educational goals, and those of society as a whole. This information about every applicant includes family, ethnic, and geographic background, activities that may reflect motivation and career aspirations, letters of recommendation, personal statements, academic records, interviews, and MCAT scores.

The selection task is further complicated by the fact that medical schools vary with respect to their educational goals. Some are dedicated to educating primary care physicians and/or physicians for specific sites or regions; many are committed to care for underserved populations. Some seek to educate academic physicians, while others educate missionaries. Various educational missions motivate schools to select students with different characteristics deemed by individual schools to be vital for their specific missions. These attributes may be academic background, geographic origin, ethnic background, career motivations, and value systems.

As an autonomous institution, each medical school has its own selection process and admissions criteria (see profiles, Chapter 6). There is considerable procedural variability among schools and one scheme cannot be applicable for all. Even the makeup of admissions committees is not fixed, although 15 seem to be the average number of members, with representatives coming from the schools' basic and clinical science departments, each serving for terms of one to three years. Some schools have appointed students (usually seniors) to their admissions committee as voting or nonvoting members.

The basic selection process takes three steps. At each step some of the variable approaches are noted.

Preliminary Screening

The first step is designed to narrow down the large pool of applications that a school receives to those who merit further serious consideration.

Screening Personnel

After your application and supplementary supporting data (in whole or in part) have been received, your folder will be screened either by two admissions officers independently or by a subcommittee of the school's admissions committee.

Screening Criteria

This is subject to variation and may include:

- Total GPA and MCAT percentile (with minimum GPA levels usually varying between 3.4 and 3.7 and MCAT levels between the 60th and the 80th percentiles).
- Total GPA, science GPA, nonscience GPA, and total MCAT scores.
- Quantitative data as well as letters of recommendation.
- Total application packet including letters of recommendation and application essay.

Supplementary Application

Certain schools have designed their own supplementary applications containing questions that they require you to answer (such as, How do you see yourself ten years from now? What will medicine be like in the next century?) or that are optional (List the medical schools that you have applied to). Receipt of a supplementary application to be completed suggests that the school is interested in you. However, not all schools have supplementary applications and not getting one should not be interpreted as a lack of interest in you.

Interview

After you have been screened, your application will be rated to determine your eligibility for an interview. You may be invited for an interview promptly if your rating is high, relative to the established numerical standard; you may be placed on an interview-eligible list making it quite likely that you will be invited in due course; you may be placed on hold for further review; or you may be put on an ineligible list. The last classification may result in your receiving a rejection, which may or may not require full committee confirmation.

Determination

After your interview, a report drafted by the interviewer will be placed in your file, which subsequently will be presented to the entire committee. It will then be discussed and rated, and depending on the rank it receives, an acceptance, hold, or rejection letter will follow.

ACCEPTANCE

Attaining an acceptance to medical school, especially the one of your choice, is your goal (see letter on page 70). In responding to an acceptance, bear in mind that the Executive Council of the AAMC has approved a set of guidelines regarding acceptance. Among the recommendations are:

1. that an applicant should not have less than two weeks in which to reply to an offer;

2. that medical schools should not notify applicants of acceptance before November 15 of each admission cycle;

3. that by April 1 any applicant holding more than one acceptance for more than two weeks (and having received all necessary financial aid information) should choose the school the applicant wishes to attend and withdraw from all others;

4. that after June 1 a medical school seeking to enroll an applicant already known to be accepted elsewhere should advise the school of its intentions;

5. that an offer of acceptance does not constitute a moral obligation to matriculate at that school.

Choosing Among the Acceptances

Naturally, if you have received only one acceptance, your course of action is restricted. If you receive multiple acceptances, then carefully consider each school so that you select the school that best meets your needs.

It is not in the best interest of the students or medical schools for an acceptee to hold on to more than one place at a time. The basic criteria in determining where to attend will be just as well known to the applicant at the time of notification of acceptance as a month or two later. If it is easy to make a choice, then it should be made promptly and a polite letter of withdrawal should be sent to the appropriate school(s). If, however, it is difficult to choose between schools, a choice should nevertheless be made rapidly (using the criteria noted below) rather than agonizing over the decision for a prolonged period. By making a decision with all deliberate speed, you can then concentrate on other important matters. At the same time, this will enable the medical school(s) you have withdrawn from to offer the place made vacant to others, perhaps even a student from your own school. (This is also the time to withdraw from schools you have not yet heard from, that you would not attend if accepted.)

In making your selection, you should bear in mind that, while all medical colleges in the country are acceptable, there are significant variations among them. Evaluate each school, keeping in mind the following criteria:

1. *Financial consideration.* You should evaluate tuition and living costs coupled with your financial means and offers of financial assistance.

2. *Location.* Consider the geographic location as well as the proximity of the school to where you wish to live.

3. *Faculty-student relationships.* What are the opportunities for informal and personal assistance and guidance in academic and general problems? What cooperation is there with the staff and administration? What is the role of the students in various policy-making organs of the school?

4. *Teaching program.* How recently has the curriculum been updated? How are the innovations working out in practice? Do the senior faculty members actively participate in teaching? Is the faculty as a whole interested in teaching or is their primary concern research and clinical services?

5. *Student performance.* Determine the current attrition rate and what percentage is due to academic failure. Of interest also is the number of students asked to repeat an academic year; compare the figure with the national average.

6. *Facilities.* Familiarize yourself with the character of the basic science teaching laboratories and what up-to-date equipment is available. How many hospital beds are available for teaching purposes? What kinds of hospitals are used (private, city, or state)?

7. *Student body.* What is the class size? What is their morale, attitude, and enthusiasm for the school? Determine the nature of student competition—is it stimulating or cut-throat?

8. *Reputation.* Speak with recent graduates about the school's standing. Find out what percentage of the school's graduates are placed as interns in prestigious teaching hospitals.

THE
GEORGE
WASHINGTON
UNIVERSITY
MEDICAL CENTER

Office of Admissions
(202) 676-3506

School of Medicine and Health Sciences / 2300 Eye Street, NW / Washington, DC 20037

February 11, 1996

Mr. Robert Brown
1234 56th Street
Belle City, MD 20000

Dear Mr. Brown:

On behalf of the George Washington University School of Medicine and Health Sciences and the Committee on Admissions, I am pleased to invite you to become a member of the First-year Class entering the Doctor of Medicine degree program starting in the fall of 1996.

You are to be congratulated on your fine record: your academic and personal qualities as assessed by a multiplicity of factors led the Committee on Admissions to believe that you will have a fine future here at George Washington and in the community of physicians.

Please read the enclosed Notice of Acceptance carefully and return the signed copy not later than the date noted. The original is enclosed for your records. I suggest that you keep it for future reference. I particularly call your attention to the need to plan your future program at the earliest possible date. Until your record is fully up to date, we cannot certify you for matriculation.

We look forward with pleasure to welcoming you next fall.

Sincerely,

Rachele I. Klein, M.D.
Associate Dean for Student
    Affairs and Admissions

RIK/pac
Encl.

There is no authoritative list of distinguished U.S. hospitals; however, an unranked sampling of 20 institutions that many would agree fall into this category is listed in Table 3.3. Other prestigious hospitals can undoubtedly be added to this list. By examining postgraduate training appointment lists, usually found in the back of medical school catalogs, one can see if any graduates were placed in these hospitals. Although the absence of placement need not be taken as reflecting negatively on a medical school's status, since the hospital sample is a very small one (20 out of 2500), the presence of placed graduates should be considered a positive sign as to the quality of its education.

RANKING OF MEDICAL SCHOOLS

There is a natural tendency to seek admission to the "best" medical school possible. The problem is identifying which medical schools are the best. It is quite possible that in reality the best school is the one that has accepted you and is also most suitable to *your own* special needs, rather than one whose only attraction is its distinguished reputation. Nevertheless, a list ranking medical schools can be useful; it may provide information that can help you decide which schools to apply to and which school to select in case of multiple acceptances.

In considering any ranking list, the following factors should be taken into consideration.

1. The ranking of a school should be only one of a number of factors affecting your final choice.

2. Formulating a ranking list that cannot be challenged is almost impossible, because there are so many variables to consider (size, curriculum, faculty, basic and clinical facilities, student services, supporting resources).

3. Since the educational philosophy of schools varies (for example, some are research oriented while others seek to train primary care physicians), one cannot objectively compare relative values. A judgment can be made only as to how well each meets its defined mission.

4. A list that ranks the schools in numerical order can be misleading, because it would suggest that a school ranked number 21 is superior to 22 when in reality the difference is based solely on minute statistical differences between the two, within the data collected.

5. A school's place on a list cannot be used as a definitive measure of the school's status, but merely serves as an estimate of its perceived reputation.

6. Any list should be considered in the context of your own observations, your advisor's opinion, and alumni comments.

Because of the absence of any recognized ranking list, an awareness of some of the most prestigious U.S. medical schools may prove helpful to prospective applicants and acceptees. To this end an *unranked* list of some of the top U.S. medical schools is provided in Table 3.2. This list correlates well with the list of the most prestigious hospitals (see Table 3.3) and the mean MCAT admission scores (see Chapter 5). Obviously, on such a short list, there may be omissions.

REJECTION

Meaning of Rejection

When you apply to medical school you obviously risk the possibility of rejection. While such a response is a major setback, it need not necessarily mean that the rejection terminates your career prospects. To a considerable degree, gaining admission lies outside of your powers to control, since it is *in part* governed by factors over which you have no control. Such factors include the total applicant pool and the ratio of men, women, and minority applicants. For a long time white males felt assured that they would stand the

Table 3.2
SOME OF THE MOST PRESTIGIOUS U.S. MEDICAL SCHOOLS

California
  Stanford University
  University of California—Los Angeles
  University of California—San Diego
  University of California—San Francisco
Connecticut
  Yale University
Illinois
  University of Chicago
Maryland
  Johns Hopkins University
Massachusetts
  Harvard University
Michigan
  University of Michigan
Minnesota
  University of Minnesota—Minneapolis

Missouri
  Washington University
New York
  Albert Einstein
  Columbia University
  Cornell University
  New York University
North Carolina
  Duke University
Pennsylvania
  University of Pennsylvania
Tennessee
  Vanderbilt University
Texas
  Baylor College of Medicine
  University of Texas—Dallas

Table 3.3
SOME OF THE MOST PRESTIGIOUS U.S. HOSPITALS

California
  Medical Center at University of California
    (San Francisco)
  University of California at Los Angeles—
    Center for Health Sciences
  Stanford University Medical Center
Connecticut
  Yale-New Haven Hospital
Florida
  Jackson Memorial Hospital
Illinois
  Northwestern University Medical Center
Maryland
  Johns Hopkins Hospital
Massachusetts
  Massachusetts General
  Brigham and Women's Hospital
Michigan
  University of Michigan Medical Center

Minnesota
  Mayo Medical Center
Missouri
  Barnes Hospital
New York
  New York Hospital–Cornell Medical Center
  The Presbyterian Hospital
North Carolina
  Duke Medical Center
Pennsylvania
  Hospital of the University of Pennsylvania
  University Health Center (Pittsburgh)
Tennessee
  Vanderbilt University Medical Center
Texas
  Baylor College of Medicine Hospital
  University of Texas Health Sciences Center
    (Dallas)

best chance of being accepted. With a larger applicant pool and a substantial female segment, the situation has changed considerably to a much more competitive one. The impact of an increasing number of minority applicants, especially those of Asian background, has made admission even more unpredictable. The uncertainty surrounding the admission process is further demonstrated by the fact that even superior applicants who apply to a number of schools will usually find that they are accepted by some and rejected by others.

The aforementioned considerations point to the fact that if you are rejected, this should not be automatically equated with being unqualified or unfit to become a physician. As noted in detail below, careful, thorough, and objective analysis of your specific situation is needed to judge possible reasons for your rejection and to determine the most appropriate response.

Further complicating the interpretation of the meaning of rejection is the fact that many such applicants may possess the qualities that make a good physician, such as compassion, listening skills, excellent judgment, a keen sense of observation, the ability to solve problems independently, and a desire to help others. The fact is that because of the large volume of applicants and the pressure to quantify the admissions process, great weight is placed on GPA, science cumulative average, and MCAT scores. Weakness in any of these areas seriously compromises one's admission potential, even when the less quantifiable elements are present. Some applicants are able to overcome grade and test score deficiencies, but many others are not, and in spite of their potential must make alternative career plans. Some applicants may clearly not merit admission. It is the rejected borderline cases that deserve special review and analysis to determine the appropriate course of action.

Responding to Rejection

Each year many thousands of applicants to medical school are rejected for one reason or another. If you unfortunately find yourself in this category, very careful examination of your future plans is needed.

Try to determine the reasons for your rejection. Weigh the advantages and disadvantages of the various alternatives that present themselves and then select a course of action that is *realistic*. Almost all rejected applicants fall into one of the six categories listed below.

1. those who plan to reapply to U.S. medical schools the following year.

2. those who plan to apply to foreign medical schools.

3. those who will apply to enter a different health profession.

4. those who will apply for admission to a graduate school to enter a career in teaching and research or in the basic medical sciences.

5. those who plan a career in science education on the high school level or lower.

6. those who will seek a nonscience-oriented career.

Seriously consider the reasons why you might have been rejected. If your academic record has been consistently poor, your SAT I and MCAT scores were low, and there were no genuine extenuating circumstances for your unimpressive performance, then you should consider either another health profession or a nonscience career. If your academic record is good, but for obvious reasons—physical or mental health—you were considered unsuitable for a medical career, consider another health career, a career in science education, or a nonscience program.

If you were a borderline candidate and you have had a consistently fair academic record at a recognized college, satisfactory test scores, a pleasant personality, and good motivation, and were probably rejected because of a very competitive admissions situation, then you should consider attending graduate school and studying for a career in teaching or research. If your test scores were low because of some unusual circumstances, you should consider retaking the examination and reapplying.

If you think that your record, as a whole, is not exceptional but does reveal the possibility of considerable capability as reflected by occasional high performance in some key courses, high test scores, and so forth, you should seriously consider reapplying to schools the following year. You should also consider applying to foreign schools or beginning a nonscience career. The schools you select to apply to the second time should be those that offer the best possibility of accepting you.

If you believe that you were rejected because of possible late applications, delay in receiving or loss of supporting data, poor selection of schools to which you applied, too few applications submitted, poor performance at the interview, or some similar explainable factor, you should consider reapplying, and think about other options open to you. A percentage of students who reapply do succeed; therefore, you should feel encouraged to do so.

A study was made of the career choices of 98 unsuccessful applicants to an entering medical class. Of that group of 57 men and 41 women, it was discovered that 52% entered occupations outside the health care field. Forty-eight percent ultimately entered health-related occupations, of which 10 men and 2 women became physicians, 7 became dentists, and 1 became an optometrist. These data indicate that a medical career is still possible if one is rejected initially and that a career in one of the many health care professions is a realistic alternative.

A later study, consistent with the aforementioned findings, showed that unsuccessful applicants to medical school tended to reapply at least once and that 51% of those employed after being rejected initially were engaged in health-related occupations (with laboratory technology being the leading choice, especially for women). This study also noted that of the respondents who were still students, 29% of the men and 20% of the women were in health-related training. The largest group among men was in dental school and among women was in the study of microbiology or other medical sciences. Women were found to be less likely than men to enter doctoral-level health science study. Careers in the new mid-level health fields such as physician's assistant and nurse practitioner attracted a few rejected premedical students. This conclusion is strongly supported by an even more recent study of a larger sampling of unaccepted applicants to the medical school class. It was found that a majority had reapplied and that 27% had gained entrance to either a U.S. or a foreign medical school. Of those still unaccepted, about half were studying or working in health-related fields or occupations. Because the state of medical school admissions is currently somewhat more competitive than it has been in the past, reapplying to U.S. schools is clearly a less attractive option than it has been in a very long time.

In any event, you should carefully consider the risks involved with medical study overseas before applying to such schools. See Chapter 12 on Foreign Medical Study for the problems involved with transferring credits, obtaining American licenses, and other difficulties of foreign study. If you should decide to undertake an alternative health profession or graduate study, you must determine if you have sufficient motivation to do so. Without sufficient motivation, the chances for success are slim.

Coping with Rejection

A second major facet of relevance to the unsuccessful applicant is the psychological impact of falling into this category.

Occupational choice results from a combination of conscious and subconscious elements involving both rational and emotional factors. The manner in which these factors are synthesized and compromised, leading to the ultimate career choice, is unclear. Although the making of a vocational choice is, for many individuals, a long-term process spanning the college years, this is not the case for most premedical students. It has been shown that about half of these had made a definite career decision before entrance to college and that 60% never changed their vocational choice once it was made.

Thus, as a group, premedical students are likely not only to enter college with a predetermined career goal, but also to insulate themselves from situations perceived as threats to their decision, as well as from faculty members who may challenge the wisdom of their career choice. Moreover, they surround themselves with peers who share their values and reinforce their beliefs.

Many premeds have, therefore, at an early (and perhaps premature) stage fixed their vocational goal irrevocably and insulated themselves from any possibility of change. Consequently, such individuals are potentially incapable of anticipatory coping with rejection to medical school. If this situation comes to pass, the potential exists for a crisis due to a thwarted career goal. Moreover, it is believed that, since our society equates self-worth with success, a career crisis becomes equivalent to an identity crisis, which can produce serious negative psychological manifestations. At the initial stage these may be evident as a sense of shame, inadequacy, and guilt-producing feelings of isolation. This phase may be followed by a second stage characterized by denial, resentment, and anger. This leads to placing the blame for failure to attain admission on others rather than oneself. A third stage may follow in which depressive behavior, instead of the rational self-appraisal that is called for, becomes apparent. Lethargy and fantasizing, as well as anxiety, dominate the individual's personality.

It is obvious, then, that students who fail to gain admission are confronted with a major crisis that easily lends itself to perception as having been brought about by others or by uncontrollable factors. Most individuals eventually work through the trauma of rejection successfully, begin a realistic appraisal, and successfully adjust to their new situation. Some, however, remain in one of the reactive stages noted above and may need help to cope with the stress produced by the circumstances in which they find themselves.

For those unable to handle the impact of admission failure, counseling by the premedical advisor may prove beneficial. The advisor, if necessary with the help of other relevant and qualified personnel, should initially seek to help the individual maintain his or her sense of self-worth and thus facilitate working through the crisis. The individual next should be made to realize that the failure should be perceived as another of life's problems that needs resolving and can be resolved successfully. Finally, the advisor should offer assistance in developing a strategy for meeting this problem.

SPECIAL EDUCATIONAL PROGRAMS

The programs discussed below will be of special interest to those seeking admission to only one specific school, minority students, high school students anxious to complete the college-medical school sequence earlier, and those interested in becoming physician-scientists.

1. **Early Decision Program (EDP)**—see page 57.
2. **Flexible Curriculum Programs**
3. **Integrated Degree Programs**
4. **Combined Programs**
5. **Interdisciplinary Programs**

Flexible Curriculum Programs

A few schools offer some minority students the possibility of completing the required courses at their own pace. Such students must meet regularly with faculty advisors to demonstrate their progress and they must pass the standard comprehensive examinations for promotion and graduation.

Integrated Degree Programs (BA-MD or BS-MD Programs)

This type of program permits selected students to participate in combined undergraduate and medical school curricula thus enabling them to obtain the MD degree in six or seven years from the time they graduate from high school. In such cases, individual students can obtain their baccalaureate degrees while enrolled in medical school. The following list includes schools presently offering such a program:

Alabama
University of South Alabama College of Medicine

California
University of California at Riverside and Los Angeles with UCLA School of Medicine
University of Southern California with School of Medicine

District of Columbia
Howard University with George Washington University School of Medicine

Florida
University of Miami

Illinois
Illinois Institute of Technology with Chicago Medical School
Northwestern University

Massachusetts
Boston University

Michigan
Michigan State University College of Human Medicine
University of Michigan

Missouri
University of Missouri—Kansas City School of Medicine

New Jersey
New Jersey Medical School
Rutgers University with Robert Wood Johnson Medical School

New York
Binghamton University—SUNY Syracuse
Brooklyn College—SUNY Brooklyn
New York University
Rensselaer Polytechnical Institute with Albany Medical College
University of Rochester School of Medical and Dentistry
Siena College and Albany Medical College
Sophie Davis School of Biomedical Education—CUNY with Mount Sinai School of
    Medicine
Union College with Albany Medical College

Ohio
Case Western Reserve University
Northeastern Ohio Universities College of Medicine

Pennsylvania
Lehigh University with Medical College of Pennsylvania and Hahnemann University
    School of Medicine
Penn State University with Jefferson Medical College
Villanova University with Medical College of Pennsylvania

Rhode Island
Brown University

Tennessee
East Tennessee State University
Fisk University with Meharry Medical College

Texas
Rice University with Baylor College of Medicine

Virginia
Eastern Virginia Medical School

Wisconsin
University of Wisconsin Medical School

Combined Programs: MD-MS, MD-PhD

These programs permit combined study for an MS or PhD degree in basic medical science, along with study for the MD degree. Average time for these programs ranges from six to seven years. A special Medical Scientist Training Program (MSTP) sponsored by the National Institutes of Health offers annual stipends and full tuition coverage for students accepted into the program at the schools offering it, listed below.

Albert Einstein College of Medicine
Baylor College of Medicine
Case Western Reserve University
Chicago-Pritzker
Columbia University
Cornell University
Duke University
Emory University
Harvard Medical School
Johns Hopkins University
Mount Sinai School of Medicine
New York University
Northwestern University
Stanford University
SUNY at Stonybrook Health Sciences Center
University of Alabama
University of California—Los Angeles
University of California—San Diego
University of California—San Francisco
University of Iowa
University of Michigan
University of Minnesota
University of Pennsylvania
University of Pittsburgh
University of Rochester
University of Texas, Dallas
University of Virginia
University of Washington
Vanderbilt University
Washington University
Yale University

Currently more than 30 medical schools receive funding and about 75 more launched MD-PhD programs on their own. All told, about 2,500 students are enrolled in such programs. The MSTP was inaugurated by the National Institute of Health (NIH) more than 30 years ago and it has supplied the nation with a significant number of its physician-scientists. Many program graduates have succeeded in securing senior administrative research appointments where they have gained access to investigative grants, laboratory staffs, and other benefits that have furthered their careers. Some have become Nobel laureates. In spite of the seven-to-ten-year length of MD-PhD programs, schools report that the program is as popular with prospective students as ever.

The changes taking place in the health care system have raised questions about the future of the program. This is because research funds are beginning to dry up due to the cutback in funding by the government and in reimbursement by the managed care system. With reduced income for academic medical centers, they have less funds to support in-house research. There has been criticism by some that combined MD-PhD programs are no longer necessary. They argue that these programs emphasize the basic rather than clinical disciplines and that the physician can perform research, as many do, without the PhD component.

The majority of graduates of combined programs ultimately end up with academic careers, being engaged in research, teaching, and perhaps some limited clinical duties. These individuals have met the goals of the original NIH concept. There still is very strong support for the MD-PhD program within the academic community as being a vital approach in generating physician-scientists.

In reaction to the existing climate, there appears to be a tendency to readjust the ratio of activities of MD-PhD candidates, with increased clinical responsibilities delegated to them. One program mandates a full month of medical work on the wards before even entering the lab. Others require a more equitable sharing of time between clinical and research work. The combined program candidates generally respond positively to this change, even when their research is far removed from patient care.

One of the negative side effects of increasing the clinical obligations of combined-degree candidates at the expense of research is that it will inevitably slow down lab work and thus lengthen the PhD phase of the program. This will further strengthen the voice of critics who claim that the program already takes up too much of the candidate's career development segment.

Besides usually interrupting the candidate's medical education with a 3- to 5-year research interlude, an additional 3 to 5 years of specialty (residency) training usually takes place after receiving the dual degrees. This brings the education-training phase to a minimum of 10 years and maybe more if a postdoctoral fellowship is elected (which can in extreme situations almost double the training time). Critics of the length of the program suggest that medical students interested in research have other options, such as taking a research elective during the school year, spending a summer or even taking off an entire year for research, or doing it on a postdoctorate (MD) level. While these options are feasible, they can't provide the solid background and training that is essential for physician-scientists.

A second major issue raised by the MD-PhD program is the disruption caused by the research phase right in the middle of medical studies. Students find themselves removed from their class (and classmates), where the social environment is supportive, and they are transferred into the relative isolation of the laboratory. Having to transfer back and forth between two radically different academic cultures—medical student, graduate student, then medical student again—can be destabilizing. The medical training is in the context of a hierarchical system, while that of graduate research is basically egalitarian. In response, some schools are allowing candidates greater flexibility in planning their program. Thus, in some cases candidates may start their research immediately or after one year of medical school, or complete either one of the degrees first, or pursue a personalized schedule. Nevertheless, there are, by the program's very nature, built-in social disadvantages that are unavoidable in a combined-degree program.

Critics of the MSTP do not deny its attractiveness in providing candidates with full funding and making them potentially very marketable. They argue that MD's can and do learn how to do sophisticated research, although the start-up time may be longer. With the dual-degree program perhaps being subjected to fiscal pressure, future candidates can anticipate a lower threshold of support.

Interdisciplinary Programs

This arrangement permits a combination medical degree program with a degree in another field such as engineering, statistics, law, physics, chemistry, administration, dentistry, or agriculture. Schools offering such programs are identified in the special features section of their profiles in Chapter 6.

The vast majority of dual degree programs are obviously linked with the biomedical sciences. There are a small number of prospective physician-scholars who set their goal to secure a doctorate in one of the humanities of social sciences. For such individuals, there are a very limited number of formal programs available. The biggest is probably the Illinois Medical Scholars program at the University of Illinois College of Medicine at Urbana-Champaign. It offers PhDs not only in the biomedical and physical sciences but also in subjects ranging from anthropology to philosophy. Similarly, the program in Medicine, Arts, and Social Sciences at the University of Chicago attracts medical students from around the country who pursue PhD's in a wide range of subjects. A third program of note is the Clinical Scholars program at the University of Michigan.

The most popular of the nonscience dual programs, relatively speaking, is the MD-JD program. There are presently at least six medical schools that offer opportunities for interested students who wish to secure a law degree along with an MD. These schools include Chicago-Pritzker, Duke, University of Pennsylvania, University of Illinois Urbana–Champaign, and Yale. Many graduates with this dual degree enter the field of medical malpractice or health policy work. Finally, it may be noted, a master's degree in Public Health is offered by Tufts University School of Medicine.

CANADIAN MEDICAL SCHOOLS

There are 16 Canadian medical schools. They are accredited jointly by the CACMS and LCME; therefore, these schools provide their students with assured high-quality medical education. They have admissions policies and procedures similar to U.S. medical schools. However, except for McGill University, Canadian schools admit very few U.S. applicants.

The basic premedical science courses plus English are usually one requirement for admission. Because the educational system in Canada differs from the United States, the prerequisite educational level requirement varies with different schools. In addition, two schools have a three-year program and three require fluency in French.

Additional information about Canadian schools can be secured from the Association of Canadian Medical Colleges, Suite 120, 151 Slater Street, Ottawa, Canada K1P 5N1. It should be noted that the five medical schools of Ontario province (identified by an asterisk in Table 5.1) belong to a common application service and that applications to them should thus be directed to OMSAS, Ontario Universities' Application Center, P.O. Box 1328, 650 Woodlawn Road West, Guelph, Ontario, Canada N1H 7P4.

THE ADMISSION PROCESS: TIMETABLE

Based on what you have read up to this point, you can see that the admission process in reality begins when you start to think you might want to become a physician. It is a complex and prolonged ordeal that all students must pass through. Doing it right is critical to success. Deadlines need to be met and careful thought and preparation is imperative. It is also a costly process. It is to your advantage to be as well informed as possible. Sources of information, aside from this book, are your advisor, upper-class students, admissions personnel, and alumni.

Table 3.4 provides you with a checklist of your activities that extend from the time you enter college until you complete the process. You can mark off each step as it is completed and thus know what you have done and what tasks lie ahead.

Table 3.4
APPLICATION PROCESS: TRACKING TABLE

(*check when complete*)

FRESHMAN YEAR

____ Joined your school's premedical society and attended its meetings.

____ Became personally acquainted with your premedical advisor.

____ Discussed your career plans with your family physician.

SOPHOMORE YEAR

____ Became familiar with the admissions process.

____ Got some hospital and/or research experience.

JUNIOR YEAR

____ November–January: Preliminary MCAT preparation

____ February. Registered to take the MCAT.

____ February–April. Intensive MCAT preparation

____ April. Took the MCAT.

____ Solicited faculty recommendation from your advisory committee.

____ May. Secured AMCAS and non-AMCAS applications.

Prepared first and revised drafts of your application essay.

____ June. Completed AMCAS and non-AMCAS applications, including essays.

____ Completed preliminary MCAT preparation for August examination.

____ Advised premedical committee where to send recommendations.

____ July–August. Completed intensive preparation for the fall MCAT.

SENIOR YEAR

____ September. Checked with premedical advisory office to see if all supporting material is complete.

____ Took or (retook) fall MCAT.

____ October. Contacted medical schools to confirm that they received application.

____ Completed and submitted supplementary applications.

____ November. Prepared for interviews.

____ December–January. Attended interviews, completed supplementary applications.

____ February. Sent lower senior year transcript (if it helps you).

____ March. Advised waiting-list schools of interest.

____ Contacted schools not heard from (by phone and/or letter), expressing interest.

____ Asked advisor to contact schools on your behalf.

____ April–August. (Affirmative reply still possible)

____ Made sure that medical schools know your summer address.

____ August. If you have still not been accepted, consider the options discussed earlier in this chapter for rejected applicants. Don't give up hope; it may be worth trying again.

4 The Medical College Admission Test (MCAT)

OVERVIEW OF THE MCAT

Essentially all applicants to the U.S. and Canadian medical schools, as well as some applicants to foreign schools, are expected to take the MCAT. It is given on a Saturday in April and in August at test centers located throughout the country and at some overseas locations. The test is administered and scored by The MCAT Program, P.O. Box 4056, Iowa City, IA 52243, (319) 337-1357. Score reporting is the responsibility of the AAMC (MCAT Operations, Association of American Medical Colleges, Section for Student Services, 2450 N Street NW, Suite 201, Washington, DC 20037, (202) 828-0600). You can arrange to take the test by filing an application (frequently obtainable at your Premedical Advisory Office), along with the examination fee (currently $155) and a recent snapshot. Special test centers are open on Sundays for students whose religious convictions prevent them from taking the exam on Saturday. An additional fee (currently $10) is required for taking the exam on Sunday.

Scores are sent automatically in mid-June or mid-October both to you and to your advisor. Your scores will also be sent automatically to AMCAS schools. You can indicate on your test application six non-AMCAS schools you wish to receive your scores; if you are applying to more than six AMCAS schools, you must pay a fee for each additional school.

The MCAT can be retaken without special permission, but it is usually advisable to do so only if there is a significant discrepancy between your college grades and MCAT scores, if the test was taken before you completed your basic biology and chemistry courses, if you were quite ill or emotionally upset at the time the test was taken, or if you are encouraged by your Premedical Committee to do so. When the MCAT is taken twice, the AAMC recommends that the initial and retest scores on the verbal reasoning tests be averaged, and the retest scores for the physical and biological sciences tests be used, unless there is evidence that unusual circumstances might have affected scores on either exam.

As a general rule, you should take the MCAT at the session at which you feel you could perform best. The overwhelming majority of students take the test in the spring and this is justified for a number of reasons:

1. Scores become available earlier and therefore prompter action on your application can be taken by admissions committees.

2. Additional knowledge accumulated between the two test periods does not significantly affect test scores.

3. Most schools interpret the scores in light of the actual coursework completed at the time the exam was taken.

4. You still have the option of retaking the examination in the fall if you missed it in the spring or if you feel that the scores, for some reason, did not reflect your true capabilities.

5. A significant number of places may already be filled by the time the schools receive the scores from the fall exam (usually after Thanksgiving).

6. You can get a necessary hurdle out of the way and you can then concentrate better on your studies.

Students who have not had basic courses in chemistry and biology and who plan to take these courses during the summer and students whose academic record is B– or less and who will have additional time to study for the examination during the summer and therefore may perform better on the exam in the fall should give serious consideration to the later test administration. In any event, the exam should not be taken in the spring as if it were a trial run, with the intention of taking it definitively in the fall since medical schools are aware that the exam is taken twice and can secure both sets of scores.

Test scores are sent to the student usually four to six weeks after the test is taken. The student also receives a copy to be given to his or her advisor. The advisor receives a computer printout of the scores from those students electing to release them.

IMPORTANCE OF THE MCAT

The MCAT scores provide admissions committees with nationally standardized measures of both academic ability and achievement. This permits comparison of applicants even though they have widely different academic backgrounds and attend different colleges. The scores attained on the MCAT do not by themselves determine admission and are supplemental in interpreting the academic record, since they help to shed light on the academic abilities of the applicant. The extent of their importance varies among medical schools because committees place different degrees of stress on the scores. In general, the MCAT scores are significant in relation to the academic record of the individual. When the scores are high or low for a student with a good or a weak record, respectively, they simply confirm the academic record. When they are significantly different from the student's record, they raise questions that can be critical in determining admissions. Thus students with poor records and high scores may have greater potential than their records indicate. In such cases, more intensive evaluation may be warranted, and the applicants may be called for an interview that they otherwise may not have been granted. At the interview, the discrepancy between the academic record and the MCAT scores can be clarified, and the applicants will have the opportunity to "sell themselves," perhaps significantly improving their chances for admission.

On the other hand, when the academic record is high and the MCAT scores are low, the applicant's interview will not be perfunctory but will be aimed at clarifying the discrepancy. He or she will have to convince the interviewer of potential ability and overcome the uncertainty that has been created. One way of doing this is to retake the test and perform significantly better.

CONTENTS OF THE MCAT

Over the past several decades, there has been a gradual but nevertheless dramatic change in the medical profession in terms of knowledge amassed, technological advances, and delivery of health care. This has brought about the belief that premedical and medical education for practitioners in the twenty-first century needs revision. This realization has similarly motivated a review of the MCAT exam for relevancy, especially since its relevance in predicting clinical success has been seriously questioned.

A study over a period of several years, including field testing, resulted in a new MCAT format that was introduced in the fall of 1991. The new format is designed to assist medical school admissions committees to identify applicants who have a broad liberal arts education as well as a solid scientific background and adequate writing skills.

The MCAT now consists of four separate subtests:

Verbal reasoning	85 minutes
Physical sciences	100 minutes
Writing sample	60 minutes
Biological sciences	100 minutes

The tests are designed so that nearly everyone will have enough time to finish each section without undue pressure, since the emphasis will be on preparation rather than on speed of response.

Timetable for the MCAT

TOTAL TIME: 5¾ hours, plus 1 hour for lunch, two 10-minute breaks

85 minutes	Verbal Reasoning	65 questions
Rest Period—10 minutes		
100 minutes	Physical Sciences	77 questions
Lunch—60 minutes		
60 minutes	Writing Sample	2 questions
Rest Period—10 minutes		
100 minutes	Biological Sciences	77 questions

Verbal Reasoning

This section consists of a 500- to 600-word selected text taken from the natural or social sciences or humanities. The source of the text will be identified. Following the text will be a set of questions presented in order from easiest to hardest. The goal of this subtest is to ascertain quantitatively the applicant's skills in several, but not necessarily all, of the following:

(a) comprehending the essence of the text,

(b) utilizing the information of the text,

(c) determining the validity of the information in the text, and

(d) integrating new data on the context of that which is in the text.

Physical Sciences

This subtest seeks to measure an applicant's comprehension of basic concepts and problem-solving ability in physics and chemistry. (This may require an understanding and ability to use basic college-level mathematical concepts to solve some of the problems in the physical sciences.) Of the 77 questions making up this subtest, 62 are based on a text that discusses a problem or situation that may be presented in a prose, graphic, tabular, or illustrative format. About ten problem sets consisting of four to eight questions each are associated with each such unit. In addition, 15 questions unrelated to the text are presented. The questions are not predicated on an ability to memorize scientific facts. Rather, they require knowledge of constants and equations commonly used in basic physics and chemistry courses.

Physics

This segment of the physical sciences subtest will judge your ability to utilize fundamental physics theories in solving problems (on a noncalculus basis). Topics that you should be familiar with include:

Mechanics: namely, concepts in equilibrium, momentum, force, motion, gravitation, translational motion, work, energy, fluids, and solids.

Wave Motion: namely, wave characteristics, periodic motion, and sound.

Electricity and Magnetism: namely, concepts in electrostatics, electromagnetism, and electric circuits.

Light and Optics: namely, concepts in visible light and geometric optics.

Modern Physics: namely, concepts in atomic and nuclear structure.

Chemistry

This segment of the physical science subtest will judge your ability to apply fundamental theories of general chemistry to solving problems. (Organic chemistry is included as part of the biological sciences subtest.) Topics you should be familiar with include:

Stoichiometry: namely, metric units, molecular weight, Avogadro number, mole concept, oxidation number, chemical equation reactions.

Electronic Structure: namely, understanding the complexities and dynamics of chemical reactions, as well as the link between quantum theories and physical and chemical properties of elements and compounds.

Bonding: namely, ionic and covalent bond formation characteristics should be understood so as to appreciate chemical and physical properties of substances.

Phases: namely, understanding the concepts involved in the dynamic phases of elements (gas, liquid, and solid) as well as phase equilibria is necessary to respond to some of the questions.

Solution Chemistry: namely, familiarity with ions in solution, solubility, and precipitation reactions.

Acids and Bases: namely, the concepts associated with acid/base equilibria and acid/base titrations.

Thermodynamics and Thermochemistry: namely, concepts associated with the evolution and absorption of heat during a reaction should be understood.

Rate of Chemical Reactions: namely, an understanding of rate concepts and reaction equilibrium is necessary.

Electrochemistry: namely, an understanding of concepts in the analysis of galvanic, electronic, or concentration cells.

Mathematics

Noncalculus prerequisite knowledge in mathematics that will permit solving some of the problems in the physical science subtests includes:

Arithmetic Computation Skills: namely, exponents, logarithms, quadratic equations, simultaneous equations, scientific notation, graphic presentation of data and functions.

Trigonometry: namely, functions (sine, cosine, tangent), the values of sines and cosines of 0°, 90°, and 180°; inverse functions ($\sin^{-1}$, $\cos^{-1}$, $\tan^{-1}$); lengths relationships of sides of right triangles containing angles of 30°, 45°, and 60°.

Vectors: namely, addition, subtraction, and right hand rule.

Probability: namely, capability to determine the mathematical probability of an event (on an elementary level).

Statistics: namely, capability to calculate the arithmetic average and range of a set of numerical data; comprehension of statistical association and correlation concepts; appreciating the value of standard deviation as a measure of variability (its calculation is not required).

Experimental Error: namely, relative magnitude as well as propagation of error, comprehension of reasonable estimates as well as the significant digits of a measurement.

Writing Sample

Written communication skills are deemed important elements for a successful medical practitioner. They provide an essential vehicle for an effective relationship with both colleagues and patients. The measure of an applicant's capability in the area is determined on the MCAT by two 30-minutes essays. Each item is made up of a short, usually one-line, statement of a policy or an opinion on a topic that can come from a broad range of issues. The applicant is then presented with three tasks: (1) to provide an in-depth interpretation of the meaning of the statement, (2) to provide a detailed rebuttal of the point of view expressed in the statement, and (3) to demonstrate how one can resolve the statement and the opposing viewpoint that was offered.

The response to all three tasks should be provided in a detailed, thoughtful, and logically expressed essay.

Biological Sciences

This subtest seeks to measure an applicant's comprehension of basic concepts of molecular biology, cell structure and function, genetics, and evolution as well as the organization of body systems. Topics in organic chemistry are also covered in the 77 questions of this subtest because it forms the bases of many biological (biochemical) reactions.

Biology

The major topics covered are:

Molecular Biology: namely, understanding enzyme regulation of cell metabolism as well as DNA and protein synthesis is necessary.

Microbiology: namely, familiarity with the structure and life histories of the bacteriophage, animal versus "fungi," and prokaryotic cell is necessary.

Eukaryotic Cell: namely, knowledge of the principal components of the typical eukaryotic cell and their functions is required.

Specialized Eukaryotic Cell: namely, the unique features of cells and tissues of connective, muscular, nervous tissues, and skin should be understood.

Body Systems: namely, the organs that compose the major body systems (skeletal, muscular, circulatory, digestive, respiratory, excretory, nervous, reproductive, and endocrine) should be known.

Genetics and Evolution: both Mendelian and modern concepts of genetics should be understood as well as concepts of evolution such as natural selection, speciation, and basic structure of chordates.

Organic Chemistry

This area requires a knowledge of organic compounds, including nomenclature, classification of functional groups, and reactions including reaction mechanisms. The major topics covered are:

Biological Molecules: namely, knowledge of the types of biologically active molecules (e.g., amino acids and proteins, carbohydrates, lipids, and phosphorus compounds) is required.

Oxygen-Containing Compounds: namely, knowledge of the principal reaction of the oxygen-containing compounds (e.g., alcohols, aldehydes, ketones, carboxylic acids, ethers, and phenols) is required.

Amines: namely, knowledge of the nitrogen-containing compounds is required.

Hydrocarbons: namely, knowledge of the alkanes, alkenes, and benzene derivatives is required.

Molecular Structure: namely, knowledge of the structure of organic compounds in terms of bonds; bond strengths, and stereochemistry of bonded molecules is necessary.

Separation and Purification: namely, familiarity with the methodology and the characteristics of different organic compounds as related to their separation and possible purification if needed. This requires knowledge of the processes of extraction, distillation, recrystallization, and chromatography.

Spectroscopy: namely, knowledge of nuclear magnetic resonance (NMR) and infrared (IR) spectroscopy is necessary.

A full description of the test is included in *The MCAT Student Manual,* obtainable from AAMC, 2450 N Street, NW, Washington, DC 20037.

PREPARING FOR THE MCAT

It can be categorically stated that your performance on the MCAT will be better if you prepare for it in an organized manner. This means that a *structured study plan* should be developed before initiating your review process.

Developing a study plan involves (1) setting a realistic starting date to begin your study program (such as one and a half to three months prior to the test date, depending on your ability, time available for study, etc.); (2) requisitioning fixed blocks of time on a weekly basis to be used exclusively for study (with alternate time-blocks if you cannot keep to your schedule); (3) proportioning your study time relative to each of the subtests, in direct proportion to your strength or weakness in each area; (4) arranging your study schedule to allow for completion of preparation for taking the exam a few days *before* the test date. This will reduce the chance or need for cramming, which would be counterproductive. Moreover, a brief interlude available just prior to the test will afford you a chance to relax physically and mentally in preparation for the examination. You can then better meet the very demanding challenge for a 5¾-hour test.

General Study Guidelines

The following nine suggestions should aid in your preparation for taking the MCAT.

1. Your first step should be to familiarize yourself with the major topics that must be mastered for each of the subtests (see pages 89–90). This will give an overview of areas that may require greater or lesser emphasis in your study schedule.

2. It is probably desirable to begin your study with the subject that you are most knowledgeable or comfortable with. Thus the learning process, which under the

circumstances should be a productive one, will also serve to reinforce your self-confidence as you prepare for more challenging segments of the exam.

3. Consider utilizing a study plan that involves a preliminary review of the material, before initiating intensive study. If areas of weakness are identified during the initial review, seek to fill in the void without excessive delay. This will lessen your anxiety due to concern over your knowledge gap. Excessive worry over your deficiencies can seriously impede preparation for and attainment of your goal.

4. Determine the inherent sequence of the information you seek to master. Try to master it within the context of a logical "framework" rather than as isolated data.

5. You should try to determine your most successful study techniques (such as repeated reading of material outlining the subject, written summary of the text, or verbalizing the highlights of the information being studied).

6. Before you commit information to memory, be certain that you comprehend it fully. It is more difficult to unlearn erroneous material and replace it with a correct version than to learn it right in the first place.

7. The length of your individual study session should be reasonable and adjusted to the state of your physical and mental well-being. If fatigue sets in during your learning period, take a break or terminate it. Pushing yourself beyond your limit will be unproductive because of inefficiency, and consequently potentially frustrating.

8. The major determinant of success on the MCAT (like any other exam) is retention of the material learned. Meaningful information—that is, knowledge associated with principles or concepts—is retained longer than nonmeaningful information—this is, isolated facts. In both cases, however, repetition at spaced intervals after initial learning will enhance retention. Thus, frequent, short, intense review periods will definitely enhance your incorporating the material for an extended interval.

9. Getting a good night's (REM) sleep after an initial intense study session in the evening is important, because (dream) sleep has been shown to consolidate long-term memory, thus enhancing retention.

Specific Study Guidelines

One can and should prepare for each of the four specific subtests. Preparation for these should be an integral part of your overall study plan.

Science Subtest Preparation

As indicated in the preceding section, a preliminary review of the major topics in the physical and biological sciences will provide you with a general assessment of your strengths and weaknesses. This can be done using well-written college textbooks or reading the Science Review chapter in *Barron's How to Prepare for the Medical College Admission Test* by Hugo R. Seibel and Kenneth E. Guyer (Barron's Educational Series, 1997). Your goal should be to refresh your memory with the general concepts and principal facts in each of the three science areas you will be tested in.

It is best that you begin intensive study only after you have completed your preliminary survey.

The major topics to be covered are summarized in the chart on pages 89–90, which is consistent with the contents of the MCAT.

Verbal Reasoning Subtest Preparation

It should be recognized that reasoning is a skill and requires practice. Some basic rules for proper reasoning are the following:

1. Strive to ascertain the meaning of the central theme of the passage under consideration.

2. Try to identify the premises upon which the passage is based, both explicit or implicit.

3. Evaluate critically the premises in terms of how strongly or poorly they support the conclusion.

4. Seek other relevant arguments to support the conclusion.

5. Be alert to being led astray in your thinking.

Newspaper or magazine articles, especially editorials, provide source material to test your verbal reasoning skills.

In responding to the paragraph under consideration, you can chose to read it first, then take note of the questions next. Conversely, you may wish to read the questions first, then read the relevant paragraph. In either case, underlining appropriate key words or phrases in the paragraph should prove helpful in your analysis of its contents.

Writing Sample Subtest Preparation

This subtest will, for some applicants, represent the greatest challenge. Meeting this challenge will depend on how successfully you have mastered the art of essay writing. Given a statement, you will have to respond to three writing tasks pertaining to the statement.

First, you must determine the meaning of the statement and do so in an orderly, thorough, and coherent manner. Second, you will have to translate the meaning of the statement in the context of some example that illustrates an opposing attitude. The third task will be to reconcile the conflict between the statement or interpretation (task 1) and its opposite viewpoint (task 2). While you may respond to the three tasks in any order, all three tasks must be met in order to maximize your credit potential.

In responding to the challenge of the writing sample, the following guidelines should prove helpful.

1. Carefully read and analyze the statement presented before you initiate your response.

2. Determine specifically what you are really being asked to do.

3. Prepare a brief outline of how you wish to respond, using key words, ideas, facts, or examples.

4. Write legibly and in direct response to the task under consideration. Focus your responses as specifically as possible.

5. Present your ideas clearly and in an organized rather than haphazard fashion.

MODEL MCAT

Some useful reference material can be found beginning on page 92.

The full-length model MCAT that follows will provide you with helpful practice. Be sure to take the model test under strict test conditions, timing each section as instructed. First, remove the answer sheets.

After you complete the test, check your answers with the explanations that begin on page 141. Then, compute your MCAT scores using the Conversion Tables and the Self-Scoring Chart on page 159. Doing this will help you to determine areas of strength and weakness. If your computed MCAT score on the model test is lower than 8 in any of the three numerically graded subtests, you should plan additional work in that area. Your writing samples should be evaluated, if possible, by an English instructor.

MCAT STUDY TOPICS

Biological Sciences

Microbiology
  Viral structure
  Prokaryotic cell
  Fungi

Molecular Biology
  Cell metabolism
  Enzyme structure
  Enzyme function
  Glycosis

The Cell
  Plasma membrane
    Ultrastructure
    Function
    Membrane transport

  Cytologic research methods
  Cytoplasmic organelles
    Mitochondria
    Golgi apparatus
    Endoplasmic reticulum
    Lysosomes and peroxisomes
    Annulate lamellae

Skeletal System
  Organization
  Bone characteristics
  Function
  Joints

Muscular Tissue
  Classification
  Terminology
  Gross and fine structure
  Function
  Control of activity

Circulatory System
  Components
  Structure
  Circulation path
  Blood
  Oxygen transport
  Lymph system
    Spleen

Cytoskeleton
  Microtubules
  Microfilaments
  Cilia

Mitosis
  Process
  Structures
  Movements and mechanisms
  Nucleus
    Nuclear envelope
    Nuclear structures

Human Body Organization
  Basic tissues
  Epithelial tissue
  Connective tissue
  Muscle tissue
  Nerve tissue

Respiratory System
  Function
  Gas exchange
  Thermoregulation
  Components
    Rib cage
    Diaphragm

Digestive System
  Organs
  Digestive glands
  Functional control
  Nutrition

Urinary System
  Organs
  Structure
  Function
  Hormonal control

Nervous System
  Components
  Central system
  Autonomic system

Immune System
  Bone marrow
  Thymus
  Function

Neuron
  Classification and groups
  Supportive cells

Special Sensory Organs
  Eyes
    Structure
    Sensory reception

  Ear
    Structure
    Mechanism of hearing

  Nose
    Structure
    Mechanism of olfaction

Endocrine System
  Major glands
  Function
  Mechanism of action

Reproductive System
  Organs

Reproductive System cont.
  Gametogenesis
  Meiotic cycle
  Menstruation
  Placenta
  Embryogenesis
    Early stages
    Germ layers
  Chordate body plan
  Vertebrate body plan

Genetics
  Mendelian concepts
  Sex-linked features
  Mutation

Evolution
  Natural selection
  Formation of species
  Origin of life

Note: While organic chemistry is covered in the biological sciences subtest, its topical outline here is given in its traditional position under chemistry.

Physical Sciences

Inorganic Chemistry

The Atom
Components of the atom
Energy levels
The Periodic Table
  Gases
  Liquids
  Solids
  Phase changes
  Chemical compounds
  Bonding
  Balanced chemical equations
  Solutions
  Acids and bases
  pH and buffers
  Electrochemistry
  Thermodynamics
  Rate of chemical reactions

Biochemistry

Enzymes
Amino acids
Proteins
Carbohydrates
Lipids
Nucleotids and nucleic acids

Organic Chemistry

Alkanes
Cycloalkanes
Alkenes
Alkynes
Aromatic compounds
Grignard reagent
Alcohols
Amines
Amides
Aldehydes
Ketones
Carboxylic acids
Esters
Ethers

Physics

Accelerated motion
Forces and motion
Projective motion
Friction
Work and power
Energy
  Momentum
  Uniform circular motion
  Fluids at rest

Energy cont.
  Gravity
  Temperature calculations
  Temperature measurements
  Heat
  Thermodynamics
  Electrostatics
  Electricity
  Electric circuits
  Electric energy
Machines
  Advantages of machines
  Harmonic motion
Waves
Sound waves
Light rays
Mirrors
Lenses
Atom composition
Radioactivity
Nuclear energy
Photons
Atomic energy units

REFERENCE DATA FOR MODEL TEST _____

Logarithms and Exponents

Logarithms

The logarithm of any number is the exponent of the power to which 10 must be raised to produce the number. The logarithm X of the number N to the base 10 is the exponent of the power to which 10 must be raised to give N (for example, $\log_{10} N = X$). Logarithms consist of two parts. First, there is the "characteristic," which is determined by the position of the first significant figure of the number in relation to the decimal point. If we count leftwards from the decimal point as positive and rightwards as negative, the characteristic is equal to the count ending at the right of the first significant figure. Thus, the characteristic of the logarithm of 2340 is 3, and of 0.00234 is –3. Second, there is the "mantissa." It is always positive, is found in logarithm tables, and depends only on the sequence of significant figures. Thus, the mantissa for the two numbers is the same, namely 0.3692. The logarithm of a number is the sum of the characteristic and the mantissa. Thus, log 2340 = 3.3692 while log 0.00234 = –3 + 0.3692 = –2.6308.

The logarithms of the whole integers 1 to 10 are given below.

log 1.0 = 0.000	log 4.0 = 0.602	log 7.0 = 0.845	log 10.0 = 1.000
log 2.0 = 0.301	log 5.0 = 0.699	log 8.0 = 0.903	
log 3.0 = 0.477	log 6.0 = 0.778	log 9.0 = 0.954	

Useful Rules in Handling Logarithms

1. The logarithm of a product is equal to the sum of the logarithm of the factors:
$$\log ab = \log a + \log b$$
(Check this out by solving for log 6, using log 2 + log 3.)

2. The logarithm of a fraction is equal to the logarithm of the numerator minus the logarithm of the denominator:
$$\log \frac{a}{b} = \log a - \log b \qquad \text{Example: } \log \frac{10}{2} = \log 10 - \log 2 = \log 5$$
How about log 2.5? The answer from the log tables is 0.398.

3. The logarithm of the reciprocal of a number is the negative logarithm of the number:
$$\log \frac{1}{a} = \log 1 - \log a$$
Since log 1 = 0, then
$$\log \frac{1}{a} = -\log a$$
Equally,
$$\log \frac{1}{2} = -\log 2 = -0.301$$

4. The logarithm of a number raised to a power is the logarithm of the number multiplied by the power:
$$\log a^b = b \log a$$
$$\log 2^2 = 0.603$$

Exponents

It is convenient to express large numbers as 10^x, where x represents the number of places that the decimal must be moved to place it after the first significant figure. This also represents $10 \cdot 10$ for x times. For example, 1,000,000 may be expressed as 1×10^6; 3663 as 3.663×10^3; and so on. To multiply, the exponents are added, but coefficients are multiplied. To divide, the exponents are subtracted but coefficients are divided.

Multiplying: $(1 \times 10^x) \cdot (1 \times 10^y) = 1 \times 10^{x+y}$ $(4 \times 10^2) \cdot (2 \times 10^3) = 8 \times 10^5$

Dividing: $(1 \times 10^x) \div (1 \times 10^y) = 1 \times 10^{x-y}$ $(4 \times 10^2) \div (2 \times 10^3) = 2 \times 10^{-1}$

Numbers less than 1 are 10^{-x}. For example, 0.000001 is 1×10^{-6}.

Multiplying: $(1 \times 10^{-x}) \cdot (1 \times 10^{-y}) = 1 \times 10^{-(x+y)}$ $(4 \times 10^{-2}) \cdot (2 \times 10^{-3}) = 8 \times 10^{-5}$

A large number multiplied by a small number: $(4 \times 10^{-2})(2 \times 10^3) = 8 \times 10^1$

(Logarithms and Exponents are reproduced through the courtesy of Dr. Richard B. Brandt, Dept. of Biochemistry, MCV, VCU, Richmond, Virginia, 23298).

Table of Common Logarithms

Numbers	0	1	2	3	4	5	6	7	8	9
10	0000	0043	0086	0128	0170	0212	0253	0294	0334	0374
11	0414	0453	0492	0531	0569	0607	0645	0682	0719	0755
12	0792	0828	0864	0899	0934	0969	1004	1038	1072	1106
13	1139	1173	1206	1239	1271	1303	1335	1367	1399	1430
14	1461	1492	1523	1553	1584	1614	1644	1673	1703	1732
15	1761	1790	1818	1847	1875	1903	1931	1959	1987	2014
16	2041	2068	2095	2122	2148	2175	2201	2227	2253	2279
17	2304	2330	2355	2380	2405	2430	2455	2480	2504	2529
18	2553	2577	2601	2625	2648	2672	2695	2718	2742	2765
19	2788	2810	2833	2856	2878	2900	2923	2945	2967	2989
20	3010	3032	3054	3075	3096	3118	3139	3160	3181	3201
21	3222	3243	3263	3284	3304	3324	3345	3365	3385	3404
22	3424	3444	3464	3483	3502	3522	3541	3560	3579	3598
23	3617	3636	3655	3674	3692	3711	3729	3747	3766	3784
24	3802	3820	3838	3856	3874	3892	3909	3927	3945	3962
25	3979	3997	4014	4031	4048	4065	4082	4099	4116	4133
26	4150	4166	4183	4200	4216	4232	4249	4265	4281	4298
27	4314	4330	4346	4362	4378	4393	4409	4425	4440	4456
28	4472	4487	4502	4518	4533	4548	4564	4579	4594	4609
29	4624	4639	4654	4669	4683	4698	4713	4728	4742	4757
30	4771	4786	4800	4814	4829	4843	4857	4871	4886	4900
31	4914	4928	4942	4955	4969	4983	4997	5011	5024	5038
32	5051	5065	5079	5092	5105	5119	5132	5145	5159	5172
33	5185	5198	5211	5224	5237	5250	5263	5276	5289	5302
34	5315	5328	5340	5353	5366	5378	5391	5403	5416	5428
35	5441	5453	5465	5478	5490	5502	5514	5527	5539	5551
36	5563	5575	5587	5599	5611	5623	5635	5647	5658	5670
37	5682	5694	5705	5717	5729	5740	5752	5763	5775	5786
38	5798	5809	5821	5832	5843	5855	5866	5877	5888	5899
39	5911	5922	5933	5944	5955	5966	5977	5988	5999	6010
40	6021	6031	6042	6053	6064	6075	6085	6096	6107	6117
41	6128	6138	6149	6160	6170	6180	6191	6201	6212	6222
42	6232	6243	6253	6263	6274	6284	6294	6304	6314	6325
43	6335	6345	6355	6365	6375	6385	6395	6405	6415	6425
44	6435	6444	6454	6464	6474	6484	6493	6503	6513	6522
45	6532	6542	6551	6561	6571	6580	6590	6599	6609	6618
46	6628	6637	6646	6656	6665	6675	6684	6693	6702	6712
47	6721	6730	6739	6749	6758	6767	6776	6785	6794	6803
48	6812	6821	6830	6839	6848	6857	6866	6875	6884	6893
49	6902	6911	6920	6928	6937	6946	6955	6964	6972	6981
50	6990	6998	7007	7016	7024	7033	7042	7050	7059	7067
51	7076	7084	7093	7101	7110	7118	7126	7135	7143	7152
52	7160	7168	7177	7185	7193	7202	7210	7218	7226	7235
53	7243	7251	7259	7267	7275	7284	7292	7300	7308	7316
54	7324	7332	7340	7348	7356	7364	7372	7380	7388	7396

Numbers	0	1	2	3	4	5	6	7	8	9
55	7404	7412	7419	7427	7435	7443	7451	7459	7466	7474
56	7482	7490	7497	7505	7513	7520	7528	7536	7543	7551
57	7559	7566	7574	7582	7589	7597	7604	7612	7619	7627
58	7634	7642	7649	7657	7664	7672	7679	7686	7694	7701
59	7709	7716	7723	7731	7738	7745	7752	7760	7767	7774
60	7782	7789	7796	7803	7810	7818	7825	7832	7839	7846
61	7853	7860	7868	7875	7882	7889	7896	7903	7910	7917
62	7924	7931	7938	7945	7952	7959	7966	7937	7980	7987
63	7993	8000	8007	8014	8021	8028	8035	8041	8048	8055
64	8062	8069	8075	8082	8089	8096	8102	8109	8116	8122
65	8129	8136	8142	8149	8156	8162	8169	8176	8182	8189
66	8195	8202	8209	8215	8222	8228	8235	8241	8248	8254
67	8261	8267	8274	8280	8287	8293	8299	8306	8312	8319
68	8325	8331	8338	8344	8351	8357	8363	8370	8376	8382
69	8388	8395	8401	8407	8414	8420	8426	8432	8439	8445
70	8451	8457	8463	8470	8476	8482	8488	8494	8500	8506
71	8513	8519	8525	8531	8537	8543	8549	8555	8561	8567
72	8573	8579	8585	8591	8597	8603	8609	8615	8621	8627
73	8633	8639	8645	8651	8657	8663	8669	8675	8681	8686
74	8692	8698	8704	8710	8716	8722	8727	8733	8739	8745
75	8751	8756	8762	8768	8774	8779	8785	8791	8797	8802
76	8808	8814	8820	8825	8831	8837	8842	8848	8854	8859
77	8865	8871	8876	8882	8887	8893	8899	8904	8910	8915
78	8921	8927	8932	8938	8943	8949	8954	8960	8965	8971
79	8976	8982	8987	8993	8998	9004	9009	9015	9020	9025
80	9031	9036	9042	9047	9053	9058	9063	9069	9074	9079
81	9085	9090	9096	9101	9106	9112	9117	9122	9128	9133
82	9138	9143	9149	9154	9159	9165	9170	9175	9180	9186
83	9191	9196	9201	9206	9212	9217	9222	9227	9232	9238
84	9243	9248	9253	9258	9263	9269	9274	9279	9284	9289
85	9294	9299	9304	9309	9315	9320	9325	9330	9335	9340
86	9345	9350	9355	9360	9365	9370	9375	9380	9385	9390
87	9395	9400	9405	9410	9415	9420	9425	9430	9435	9440
88	9445	9450	9455	9460	9465	9469	9474	9479	9484	9489
89	9494	9499	9504	9509	9513	9518	9523	9528	9533	9538
90	9542	9547	9552	9557	9562	9566	9571	9576	9581	9586
91	9590	9595	9600	9605	9609	9614	9619	9624	9628	9633
92	9638	9643	9647	9652	9657	9661	9666	9671	9675	9680
93	9685	9689	9694	9699	9703	9708	9713	9717	9722	9727
94	9731	9736	9741	9745	9750	9754	9759	9763	9768	9773
95	9777	9782	9786	9791	9795	9800	9805	9809	9814	9818
96	9823	9827	9832	9836	9841	9845	9850	9854	9859	9863
97	9868	9872	9877	9881	9886	9890	9894	9899	9903	9908
98	9912	9917	9921	9926	9930	9934	9939	9943	9948	9952
99	9956	9961	9965	9969	9974	9978	9983	9987	9991	9996

Periodic Table of the Elements

KEY

Relative atomic masses are based on $^{12}C = 12.00000$

Selected Oxidation States

Atomic Mass → 12.0111

$$\begin{array}{c} -4 \\ +2 \\ +4 \end{array}$$

C

Symbol

Atomic Number → 6

Electron Configuration → $1s^2 2s^2 2p^2$

New Designation

Former Designation
(prior to 1994 IUPAC decision)

Transition Elements

d-block

Note: The Periodic Table that appears in the MCAT Examination Booklet provides only the Atomic Mass and the Atomic Number.

* The systematic names and symbols for elements of atomic numbers greater than 103 will be used until the approval of trivial names by IUPAC.

MASS NUMBERS IN PARENTHESIS ARE MASS NUMBERS OF THE MOST STABLE OR COMMON ISOTOPE.

s-block

GROUP

p-block GROUP

d-block GROUP

f-block

Lanthanoid Series

Actinoid Series

List of Elements with Their Symbols

Element	Symbol	Element	Symbol
Actinium	Ac	Mendelevium	Md
Aluminum	Al	Mercury	Hg
Americium	Am	Molybdenum	Mo
Antimony	Sb	Neodymium	Nd
Argon	Ar	Neon	Ne
Arsenic	As	Neptunium	Np
Astatine	At	Nickel	Ni
Barium	Ba	Niobium	Nb
Berkelium	Bk	Nitrogen	N
Beryllium	Be	Nobelium	No
Bismuth	Bi	Osmium	Os
Boron	B	Oxygen	O
Bromine	Br	Palladium	Pd
Cadmium	Cd	Phosphorus	P
Calcium	Ca	Platinum	Pt
Californium	Cf	Plutonium	Pu
Carbon	C	Polonium	Po
Cerium	Ce	Potassium	K
Cesium	Cs	Praseodymium	Pr
Chlorine	Cl	Promethium	Pm
Chromium	Cr	Protactinium	Pa
Cobalt	Co	Radium	Ra
Copper	Cu	Radon	Rn
Curium	Cm	Rhenium	Re
Dysprosium	Dy	Rhodium	Rh
Einsteinium	Es	Rubidium	Rb
Element 106		Ruthenium	Ru
Erbium	Er	Samarium	Sm
Europium	Eu	Scandium	Sc
Fermium	Fm	Selenium	Se
Fluorine	F	Silicon	Si
Francium	Fr	Silver	Ag
Gadolinium	Gd	Sodium	Na
Gallium	Ga	Strontium	Sr
Germanium	Ge	Sulfur	S
Gold	Au	Tantalum	Ta
Hafnium	Hf	Technetium	Tc
Helium	He	Tellurium	Te
Holmium	Ho	Terbium	Tb
Hydrogen	H	Thallium	Tl
Indium	In	Thorium	Th
Iodine	I	Thulium	Tm
Iridium	Ir	Tin	Sn
Iron	Fe	Titanium	Ti
Krypton	Kr	Tungsten	W
Lanthanum	La	Uranium	U
Lawrencium	Lr	Vanadium	V
Lead	Pb	Xenon	Xe
Lithium	Li	Ytterbium	Yb
Lutetium	Lu	Yttrium	Y
Magnesium	Mg	Zinc	Zn
Manganese	Mn	Zirconium	Zr

Reference Tables for Chemistry

PHYSICAL CONSTANTS AND CONVERSION FACTORS

Name	Symbol	Value(s)	Units
Angstrom unit	Å	1×10^{-10} m	meter
Avogadro number	N_A	6.02×10^{23} per mol	
Charge of electron	e	1.60×10^{-19} C	coulomb
Electron volt	eV	1.60×10^{-19} J	joule
Speed of light	c	3.00×10^8 m/s	meters/second
Planck's constant	h	6.63×10^{-34} J·s	joule-second
		1.58×10^{-37} kcal·s	kilocalorie-second
Universal gas constant	R	0.0821 L·atm/mol·K	liter-atmosphere/mole-kelvin
		1.98 cal/mol·K	calories/mole-kelvin
		8.31 J/mol·K	joules/mole-kelvin
Atomic mass unit	μ(amu)	1.66×10^{-24} g	gram
Volume standard, liter	L	1×10^3 cm^3 = 1 dm^3	cubic centimeters, cubic decimeter
Standard pressure, atmosphere	atm	101.3 kPa	kilopascals
		760 mmHg	millimeters of mercury
		760 torr	torr
Heat equivalent, kilocalorie	kcal	4.18×10^3 J	joules

Physical Constants for H_2O

Molal freezing point depression	1.86°C
Molal boiling point elevation	0.52°C
Heat of fusion	79.72 cal/g
Heat of vaporization	539.4 cal/g

STANDARD UNITS

Symbol	Name	Quantity
m	meter	length
kg	kilogram	mass
Pa	pascal	pressure
K	kelvin	thermodynamic temperature
mol	mole	amount of substance
J	joule	energy, work, quantity of heat
sec	second	time
C	coulomb	quantity of electricity
V	volt	electric potential, potential difference
L	liter	volume

Selected Prefixes

Factor	Prefix	Symbol
10^6	mega	M
10^3	kilo	k
10^{-1}	deci	d
10^{-2}	centi	c
10^{-3}	milli	m
10^{-6}	micro	μ
10^{-9}	nano	n

RELATIVE STRENGTHS OF ACIDS IN AQUEOUS SOLUTION AT 1 atm AND 298 K

Conjugate Pairs		K_a
ACID	BASE	
$HI = H^+ + I^-$		very large
$HBr = H^+ + Br^-$		very large
$HCl = H^+ + Cl^-$		very large
$HNO_3 = H^+ + NO_3^-$		very large
$H_2SO_4 = H^+ + HSO_4^-$		large
$H_2O + SO_2 = H^+ + HSO_3^-$		1.5×10^{-2}
$HSO_4^- = H^+ + SO_4^{2-}$		1.2×10^{-2}
$H_3PO_4 = H^+ + H_2PO_4^-$		7.5×10^{-3}
$Fe(H_2O)_6^{3+} = H^+ + Fe(H_2O)_5(OH)^{2+}$		8.9×10^{-4}
$HNO_2 = H^+ + NO_2^-$		4.6×10^{-4}
$HF = H^+ + F^-$		3.5×10^{-4}
$Cr(H_2O)_6^{3+} = H^+ + Cr(H_2O)_5(OH)^{2+}$		1.0×10^{-4}
$CH_3COOH = H^+ + CH_3COO^-$		1.8×10^{-5}
$Al(H_2O)_6^{3+} = H^+ + Al(H_2O)_5(OH)^{2+}$		1.1×10^{-5}
$H_2O + CO_2 = H^+ + HCO_3^-$		4.3×10^{-7}
$HSO_3^- = H^+ + SO_3^{2-}$		1.1×10^{-7}
$H_2S = H^+ + HS^-$		9.5×10^{-8}
$H_2PO_4^- = H^+ + HPO_4^{2-}$		6.2×10^{-8}
$NH_4^+ = H^+ + NH_3$		5.7×10^{-10}
$HCO_3^- = H^+ + CO_3^{2-}$		5.6×10^{-11}
$HPO_4^{2-} = H^+ + PO_4^{3-}$		2.2×10^{-13}
$HS^- = H^+ + S^{2-}$		1.3×10^{-14}
$H_2O = H^+ + OH^-$		1.0×10^{-14}

Note: $H^+(aq) = H_3O^+$

Sample equation: $HI + H_2O = H_3O^+ + I^-$

CONSTANTS FOR VARIOUS EQUILIBRIA AT 1 atm AND 298 K

$H_2O(\ell) = H^+(aq) + OH^-(aq)$	$K_w = 1.0 \times 10^{-14}$
$H_2O(\ell) + H_2O(\ell) = H_3O^+(aq) + OH^-(aq)$	$K_w = 1.0 \times 10^{-14}$
$CH_3COO^-(aq) + H_2O(\ell) = CH_3COOH(aq) + OH^-(aq)$	$K_b = 5.6 \times 10^{-10}$
$Na^+F^-(aq) + H_2O(\ell) = Na^+(OH)^- + HF(aq)$	$K_b = 1.5 \times 10^{-11}$
$NH_3(aq) + H_2O(\ell) = NH_4^+(aq) + OH^-(aq)$	$K_b = 1.8 \times 10^{-5}$
$CO_3^{2-}(aq) + H_2O(\ell) = HCO_3^-(aq) + OH^-(aq)$	$K_b = 1.8 \times 10^{-4}$
$Ag(NH_3)_2^+(aq) = Ag^+(aq) + 2NH_3(aq)$	$K_{eq} = 8.9 \times 10^{-8}$
$N_2(g) + 3H_2(g) = 2NH_3(g)$	$K_{eq} = 6.7 \times 10^{5}$
$H_2(g) + I_2(g) = 2HI(g)$	$K_{eq} = 3.5 \times 10^{-1}$

Compound	K_{sp}	Compound	K_{sp}
AgBr	5.0×10^{-13}	Li_2CO_3	2.5×10^{-2}
AgCl	1.8×10^{-10}	$PbCl_2$	1.6×10^{-5}
Ag_2CrO_4	1.1×10^{-12}	$PbCO_3$	7.4×10^{-14}
AgI	8.3×10^{-17}	$PbCrO_4$	2.8×10^{-13}
$BaSO_4$	1.1×10^{-10}	PbI_2	7.1×10^{-9}
$CaSO_4$	9.1×10^{-6}	$ZnCO_3$	1.4×10^{-11}

**STANDARD ENERGIES OF FORMATION
OF COMPOUNDS AT 1 atm AND 298 K**

Compound	Heat (Enthalpy) of Formation* kcal/mol (ΔH_f°)	Free Energy of Formation* kcal/mol (ΔG_f°)
Aluminum oxide Al_2O_3(s)	−400.5	−378.2
Ammonia NH_3(g)	−11.0	−3.9
Barium sulfate $BaSo_4$(s)	−352.1	−325.6
Calcium hydroxide $Ca(OH)_2$(s)	−235.7	−214.8
Carbon dioxide CO_2(g)	−94.1	−94.3
Carbon monoxide CO(g)	−26.4	−32.8
Copper (II) sulfate $CuSO_4$(s)	−184.4	−158.2
Ethane C_2H_6(g)	−20.2	−7.9
Ethene (ethylene) C_2H_4(g)	12.5	16.3
Ethyne (acetylene) C_2H_2(g)	54.2	50.0
Hydrogen fluoride HF(g)	−64.8	−65.3
Hydrogen iodide HI(g)	6.3	0.4
Iodine chloride ICl(g)	4.3	−1.3
Lead (II) oxide PbO(s)	−51.5	−45.0
Magnesium oxide MgO(s)	−143.8	−136.1
Nitrogen (II) oxide NO(g)	21.6	20.7
Nitrogen (IV) oxide NO_2(g)	7.9	12.3
Potassium chloride KCl(s)	−104.4	−97.8
Sodium chloride $NaCl$(s)	−98.3	−91.8
Sulfur dioxide SO_2(g)	−70.9	−71.7
Water H_2O(g)	−57.8	−54.6
Water H_2O(ℓ)	−68.3	−56.7

*Minus sign indicates an exothermic reaction.

Sample equations:

$$2Al(s) + \frac{3}{2} O_2(g) \rightarrow Al_2O_3(s) + 400.5 \text{ kcal}$$

$$2Al(s) + \frac{3}{2} O_2(g) \rightarrow Al_2O_3(s) \quad \Delta H = -400.5 \text{ kcal/mol}$$

The MCAT
Model Examination

From *How to Prepare for the Medical College Admission Test,* 8th ed., by Hugo R. Seibel, Kenneth E. Guyer, et al. (Barron's Educational Series, 1997).

ANSWER SHEET

DIRECTIONS: After locating the number of the question to which you are responding, fill in the circle containing the letter of the answer you have selected. Use pencil (not a ballpoint pen) to completely blacken the circle.

VERBAL REASONING

1. Ⓐ Ⓑ Ⓒ Ⓓ
2. Ⓐ Ⓑ Ⓒ Ⓓ
3. Ⓐ Ⓑ Ⓒ Ⓓ
4. Ⓐ Ⓑ Ⓒ Ⓓ
5. Ⓐ Ⓑ Ⓒ Ⓓ
6. Ⓐ Ⓑ Ⓒ Ⓓ
7. Ⓐ Ⓑ Ⓒ Ⓓ
8. Ⓐ Ⓑ Ⓒ Ⓓ
9. Ⓐ Ⓑ Ⓒ Ⓓ
10. Ⓐ Ⓑ Ⓒ Ⓓ
11. Ⓐ Ⓑ Ⓒ Ⓓ
12. Ⓐ Ⓑ Ⓒ Ⓓ
13. Ⓐ Ⓑ Ⓒ Ⓓ
14. Ⓐ Ⓑ Ⓒ Ⓓ
15. Ⓐ Ⓑ Ⓒ Ⓓ
16. Ⓐ Ⓑ Ⓒ Ⓓ
17. Ⓐ Ⓑ Ⓒ Ⓓ
18. Ⓐ Ⓑ Ⓒ Ⓓ
19. Ⓐ Ⓑ Ⓒ Ⓓ
20. Ⓐ Ⓑ Ⓒ Ⓓ
21. Ⓐ Ⓑ Ⓒ Ⓓ
22. Ⓐ Ⓑ Ⓒ Ⓓ
23. Ⓐ Ⓑ Ⓒ Ⓓ
24. Ⓐ Ⓑ Ⓒ Ⓓ
25. Ⓐ Ⓑ Ⓒ Ⓓ
26. Ⓐ Ⓑ Ⓒ Ⓓ
27. Ⓐ Ⓑ Ⓒ Ⓓ
28. Ⓐ Ⓑ Ⓒ Ⓓ
29. Ⓐ Ⓑ Ⓒ Ⓓ
30. Ⓐ Ⓑ Ⓒ Ⓓ

31. Ⓐ Ⓑ Ⓒ Ⓓ
32. Ⓐ Ⓑ Ⓒ Ⓓ
33. Ⓐ Ⓑ Ⓒ Ⓓ
34. Ⓐ Ⓑ Ⓒ Ⓓ
35. Ⓐ Ⓑ Ⓒ Ⓓ
36. Ⓐ Ⓑ Ⓒ Ⓓ
37. Ⓐ Ⓑ Ⓒ Ⓓ
38. Ⓐ Ⓑ Ⓒ Ⓓ
39. Ⓐ Ⓑ Ⓒ Ⓓ
40. Ⓐ Ⓑ Ⓒ Ⓓ
41. Ⓐ Ⓑ Ⓒ Ⓓ
42. Ⓐ Ⓑ Ⓒ Ⓓ
43. Ⓐ Ⓑ Ⓒ Ⓓ
44. Ⓐ Ⓑ Ⓒ Ⓓ
45. Ⓐ Ⓑ Ⓒ Ⓓ
46. Ⓐ Ⓑ Ⓒ Ⓓ
47. Ⓐ Ⓑ Ⓒ Ⓓ
48. Ⓐ Ⓑ Ⓒ Ⓓ
49. Ⓐ Ⓑ Ⓒ Ⓓ
50. Ⓐ Ⓑ Ⓒ Ⓓ
51. Ⓐ Ⓑ Ⓒ Ⓓ
52. Ⓐ Ⓑ Ⓒ Ⓓ
53. Ⓐ Ⓑ Ⓒ Ⓓ
54. Ⓐ Ⓑ Ⓒ Ⓓ
55. Ⓐ Ⓑ Ⓒ Ⓓ
56. Ⓐ Ⓑ Ⓒ Ⓓ
57. Ⓐ Ⓑ Ⓒ Ⓓ
58. Ⓐ Ⓑ Ⓒ Ⓓ
59. Ⓐ Ⓑ Ⓒ Ⓓ
60. Ⓐ Ⓑ Ⓒ Ⓓ

61. Ⓐ Ⓑ Ⓒ Ⓓ
62. Ⓐ Ⓑ Ⓒ Ⓓ
63. Ⓐ Ⓑ Ⓒ Ⓓ
64. Ⓐ Ⓑ Ⓒ Ⓓ
65. Ⓐ Ⓑ Ⓒ Ⓓ

PHYSICAL SCIENCES

66. Ⓐ Ⓑ Ⓒ Ⓓ
67. Ⓐ Ⓑ Ⓒ Ⓓ
68. Ⓐ Ⓑ Ⓒ Ⓓ
69. Ⓐ Ⓑ Ⓒ Ⓓ
70. Ⓐ Ⓑ Ⓒ Ⓓ
71. Ⓐ Ⓑ Ⓒ Ⓓ
72. Ⓐ Ⓑ Ⓒ Ⓓ
73. Ⓐ Ⓑ Ⓒ Ⓓ
74. Ⓐ Ⓑ Ⓒ Ⓓ
75. Ⓐ Ⓑ Ⓒ Ⓓ
76. Ⓐ Ⓑ Ⓒ Ⓓ
77. Ⓐ Ⓑ Ⓒ Ⓓ
78. Ⓐ Ⓑ Ⓒ Ⓓ
79. Ⓐ Ⓑ Ⓒ Ⓓ
80. Ⓐ Ⓑ Ⓒ Ⓓ
81. Ⓐ Ⓑ Ⓒ Ⓓ
82. Ⓐ Ⓑ Ⓒ Ⓓ
83. Ⓐ Ⓑ Ⓒ Ⓓ
84. Ⓐ Ⓑ Ⓒ Ⓓ
85. Ⓐ Ⓑ Ⓒ Ⓓ
86. Ⓐ Ⓑ Ⓒ Ⓓ
87. Ⓐ Ⓑ Ⓒ Ⓓ
88. Ⓐ Ⓑ Ⓒ Ⓓ

89. Ⓐ Ⓑ Ⓒ Ⓓ
90. Ⓐ Ⓑ Ⓒ Ⓓ
91. Ⓐ Ⓑ Ⓒ Ⓓ
92. Ⓐ Ⓑ Ⓒ Ⓓ
93. Ⓐ Ⓑ Ⓒ Ⓓ
94. Ⓐ Ⓑ Ⓒ Ⓓ
95. Ⓐ Ⓑ Ⓒ Ⓓ
96. Ⓐ Ⓑ Ⓒ Ⓓ
97. Ⓐ Ⓑ Ⓒ Ⓓ
98. Ⓐ Ⓑ Ⓒ Ⓓ
99. Ⓐ Ⓑ Ⓒ Ⓓ
100. Ⓐ Ⓑ Ⓒ Ⓓ
101. Ⓐ Ⓑ Ⓒ Ⓓ
102. Ⓐ Ⓑ Ⓒ Ⓓ
103. Ⓐ Ⓑ Ⓒ Ⓓ
104. Ⓐ Ⓑ Ⓒ Ⓓ
105. Ⓐ Ⓑ Ⓒ Ⓓ
106. Ⓐ Ⓑ Ⓒ Ⓓ
107. Ⓐ Ⓑ Ⓒ Ⓓ
108. Ⓐ Ⓑ Ⓒ Ⓓ
109. Ⓐ Ⓑ Ⓒ Ⓓ
110. Ⓐ Ⓑ Ⓒ Ⓓ
111. Ⓐ Ⓑ Ⓒ Ⓓ
112. Ⓐ Ⓑ Ⓒ Ⓓ
113. Ⓐ Ⓑ Ⓒ Ⓓ
114. Ⓐ Ⓑ Ⓒ Ⓓ
115. Ⓐ Ⓑ Ⓒ Ⓓ
116. Ⓐ Ⓑ Ⓒ Ⓓ
117. Ⓐ Ⓑ Ⓒ Ⓓ
118. Ⓐ Ⓑ Ⓒ Ⓓ

119. Ⓐ Ⓑ Ⓒ Ⓓ

120. Ⓐ Ⓑ Ⓒ Ⓓ

121. Ⓐ Ⓑ Ⓒ Ⓓ

122. Ⓐ Ⓑ Ⓒ Ⓓ

123. Ⓐ Ⓑ Ⓒ Ⓓ

124. Ⓐ Ⓑ Ⓒ Ⓓ

125. Ⓐ Ⓑ Ⓒ Ⓓ

126. Ⓐ Ⓑ Ⓒ Ⓓ

127. Ⓐ Ⓑ Ⓒ Ⓓ

128. Ⓐ Ⓑ Ⓒ Ⓓ

129. Ⓐ Ⓑ Ⓒ Ⓓ

130. Ⓐ Ⓑ Ⓒ Ⓓ

131. Ⓐ Ⓑ Ⓒ Ⓓ

132. Ⓐ Ⓑ Ⓒ Ⓓ

133. Ⓐ Ⓑ Ⓒ Ⓓ

134. Ⓐ Ⓑ Ⓒ Ⓓ

135. Ⓐ Ⓑ Ⓒ Ⓓ

136. Ⓐ Ⓑ Ⓒ Ⓓ

137. Ⓐ Ⓑ Ⓒ Ⓓ

138. Ⓐ Ⓑ Ⓒ Ⓓ

139. Ⓐ Ⓑ Ⓒ Ⓓ

140. Ⓐ Ⓑ Ⓒ Ⓓ

141. Ⓐ Ⓑ Ⓒ Ⓓ

142. Ⓐ Ⓑ Ⓒ Ⓓ

WRITING SAMPLE
Use separate ruled sheets of paper.

BIOLOGICAL SCIENCES

143. Ⓐ Ⓑ Ⓒ Ⓓ

144. Ⓐ Ⓑ Ⓒ Ⓓ

145. Ⓐ Ⓑ Ⓒ Ⓓ

146. Ⓐ Ⓑ Ⓒ Ⓓ

147. Ⓐ Ⓑ Ⓒ Ⓓ

148. Ⓐ Ⓑ Ⓒ Ⓓ

149. Ⓐ Ⓑ Ⓒ Ⓓ

150. Ⓐ Ⓑ Ⓒ Ⓓ

151. Ⓐ Ⓑ Ⓒ Ⓓ

152. Ⓐ Ⓑ Ⓒ Ⓓ

153. Ⓐ Ⓑ Ⓒ Ⓓ

154. Ⓐ Ⓑ Ⓒ Ⓓ

155. Ⓐ Ⓑ Ⓒ Ⓓ

156. Ⓐ Ⓑ Ⓒ Ⓓ

157. Ⓐ Ⓑ Ⓒ Ⓓ

158. Ⓐ Ⓑ Ⓒ Ⓓ

159. Ⓐ Ⓑ Ⓒ Ⓓ

160. Ⓐ Ⓑ Ⓒ Ⓓ

161. Ⓐ Ⓑ Ⓒ Ⓓ

162. Ⓐ Ⓑ Ⓒ Ⓓ

163. Ⓐ Ⓑ Ⓒ Ⓓ

164. Ⓐ Ⓑ Ⓒ Ⓓ

165. Ⓐ Ⓑ Ⓒ Ⓓ

166. Ⓐ Ⓑ Ⓒ Ⓓ

167. Ⓐ Ⓑ Ⓒ Ⓓ

168. Ⓐ Ⓑ Ⓒ Ⓓ

169. Ⓐ Ⓑ Ⓒ Ⓓ

170. Ⓐ Ⓑ Ⓒ Ⓓ

171. Ⓐ Ⓑ Ⓒ Ⓓ

172. Ⓐ Ⓑ Ⓒ Ⓓ

173. Ⓐ Ⓑ Ⓒ Ⓓ

174. Ⓐ Ⓑ Ⓒ Ⓓ

175. Ⓐ Ⓑ Ⓒ Ⓓ

176. Ⓐ Ⓑ Ⓒ Ⓓ

177. Ⓐ Ⓑ Ⓒ Ⓓ

178. Ⓐ Ⓑ Ⓒ Ⓓ

179. Ⓐ Ⓑ Ⓒ Ⓓ

180. Ⓐ Ⓑ Ⓒ Ⓓ

181. Ⓐ Ⓑ Ⓒ Ⓓ

182. Ⓐ Ⓑ Ⓒ Ⓓ

183. Ⓐ Ⓑ Ⓒ Ⓓ

184. Ⓐ Ⓑ Ⓒ Ⓓ

185. Ⓐ Ⓑ Ⓒ Ⓓ

186. Ⓐ Ⓑ Ⓒ Ⓓ

187. Ⓐ Ⓑ Ⓒ Ⓓ

188. Ⓐ Ⓑ Ⓒ Ⓓ

189. Ⓐ Ⓑ Ⓒ Ⓓ

190. Ⓐ Ⓑ Ⓒ Ⓓ

191. Ⓐ Ⓑ Ⓒ Ⓓ

192. Ⓐ Ⓑ Ⓒ Ⓓ

193. Ⓐ Ⓑ Ⓒ Ⓓ

194. Ⓐ Ⓑ Ⓒ Ⓓ

195. Ⓐ Ⓑ Ⓒ Ⓓ

196. Ⓐ Ⓑ Ⓒ Ⓓ

197. Ⓐ Ⓑ Ⓒ Ⓓ

198. Ⓐ Ⓑ Ⓒ Ⓓ

199. Ⓐ Ⓑ Ⓒ Ⓓ

200. Ⓐ Ⓑ Ⓒ Ⓓ

201. Ⓐ Ⓑ Ⓒ Ⓓ

202. Ⓐ Ⓑ Ⓒ Ⓓ

203. Ⓐ Ⓑ Ⓒ Ⓓ

204. Ⓐ Ⓑ Ⓒ Ⓓ

205. Ⓐ Ⓑ Ⓒ Ⓓ

206. Ⓐ Ⓑ Ⓒ Ⓓ

207. Ⓐ Ⓑ Ⓒ Ⓓ

208. Ⓐ Ⓑ Ⓒ Ⓓ

209. Ⓐ Ⓑ Ⓒ Ⓓ

210. Ⓐ Ⓑ Ⓒ Ⓓ

211. Ⓐ Ⓑ Ⓒ Ⓓ

212. Ⓐ Ⓑ Ⓒ Ⓓ

213. Ⓐ Ⓑ Ⓒ Ⓓ

214. Ⓐ Ⓑ Ⓒ Ⓓ

215. Ⓐ Ⓑ Ⓒ Ⓓ

216. Ⓐ Ⓑ Ⓒ Ⓓ

217. Ⓐ Ⓑ Ⓒ Ⓓ

218. Ⓐ Ⓑ Ⓒ Ⓓ

219. Ⓐ Ⓑ Ⓒ Ⓓ

The MCAT Model Examination

VERBAL REASONING

9 PASSAGES
65 QUESTIONS
85 MINUTES

DIRECTIONS: The questions are based on the accompanying passages. Read each passage carefully, then answer the following questions. Consider only the material within the passage. For each question, select the *ONE BEST ANSWER* and indicate your selection by marking the corresponding letter on the Answer Form.

Passage I (Questions 1–7)

In the fall of 1990, a vigorous debate broke out at the University of Texas at Austin, a debate that turned into a heated national conversation on the purpose of the writing classroom and, to some extent, the purpose of liberal education. Among composition specialists the debate delineated two separate ways of thinking about freshman composition and the field of composition studies.

The debate focused on a proposed curriculum for the freshman composition program at the University of Texas, English 306, a curriculum which required students to produce approximately 3,900 words of writing and taught students to conduct and sustain rhetorical inquiry into a single topic. Some of the goals of the curriculum were to introduce undergraduates to the intellectual demands of college through the teaching of skills such as analysis, research, and synthesis, to create an intimate, participatory classroom experience for the students whose freshman schedules are often otherwise confined to huge lecture halls, and to help the new graduate student teachers focus on the teaching of writing by creating a bridge between skills learned in the study of literature and the teaching of freshman composition. All seemingly laudable, standard goals for freshman composition. The problem, the reason for the violent debate, was the topic chosen for the class: difference, specifically difference related to legal opinions given in court cases involving issues such as race, gender, bilingualism, and sexual orientation. The debate that followed the submission and ultimate rejection of the program in many ways disregarded the course itself; the discussion became a forum for stating the purpose of composition and liberal education.

One group, that I will call the traditionalists, view the writing classroom as the place to focus on process, a place where students write, primarily, personal essays to engage in the writing process. The other group, the radical pedagogists, believe that the purpose of the writing classroom is to engage the student as critical thinker, often defined as one who rethinks cultural assumptions and becomes committed to social change. There are varying views among radical pedagogists of the ways and means of teaching critical thinking....

....The traditionalist point of view is, relatively speaking, fairly new. It arose in the past 25 years or so, in tandem with the advent of composition studies as a legitimate academic discipline. The traditionalist approach focuses on process, and states that a primary way to engage the student is to have the student determine essay topics. As Richard Graves says, "the first lesson in teaching composition is that the writer must find his or her own subject." This student-centered approach assumes that the student will not only be more invested in the essay if the idea originates with her, but that the student learns that she has a wealth of information inside her, information that once organized not only reflects her knowledge base but proves interesting to others. This new knowledge engages the student in her own writing, making it a forum for her voice, thus giving her a sense of legitimacy to her own experiences and reflections. Although aware of the powerful effects of writing on the student as thinker, the primary concern for the traditionalists is the student as writer, as they seek to engage the students in the process and act of writing.

The radical pedagogists are more concerned with the student as thinker and want to use the mind power generated in the writing process to foster social change. Patricia Bizzell states that "we rhetoricians like to see ourselves as social reformers, if not revolutionaries."....
This concern with social and political change is prevalent among the radical pedagogists. Sharon Crowley

Adapted from a paper by Abby Arnold, "Empowerment Pedagogy and the Writing Classroom," English 636, VCU, 1996 and used with permission of the author.

states that "freshman composition can be radicalized in the service of social justice" and commends writers who "would put literacy to work with the specific goal of effecting social change." There is little mention among these highly political pedagogists of the student as writer, or of developing writing skills in a student for the sake of individual education.

Donald Lazere, a committed leftist educator and radical pedagogist, offers an alternative to both schools of composition theory. He sees student empowerment and social change as coming through the student's learning to write, thus learning to access and manipulate the dialogue of mainstream culture. He criticizes both the "process" contention that skills are less important than the act of writing and the "radical" determination to focus on critical thinking at the expense of writing instruction. He states that "the lack of basic skills and factual knowledge is an obstacle to autonomous critical thinking" and that "a sophisticated level of literacy is virtually necessary, or at least highly advantageous, for effective opposition to the dominant culture in today's society."

Although committed to his view of social change, Lazere is also committed to the growth of the student. He recognizes the coercive nature of some radical pedagogy, the kind of belief in one's agenda which led Sharon Crowley to state that composition teachers "must give up our traditional subscription to liberal tolerance if we are to bring about social change through [our students.]" Lazere believes that to force any ideology on students "is only to replace the coercion...in mainstream education with coercion into accord with an opposing ideology."

1. Which of the following was **not** a stated goal of the freshman curriculum at the University of Texas when the debate over English 306 broke out?

   A. to create a smaller, more intimate classroom experience than freshmen typically have

   B. to help new graduate student teachers focus on the teaching of writing

   C. to teach freshmen how to bring about social change through their writing

   D. to introduce freshmen to the intellectual demands of college by teaching various skills

2. Of the two main groups in opposition with each other in the University of Texas debate, which of the following groups have as a goal the use of writing and the teaching of writing to bring about social change?

   A. the traditionalists

   B. the pragmatists
   C. the radical pedagogists
   D. the purists

3. According to the passage, Donald Lazere could best be characterized as

   A. a leftist educator.
   B. a person who would disagree with the methods proposed by Sharon Crowley.
   C. a radical pedagogist.
   D. all of the above.

4. The proposed topic for English 306 was to include

   A. a study of world literature.
   B. an examination of the relationship between writing for the mass media and writing for scholarly journals.
   C. a study of legal opinions from court cases involving, among other things, sexual orientation.
   D. an analysis of fiction and creative nonfiction.

5. Based on the quotations attributed to Sharon Crowley in the passage, we can deduce that she belongs to the group referred to as

   A. the traditionalists.
   B. the radical pedagogists.
   C. the free thinkers.
   D. the grammar advocates.

6. Though the University of Texas debate originated as a response to a proposed course in the curriculum, it evolved into something larger. Which of the following best describes what the debate became?

   A. a referendum on the role of the teaching of literature in composition classes
   B. an examination of the positive and negative factors in using graduate teaching assistants in the freshman classroom
   C. a forum on the teaching of grammar and usage in freshman composition classes
   D. a forum for stating the purpose of composition and liberal education

7. The proposed curriculum, which involved English 306, was ultimately

   A. defeated.
   B. passed by a slim majority.
   C. deferred for a year.
   D. approved, but only for one year.

Passage II (Questions 8–15)

To establish a prima facie case of sex discrimination in compensation, an employee must present data that compare her salary to that of male coworkers doing the same job under the same circumstances. The standard or test that has emerged from case law is called the equal pay for equal work standard. Not to be confused with the idea that one must hold a job identical to that of someone else, the standard is built on a concept that evaluates jobs within a context of substantial equivalency. The issue to probe thus becomes: Is complainant's job equal in effort and responsibility to that of a male counterpart? A corollary question also is asked. Do the two incumbents in these jobs (the male and the female) possess comparable skills?

On March 11, 1974, the Secretary of Labor took action against Columbia University and its president, seeking to enjoin the University from discriminating against its female custodial workers (classified as light cleaners). Alleging a violation of the Equal Pay Act on the basis of sex, the evidence showed that female light cleaners were paid a lower hourly rate than male heavy cleaners. At trial, the court came to the conclusion that the jobs of light cleaners and heavy cleaners were different. And, because the job of heavy cleaners involved greater effort than that of light cleaners, the plantiff had failed to sustain the burden of establishing the idea of equal work within the meaning of the Act.

On appeal, the Second Circuit Court of Appeals focused its attention on the "equal effort" criteria in connection with the workers' primary duties. The Court stated:

> The concept of "effort" in the act is straightforward. It calls for a direct comparison of the amount of physical exertion required by the jobs; there is no factor added to compensate for physiological differences between men and women. Based on our careful review of the record before us we cannot say that the district court was clearly erroneous in making this direct comparison and in finding as a fact that heavy cleaning involves "greater effort."

The court also noted that the differences between the heavy cleaner and light cleaner jobs were known by the employees. Furthermore, no heavy cleaner job had ever been denied to a woman. In fact, in 1972, Columbia opened a heavy cleaner category to women, and seven light cleaners were accepted into

Adapted from Richard S. Vacca: "Sex Discrimination in Public School Employment." In S. B. Thomas, N. H. Cambron-McCabe, and M. M. McCarthy, Eds, *Education and the Law*. New York: Institute for School Law and Finance, 1983.

on-the-job training for that position. However, after seven weeks, four of the seven workers transferred back to light cleaning.

In conclusion, the circuit court held that based on the evidence of the understanding and experience of the individuals most closely involved, together with the undisputed fact that heavy cleaning called for greater effort, there was no valid claim of unequal pay for substantially equivalent work within the meaning of the Equal Pay Act.

A new and more controversial standard in sex discrimination cases involves the notion of comparable worth. Under the theory of comparable worth, one must look beyond the equal pay for equal work criterion. In such cases, the female plaintiff argues the intrinsic worth, or the intrinsic difficulty of her job, as compared to other jobs in the same organization. Such an argument thus carries the complaint beyond the confines of an equal wage matter and places it under the broader umbrella protection of Title VII.

The judiciary has not yet endorsed the notion of comparable worth, but the Supreme Court has ruled that Title VII provides a remedy for sex discrimination in compensation beyond that covered by the Equal Pay Act. The matter arose in Washington County, Oregon, when four women guards in the female section of the county jail alleged that they were paid unequal wages for work substantially equal to that performed by male guards. In their complaint, the women guards charged that because of intentional discrimination, the county set the pay scale of female guards (but not male guards) "at a level lower than that warranted by its own survey of outside markets and the worth of the jobs."

After an adverse decision at trial, the female guards appealed to the Eighth Circuit Court of Appeals. The appellate court reversed the trial court and held that petitioners were not precluded from suing under Title VII, solely because their jobs were not substantially equal to higher-paying jobs held by male employees. The Supreme Court agreed and ruled in *County of Washington v. Gunther* that the wage differentials were based on intentional sex discrimination even though female guards did not actually perform work equal to that of male guards. Although not adopting the controversial concept of comparable worth, the Court left the door open for a comparable worth argument to be raised in future litigation.

It is significant to note that Justice Rehnquist for the four dissenters in *Gunther* strongly stated that this decision could spell the nullification of the Equal Pay Act if future plantiffs are allowed to substitute the comparable worth standard for that of the equal pay for equal work standard. He asserted that the majority's opinion must be read narrowly ("the opinion does not endorse the so-called 'comparable worth' theory): though the Court does not indicate how a plaintiff might establish a prima facie case under Title VII, the Court does suggest that allegations of unequal pay for unequal, but comparable, work will not state a claim on which relief may be granted.''

Others would argue that the Supreme Court's decision in *Gunther* establishes a possibility for plantiffs in future cases to be given the opportunity to produce evidence showing a Title VII violation based on a comparable worth, rather than on an equal work basis. For example, female teachers might argue that over the years the historical pattern and practice in public school systems have inflated the value and salaries of certain jobs simply because they were held by men, while depressing the value and salaries of other jobs because they were held by women, even though each of the jobs is of comparable worth to the school system.

8. When one investigates an equal pay issue, attention must be given to:

    I.   equal worth.
    II. equal effort.
    III. equal length of employment.
    IV. equal responsibility.

    A. I, II, and III   C. II and IV
    B. I and III   D. I, II, III, and IV

9. Which of the following statement(s) is/are *sup ported by* the passage?

    A. Identical jobs should receive equal reimbursement.
    B. Substantial equivalency is at the bottom of the issue.
    C. The question also to be asked is whether the concerned possess equal levels of education.
    D. Effort, attitude, drive, and determination are important considerations in equal pay for equal work cases.

10. In sex discrimination cases the courts:

    I.   have considered the fact that women bear children.
    II. have decided that maternity leave is a constitutional right.
    III. have allowed the notion of physical and physiological differences.

    IV. view the Equal Pay Act and the Title VII laws as equal in impact.

    A. I, II, and III   C. II and IV
    B. I and III   D. neither I, II, III, nor IV

11. The Columbia University case illustrates:

    A. that on-the-job training is essential in avoiding problems.
    B. the haphazard approach used by the Department of Labor in filing suit.
    C. that employees are not always aware of differences in their jobs.
    D. the well-defined limits of the Equal Pay Act in regard to the equal effort interpretation.

12. Which of the following statement(s) is/are *supported by* the passage?

    I.   Comparable worth is a complex issue.
    II. In comparable worth issues one must probe well beyond the equal pay for equal work issues.
    III. The Supreme Court considers Title VII as a remedy for sex discrimination.
    IV. The judiciary has endorsed Title VII.

    A. I, II, and III   C. II and IV
    B. I and III   D. I, II, III, and IV

13. In the Oregon case:

    I.   the first trial ended with a ruling for the county.
    II. the first trial resulted in no definitive decision.
    III. the appellate court did not preclude a suit based on job unequality.
    IV. the Supreme Court adopted the concept of comparable worth.

    A. I, II, and III   C. II and IV
    B. I and III   D. I, II, III, and IV

14. Which of the following is/are *supported by* the passage?

    I.   There were four dissenters to the Supreme Court decision.
    II. Concern was voiced about the future effectiveness of the Equal Pay Act.

III. It is anticipated that litigation might substitute the principle of comparable worth for the argument equal pay and equal work.

IV. The majority opinion clearly defined the limits of the decision in the *County of Washington v. Gunther* case.

A. I, II, and III   C. IV only
B. I and III   D. I, II, III, and IV

15. The main theme of this passage can be considered to be:

A. Equal Pay Act v. Title VII.
B. comparable worth.
C. sex discrimination.
D. judiciary policy making.

Passage III (Questions 16–24)

There have been two controversies over Eoanthopus, and it is the first of them that has the incongruous mandible for its theme. The question at issue was whether this specimen represents a single creature or two different ones. Scientists made reconstructions reconciling jaw and skull; however, one group described the jaw as an ape's separately from the skull that was assigned to Homo sapiens. The finder's argument ran as follows: All of the remains were found very close together. The lower jaw and brain case were both of a similar brown color and apparently in the same state of fossilization. The jaw, even though ape-like, did have human features, particularly in the teeth. The molar teeth had apparently been worn to a flatness never seen in apes, and only expected if the jaw had belonged to a type of human being. The roots of the teeth seen radiologically also resembled human teeth. The appearance of this ape-like man at the beginning of the Ice Age was just what many authorities expected to find. Shortly thereafter, a canine tooth, ape-like, but worn in a way never found in modern apes, was found. This was strong support for the missing link interpretation and man's ape-like ancestry. Questions remained concerning how anatomically the jaw could have worked as part of a human skull, and the wear of the teeth.

Three years later, about two miles away from the first site, pieces of a thick braincase and a molar tooth (both similar to the first find) were unearthed. The

climate was ripe for the view that the human ancestor would show a combination of ape and man. However, as more human fossils were found in other parts of the world, this particular specimen differed from all in regard to skull characteristics. Their braincases were far more ape-like and their jaws less so, and a consistent line of evolution was found. Restorations of the cranium resulted in the revisions of brain volume, but in the end the controversial specimen had a brain of modern size to go with its modern skull.

If the remains were old, they could be accepted even though odd and isolated. When the fluorine method was applied, it was found that neither jawbone nor braincase contained more than small traces of fluorine meaning that the specimen did not date before the Ice Age. The specimen was now believed to be 50,000 and not 500,000 years old, making it an evolutionary absurdity with no known ancestor or descendants. An explanation was to suppose that a piece of modern ape jaw had been deliberately placed with an ancient braincase and both suitably stained. Another fluorine analysis placed the braincase as ancient, but the jaw and teeth in modern times. In fact, chemical analysis showed that the jaw and teeth contained the same amount of nitrogen and organic carbon as modern specimens, the calvarium, however, much less. Ruling out that the organic matter was not gelatin or glue with which the specimen had been impregnated as a means of hardening was accomplished with electron microscopy because the jaw showed preserved fibers of organic tissue and the calvarium lacked this feature. Besides this, it was established that the jaw had been colored artificially with iron to match the calvarium.

The first specimen was apparently made up by placement of an artificially abraded molar tooth of an orangutan with a piece of thick frontal bone; the last fragment found duplicated the thinnest part of the first skull. Chromium detected in the jaw indicates that a dichromate solution was used in an attempt to assist the oxidation of iron salts used to stain these specimens.

From H. R. Seibel, "The Piltdown Hoax," *Bioscope*, 1962.

16. The skull was classified to belong to:

I. a vertebrate.
II. a mammal.
III. a man.
IV. an ape.

A. I, II, and III   C. II and IV
B. I and III   D. I, II, III, and IV

17. This passage was probably written by:

    A. a historian.   C. a sociologist.
    B. an anthropologist.   D. an archeologist.

18. From the passage one could surmise that fluorine:

    A. was obtained from drinking water.
    B. was absorbed from the soil.
    C. becomes more concentrated.
    D. is a by-product of the decay process.

19. If the jawbone was modern, its fluorine content in relation to the braincase would have been:

    A. the same.
    B. more.
    C. less.
    D. not important in the solution.

20. The analysis of iron was used to establish:

    A. a color comparison.
    B. the organic matrix pattern.
    C. the age of the specimens.
    D. none of the above.

21. The piece of fossil found last was:

    A. not unusual in size.
    B. thick.
    C. thin.
    D. none of the above.

22. With age iron salts:

    A. are reduced.   C. deteriorate.
    B. are halogenated.   D. are oxidized.

23. Chromium:

    A. is naturally found in bones.
    B. is absorbed from the surrounding areas by a specimen.
    C. is used as a parameter in testing fossils.
    D. none of the above.

24. The passage mainly deals with:

    A. the development of experimental methods of studying fossils.
    B. the verification of the missing link.
    C. a valuable fossil find.
    D. a brilliantly devised falsification.

Passage IV (Questions 25–32)

Many who have seen photographs of Zelda Sayre Fitzgerald note that no two images of her resemble each other. She had many different, unforgettable faces, among them the polished and strikingly beautiful one which appeared on the cover of *Hearst's International* magazine in the early 1920s and which she referred to as her Elizabeth Arden face. But the different faces of Zelda, as the Fitzgeralds' friend Sara Murphy observed shortly after Zelda's first mental breakdown, had much less to do with subtle changes in makeup or lighting than with inner complexity and mystery that no one, not even her husband Scott, ever touched. There have been many constructions of Zelda Fitzgerald, all hinting at the complexity that Sara Murphy noted. But, not surprisingly, the various constructions like the various photographs of Zelda's face rarely resemble each other.

From the actual Zelda Sayre of Montgomery, Alabama, Scott Fitzgerald constructed a fairy princess, hidden away in a tower to be rescued from her provincial surroundings and taken by him into the more sophisticated world of Princeton and New York. She had been born July 24, 1900, the sixth child of Alabama Judge Anthony Sayre and his wife Minnie, who named Zelda after a gypsy queen in a novel she had read and who spoiled her from the beginning, nursing her, some say, until she was 4 years old. By the time Fitzgerald arrived at Fort Sheridan, near Montgomery, in his tailored Brooks Brothers uniform Zelda was, at 18, thought of as an original, a daring local beauty who was known not only in Montgomery but in most college towns in Alabama. She became not only Scott's idealized version of the Southern Belle but also the incarnation of all that was desirable in woman. He went back to New York from Montgomery after the war was over, finished the novel that was to become *This Side of Paradise,* sent for Zelda, and married her in the rectory of St. Patrick's Cathedral.

The process of Scott's invention and reinvention of Zelda, which had already begun with his creation of the heroine of "The Ice Palace," set in a small southern town, would be repeated numerous times in the next two decades, among other places in Gloria in *The Beautiful and Damned* and in Daisy in *The Great Gatsby.* His two final fictional recreations of Zelda in fiction, as Nicole Diver in *Tender Is the Night* and as Ailie Calhoun in "The Last of the Belles," remain strong at the end, though the hero has lost the ability to sustain a romantic vision of her. Fitzgerald constructed and reconstructed Zelda for as long as he had the emotional vitality to do so. But after Zelda's mental collapse, precipitated in part by her obsessive pursuit of ballet—in effect her obsessive pursuit of an artistic identity of her own that she

Adapted from "Zelda," VCU, 1995 and used with permission of Dr. Bryant Mangum.

could have separate from Scott's imagined version of her—Scott began his descent into alcoholism. He left his capacity for hope, he said, on the road leading away from Zelda's sanitarium.

Nancy Milford, Zelda's first major biographer, constructs a Zelda shaped in large part by Scott's exploitation of her, by his appropriation of her image and even of the prose from her diaries for the purpose of enhancing his own literary reputation. There was no room for two artists in the Fitzgerald household, as Milford's description of the bitter conflict that surrounded the publication of Zelda's 1932 novel *Save Me the Waltz* demonstrates. She was, as Scott reminded her, a third-rate talent. But his assault on Zelda's self-esteem is only part of Milford's picture of a self divided by internal forces beyond her control. Her entrapment in a world with little understanding or appreciation of her predicament makes Milford's Zelda a symbol for our time, her death in 1948 by fire while locked away in the upper reaches of a mental institution dramatically underscoring the powerlessness of her plight. Sara Mayfield's competing portrait of Zelda, who was Mayfield's girlhood friend, depicts a southern belle whose major misfortune was her loss of the traditions of the genteel South at the hands of Scott, who took Zelda from her home and set in motion the tragedy of two "exiles from paradise." These are only two of many recreations of Zelda.

The actual Zelda Sayre Fitzgerald is fragmented in the many constructions of her life that we have. Once, in an attempt to establish the historical truth about Zelda's role in Scott's life and his role in hers, someone asked Scott for his analysis. He replied that if one asked Zelda's friends, they would say that his drinking drove her to insanity. His friends would say that her insanity drove him to drink. But the truth, he noted, is that "liquor on my mouth is sweet to her and I cherish her wildest hallucinations." And here we are back where we began. Historically, Scott did cherish, celebrate, and enshrine as art Zelda's wildest hallucinations, particularly during the decade of the Roaring Twenties, which marked the high point of their lives together. After the stock market crash of 1929 and Zelda's first mental collapse which shortly followed it, Scott went through the motions of supporting her, among other things by paying her hospital bills, until his death in 1940.

But, in effect, Scott left Zelda in the mid-1930s to herself and to the biographers, poets, and playwrights who continue to create versions of her from the known facts of her life, from the gallery of her paintings, from her scrapbooks, from her published and unpublished novels, stories, essays, and letters—and from their own imaginations.

25. According to the passage, Zelda Fitzgerald rarely looked the same in any two of the many pictures taken of her. Sara Murphy attributed this to

   A. Zelda's inner complexity.
   B. the unpredictable quality of photographic equipment in the 1920s and 1930s, during which most of the photographs were taken.
   C. Zelda's careful use of makeup.
   D. Zelda's insistence that photographers take her picture from unusual angles.

26. Zelda Fitzgerald's first major biographer, according to the passage, was

   A. Sara Mayfield.   C. Arthur Mizener.
   B. Sara Murphy.   D. Nancy Milford.

27. One could deduce from the passage that Zelda Fitzgerald's husband, F. Scott Fitzgerald,

   A. married Zelda on the rebound from his first love, Ginevra King.
   B. had known Zelda all of his life and became romantically interested in her only after he had gone off to college.
   C. met her when he was stationed near her home in Alabama during the war.
   D. agreed to marry Zelda only if she would not pursue her career as a ballet dancer.

28. Minnie Sayre, Zelda's mother, the passage states, named her daughter after

   A. a gypsy queen in a novel she was reading.
   B. a distant relative who had agreed to remember Zelda in her will.
   C. her maternal grandmother.
   D. a character in a popular radio drama of the time.

29. The passage would support the following conclusion:

   A. Insanity ran in Zelda's family according to family medical records.
   B. Zelda was exploited by Scott, but she also suffered from internal conflicts probably not attributable to her husband, according to a major biographer.
   C. Zelda was unpopular in her hometown of Montgomery, Alabama, one of her high school friends maintained.
   D. Zelda had always wanted to marry a popular author, she told her brother many years after her marriage to Scott.

30. According to the passage, when asked about his role in Zelda's life and her role in his, Scott made an observation that revealed his own belief about their relationship:

    A. Their mutual friends were better qualified to comment on this than he was.
    B. They were mutually destructive of each other.
    C. Zelda was to blame for driving him to drink.
    D. His drinking was responsible for driving her to insanity.

31. In which of the following works by F. Scott Fitzgerald, according to the passage, was his wife *not* the model for a main character in the work?

    A. *This Side of Paradise*
    B. "The Last of the Belles"
    C. *Tender Is the Night*
    D. *The Last Tycoon*

32. The passage asserts that Zelda's death occurred

    A. while she was at work on her novel, *Save Me the Waltz.*
    B. when she attempted to drive a car down an embankment in the south of France.
    C. while she was locked away during a fire in a mental institution.
    D. as a result of diving into a dark stairwell.

Passage V (Questions 33–38)

"In this way you shall set the fiftieth year apart and proclaim freedom to all the inhabitants of the land." In this way the ancient writer of *Leviticus* had God speak through Moses for the purpose of commemorating the entrance of the people of Israel into the "Promised Land." This is not the oldest reference to the celebration of an "anniversary," but it does show that celebrating anniversaries is a very old practice, and it also illustrates the role of round numbers in such celebrations.

Thus, the institution's celebration of its one hundred fiftieth year of existence adheres to a very old tradition. We celebrate birthdays and wedding anniversaries annually, whereas we usually commemorate the formation of institutions, businesses, churches, nations and schools on the round-num-

From Dr. William E. Blake, Jr., VCU's Sesquicentennial Celebration, 1989.

bered years. (Even with birthdays and weddings we call special attention to the "big" years—tenth, twenty-fifth, fiftieth, and so on.) That we do so, may have something to do with the fact that our numbering is on the base ten system, and the round numbers are those that finish the pattern. Although that explains why we pick the round numbers for our large celebrations, it does not explain why we think it important to celebrate such occasions. A brief discussion of why we *do* observe anniversaries is also an argument for why we *should* do so.

Perhaps the most obvious reason for celebrating the birth of an institution or the commemoration of some dramatic event is our belief that there was a good in it worth perpetuating. Thus, John Adams said of the 1776 Resolution of Independence:

I am apt to believe that it will be celebrated by succeeding generations as the great anniversary festival. It ought to be commemorated as the day of deliverance, by solemn acts of devotion to God Almighty. It ought to be solemnized with pomp and parade, with shows, games, sports, guns, bells, bonfires, and illuminations, from one end of this continent to the other, from this time forward for evermore.

Quite obviously, Adams believed that the launching of a free and independent nation was an act of such worth as to warrant regular celebration. It might be noted in passing that the inauguration of a new enterprise is always an act of hope. It is only at some future time, when folk have seen how an organization, institution, or nation has turned out—when growth and achievement became history—that there can be a confident celebration of the founding day.

But there is also an almost contradictory reason for anniversary celebrations. Instead of perpetuating ancient values they are often viewed as the occasion for a new beginning. As James Russell Lowell wrote, "New occasions teach new duties; time makes ancient good uncouth." So, anniversaries offer the opportunity to reflect on the path traveled, where a people are, where they wish to go next, and what's the best way to get there.

Anniversaries are also a time to honor the people who started the enterprise. Even if it is a romantic conception, we usually think of these pioneers as the hardier sort, whose lives and efforts are worthy of emulation.

Perhaps there is in anniversary celebrations something of an attempt to recapture or to *capture* the drama and emotion of the founding days. Nostalgia, even if it is variously felt, seems to be pleasant to the human spirit. Even if it is tinged with sadness, it is still treasured. Just call to mind (if you can) the lyrics of "Love's Old Sweet Song."

We must confess that part of the motivation for celebrating anniversaries is just plain, human pride. It doesn't matter whether one was among the founding party or joined the institution much later. If the organization has had a long, distinctive history, one may say, "I helped put that together" or "That eminent institution values me enough to make me a part of it." The power of human pride cannot be underestimated as the motor of an institutional machine.

And we cannot ignore the commercial motivation behind anniversary celebrations. It is not just business organizations that stress, "One Hundred and Fifty Years of Faithful Service to the Community." Organizations of all varieties—churches, clubs, social and humane societies, *and* schools—use anniversaries to emphasize their legitimacy, durability, and trustworthiness and use the occasion to appeal for continued—and expanded—patronage by the public. All of these motivations are *implicit* in a celebration. There is real value in making them *explicit*. To be consciously aware of *why* we're celebrating would make the occasion more meaningful and enjoyable.

33. Which of the following statements are *neither supported nor contradicted by* the passage?

    A. After 50 years, the Jews celebrated their leaving Egypt.
    B. God spoke to Moses to initiate the celebration.
    C. Most celebrations are joyous events.
    D. Celebrations are a part of civilizations.

34. Which of the following statements is/are *supported by* the passage?

    I. There is a logical reason for celebrating.
    II. Round-numbered year festivities are usually special.
    III. Our mathematical system depends on round numbers that enhance remembering events.
    IV. Independence Day should be observed for always.

    A. I, II, and III   C. II and IV
    B. I and III   D. IV only

35. The passage supports the notion(s):

    A. that Founding Day is an act of hope.
    B. that history will be the determining factor.
    C. that a celebration is a renewal.
    D. that all of the above are valid.

36. Which of the following statements is/are *supported by* the passage?

    A. Nostalgia is good for mankind.
    B. Pioneers are usually worthy of emulating.
    C. People need a time to reflect.
    D. All of the above are viewed positively by the author.

37. The author believes:

    A. that a sense of being a part of history is productive.
    B. entrepreneurship is part and parcel of a festival.
    C. justification for existence is a motive for anniversary celebrations.
    D. all of the above statements.

38. The passage could properly be titled:

    A. Our One Hundred Fiftieth-Year Celebration.
    B. Why We Celebrate.
    C. Founding Day.
    D. A History of Anniversary Celebrations.

Passage VI (Questions 39–44)

Myths and fairy tales are most often told and remembered as plots (who did what to whom and what happened). But they actually endure in our continuing imaginations because of the "character" of the characters involved. If you place Oedipus into Daedalus's story, or Narcissus into Odysseus's story, you won't have the same story. Cinderella wouldn't do what Red Riding Hood does, nor would Jack-in-the-Beanstalk do what Hansel does. The character doesn't merely *follow* a plot line—the plot happens *because* of the particular human weaknesses and strengths of the particular character.

Underlying all these characters, of course, are larger issues, such as greed and selfishness, pride, acceptance of fate, compassion, cleverness, and risk. But what distinguishes one character from another are the choices, actions, and consequences of those choices peculiar to the individual character. When a teenager (like Theseus) is faced with a dilemma of State (his country must pay human sacrifice tribute in the form of seven youths and seven maidens to a more power-

Adapted from Sally V. Doud, "Essay Test Introduction," VCU, Spring 1990.

ful country), there are a number of choices or decisions he can make. He can ignore the whole problem (it's not his fault, after all); he can take personal responsibility for solving the problem, either because he wants to be a Big Hero or because (as son of the King) he must learn to face problems if he expects to inherit the throne; or he might simply be in a boastful or adventuresome mood when the idea crosses his mind. Once Theseus commits himself to the task (destroying the Minotaur, symbol of the opposing country's power), there are further choices: He can take all the credit but allow his underlings to do all the hard work; he can sacrifice himself on a seemingly impossible task (finding and destroying the Minotaur in its Labyrinth); or he can take advantage of a girl's love for him (agreeing to take Ariadne away with him if she gives him the secret of the Labyrinth). And once he's solved the primary problem of the Minotaur, there are even more choices: does he really want to take Ariadne back with him as he promised? Should he take time out to change the color of his ship's sails (as he promised his father) when he's being pursued by an angry enemy? Because he doesn't change the sails, he directly causes his father's suicide; because he chooses to leave Ariadne behind, he indirectly sets up an even more tragic chain of events in his own life that won't become apparent for a number of years. The series of choices and consequent actions that Theseus takes thus becomes the plot we know, only after we look back on it.

Young people still face seemingly impossible tasks today. These might involve the State (expose corruption, act on one's conscience, protest the military draft), or they might involve other people and relationships (whether to live up to an agreement made under different circumstances, such as an engagement, marriage, contract, job, project). People still have to decide whether to try and save a sinking ship, or whether to catch the first lifeboat; whether to admit a harsh truth or to avoid it (lie, exaggerate, use diplomacy, pass blame, run away). Can or should one be loyal to a person or way of life one no longer cares about? What are the risks and benefits of any decision? Does it still "pay" to be a hero, or do other occupations seem more lucrative? Is the difference between a hero and a fool merely success? Should you get involved with someone else's problem or shrug it off? Should you take a stance or merely cast your eyes to heaven and wait for divine intervention and fate? Also, it isn't always easy to separate personal ego or animal needs from more "noble" desires to bring about social or human justice, and often the two run along together for a considerable distance before they part ways. These are matters for contemporary characters in contemporary stories, but these are the same matters Theseus dealt with. We still have our Minotaurs, escape ships, labyrinths, tasks, Ariadnes, and Theseuses, though the forms are different each time. That's why myth and fairy tales (based on folktales or myths) are called Universal.

39. The most appropriate title for this essay would be:

   A. The Role of Fate in Contemporary Life.
   B. Red Riding Hood and Theseus: Two Versions of the Same Character.
   C. Universal Aspects of Everyday Experience.
   D. Myth is Dead.

40. According to the author of the passage:

   A. people today do not face impossible tasks as did the characters in the Greek myths.
   B. the outcomes of fairy tales and myths are rarely determined by choices the characters have made.
   C. myths and fairy tales are universal because the choices that are faced by characters in them are similar to the ones faced by people of all times.
   D. there are fewer choices for heroes today than there were for the heroes of Greek myths.

41. One might infer from this passage that:

   A. Theseus is responsible for the death of his father.
   B. one should not sacrifice himself to a seemingly impossible task.
   C. Theseus should not be blamed for the suicide of his father.
   D. in making decisions, individuals should wait for divine intervention.

42. According to the author of the passage:

   A. plots proceed as a pattern of cause and effect events.
   B. plots are always the same from one story to the next.
   C. plots are merely an accumulated series of events.
   D. plots are the most important part of any story.

43. The most important part of the passage is:

   A. that we not forget the story of Theseus and his adventures surrounding the Labyrinth.

B. stories change, but the realm of human choices remains the same.

C. universality deals with language.

D. we are always punished for our misdoing.

44. According to the passage, the primary problem facing Theseus is:

A. how he can reward Ariadne for giving him the secret of the Labyrinth.

B. the killing of the Minotaur.

C. the changing of his ship's sails so as to inform his father of his fate.

D. how he will rid himself of guilt after he has killed the Minotaur.

Passage VII (Questions 45–50)

Caricature is a device satirists commonly use in their work. Why is it so common? Caricatures grab readers' or viewers' attention; moreover, they are funny. Caricatures distort reality and that distortion is often hilarious. An audience that will appreciate the caricature recognizes the incongruity between the real object and the satirist's portrayal of it. They also understand why the satirist is attacking this object. In effect, the appreciative audience says, "Of course, this is all out of proportion. But, you know, he's got a point there. This person (place, thing) really does have a weak spot." Meanwhile, as they muse on the message, they are reacting to the incongruities, the exaggeration, with anything from a wry smile to convulsive laughter.

What exactly is a caricature? I would define it as a pictorial (drawing, painting, sculpture, collage, mask, dramatization) or verbal (poem, essay, descriptive sketch in fiction or nonfiction) exaggeration of an object (person, place, thing, situation, organization). The distortion must be based on a fact about the object, for example, bushy eyebrows. The artist or writer just stretches that fact all out of shape; the politician's eyebrows are not *that* bushy. He plays with his object as if it were a glob of silly putty or bread dough. He kneads it, rolls it up, flattens it, stretches it out, shapes it any way to suit his fancy. He must not go so far as to make the object completely unrecognizable, but he has a lot of room to play with his object.

One thing that happens when an object becomes so pliable in the hands of an artist or writer is that the object instantly plummets in value. It becomes ridic-

ulous, at least to some extent, and not as important as it had been. Often the satirist's purpose is to show that the object, because of people's vanity or hypocrisy, is considered more valuable than it really is. By doing a caricature of it, he deflates its value. Furthermore, the artist or writer shows that he has control over the object, at least temporarily. He is exerting his power by the way he portrays the object. It's as if he's saying, "Ah ha! You thought you were so important. But look at you now, the way *I*'ve made you. I'm calling the shots for now." Needless to say, the people being caricatured rarely think kindly about the creators of the satire—not only do the caricatures deflate their importance, but also the caricatures show that the people who are being satirized don't have control over their image.

It's important to note that one of the effects of caricature is to dehumanize the person being caricatured. This dehumanization is even there in the language of how we discuss satire: the word "object." As the audience, we often enjoy seeing a vaunted person being devalued by caricature and agree that the devaluation is often deserved. But does the means justify the end? Caricatures certainly work, and creators and audience have a lot of fun while criticizing the object. However, a side effect is that caricatures serve as one out of many ways we tend in our society to dehumanize each other. Rarely does the creator or the audience notice this; we're caught up in the laughter and disregard any objections to a caricature by saying, "It's just a joke. Don't you have a sense of humor? He (object of caricature) deserved it anyway." Yes, it's just a joke. But also, yes, it makes it easier for us to view people as objects to be manipulated, vilified, destroyed. Think back to the caricatures we did of the Japanese in World War II. It is much easier to work up enthusiasm for killing people when they are depicted as hideous monsters. Hitler readily used caricature to depict Jews as less-than-human animals.

Exaggeration, playing the extremes against each other, distortion—these are all elements of caricature. Caricatures are a quite effective means for satire—creators enjoy creating them, audiences respond eagerly to them, they make their point. However, they are not innocuous little creatures; they can be used to stereotype and dehumanize people. Also, as we use them casually day after day, we sometimes don't even notice anymore that they are caricatures. The cartoon character becomes the norm. Wiley the Coyote makes falling off cliffs, holding an exploding piece of dynamite, or being crushed with huge stones seem like normal, everyday events; he is just a little frazzled after each episode. Numbed day after day with caricatures, might we begin to think of life as a cartoon?

Adapted from Rebecca Dale, "Caricature," VCU, Spring 1989.

45. Which of the following statements about caricatures is NOT *supported by* the passage?

A. Caricatures do not have to be pictures.
B. People who are satirized often lose the public's respect.
C. People who are satirized often deserve the ridicule.
D. Caricatures can be based on falsehoods.

46. According to the passage, people laugh at caricatures because:

A. bushy eyebrows and other such facial quirks are naturally funny.
B. we laugh at people who are vain and hypocritical.
C. we recognize the incongruities between the object and the caricature of it.
D. the people who create caricatures have a good sense of humor.

47. Which of the following statements best sums up the author's opinion of caricatures?

A. Caricatures are hilarious.
B. Caricatures reveal the hypocrisies of our society.
C. Caricatures have insidious effects.
D. People who do not appreciate caricatures have no sense of humor.

48. According to the passage, caricatures are effective forms of satire because:

I. ridicule devalues an object.
II. caricatures appeal to many kinds of audiences.
III. the satirist controls his object's public image.

A. I and II   C. I and III
B. II and III   D. I, II, and III

49. According to the passage, caricatures can be dangerous because:

A. people satiated with exaggeration may not recognize the norm.
B. a person who is satirized may not deserve the ridicule.
C. caricatures divert our attention from real problems.
D. caricatures give satirists too much power over society.

50. Of the following titles, which is most appropriate for the passage?

A. The Cruel Art of Caricature
B. Caricature and Understatement
C. Caricature: Exaggeration as a Satirist's Tool
D. Cartoon Art

Passage VIII (Questions 51–59)

On a physiological level, aggression is a neurochemical impulse, causing tension that necessitates a physical release. According to the evolutionist position, aggression as instinct can be traced from some of the earliest primitive animal forms from which we humans draw a common ancestor, and must therefore, by reason of evolution as well as observed behavioral patterns, be attributable to man. If conflict is the father of all things, it may be the activating force behind all human behavior (love as well as hate), and its ritual forms of appeasement and redirected activity provide a basis for culture.

In order that aggression be considered an element of man's genetic inheritance, some explanation must be offered for its existence in his past. Ethologists maintain that aggression in earliest man, as in all of the lower animals, had a distinct survival advantage, most commonly linked to the defense of territory. "What directly threatens the existence of an animal species," says Konrad Lorenz, "is never the 'eating enemy' but competition" within the species. In this sense, intraspecies aggression provides for the even distribution of a particular species over an inhabitable area; a form of population control as well as quality control. The stronger animal will control the more advantageous territory and subsequently corner the hardier breeding population. Man's traditional attachment to his land is seen as a modern refinement of his territoriality; most human conflicts can be traced back to dispute over land itself or to his sense of independence concerning his property.

According to Robert Ardrey, the defense of the territory holds animals together in breeding pairs or larger groups; but the most powerful defense is offered by the pair, thereby encourages bonding, to even further selective advantage. Territoriality is also psychological, providing the three basic animal needs: security, identity, and stimulation. The first two are self-explanatory; with the third we are more concerned, for stimulation—by other animals of one's kind—is accomplished through aggression. This may take the

Adapted from Sally V. Doud, "Aggression and Human Nature," VCU, 1976.

form of *inward antagonism,* bickering among one's closest neighbors, which serves no apparent purpose except perhaps sheer stimulation; yet this is considered responsible for socialization. The growth of population into congested cities instead of more evenly spacing out has even been interpreted in this context to be a reaction of man's aggressive needs rather than a practical understanding of cooperation.

Stimulation through aggression can also take the form of *outward antagonism,* the defense of a species group of its territory against outsiders; uniting its members in a common cause and often considered the basis for the human Nation.

Another important aspect of aggression, says Lorenz, is its role in securing the personal bond. "The danger in aggression is its spontaneity..." therefore, "...aggression of animals toward their own kind is held in check by inhibiting mechanisms" such as ritualization of fighting, appeasement gestures, and redirected activity. As each relationship between two members of the species must be individually negotiated, this constitutes the beginnings of personality. Various forms of greeting as well as many human emotional expressions, such as laughter, are considered ceremonies of redirected activity or appeasement; Lorenz notes that everyone is aware of how laughter tends to create a bond.

Lionel Tiger provides an example of aggression's role in establishing order and custom within a human society: competition between several age groups of males (for females, for prestige) is often responsible for rigid initiatory tradition, along with other political measures prohibitive to one group while enhancing the chances of a second.

The human being who voluntarily places himself within the power of the law embodies the theory of inhibiting mechanisms. Members of the Cheyenne tribe who broke the law during a hunt willingly submitted to the authority of the Shield Soldiers, a gesture of ritual appeasement. In turn, the Shield Soldiers rendered only token punishment, and that on the property of the offenders, acknowledging the appeasement gesture by a redirected activity.

The theory of innate aggression carried to its ultimate climax presents us with the uncomforting image of man with "killer instincts." Although Ardrey points out that territoriality is defensive, that early man hunted because he was hungry, still others point to cannibalism as human acts of aggression as well as a cultural phenomenon.

The more dangerously aggressive the particular species is, the firmer is the bond necessary to prevent intraspecies destruction. Here is man's anomaly: he is devoid of the more elaborate safety devices to prevent the abuse of his killing power, because these devices were unnecessary in the harmless protohuman for whom quick and easy killing was impossible. The acquisition of weapons threw off the natural balance, for now he is capable of great destruction without the accompanying mechanics of inhibition; the Cain and Abel, the master of war, the deadly predator who kills for enjoyment.

"It is true," says Morton Hunt, "like other animals, we are impelled to action by hunger, fear, anger, sexual desires... but are not directed by instinct to take specific actions in order to satisfy those desires.... Man may be innately aggressive... but he is not programmed... the drive can be directed to many different ends." The apparatus with which we are equipped to speak is a product of our evolution, and the particular language is culturally transmitted.

The emphasis then is on interdependence of instinct and culture; no longer is man at the mere beck and call of his instincts, but capable of exercising control over them. His intelligence permits him the conscious choice of goals.

51. The passage suggests that:

    A. aggression has not yet been traced to earlier evolutionary forms than man.
    B. aggression is a neurochemical impulse.
    C. unlike hunger, aggression does not require release.
    D. aggression seeks direct expression or appeasement and therefore is not redirected into culture building activities.

52. According to Lorenz, the greatest threat to the survival of an animal species is:

    A. what he calls the "eating enemy."
    B. natural disaster.
    C. various forms of pollution.
    D. competition within the species.

53. The passage suggests that of the three basic animal needs, the one that is thought to account for bickering among one's closest neighbors is:

    A. identity.
    B. security.
    C. stimulation.
    D. structure.

54. The passage asserts that one of man's greatest anomalies is that:

    A. he instinctively pairs with or bonds to another human being, but that he cannot remain monogamous throughout his life cycle.

B. he possesses the "killer instinct" but lacks the internal controls or safety devices that restrict this instinct.

C. he has free access to weapons but lacks the "killer instinct" to take full advantage of them.

D. man is territorial and nomadic at the same time.

55. Morton Hunt, who is quoted in the essay, asserts that:

A. man is innately aggressive, but he is not biologically programmed as to how to direct his aggression.

B. cultural transmission plays only a minor role in determining how aggression is channeled from generation to generation.

C. it is a mistake to think of man as innately aggressive.

D. the existence of anger in man differentiates him from other animals.

56. One might infer from this passage that:

A. the existence of aggression in lower animals is unimportant in the study of aggression in man.

B. aggression plays a very important role in determining the ways in which human beings interact in social groups.

C. humans are not territorial.

D. people live in cities because of innate cooperativeness.

57. The most appropriate title for this essay would be:

A. Lorenz On Aggression.

B. The "Killer Instinct" in Man.

C. Man as Pure Instinct.

D. Aggression as the Basis for Culture.

58. The growth of population into congested cities rather than an even spacing out has been interpreted in the context of Ardrey's ideas as:

A. a natural need in man to cooperate.

B. the herding instinct.

C. a need for sharing material goods.

D. a reaction of man's aggressive needs.

59. Members of the Cheyenne tribe who broke the law during a hunt:

A. rebelled against punishment, thus exhibiting aggression.

B. willingly submitted in a gesture of ritual appeasement.

C. insisted that their punishment be on their own land.

D. never broke the same law twice, thus suppressing aggression.

Passage IX (Questions 60–65)

Because the ability to write well is so crucial to success in school, educators are paying more attention to assessments of writing. States have begun requiring students to take minimum competency tests before graduation or before entering high school. Colleges want to limit admissions to students who have shown a certain level of competency in writing. Or they want to place students in an appropriate level of freshman English. How are all these decisions on proficiency, admissions, placement, and exemption made? Tests. Because decisions have to be made on large numbers of students, the tests are large scale assessments, tests that *everyone* in the group (school, state, nation) takes.

There are two major types of tests—direct assessments and indirect assessments. Direct assessments are tests that use readers to judge actual samples of students' writing, writing done in timed in-class sessions on a common topic. Indirect assessments are tests that use answers to multiple-choice questions to judge students' knowledge about certain aspects of writing, such as mechanics or grammar.

Statistics show that multiple-choice tests are very reliable, meaning that students' scores are consistent (if Johnny retakes the test, he is likely to receive about the same score), but how valid they are is speculative (validity refers to what extent a test actually tests what it purports to test). Because multiple-choice questions can test only reading and editing skills for the most part, the scores have meaning only about a student's knowledge of those areas tested. G. Conlan points out that multiple-choice questions have become more sophisticated recently in the types of knowledge tested and can test such things as principles of organization, logic, ability to shift parts of sentences, and sensitivity to idioms. But still it is someone else's text. Does ability to edit someone else's text necessarily mean ability to *create* texts of one's own?

If we want to measure writing skills, a test that requires a person to write would likely be a more valid test than one that doesn't. However, direct assess-

Adapted from Rebecca Dale, "Direct-Indirect Assessment of Writing," Capitol Writing Project, VCU, Summer 1989.

ment is not proving to be a panacea either. A valid test must necessarily be reliable also; many of the problems with direct assessment testing have to do with reliability. If we change the wording of test topics, the testing conditions, or the readers scoring essays, scores can change dramatically.

Reliability problems are most conspicuous in the scoring process. Here is the main objection to direct assessment—different readers have different reactions to the same essay. How can we determine if an essay has been scored accurately? Reader-response theory has pointed out that readers "recreate" a text when they read it, that interpretation depends on what readers bring to the experience of reading a text as well as what writers put into the text.

Administrators of these tests try to cope with this problem in several ways. One, they develop scoring guides that specify the criteria to be used in evaluating the student papers. Whether they use holistic scoring (scoring an essay as a whole), primary trait scoring (a type of holistic scoring focusing on certain traits found in the particular mode of discourse tested), or analytic scoring (scoring subcategories, such as content, organization, mechanics, and adding the scores up), they all specify in the scoring guides the characteristics of a paper for each score in the scoring range.

Secondly, test administrators train readers with "anchor" papers and trial grading runs. This is sometimes referred to as "calibrating the readers." Readers need to internalize the criteria in the scoring guide, and by comparing their judgments on an essay to an anchor paper whose score has been predetermined, they can get a feel for how lenient or rigorous the scoring should be. The trial grading runs, where each of the readers grades some sample essays, give additional calibration. After grading the samples, the readers discuss the scores they gave, along with their reasons for assigning those scores. The discussion of discrepancies brings up issues in how to apply the criteria and allow the group to reach greater consensus on what the various scores mean.

Thirdly, each essay is read by two readers, each unaware of the score the other reader has given it. If the scores differ by more than one point, a third reader reads the essay. White considers the practice of multiple readings essential:

Although there is a constant temptation to reduce the costs by reducing the second reading to samples or by eliminating second readings altogether, such an economy renders the reading unaccountable and unprofessional.

Scores do vary. "Most papers, if rescored by the same readers at the same reading, would probably receive different scores."

These measures in administering tests help increase reliability in scoring essays, but they do not solve the problem. Readers react to the topic and unintentionally may bring some bias to their grading. In cases where readers are aware of their own bias, they even may try to compensate for their bias and be too lenient in grading essays that offend them.

Another problem is reader drift. Readers who are reading hundreds of essays at a time may be more or less lenient at some times than at others. For example, a paper read right after a brilliant one is more likely to receive a lower score than if it's read after an average one. Barritt, Stock, and Clark have raised a provocative question in their study of how expertly trained readers of students' texts can disagree widely in scoring: They found that readers expected to find "average" student papers, and they could agree on scores for papers that met their expectations. But when they read papers that did not fit their expectations of an "average" student, their scores differed widely. S. Freedman had a similar finding in a comparison of student and professional writers: Evaluators gave student work fairly consistent scores, but in scoring the professional essays, "the raters disagreed violently with one another."

60. According to the passage, indirect assessments of writing have been criticized because:

   A. scores are unreliable.
   B. only reading and editing skills are tested.
   C. the tests are biased.
   D. evaluators cannot agree on the criteria for scoring.

61. Which of the following statements does the passage state or imply is/are true?

   I.   A reliable test is necessarily valid.
   II. A valid test is necessarily reliable.
   III. A test may be reliable, but not valid.
   IV. A test may be valid, but not reliable.

   A. I and II   C. II and III
   B. III and IV   D. II only

62. Which of the following statements best sums up the importance of reader-response theory to the problems of evaluating essays on large-scale assessments?

   A. Scoring guides are necessary to set the criteria by which essays are judged.
   B. Evaluators are influenced by their own ideas.

C. Evaluators need to be calibrated.

D. Evaluators give inconsistent scores to professional essays.

63. According to the passage, administrators deal with the reliability problems in scoring direct assessments by all EXCEPT which of the following?

A. essays are scored by multiple readers.

B. evaluators must use specific criteria in judging essays.

C. holistic scoring, primary trait scoring, or analytic scoring is used.

D. evaluators are trained with "anchor papers."

64. According to the passage, which of the following affects the reliability of scores on essays?

A. Multiple readings mean that scores will likely differ.

B. Evaluators may not agree on which criteria are the most important.

C. An average paper read after an outstanding one may receive a lower score than if it's read after another average one.

D. Trial grading runs do not give sufficient calibration.

65. Which statement probably best sums up the author's evaluation of the ways to test writing in large-scale assessments?

A. Indirect assessments are better than direct assessments because of the reliability problems involved in direct assessments.

B. Direct assessments are better than indirect assessments because they test a student's ability to create a text.

C. Evaluators of essays in direct assessments need to be carefully trained.

D. Both indirect assessments and direct assessments have only limited value.

PHYSICAL SCIENCES

10 PROBLEM SETS OF 5–10 QUESTIONS EACH
15 PROBLEMS FOLLOWED BY A SINGLE QUESTION
77 QUESTIONS
100 MINUTES

DIRECTIONS: The following questions or incomplete statements are in groups. Preceding each series of questions or statements is a paragraph or a short explanatory statement, a formula or set of formulas, or a definition. Read the written material and then answer the questions or complete the statements. Select the ONE BEST ANSWER for each question and indicate your selection by marking the corresponding letter of your choice on the Answer Form. Eliminate those alternatives you know to be incorrect and then select an answer from among the remaining alternatives. A periodic table is provided (see p. 506). You may consult it whenever you wish to do so.

Passage I (Questions 66–70)

In a physics class, an experimental motion experiment is devised to allow the study of the motion of a number of objects under a variety of conditions. One part involves projecting identical steel or wooden balls at a variety of initial angles and speeds, starting at various heights above the floor. Equipment, such as protractors and photogate timers, is available so the angles and speeds are known. Rectangular metal blocks of various masses can be slid across horizontal surfaces and also down inclined planes. The surfaces vary from essentially frictionless to quite rough surfaces. The balls can be rolled down the inclined planes also. The masses of each object are measured in advance and the velocities can be measured at any point of the motion with the photogate timers.

66. One of the identical balls is dropped from the edge of a lab table 1.1 m high at the same instant another one is projected horizontally with an initial velocity of 2 m/sec. If there is no air resistance, what are the times for the two balls, respectively, to strike the floor?

    A. 0.11 sec, 0.11 sec   C. 0.47 sec, 0.95 sec
    B. 0.47 sec, 0.47 sec   D. 1.2 sec, 2.3 sec

67. One ball is projected horizontally with an initial horizontal velocity of 10 m/sec while the second is projected at an angle of 30° *above* the horizontal with the same initial speed. Both balls strike a vertical wall that is exactly 10 m away. How long does it take each ball, respectively, to hit the wall?

    A. 0.87 sec, 1.5 sec   C. 1 sec, 1 sec
    B. 1 sec, 0.87 sec   D. 1 sec, 1.5 sec

68. A rectangular block of mass 1 kg and one of mass 3 kg are projected across a rough surface with the same starting speed of 4 m/sec. The coefficient of friction is 0.4. How far do the blocks slide, respectively?

    A. 2 m, 2 m
    B. 3 m, 2 m
    C. 4 m, 4 m
    D. 6 m, 2 m

69. One of the balls is released from rest at the top of an inclined plane 0.5 m high and rolls down without slipping. At the same instant a rectangular block is released and slides down a frictionless plane which is also 0.5 m high. Which of the two objects has the greater speed at the bottom of the inclines?

    A. The ball.
    B. The block.
    C. Both have the same speed.
    D. The question cannot be answered because there is not enough information given.

70. A wooden ball of mass 0.4 kg is dropped down a circular stairwell. It is observed to reach a terminal velocity of 35 m/sec and continues falling at that speed. What is the force of air friction acting on the ball?

    A. 3.9 N
    B. 7.8 N
    C. 14 N
    D. 28 N

Passage II (Questions 71–76)

The students in an introductory physics class are nearly all in premedicine, so the instructor decides to have one lab session in which all the topics are related to the human body and its physiology. The students' blood pressures, temperatures, weights (masses), height, and so on can be measured. The instructor has obtained clinical equipment to test hearing, sight, pulmonary function, metabolic rates, and so on with reasonable accuracy.

71. The lab instructor weighs 205 pounds. If 1 kg weighs 2.2 pounds, what is the instructor's mass in kg. and his weight in newtons?

    A. 45.5 kg and 446 N
    B. 78 kg and 674 N
    C. 93.2 kg and 913 N
    D. 451 kg and 46 N

72. The average aortic pressure for a student is determined to be 100 mmHg. What is the gauge pressure in the foot artery, which is 1.35 m below the aorta? (The density of blood is 1,050 kg/m^3.)

    A. 120 mmHg   C. 405 mmHg
    B. 205 mmHg   D. 660 mmHg

73. The metabolism for one of the women in the class requires about 2,000 kcal per day. Given a food intake of 3,200 kcal per day for a period of two weeks, what mass of fat corresponds to the excess food intake? The energy of oxidation for fats and oils is 9.5 kcal per gram.

    A. 440 g   C. 1,240 g
    B. 860 g   D. 1,700 g

74. It is known that in human metabolic processes, the ratio of energy released to oxygen consumed is about 20,000 joules/liter. A student with a basal metabolic rate of 95 W steps up and down repeatedly on a step for 10 minutes. The student's metabolic rate rises to an average of 630 W during the 10 minutes. What is the approximate number of liters of oxygen the student consumes during the exercise period?

    A. 9 L   C. 45 L
    B. 19 L   D. 134 L

75. A simple experiment in static equilibrium can determine the vertical position of a student's center-of-mass above the soles of the feet. The student lies on a board resting on two bathroom scales set on zero. The centers of the scales are 1.83 m apart. The head scale reads 90 pounds whereas the scale at his feet reads 100 pounds. What is the location of the center-of-mass above the soles of his feet?

    A. 0.60 m   C. 1.03 m
    B. 0.87 m   D. 1.23 m

76. A student wants to lose 1 pound of fat (0.4545 kg) by exercising as above. (1 kcal = 4186 joules.) The average rate of energy expended is 500 watts (above that required for ordinary metabolism). For how many hours will the student have to exercise continuously?

    A. 0.5 hours   C. 23.5 hours
    B. 10.0 hours   D. 455 hours

Passage III (Questions 77–81)

A set of experiments in the physics lab is designed to develop understanding of simple electrical circuit principles for direct current circuits. The student is given a variety of batteries, resistors, and DC meters; and is directed to wire series and parallel combinations of resistors and batteries making measurements of the currents and voltage drops using the ammeters and voltmeters. The student calculates expected current and voltage values using Ohm's law and Kirchhoff's circuit rules and then checks the results with the meters.

77. A student connects a 6-volt battery and a 12-volt battery in series and then connects this combination across a 10-ohm resistor. What is the current in the resistor?

    A. 0.8 A   C. 1.8 A
    B. 0.9 A   D. 3.6 A

78. Resistors of 4 ohms and 8 ohms are connected in series. A battery of 6 volts is connected across the series combination. How much power, in watts, is consumed in the 8-ohm resistor?

    A. 0.67 W   C. 12 W
    B. 2 W   D. 24 W

79. Two 4-ohm resistors are connected in series and this pair is connected in parallel with an 8-ohm resistor. A 12-volt battery is connected across the ends of this parallel set. What power, in watts, is consumed in the 8-ohm resistor in this case?

    A. 0.9 W   C. 4.4 W
    B. 2.0 W   D. 18 W

80. A 6-volt battery is connected across a 2-ohm resistor. What is the heat energy dissipated in the resistor in 5 minutes?

    A. 430 joules   C. 4300 joules
    B. 560 joules   D. 5400 joules

81. A 12-volt battery is connected across a 4-ohm resistor and the heat energy dissipated in the resistor in 10 minutes is used to heat 2 kg of water (which is thermally insulated so that no heat escapes). The initial temperature of the water is 20°C and the specific heat of the water is 4184 joule/kg-°C. What is the final temperature of the water at the end of the 10 minutes of heating?

    A. 22.6 °C   C. 34.2 °C
    B. 28.4 °C   D. 56.4 °C

Passage IV (Questions 82–87)

A set of introductory physics experiments is for the purpose of studying different types of wave motion in different aspects. The student can generate mechanical waves on strings, sound waves in different media, light waves, and water waves in ripple tanks. The plan is to show the similarities (and differences) between different kinds of waves, and to study the propagation of waves through differing materials.

82. A small loudspeaker sends a sound wave into a tube, which is closed on the other end, and a loud resonance is obtained at a frequency of 340 Hz. The tube is 25 cm long. It is known that the open end is an antinode of the standing wave and the closed end is a node. If the 340 Hz resonance is the lowest frequency resonance (the fundamental frequency), what is the speed of sound in the air?

    A. 120 m/sec   C. 340 m/sec
    B. 280 m/sec   D. 680 m/sec

83. The highest sound frequency a student can hear is 20,000 Hz at a wavelength of 1.7 cm. If the highest frequency the instructor can hear is 15,000 Hz; about what wavelength is this in cm?

    A. 1.6 cm   C. 2.6 cm
    B. 2.3 cm   D. 34.0 cm

84. Suppose the amplitudes of a 15,000 Hz sound wave and a 20,000 Hz sound wave are the same. It is known that the energy in a wave is proportional to the square of the frequency and the square of the amplitude. ($W = Kf^2A^2$). What is the ratio of the energy in the 20,000 Hz wave to the energy of the lower frequency wave?

    A. 1.8   C. 6.8
    B. 2.4   D. 8.6

85. Some properties of longitudinal waves are similar to those of transverse waves. For example, the speed that both types of waves travel does not usually depend on the frequency. What experimental fact clearly distinguishes longitudinal waves from transverse waves?

    A. Longitudinal waves always have longer wavelengths than transverse waves.
    B. Transverse waves can be polarized.
    C. Transverse waves vibrate parallel to the direction the wave travels.
    D. Transverse waves have a higher frequency than longitudinal waves.

86. The students measure the shortest and longest wavelengths of visible light that they can see and find the range to be 400 nm (violet) to about 750 nm (deep red). (1 nm = 10^{-9} m.) They know that light of all wavelengths travels with the same speed, c. The Planck Quantum hypothesis states that the energy of a photon of light is proportional to the frequency, $E = hf$, where h is Planck's Constant. What is the ratio of the energy of 400 nm light to the energy of 750 nm light?

    A. 1.88   C. 34.4
    B. 2.66   D. 45.6

87. Consider the two sound waves of 20,000 Hz and 15,000 Hz that are heard by the student and instructor. What is the ratio of the speed of

sound for the 20,000 Hz wave to the speed of sound for the 15,000 Hz wave?

A. 0.75   C. 1.2
B. 1.0   D. 1.33

Questions 88–95 are independent of any passages and of each other.

88. A car of mass 1,000 kg traveling due East and a truck of mass 3,000 kg traveling due West crash head-on and stick together. They both had speeds of 21 m/sec (47 mi/hr) before the impact. Give the magnitude and direction of their common velocity after impact?

A. 10.5 m/sec, West   C. 3.1 m/sec, East
B. 14.2 m/sec, Wes   D. 9.4 m/sec, West

89. An ultrasound wave of frequency 5 MHz and a radio wave of the same frequency travel in air. What is the ratio of the wavelength of the radio wave to the wavelength of the sound wave. (Assume the speed of sound in air is 340 m/sec and the speed of light is $c = 3 \times 10^8$ m/sec.)

A. 3   C. 114
B. 14   D. 882,353

90. A mass of 4 kg oscillates in Simple Harmonic Motion with a frequency of 2.0 Hz. The 4-kg mass is replaced with an unknown mass for which the oscillation frequency is 4 Hz. The unknown mass is equal to:

A. 8 kg   C. 1 kg
B. 2 kg   D. 0.5 kg

91. A centrifuge rotates initially at 60,000 rev/min and takes 100 sec to come to rest. What is the angular acceleration of the centrifuge in rad/sec^2? (Recall that 1 rev = 2π radians.)

A. 12π rad/sec^2 C. 20π rad/sec^2
B. 42π rad/sec^2 D. 5π rad/sec^2

92. A proton and an electron have the same velocity. Their velocity vectors are perpendicular to a uniform magnetic field of 1.0 Tesla. They travel (in opposite directions) in circular paths of radii r_p and r_e in the magnetic field. What is the ratio, r_p/r_e? (The masses in unified mass units, u, are: $m_p = 1.007276$ u and $m_e = 0.0005486$ u.)

A. 1.0   C. 0.00055
B. 1836   D. 256.4

93. A lens of focal length +12 cm is used to view an object placed 6 cm in front of the lens. The *image* is 8 cm tall ($h_i = 8$ cm). How tall (h_o) is the original object?

A. 8.2 cm   C. 2.5 cm
B. 4.0 cm   D. 3.3 cm

94. A box of mass 2 kg is given an initial speed of 3 m/sec. It slides horizontally across a rough floor a distance of 3.4 m. What is the coefficient of friction, μ, between box and floor?

A. 0.45   C. 0.14
B. 0.24   D. 0.60

95. A ball of mass 1 kg is thrown horizontally with a speed of 20 m/sec from the edge of a building 5.1 m high. Another ball of mass 2 kg is thrown with the *same speed* at an angle of 30° above the horizontal. Use *Conservation of Mechanical Energy* to find the ratio of the final speeds of the two balls when they strike the ground 5.1 m below.

A. $V_2/V_1 = 1.0$ C. $V_2/V_1 = 4.0$
B. $V_2/V_1 = 2.0$ D. $V_2/V_1 = 1.5$

Passage V (Questions 96–105)

Students are given a variety of lenses and optics equipment, such as lens holders, lighted object sources, optical benches, meter sticks and tapes, image screens, and several examples of commercial optical equipment, such as microscopes and telescopes. They are to work in an open-ended optics lab in order to learn the general principles of lenses and the optical devices that can be constructed using lenses.

96. A student is given a short focal length converging lens and a long focal length converging lens. One lens is placed in a holder. A lighted object is placed 18 cm in front of the lens and it is found that a clear image can be focused on a screen placed 36 cm behind the lens. What is the focal length of this lens?

A. 8 cm   C. 27 cm
B. 12 cm   D. 46 cm

97. What magnification is produced by the above lens when the object is 18 cm in front of the lens and the image is 36 cm behind the lens?

   A. 2 ×   C. 4 ×
   B. 3 ×   D. 6 ×

98. A lighted object is placed 6 cm in front of the second lens, which has a focal length of +24 cm. Where is the image and which kind of image is it?

   A. 8 cm in front of the lens; a virtual image
   B. 8 cm behind the lens; a real image
   C. 16 cm in front of the lens; a real image
   D. 16 cm behind the lens; a virtual image

99. The 24 cm focal length lens is used as the objective of a simple refracting telescope and a third converging lens of focal length +8 cm is used as the eyepiece. What is the magnification of this simple refractor?

   A. 0.6 ×   C. 4 ×
   B. 3 ×   D. 6 ×

100. A commercial microscope is examined by the student. The objective is marked 20 × and the eyepiece is marked 10 ×. What power objective should replace the above objective so that the microscope's magnification will be 400 ×?

   A. 5 ×   C. 40 ×
   B. 10 ×   D. 100 ×

101. A lighted object is placed 24 cm in front of a +12 cm focal length lens. The image formed by this lens is the object for a second lens of +24 cm focal length. The second lens is placed 72 cm behind the first lens. Where is the final image with respect to the second lens?

   A. 24 cm in front of #2
   B. 24 cm behind #2
   C. 36 cm in front of #2
   D. 48 cm behind #2

102. A lens of focal length +24 cm is used to view an object placed 12 cm in front of the lens. The object is 5 cm tall. How tall is the image?

   A. 2.5 cm   C. 7.5 cm
   B. 3.3 cm   D. 10 cm

103. A diverging lens of focal length −24 cm is now used with the object 12 cm in front of the lens. How tall is the image if the object is 5 cm tall?

   A. 2.5 cm   C. 8 cm
   B. 3.3 cm   D. 10 cm

104. A nearsighted student cannot see objects clearly unless they are as close as 80 cm (his "far-point"). The image that he sees through his new contact lens is a virtual image because he looks through the lens to see the image. What focal length lenses does he need in order to see very distant objects, such as the stars?

   A. −20 cm   C. −80 cm
   B. −30 cm   D. +40 cm

105. A student uses a lens marked "− 4 D," where D stands for diopters. What is the focal length of this lens in cm?

   A. −0.04 cm   C. −4 cm
   B. −0.25 cm   D. −25 cm

Passage VI (Questions 106–110)

Phases include solid, liquid, and gas. Many materials can exist in any of these depending upon conditions. There is, however, usually a gain or loss of heat in the transition.

106. A mechanical refrigerator is cooled by:

   A. conversion of a liquid to a gas.
   B. conversion of a solid to a liquid.
   C. conversion of a solid to a gas.
   D. conversion of a gas to a solid.

107. The freezing point of a crystalline solid is:

   A. several °C lower than the melting point.
   B. equal to the melting point.
   C. several °C higher than the melting point.
   D. not directly related to the melting point.

108. Transition of a material directly from solid to gas:

   A. is not known.
   B. is known as evaporation.
   C. is known as expiration.
   D. is known as sublimation.

109. Boiling point of a pure liquid is:

A. usually increased by increased pressure.
B. not usually affected by changes in pressure.
C. usually decreased by increased pressure.
D. affected by pressure but in a fairly unpredictable direction.

110. Conversion of oxygen from a gas to a liquid is possible only below −118°C, no matter what pressure is imposed. This temperature is known as the:

A. boiling point.
B. critical temperature.
C. condensation temperature.
D. Clausius temperature.

Passage VII (Questions 111–115)

An enzyme is a special kind of biological catalyst. In many ways it can be considered much as other catalysts.

A series of experiments gave results on the velocity (V) of an enzyme reaction (i.e., rate of formation of products) while keeping the enzyme concentration constant but varying substrate (S). The results were graphed as below:

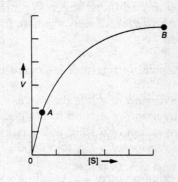

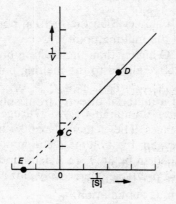

111. Point A is an area where the reaction is _____ order with respect to the substrate.

A. zero   C. second
B. first   D. third

112. Point B is in an area where the reaction is _____ order with respect to the substrate.

A. zero   C. second
B. first   D. third

113. The substrate concentration of point C is:

A. zero.
B. the maximum soluble.
C. infinite.
D. the minimum amount that will give a measurable product.

114. The reciprocal of the ordinate at point C is:

A. the minimum velocity at minimum substrate.
B. the maximum velocity.
C. the minimum velocity at maximum substrate.
D. zero velocity.

115. Considering the two graphs, maximum velocity would be shown (or could be readily computed from):

A. point B.   C. point E.
B. point C.   D. point B or point C.

Passage VIII (Questions 116–120)

By varying the temperature and pressure for Substance X, the following phase diagram is obtained. It indicates the phase(s) that will be found at a variety of temperatures and pressures.

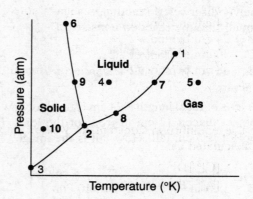

116. Liquid, solid, and gas may be found in equilibrium at the temperature and pressure indicated by:

    A. point 1.   C. point 3.
    B. point 2.   D. point 4.

117. Starting at a temperature and pressure indicated by point 4 and heating the material without change of pressure, one would reach a phase change at:

    A. point 6.   C. point 8.
    B. point 7.   D. point 9.

118. Starting at a temperature and pressure indicated by point 10 and increasing the pressure as much as possible without changing temperature, one would:

    A. pass through the point where gas, liquid, and solid are in equilibrium.
    B. reach a point where solid is in equilibrium with gas.
    C. reach a point where solid is in equilibrium with liquid.
    D. note no phase change.

119. The critical temperature is indicated at:

    A. point 1.   C. point 3.
    B. point 2.   D. point 4.

120. The temperature at point 7, at the indicated pressure, is called the:

    A. freezing temperature.
    B. sublimation temperature.
    C. boiling temperature.
    D. allotropic temperature.

Passage IX (Questions 121–125)

A newly discovered reaction is being studied. It is concluded that the reaction consists of

$$2A + 3B \rightleftharpoons 3C + 2D$$

(The letters A, B, C, and D represent hypothetical compounds.)

121. The equilibrium constant as written may be calculated as:

    A. $\dfrac{[C]^3 [D]^2}{[A]^2 [B]^3}$

    B. $\dfrac{3[C]\ 2[D]}{2[A]\ 3[B]}$

    C. $\dfrac{[A]^2 [B]^3}{[C]^3 [D]^2}$

    D. $\dfrac{[C]\ [D]}{[A]\ [B]}$

122. If the equilibrium constant is 0.001:

    A. reaction to the right will be favored.
    B. reaction to the left will be favored.
    C. the reaction rate is fast.
    D. the reaction rate is slow.

123. If *A, B,* and *D* are gases and *C* is a solid, the reaction will:

    A. be improved toward the right with increased pressure.
    B. be improved toward the left with increased pressure.
    C. be unaffected by increased pressure.
    D. not proceed in either direction in the presence of increased pressure.

124. At standard temperature and pressure, the volume represented by 3 moles of C is about:

    A. 22 liters.
    B. 45 liters.
    C. 67 liters.
    D. more than 80 liters.

125. A small equilibrium constant is indicative of:

    A. a fast reaction rate.
    B. a slow reaction rate.
    C. no reaction.
    D. none of the above.

Passage X (Questions 126–135)

A liquid is isolated, containing 5.9% hydrogen and 94.1% oxygen by mass. The elements are 50% hydrogen and 50% oxygen by volume. The molecular weight is determined to be 34.0. In a decomposition reaction this liquid produces water, oxygen, and no other products.

126. The empirical formula is:

   A. HO.
   B. H_2O_2.
   C. H_3O_3.
   D. H_3O_4.

127. The molecular formula is:

   A. HO.
   B. H_2O_2.
   C. H_3O_3.
   D. H_3O_4.

128. The balanced equation for the decomposition indicates that one mole of the liquid will produce _____ moles of oxygen.

   A. 0.25
   B. 0.50
   C. 1.0
   D. 2.0

129. The balanced equation for the decomposition indicates that one mole of the liquid will produce _____ moles of water.

   A. 0.25
   B. 0.50
   C. 1.0
   D. 2.0

130. The balanced equation for the decomposition of the liquid indicates the formation of _____ liters of oxygen at S.T.P. from one mole of the liquid.

   A. 1.12
   B. 2.24
   C. 11.2
   D. 22.4

131. The balanced equation for the decomposition of the liquid indicates the formation of _____ g of water from 34 g of the liquid.

   A. 16
   B. 18
   C. 30
   D. 32

132. For an equilibrium reaction at 25°C, the decomposition we have been considering would be _____ by an increase in pressure.

   A. favored
   B. unaffected
   C. adversely affected
   D. affected, but in an unpredictable direction

133. For an equilibrium reaction at 25°C, the decomposition would be _____ by an increase in oxygen without an increase in pressure.

   A. favored
   B. unaffected
   C. adversely affected
   D. affected, but in an unpredictable direction

134. In the above question, the equilibrium constant would be:

   A. increased.
   B. unaffected.
   C. decreased.
   D. affected, but in an unpredictable direction.

135. The order of the reaction, from information given above, will be definitely

   A. zero.
   B. first.
   C. second.
   D. unpredictable.

Questions 136–142 are independent of any passages and of each other.

136. Catalysts:

   A. are changed and consumed during a reaction.
   B. have virtually no effect on the overall rate of the reaction.
   C. are changed but not consumed during a reaction.
   D. speed up the rate of the reaction.

137. If solution A is less concentrated in dissolved particle content than solution B, then solution B is said to be:

   A. hypertonic.
   B. hypotonic.
   C. isoosmotic.
   D. isotonic.

138. Compared to one mole of oxygen, how many more molecules do two moles of carbon dioxide contain?

   A. 25×10^6
   B. 12.04×10^{46}
   C. 6.02×10^{23}
   D. 12.04×10^{23}

139. Which one of the following acids does not commonly form acid salts?

   A. $HC_2H_3O_2$
   B. H_2SO_4
   C. H_2CO_3
   D. H_3PO_4

140. Which of the statements listed below is false?

    A. An aqueous solution in which $[H^+] > 1 \times 10^{-7}$ is said to be acidic.

    B. Ions are atoms or groups of atoms that have lost or gained one or more electrons.

    C. HCl is a Bronsted acid because it furnishes H^+ ion in solution.

    D. NaOH is called a base because it furnishes Na^+ ions in solution.

141. In the decomposition of $KClO_3$ to generate oxygen gas, MnO_2 is added in order to:

    A. increase the volume of oxygen obtained from the $KClO_3$.

    B. produce oxygen of higher purity.

    C. reduce the temperature at which decomposition of $KClO_3$ takes place.

    D. increase the temperature at which decomposition of $KClO_3$ takes place.

142. The name applied to a substance such as MnO_2 used in the reaction above is a (an):

    A. enzyme.

    B. catalyst.

    C. isotope.

    D. free radical scavenger.

WRITING SAMPLE

2 ESSAYS - TOPICS
60 MINUTES (30 MINUTES/TOPIC)

DIRECTIONS: Your response must be a unified, organized essay; it should contain fully developed, logically constructed paragraphs. Remember quality is more important than length. Before you begin writing, make sure you have read the item carefully and understand what is being asked. Write as legibly as possible. Because your essays will be scored as first-draft compositions, you may cross out and make corrections on your response booklet as necessary. It is not necessary to recopy your essay.

Part 1

Consider this statement:

A wise man sees as much as he ought, not as much as he can.

Montaigne

Write a unified essay in which you perform the following tasks. Explain what the above quotation means. Describe a specific situation in which a wise man sees as much as he can, not as much as he ought. Discuss what you think determines the limits that should and should not be placed on vision.

Part 2

Consider this statement:

There is properly no history; only biography.

Emerson

Write a unified essay in which you perform the following tasks. Explain what you think the above quotation means. Describe a specific situation in which there would, in fact, be history, whether or not there were biography. Discuss what you think determines the relationship between history and biography.

BIOLOGICAL SCIENCES

10 PROBLEM SETS OF 5–10 QUESTIONS EACH
15 PROBLEMS FOLLOWED BY A SINGLE QUESTION
77 QUESTIONS
100 MINUTES

DIRECTIONS: The following questions or incomplete statements are in groups. Preceding each series of questions or statements is a paragraph or a short explanatory statement, a formula or set of formulas, or a definition. Read the written material and then answer the questions or complete the statements. Select the ONE BEST ANSWER for each question and indicate your selection by marking the corresponding letter of your choice on the Answer Form. Eliminate those alternatives you know to be incorrect and then select an answer from among the remaining alternatives.

Passage I (Questions 143–148)

The diagram illustrates a typical neuron, the basic unit of the nervous system, located in a spinal (dorsal root) ganglion. Neurons connect with each other and in that manner an impulse is conducted and transmitted throughout the body. Two types of cell processes are indicated.

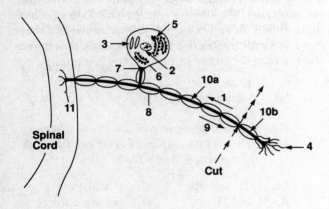

143. An impulse on the skin will be picked up by:

A. 4.   C. 7.
B. 6.   D. 10.

144. The genetic material of the cell is located in:

A. 2.   C. 5.
B. 3.   D. 7.

145. Protein synthesis is carried out under the direction of:

A. 3 in 5.   C. 2 in 5.
B. 2 in 3.   D. 2 in 7.

A person has been in an accident and the physician is conducting a neurological examination. Sensation is lost over several fingers and the examiner fears that a nerve has been cut. Note the cut indication on the diagram preceeding question 143.

146. Which process would completely degenerate?

A. 11   C. 10a
B. 8   D. 10b

147. Retrograde degeneration would be visible in:

A. 2.   C. 6.
B. 3.   D. 10b.

148. The impulse in the neuron is normally conducted in which direction?

A. 9   C. Neither 9 nor 1
B. 1   D. Both 9 and 1

Passage II (Questions 149–154)

The purpose of these experiments is to illustrate the action of both active and passive driving forces on the absorption of solutions of hemoglobin, Ringer's solution, $MgSO_4$, xylose, and glucose from the lumen of the small intestines *in vivo*.

Fluid can be absorbed from the small intestine even when the luminal solution is isotonic Ringer's. The absence of a net passive driving force for water uptake between lumen and blood indicates that active processes are involved. The active transport is *not* on the water itself but rather on sodium chloride. Active sodium transport from the epithelial cells renders the intercellular spaces sufficiently hypertonic to create osmotic driving forces for water movement out of the lumen.

Glucose is transported from the lumen by means of a specific carrier. The carrier has a site for the sugar and for sodium. It is the sodium gradient across the apical cell membrane that provides the energy for glucose entry. The sodium gradient is maintained by the active extrusion of sodium from the cells. The carrier shows typical saturation kinetics. In the case of glucose, the Km for absorption is 2mM, when sodium levels are 145mM. By contrast, the pentose, xylose, is far less effective as a substrate for this carrier. At the same level of Na, its Km is about 100 mM.

Ions such as Mg^{2+} and SO^{2-}_4, which are poorly absorbed, behave toward the intestinal epithelium almost as if it were a semipermeable membrane. Thus passive osmotic forces play a predominant role in determining the magnitude and direction of fluid movement. A similar statement can be made about intact proteins such as hemoglobin. These are ordinarily impermeable solutes.

By measuring the changes in fluid volume due to the presence of the test substances and by chemically analyzing for changes in the glucose, xylose, and hemoglobin concentration, data on how the *in vivo* intestine treats each substance will be obtained.

Experiment

In two rats, three successive 10 cm segments of intestine are tied off. Injected into the segments of one rat from proximal to distal were solutions of hemoglobin, Ringer's, and MgSO$_4$.

Injected into the segments of rat two from proximal to distal were solutions of xylose, Ringer's, and glucose. After one hour whatever fluid was present in the respective segments was withdrawn, and volumes recorded. Analysis for solutes present were conducted and percentage of absorption and recovery recorded.

149. From the "absorption from the intestine laboratory: when equal volumes of 100 mM of D-glucose or D-xylose are added in isotonic Ringer's solutions to isolated intestinal segments, the following would be expected (Km, glucose 2mM, xylose 100 mM).

   A. Equal volumes would be absorbed in a one-hour incubation.
   B. A greater volume absorbed from the xylose segment than for glucose.
   C. A greater volume absorbed from the glucose segment than for xylose.
   D. No volume change for either.

150. When 1 ml of a 1.8% solution of D-glucose was added to an intestinal segment in isotonic Ring-

er's solution and the total glucose analyzed at one hour, it was found that 1.8 mg was recovered. What percent of the D-glucose injected was absorbed or metabolized?

   A. 1.8%   **C.** 10%
   B. 1%   **D.** 90%

151. For the "absorption from the intestine laboratory," when a hemoglobin solution in water was injected into the isolated small intestine, at the end of one hour:

   A. more hemoglobin would be recovered than injected because proteins are secreted into the intestine.
   B. less hemoglobin was recovered because intact proteins are normally absorbed.
   C. less hemoglobin was recovered because bleeding into the intestine would normally occur.
   D. less hemoglobin was recovered because some hemoglobin was adsorbed on the surface of the mucosal lumen.

152. For the "absorption from the intestine laboratory," for injection of D-glucose in isotonic Ringer's solution, inhibition of glucose transport would occur when:

   I.   D-galactose was also added to the segment.
   II. sodium ion was replaced by a large cation.
   III. when L-glucose replaced D-glucose.
   IV. when an uncoupler of ATP synthesis (dinitrophenol) was added.

   A. I, II, and III   **C.** II and IV
   B. I and III   **D.** All are correct

153. For the "absorption from the intestine laboratory," when 25% MgSO$_4$ was injected into the isolated small intestine, the expected change was:

   A. an increase in volume.
   B. a decrease in volume.
   C. no change in volume.

154. For the "absorption from the intestine laboratory," when a hemoglobin solution in water was injected into the isolated small intestine, the expected change was:

   A. an increase in volume.
   B. a decrease in volume.
   C. no change in volume.

Passage III (Questions 155–161)

The schema of thyroxine formation is outlined below:

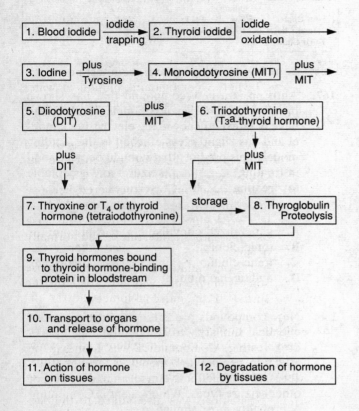

155. Chemically, thyroid hormones are:

- A. iodotyrosines.
- B. iodothyronines.
- C. iodides.
- D. iodines.

156. In proceeding from compound 3 to compound 4, the amino acid tyrosine is:

- A. oxidized.
- B. reduced.
- C. iodinated.
- D. synthesized.

157. During transport thyroid hormones are inactive because they are:

- A. in the form of thyroglobulin.
- B. free hormones.
- C. protein-bound.
- D. on red blood cells.

158. Untreated goiter is associated with:

- A. hyperthyroidism.
- B. hypothyroidism.
- C. euthyroidism.
- D. A, B, and C.

159. TSH:

- A. is made up of two peptide chains (alpha and beta).
- B. is released by the hypothalamus.
- C. binds tightly to thyroid binding globulin (TBG).
- D. secretion decreases upon exposure to the cold.

160. Involved in the regulation of the synthesis of thyroid hormone are

- A. availability of iodide ions.
- B. TSH.
- C. negative feedback of circulating T_3 and T_4 at the level of the anterior pituitary (by down regulation of TRH receptors).
- D. all of the above.

161. Which of the following describes the metabolic effect of thyroid hormone?

- A. decreased myocardial beta adrenergic receptors
- B. decreased BMR
- C. increased oxygen consumption
- D. increased plasma cholesterol

Passage IV (Questions 162–166)

The following graph illustrates several phenomena that develop while a muscle is being repetitively stimulated:

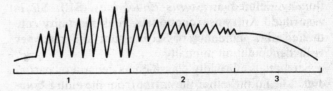

162. In the diagram above, region 1 represents:

- A. summation.
- B. complete or fused tetanus.
- C. repeated identical twitches.
- D. hyperpolarization.

163. What is the most likely cause of the event in region 3?

- A. consumption of ATP stored in the muscle
- B. loss of myosin from the muscle
- C. gradual failure to transmit the stimulus to the contraction apparatus
- D. loss of elasticity within the muscle

164. What is the major difference between regions 1 and 2?

A. Elastic elements have become fully stretched in region 1, but not in region 2.

B. Elastic elements have become fully stretched in region 2, but not in region 1.

C. The stimulus strength is greater in region 2.

D. The stimulus strength is greater in region 1.

165. In the diagram, region 2 represents:

A. incomplete tetanus.
B. muscle fatigue.
C. relaxation.
D. an absolute refractory period.

166. If a muscle is stimulated to contract, allowed to develop force, but not allowed to shorten, then the contraction is called:

A. spasmodic.   C. tetanic.
B. isotonic.   D. isometric.

Passage V (Questions 167–171)

Epilepsy affects approximately one in 200 people or about 1.2 million persons in the United States alone. Despite pharmacologic treatment, 25% of patients continue to have intermittent seizures, and one-quarter million persons have seizures more frequently than once per month. A form of continuous or recurrent seizures persisting for over 30 minutes is operationally defined as *Status Epilepticus* (SE). SE is associated with an exceptionally high mortality rate of 25%. The incidence of SE is about 250 cases per million population annually.

Seizures are broadly classified as general or partial depending on whether they arise from the entire brain simultaneously or just from a restricted region respectively. They are subclassified on the basis of the presence or absence of associated convulsive activity.

Because of the significance of epilepsy as a public health issue and present inadequacies in drug therapy, better pharmacologic strategies for the treatment of epilepsy are currently being sought. Toward this end, a number of animal models have been developed that can predict the success of new and potentially useful anticonvulsant compounds. These predictions are based on the correlation between the recognized clinical success in treating certain classes of seizures with present anticonvulsants and the degree of efficacy (effectiveness) of these same medications against seizures generated in each of the different animal models.

Class	Generalized			Partial
Subclass	Absence	Tonic-Clonic	Myoclonic	Complex
Convulsive?	No	Yes	Yes	Usually
Animal Model	GABA challenge	Electroshock	Audiogenic mouse	Kindling
First Choice	ESM	PHT	VPA	CBZ
Second Choice	VPA	VPA	PB	PHT
Third Choice				VPA

Abbreviations: CBZ—carbamazepine, ESM—ethosuximide, GABA—gamma amino butyric acid, PB—phenobarbital, PHT—phenytoin, VPA—valproic acid

167. AntiEpp is a new compound that has shown promise in animal seizure models. It is found to have greatest efficacy in the electroshock model and has slightly less efficacy in the kindling model. This predicts that it might be very good in treating ____i____ seizures and acceptable for treating ____ii____ seizures.

	i	ii
A.	generalized convulsive	partial complex
B.	tonic-clonic	no other
C.	tonic-clonic	partial complex
D.	audiogenic mouse	electro shock

168. New compounds are often tested because of chemical similarity to conventional agents. In drug testing, Compound X was found to be effective against the model of absence seizures. It was ineffective in all animal models of other seizure types. Which agent is Compound X probably most similar to?

A. carbamazepine
B. ethosuximide
C. valproic acid
D. not enough information is available to answer the question

169. The 1990 population of New York City is about 7 million persons. How many persons are statistically likely to suffer from epilepsy?

A. 3,500 persons   C. 35,000 persons
B. 1,750 persons   D. 17,500 persons

170. A patient is found to have been seizing for over an hour. Electrical activity from her brain recorded on an electroencephalogram reveals that the abnormal activity is localized only to a restricted region. The best description of her condition is:

A. status epilepticus.
B. generalized status epilepticus.
C. partial status epilepticus.
D. partial complex seizure.

171. From information provided in the reading passage, please indicate the approximate number of patients with epilepsy who continue to have seizure at least once per month despite pharmacologic (drug) therapy.

A. 30,000   C. ¼ million
B. 300,000   D. 250,000

Passage VI (Questions 172–179)

Using a syringe containing heparin, 50 milliliters of blood were drawn from a healthy male volunteer. Following centrifugation, the "buffy coat" was removed and a lymphocyte-rich cell population was obtained by sedimentation through 2% Dextran. After washing in 0.9% saline the lymphocytes were placed in cell culture tubes at a concentration of 5×10^6 cells/ml cell culture medium/tube. To one-half of the tubes was added 5 µg of phytohemagglutinin, a substance which causes lymphocytes to undergo mitosis. The other half of the tubes received no phytohemagglutinin. Radioactive tracers for RNA, DNA, and protein synthesis were then added to all tubes and aliquots removed at selected intervals. The following data were obtained:

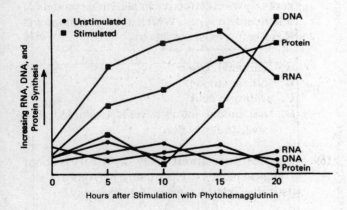

172. The purpose of this experiment was to:

A. determine the role of heparin in blood clotting.
B. determine the sequence of events in cells stimulated to undergo mitosis, and to compare these data to those gathered from unstimulated cells.
C. isolate a pure population of lymphocytes.
D. determine the lifespan of lymphocytes.

173. From these data it can be seen that increased:

A. RNA synthesis precedes increased protein synthesis.
B. DNA synthesis precedes increased protein synthesis.
C. protein synthesis precedes increased RNA synthesis.
D. DNA synthesis precedes increased RNA synthesis.

174. It may also be assumed that:

A. DNA synthesis is dependent on previous RNA synthesis.
B. protein synthesis is dependent on previous DNA synthesis.
C. RNA synthesis is dependent on previous protein synthesis.
D. unstimulated lymphocytes synthesize RNA, DNA, and protein at a low rate.

175. The smallest unit possessing the capability to maintain life and to reproduce is:

A. an organ.   C. DNA.
B. a cell.   D. RNA.

176. Normally, a complete set of chromosomes ($2n$) is passed on to each daughter cell as a result of:

A. reduction division.
B. mitotic cell division.
C. meiotic cell division.
D. nondisjunction.

177. Messenger RNA receives its instructions from:

A. ribosomes.
B. endoplasmic reticulum.
C. DNA in the nucleus.
D. cytoplasm.

178. During which phase of the mitotic cycle do the two chromatids split apart and start migration toward the poles of the spindle?

A. prophase   C. anaphase
B. metaphase   D. telophase

179. During metaphase of mitosis:

A. there is a dissolution of the chromosomal material.
B. the centrioles with asters are at the opposite poles.
C. the cell membrane starts to reappear.
D. the nuclear membrane disappears.

Passage VII (Questions 180–189)

The liver from a rat was gently homogenized in buffered sucrose solution using a Dounce homogenizer (which does not break most membranous organelles in cells). The homogenate was layered over a sucrose gradient and centrifuged for four hours at 100,000 xg. The sucrose gradient was then collected as a series of fractions. Each fraction was analyzed for DNA concentration, RNA concentration, cytochrome oxidase activity, acid phosphatase activity, and cytochrome P-450 concentration. Concentrations and enzyme activities are given as relative values, with the fraction giving the highest value for each component being shown as 100 and all other values for that component being scaled relative to the highest value.

180. Which fraction contains most of the nuclei from the hepatocytes?

    A. fraction 1   C. fraction 3
    B. fraction 2   D. fraction 4

181. Which fraction contains most of the mitochonria from the hepatocytes?

    A. fraction 1   C. fraction 3
    B. fraction 2   D. fraction 4

182. Which fraction contains most of the rough endoplasmic reticulum from the hepatocytes?

    A. fraction 1   C. fraction 3
    B. fraction 2   D. fraction 4

183. Which fraction contains most of the lysosomes from the hepatocytes?

    A. fraction 1   C. fraction 3
    B. fraction 2   D. fraction 4

184. Which fraction contains most of the smooth endoplasmic reticulum from the hepatocytes?

    A. fraction 1   C. fraction 3
    B. fraction 2   D. fraction 4

185. Which fraction contains most of the Krebs cycle enzymes from the hepatocytes?

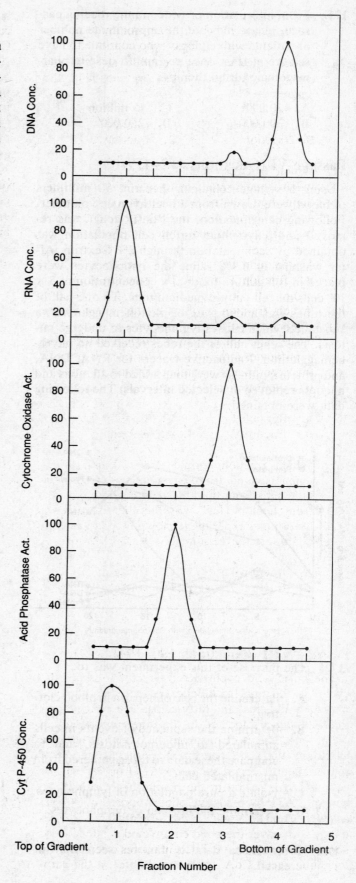

A. fraction 1   C. fraction 3
B. fraction 2   D. fraction 4

186. Which fraction should contain most of the newly synthesized plasma proteins from the hepatocytes?

A. fraction 1   C. fraction 3
B. fraction 2   D. fraction 4

187. Which fraction should appear much larger when isolated from pancreatic exocrine cells than when isolated from hepatocytes? Assume that the assays used in the experiment shown here are used to quantitate the fractions.

A. fraction 1   C. fraction 3
B. fraction 2   D. fraction 4

188. Which fraction should appear much larger when isolated from monocytes or connective tissue macrophages than when isolated from hepatocytes? Assume that the assays used in the experiment shown here are used to quantitate the fractions.

A. fraction 1   C. fraction 3
B. fraction 2   D. fraction 4

189. Which fraction should appear much larger when isolated from proximal convoluted tubule cells from the kidney than when isolated from hepatocytes? Assume that the assays used in the experiment shown here are used to quantitate the fractions.

A. fraction 1   C. fraction 3
B. fraction 2   D. fraction 4

Passage VIII (Questions 190–194)

The citric acid cycle (Krebs cycle, tricarboxylic cycle) is the final metabolic pathway for glucose, many amino acids, and fatty acids. The enzymes for the pathway are located in the inner mitochondrial membrane. The electrons from the oxidation of these metabolic fuels are conserved in the formation of reducing equivalents, such as NADH or $FADH_2$ for eventual reoxidation in the respiratory assembly to generate ATP by oxidative phosphorylation. Whereas glucose and fatty acids produce acetyl CoA for oxidation to recover the bond energy and produce CO_2, some amino acids have different routes of catabolism including acetyl CoA, other metabolites of the path-

way, and pyruvate formation. The citric acid cycle can accept metabolites at places other than acetyl CoA and is able to supply metabolites for biosynthesis such as in the synthesis of porphyrins or amino acids. However, net glucose cannot be synthesized from acetyl CoA entering the cycle. The reactions have many similarities such as hydration—dehydration or oxidation, particularly of secondary alcohols to ketone. For every mole of acetyl CoA entering the cycle and condensing with oxaloacetate, 12 moles of ATP and two moles of CO_2 are formed and a mole of oxaloacetate is recovered. The rate of the cycle is controlled by energy levels of the cell at specific enzymatic points including the formation of citric acid and the formation of α-ketoglutarate.

190. For one mole of acetyl CoA entering the Krebs (TCA) cycle (coupled to oxidative phosphorylation):

A. one mole of carbon dioxide and 38 ATP are formed.
B. two moles of carbon dioxide and 38 ATP are formed.
C. two moles of carbon dioxide and 24 ATP are formed.
D. two moles of carbon dioxide and 12 ATP are formed.

191. All of the following are similar pairs of types of reactions starting with pyruvate EXCEPT:

A. isocitrate to oxalosuccinate; malate to oxaloacetate.
B. alpha ketoglutarate to succinyl CoA; acetyl CoA to pyruvate.
C. cis-aconitase to isocitrate; fumarate to malate.
D. pyruvate to acetyl CoA; alpha ketoglutarate to succinyl CoA.

192. The citric acid cycle provides biosynthetic intermediates (net) for the following EXCEPT:

A. acetyl CoA to oxaloacetate.
B. acetyl CoA to malonyl CoA.
C. succinyl CoA to porphyrins.
D. oxaloacetate to aspartate.

193. All of the following are metabolic functions or possible interactions of the tricarboxylic acid cycle EXCEPT:

A. decreased activity when ATP levels are high.

B. control of glycolysis.

C. accepting acetyl CoA from fatty acids, glucose, and some amino acids.

D. net synthesis of glucose occurs from acetyl CoA.

194. All of the following are correct about the citric acid cycle EXCEPT:

A. active in the mature red blood cell in humans.

B. occurs in the mitochondria.

C. provides about 24 ATP/moles of glucose (coupled to ox-phos).

D. when acetyl CoA amount increases it may increase gluconeogenesis from other carbon atoms.

Passage IX (Questions 195–199)

The carbon atom can have four different substituted groups. Because these molecules are not flat, but occupy a three-dimensional shape, they become chiral (handedness, like your right and left hand). The basal molecule that originally all other molecules were compared to was $D(+)$ glyceraldehyde. It has a mirror image $L(-)$ glyceraldehyde with the same chemical and physical properties (with special exceptions) but different biological properties. The D isomer has the OH group on the right side, whereas the L isomer has the OH on the left side. These are enantiomers. The next higher homolog of this aldotriose is an aldotetrose. The family of the aldosugars for trioses and tetroses is shown below. Note that the D tetroses (erythrose and threose) are not entiomers (not mirror images) but are diastereoisomers with different chemical, physical, and biological properties. These D tetroses are also epimers, because they differ only by the configuration around a single carbon atom. The stability of certain stereoforms has allowed them to predominate in nature (D-glucose, for example). The specificity of enzymes allows them to recognize three dimensional stereodifferences. For example, D-glucose and an epimer at the C4 carbon D-galactose. The translation of amino acids in proteins in humans is for the L-form.

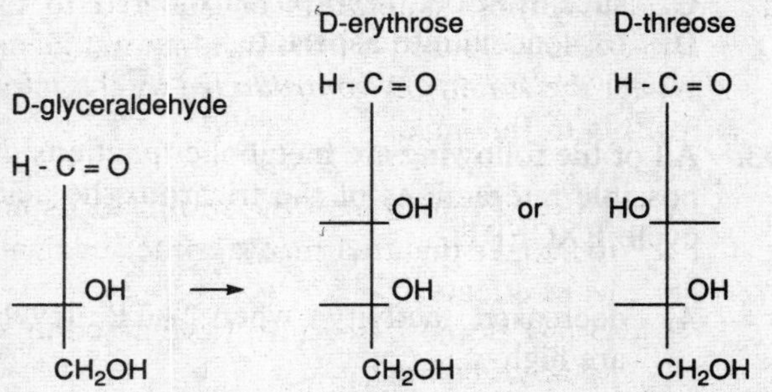

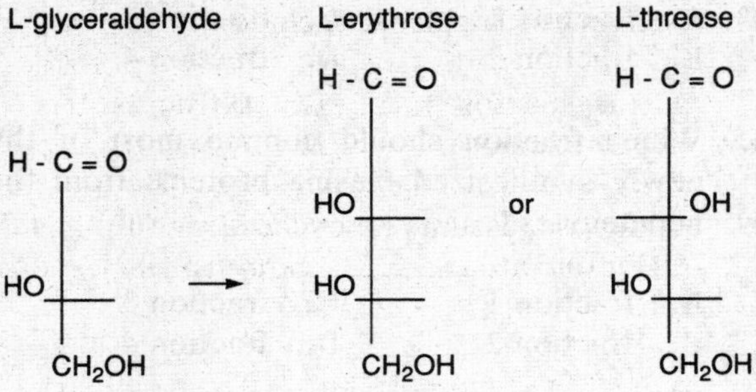

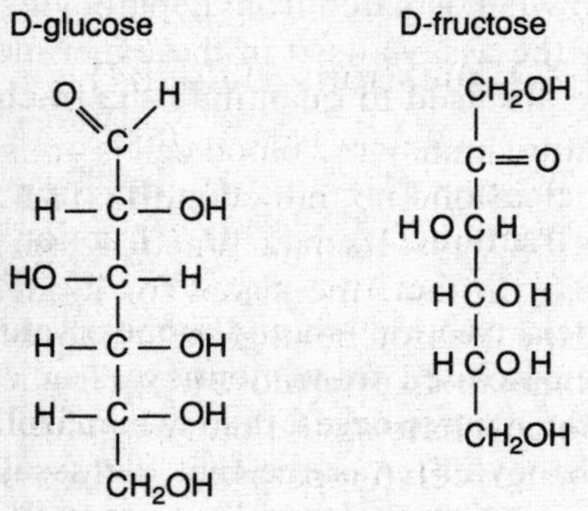

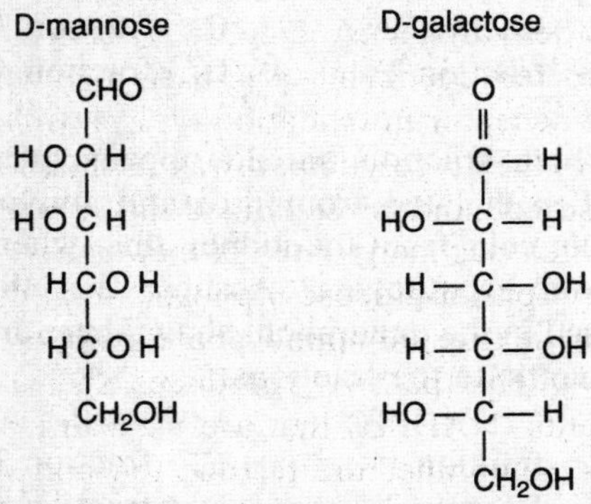

L-glyceraldehyde   L-erythrose   L-threose

D-glyceraldehyde   D-erythrose   D-threose

D-glucose   D-fructose

D-mannose   D-galactose

195. Amino acids found in humans are usually:

A. optically inactive.

B. of the L-series.

C. of the D-series.

D. a racemic mixture.

196. Carbohydrates in humans (glucose, galactose, fructose, mannose, for example) are usually:

A. optically inactive.

B. of the L-series.

C. of the D-series.

D. a racemic mixture.

197. D-glucose and L-galactose are:

A. epimers.   C. enantiomers.

B. diastereomers.   D. A and B.

198. Epimers of D-glucose include:

A. D-galactose.
B. D-mannose.
C. D-fructose.
D. A and B.

199. D-glucose (assume no cyclic structure) has the OH group at _____ carbon as its D indicator.

A. 1
B. 2
C. 3
D. 5

Passage X (Questions 200–204)

The mature human red blood cell is unique in that it has no nucleus and no mitochondria, and has a finite lifetime of 120 days. Its main function is as a carrier of hemoglobin. In fact, the signal for its death is triggered by the loss of hemoglobin function. The red blood cell metabolizes glucose by two pathways with glucose-6-phosphate as the branch point. One direction is the glycolytic pathway to provide energy through substrate level phosphorylation and to produce pyruvate. In order to maintain the glycolytic pathway, the pyruvate is reduced enzymatically using L-lactic dehydrogenase and the coenzyme NADH. The oxidized coenzyme NAD^+ is then used as an electron acceptor in oxidation of 3-phosphoglyceraldehyde in the glycolytic pathway. Lactate leaves the red blood cell and is reoxidized in the liver to pyruvate, which has many fates in metabolism. The second direction for glucose-6-phosphate in metabolism is in the hexose monophosphate pathway (pentose pathway). This pathway produces special reducing equivalents (NADPH) that are used to maintain the red cell membrane, the ferrous ion and molecules, that are the cells' reservoir of -SH groups (glutathione). Drug metabolism frequently requires NADPH so that a deficit in the first enzyme directing this pathway (glucose-6-phosphate dehydrogenase) results in a premature hemolysis of the red blood cell.

200. The end product(s) of catabolism of glucose in the red blood cell by the glycolytic pathway is/are:

A. glucose-6-phosphate.
B. carbon dioxide.
C. acetyl CoA.
D. pyruvate and lactate.

201. The first step in the metabolism of glucose:

A. occurs in the cytoplasm.

B. requires ATP.
C. produces glucose-6-phosphate.
D. all are correct.

202. ATP producing steps in glycolysis include:

A. glucose to glucose-6-phosphate.
B. phosphoenol pyruvate to pyruvate.
C. 1,3 bis phosphoglycerate to 3-phosphoglycerate.
D. B and C.

203. A genetic defect in the red blood cell enzyme glucose-6-phosphate dehydrogenase will result in all of the following EXCEPT:

A. decrease in the formation of NADPH.
B. increase in the hemolysis of red blood cells.
C. failure to reduce pyruvate to lactate.
D. A and B are correct.

204. Glycolysis and the hexose monophosphate shunt:

A. have no common places of interaction.
B. only interface through glucose-6-phosphate.
C. both produce CO_2 in the red blood cell.
D. interact through common intermediates, such as glyceraldehyde-3-phosphate.

DIRECTIONS: Read each passage carefully, study each table, chart, or formula, then answer the question following it. Eliminate those choices that you think to be incorrect and mark the letter of your choice on the answer sheet.

EFFECT OF VARIOUS TREATMENTS ON ORGAN WEIGHTS

Treatments	No. of Animals	Body Weight Grams	Organ Weight (mg/100 g Body Weight)		
			Organ 1	Organ 2	Organ 3
Control	8	70	1509 ± 34	223 ± 20	22 ± 0.8
Drug A	8	66	1044 ± 30	87 ± 14	23 ± 1.0
Drug B	8	73	1432 ± 51	224 ± 24	26 ± 0.9
Drug A + B	8	71	1586 ± 68	208 ± 28	25 ± 1.2
Drug C	8	73	1383 ± 80	146 ± 19	31 ± 1.3
Drug B + C	8	65	954 ± 50	61 ± 3	26 ± 2.0

205. The following statements are related to the table above. Based on the information given, select the statement *contradicted by* the information in the table.

A. Causal evaluation of the results leads one to believe that treatment resulted in significant effects.
B. Drugs B and C seem to have acted in an additive manner.

C. The experimenters should have paid closer attention to body weights.

D. Drug C affects all parameters under investigation.

Diet	Losing Weight	Mortality
Balanced Diet	4%	2%
Diet A	90%	74%
Diet A + Vitamin C	84%	72%
Diet A + Vitamin B	4%	2%
Diet A + Vitamin A	88%	76%

Groups of 50 mice were fed the diets listed in the table, and the percentage losing more than 10% of their initial body weight and the percentage mortality after 30 days were recorded.

206. The best conclusion to be drawn from this study is that:

A. diet A is a good reducing diet.
B. diet A lacks B vitamins.
C. vitamin C is not necessary for life.
D. vitamin A is necessary for life.

The epiphyseal cartilage plate is very sensitive to somatotrophin (growth hormone) and, therefore, can be used as an assay for this compound. Species variations exist and other hormones such as estrogen, thyroxine, and several antibiotics also have an effect upon cartilage growth. The assay must be carried out on hypophysectomized animals.

The following experiments were conducted as can be seen from the table:

Test Groups	No. of Animals	Cartilage Growth in μ	
		1 Injection Daily	2 Injections/Day (½ amount each time)
Control (normal) (saline)	20 (10/injecting group)	100	100
Hypophysectomized (saline)	20	60	60
Hypox + 100 mg STH	20	150	160
Hypox + 300 mg STH	20	180	195
Stressed normal animals (saline)	20	175	190
Hypox & stressed (saline)	20	50	50
Stressed normal + 100 mg STH	20	200	210
Hypox, stressed + 100 mg STH	20	110	120

207. The reason the assay must be carried out on hypophysectomized rats is:

A. just to add another sophisticated method to the experiment.
B. because the pituitary produces its own growth hormone and it might interfere with the assay.

C. to study the pituitary composition of growth hormone.
D. to obtain the animals' own growth hormone.

The following experimental protocol was carried out. Bean seeds were picked for their uniformity and 20 were planted/pot. One hundred percent germination was observed; and when the seedlings were nine days old, the seedlings of uniform growth were selected for treatment with X rays. Four hundred r units/minute were applied at a distance of 30 cm from the object. Seedlings were exposed up to 60 minutes with up to 24,000 r. After exposure, seedlings were placed in a greenhouse and kept at uniform light, temperature, and moisture conditions. Seedlings were measured as indicated in the table.

	CODE	
	I	II
1	From ground to cotyledon (a mark was made on the seedling near the ground with india ink)	A 0 minutes—control
2	Cotyledon to 1st node	B 7.5 minutes—3,000 r
3	Petiole length of 1st leaf	C 15 minutes—6,000 r
4	Midrib of 1st leaf	D 30 minutes—12,000 r
5	From 1st node to tip of the plant (when included).	E 60 minutes—24,000 r

EXPERIMENTAL RESULTS

10 Days

	A	B	C	D	E
1	6.20	6.58	7.30	5.45	4.43
2	2.17	2.16	2.30	1.15	.76
3	.87	1.11	1.10	0.65	.53
4	3.00	3.23	3.02	2.03	1.86
5					

17 Days

	A	B	C	D	E
1	7.08	6.73	8.00	6.99	5.82
2	8.06	7.11	5.36	2.50	1.63
3	4.12	4.50	4.15	2.13	1.70
4	5.44	5.27	5.68	5.33	4.97
5					

33 Days

	A	B	C	D	E
1	7.21	6.73	8.00	7.00	6.05
2	8.07	7.11	5.48	2.65	1.65
3	4.33	4.61	4.86	2.30	1.90
4	5.50	5.50	6.13	5.91	5.25
5	12.56	11.38	5.27		

208. The purpose of this experiment was:

    A. to observe the germination rate.
    B. to check for uniform growth rate
    C. test output and scatter of the X ray machine.
    D. observe X ray effect on growth.

Both sexes carry a complete complement of sex-linked genes. A female, however, with the XX arrangement will only exhibit a recessive gene if she has received it from both parents (a rare event if we are dealing with an uncommon gene of the population); while in the male with the XY arrangement the recessive gene cannot be masked since there is no partner X chromosome and, therefore, a larger number of recessive genes are expressed (examples are hemophilia and color blindness). A man receives his X chromosome from his mother and passes it on to his daughters not his sons. His daughters in this respect are the carriers of his sex-linked traits and their sons will be the affected ones. Let us illustrate with an example. The normal czarina of Russia produced sons suffering from hemophilia, a disease that is caused by a sex-linked recessive gene, h. The more dominant gene, H, produces normal blood clotting. Genotypically, these women must have carried Hh (X_H and X_h). A daughter, depending on the father (X_HY or X_hY), could have carried X_HX_h or X_HX_H while a son could have been born either with an X_HY or an X_hY (hemophilic) chromosomal complement.

209. The following statements are related to the information presented above. Select the statement *supported by* the information given.

    A. A cattle breeder has in a herd a dominant Y-linked trait. A calf sired by a bull carrying this trait is born. The chances of the inheritance of the trait are 50%.
    B. A female calf was born; the chances of exhibiting the trait are zero.
    C. If the sex in the above cross is known, there is no doubt about whether a calf has the trait.
    D. All of the above.

Melanoma tumors were implanted into three strains of mice. Experiments were then performed to determine the types and amounts of host serum antibodies produced against the lipid components of the virus contained in the melanoma cells. The results are summarized in the table below.

Host	Ag A Phenotype	Antilipid Antibody Day 40 Post Implant	Antilipid Antibody Day 60 Post Implant
Strain 1	3/3	4.5 ± 0.3	6.3 ± 1.7
Strain 2	1/3	3.4 ± 0.4	5.5 ± 1.3
Strain 3	1/1	1.3 ± 0.1	1.3 ± 0.3

210. The following statements are related to the information presented above. Select the statement *supported by* the information given.

    A. Strain 1 produced less antilipid antibody at both time periods measured than the other two hosts.
    B. On the basis of this information, Strain 1 animals are less resistant to melanoma-type cancers than either Strain 2 or 3 animals.
    C. All three hosts produced more antibody at 60 days than they did at 40 days.
    D. An Ag A phenotype containing three seems to be related to higher antibody production.

During wound healing, proliferation of cells in epithelial tissues, connective tissues, and vascular tissues occurs in order to fill in and resurface the defect caused by necrotic (dead) tissue. In experimental studies of the cellular kinetics of wound healing, it is often necessary to assess the amount of proliferation in various cell populations. Because cells replicate DNA within 8 to 12 hours before dividing, determination of the frequency of DNA synthesis at a particular time among cells in a population is a good index of the rate of cell division. DNA synthesis can be determined by tagging replicating DNA with radioactive thymidine. By the procedure of autoradiography, the nuclei of cells which have incorporated radioactive thymidine can be identified on histological sections. The percentage of cells labeled with radioactive thymidine is called the labeling index.

The following table includes data on the labeling index of endothelial cells which form the lining of blood vessels.

[3]H-THYMIDINE INDEX IN WOUND HEALING

Wound Age	Amount of Epidermal Resurfacing	Endothelial Labeling Index
1 day	0%	3.5%
2 days	0%	13.3%
3 days	0-5%	10.5%
6 days	60-70%	5.6%
10 days	90-100%	2.5%

211. The following statements are related to the information presented. Select the statement *not supported by* the information given.

A. The ^{3}H-thymidine labeling index, and hence the amount of endothelial proliferation, increased before epidermal resurfacing had become evident.

B. The endothelial labeling index, after 2 days, decreased both with advancing wound age and with advancing surface coverage.

C. The increased endothelial proliferation at 2 and 3 days led to the formation of new blood vessels, which then induced epidermal resurfacing.

D. Endothelial proliferation ceases when the wounds are 90–100% resurfaced with epidermis.

Androgen compounds are responsible for maintaining the secondary sex organs and characteristics of organisms. An endocrinology class was divided into 4 groups to conduct a blind experiment and at the end was asked to compare results. Each group received a compound and injected a similar amount. The experimental protocol in male animals was: 1) Unoperated control animals; 2) Unoperated control animals receiving vehicle only; 3) Bilaterally castrated (testes removed) animals; and 4) Bilaterally castrated animals receiving unknown. The results were summarized in table form.

Experimental Groups	Prostate Weight-mg Student Groups				Seminal Vesicle Weight-mg Student Groups			
	1	2	3	4	1	2	3	4
Unoperated Control	33	31	29	34	68	65	63	67
Unoperated Control and Vehicle	31	32	30	31	69	70	65	64
Bilaterally Castrated	10	9	7	8	12	14	10	15
Bilaterally Castrated and Unknown	37	33	28	31	70	64	61	59

212. The following statements are related to the information presented above. Select the statement *supported by* the information given.

A. The prostate gland is more sensitive than the seminal vesicle to a lack of androgens.

B. These experiments were properly controlled.

C. The results obtained are probably not statistically significant.

D. Bilateral castration removes a major source of sex hormones.

Gerbils were used for this experiment. One group served as a control; one group was thyroidectomized and maintained on 1% calcium gluconate since the parathyroids were probably removed also; one group received daily injections of thyroxin; and one group that was thyroidectomized and maintained as described above also received daily injections of thyroxin. Oxygen was measured in a standard manner. The following were the results.

Groups	Initial Body Weight gm	Final Body Weight gm	Thyroid Gland Weight mg	Liter of O_2 Consumed hour/meter^2
Normal	143	150	5.0	1.54
Hypothyroid	160	174	0.0	0.16
Hyperthyroid	123	120	8.0	7.33
Hypothyroid + thyroxin	164	158	4.9	1.23

213. The following statements are based on the information presented above. Select the statement(s) *consistent with* the information given.

A. The quantity of heat liberated by an organism as calculated on the basis of respiratory exchange is decreased by deficiencies and elevated by excesses of the active thyroid principle.

B. After total thyroidectomy, the basal metabolic rate falls to 10% of its normal value.

C. Hypothyroid animals probably exhibited sluggishness.

D. All of the above.

A manufacturer is testing a newly designed line of autoclaves that will be marketed. Calibration of timers and temperature controls is critical to insure destruction of bacteria.

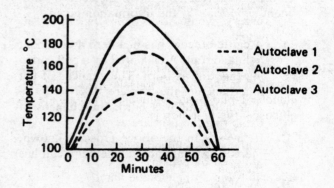

214. Bacteria Z will grow following exposure to temperature below 160°C. Which autoclave will fail to inactivate bacteria Z?

A. autoclave 1.

B. autoclave 1 and 2.

C. autoclave 2 and 3.

D. autoclave 3.

The pineal complex is implicated in the modulation of reproductive functions of the golden hamster. Surgical removal of the eyes produced atrophy of the testes and seminal vesicles within four to six weeks, and simultaneous pinealectomy prevented the atrophy. In the following experiment the drug MTPH was injected subcutaneously daily for 30 days to learn if there was an enhancement of atrophy. The results are summarized below.

Treatment	Number of Hamsters Treated	Organ Weight (mg/100g body weight)	
		Testes	Seminal Vesicles
Untreated Control	6	2884	722
Blinding	6	1695[a]	396[a]
Pinealectomy	6	2600	544
Blinding, Pinealectomy	6	2580	577
MTPH, No Surgery	6	3069	699
MTPH, Blinding	6	1419[a]	398[a]
MTPH, Pinealectomy	6	2875	591
MTPH, Blinding, Pinealectomy	6	2635	577

[a]($p < 0.05$)

215. The following statements are related to the information presented above. Select the statement *supported by* the information given.

   A. Drug MTPH increased the testicular atrophy in blinded hamsters when compared with blinded hamsters not receiving MTPH.
   B. Drug MTPH increased the seminal vesicle atrophy in blinded hamsters when compared with blinded hamsters not receiving MTPH.
   C. Drug MTPH had no effect on atrophy, either testicular or seminal vesicles.
   D. Drug MTPH, when administered without surgery, would affect reproductive organ weight.

216. In the reaction sequence used in breakdown of glycogen in the liver or muscle—glycogen → glucose-1-phosphate→glucose-6-phosphate→ glucose—the first step is:

   A. catalyzed by phosphorylase.
   B. catalyzed by pepsin.
   C. catalyzed by pancreatic amylase.
   D. nonenzymatic.

217. A metabolic process that produces energy to convert ADP + phosphate into ATP is the:

   A. production of fructose and glucose from sucrose.
   B. production of fatty acids and glycerol from triglycerides.
   C. production of CO_2 and water from fatty acids.
   D. production of steroids from acetate.

218. A negative iodoform test (i.e., no yellow precipitate) will be the result when $NaOH + I_2$ is reacted with:

   A. $CH_3{-}CH{-}CH_3$
   $\qquad\quad |$
   $\qquad\ \ \ OH$

   B. $CH_3{-}C{-}CH_2{-}CH_3$
   $\qquad\quad \|$
   $\qquad\quad O$

   C. $\emptyset{-}\overset{\overset{\textstyle O}{\|}}{C}{-}CH_3$

   D. $CH_3{-}CH_2{-}CH_2{-}\overset{\overset{\textstyle H}{|}}{C}{=}O$

Phenylamine is cooled to 0°C and treated with HCl and $NaNO_2$. After a few minutes of reaction time cuprous bromide is added, and the solution is heated.

219. The final product would primarily be a (an):

   A. azo dye.
   B. organometallic compound.
   C. monosubstituted benzene containing no metal.
   D. disubstituted benzene.

Model Examination Answer Key

Verbal Reasoning

1.	C	14.	A	27.	C	40.	C	53.	C
2.	C	15.	C	28.	A	41.	A	54.	B
3.	D	16.	A	29.	B	42.	A	55.	A
4.	C	17.	D	30.	B	43.	B	56.	B
5.	B	18.	B	31.	D	44.	B	57.	D
6.	D	19.	C	32.	C	45.	D	58.	D
7.	D	20.	D	33.	C	46.	C	59.	B
8.	C	21.	C	34.	C	47.	C	60.	B
9.	B	22.	D	35.	D	48.	C	61.	C
10.	D	23.	D	36.	D	49.	A	62.	B
11.	D	24.	D	37.	D	50.	B	63.	C
12.	A	25.	A	38.	B	51.	B	64.	C
13.	B	26.	D	39.	C	52.	D	65.	D

Physical Sciences

66.	B	82.	C	98.	A	113.	C	128.	B
67.	D	83.	B	99.	B	114.	B	129.	C
68.	A	84.	A	100.	C	115.	D	130.	C
69.	B	85.	B	101.	D	116.	B	131.	B
70.	A	86.	A	102.	D	117.	B	132.	C
71.	C	87.	B	103.	B	118.	D	133.	C
72.	B	88.	A	104.	C	119.	A	134.	B
73.	D	89.	D	105.	D	120.	C	135.	D
74.	B	90.	C	106.	A	121.	A	136.	D
75.	B	91.	C	107.	B	122.	B	137.	A
76.	B	92.	B	108.	D	123.	A	138.	C
77.	C	93.	B	109.	A	124.	C	139.	A
78.	B	94.	C	110.	B	125.	D	140.	D
79.	D	95.	A	111.	B	126.	A	141.	C
80.	D	96.	B	112.	A	127.	B	142.	B
81.	A	97.	A						

Biological Sciences

143.	A	159.	A	175.	B	190.	D	205.	C
144.	A	160.	D	176.	B	191.	B	206.	B
145.	C	161.	C	177.	C	192.	A	207.	B
146.	D	162.	A	178.	C	193.	D	208.	D
147.	A	163.	C	179.	B	194.	A	209.	D
148.	B	164.	B	180.	D	195.	B	210.	D
149.	C	165.	A	181.	C	196.	C	211.	D
150.	D	166.	D	182.	A	197.	B	212.	D
151.	D	167.	C	183.	B	198.	D	213.	D
152.	D	168.	B	184.	A	199.	D	214.	A
153.	A	169.	C	185.	C	200.	D	215.	A
154.	B	170.	C	186.	A	201.	D	216.	A
155.	B	171.	B	187.	A	202.	D	217.	C
156.	C	172.	B	188.	B	203.	C	218.	D
157.	C	173.	A	189.	C	204.	D	219.	C
158.	D	174.	D						

Explanation of Answers for Model Examination

VERBAL REASONING

1. **C.** The author characterizes the goals for freshman composition at the University of Texas as "standard" (three of them are listed in **A**, **B**, and **D**) and enumerates them in paragraph two. The goal not listed is **C**, the goal of teaching freshmen to bring about social change, an objective of the radical pedagogists.

2. **C.** See the explanation of question 1 (above). Bringing about social change is the goal of the radical pedagogists, according to paragraph five.

3. **D.** In paragraph six, Lazere is described as a "leftist educator and radical pedagogist" (**A** and **C**); in paragraph seven the passage clearly suggests that he would be in disagreement with the methods proposed by Sharon Crowley's because it would force ideology on the student. The correct answer, therefore, would be **D**, all of the above.

4. **C.** The course, described in paragraph two, would examine the subject of "difference, specifically difference related to legal opinions given in court cases involving issues such as race, gender, bilingualism, and sexual orientation." Answer **C** partially describes the content of the course and is the correct response.

5. **B.** One can easily infer from the statements attributed to her in the passage that Crowley fits the definition for a radical pedagogist given in paragraph three. Among other things, she asserts that composition teachers "must give up our traditional subscription to liberal tolerance if we are to bring about social change through [our students]" (see paragraph seven).

6. **D.** Though **A**, **B**, and **C** are certainly logical areas for study in establishing a curriculum, they were not the endpoints for discussion sparked by the University of Texas debate. As the passage states in paragraph two, "the discussion became a forum for stating the purpose of composition and liberal education," the answer provided by **D**.

7. **D.** Early in the passage (in paragraph two), the author observes that the "debate that followed the submission and ultimate rejection of the program in many ways disregarded the course itself," a statement that provides the only evidence in the passage of the outcome of the specific curriculum proposal.

8. **C.** Paragraph one makes it clear that the investigator must focus on the question: "is complainant's job equal in effort and responsibility to that of a male counterpart?" Paragraph seven indicates that the judiciary has not yet endorsed the notion of comparable worth, and the length of employment is not addressed in the reading passage.

9. **B.** Paragraph one makes the point that identical jobs are not necessary because the standard is built on the concept that jobs must be evaluated within a context of substantial equivalency. None of the other statements is supported.

10. **D.** Statements **A** and **B** are not discussed in the passage. Paragraph three contradicts statement **C**, whereas paragraph five implies that Title VII encompasses very broad aspects and reaches beyond the confines of equal wage matters.

11. **D.** Although we might assume that the program of on-the-job training was a positive factor, the law does not address the issue. We could argue that the Department of Labor acted irresponsibly; however, we have no data to substantiate our claim. In the Columbia case, employees were aware of the differences in their positions. Paragraph five supports statement **D** because the court took into consideration the fact that heavy cleaning called for greater effort.

12. **A.** Paragraphs six and seven support statements I, II, and III, however; paragraph seven makes it clear that although the Supreme Court

has ruled that Title VII provides a remedy for sex discrimination, the judiciary has not yet endorsed the notion of comparable worth.

13. **B.**   Paragraph eight mentions the adverse decision the female guards received during the initial trial, and statement I is supported. It also makes it clear that the appellate court reversed the trial court and held that one could sue even though jobs were not substantially equal; statement III is supported. The paragraph also states that although the Supreme Court did not adopt the concept of comparable worth, it left the door open for further litigation.

14. **A.**   Paragraphs nine and ten clearly substantiate statements I, II, and III. Paragraph nine also indicates that the Supreme Court did not indicate how a plaintiff might establish a prima facie case under Title VII, and so statement IV is not supported.

15. **C.**   It should be clear to the reader that the issue under consideration is sex discrimination and its resolution.

16. **A.**   Paragraph one assigns the skull to Homo sapiens. Man is a vertebrate (subphylum); a mammal (class); Homo is the genus and sapiens is denoted as the species.

17. **D.**   Because we are dealing with a fossil, the best answer is an archeologist.

18. **B.**   The specimen was found in soil. The fluorine method of dating fossils was developed in 1949 and is based on the fact that buried bones absorb fluorine from the soil, and the amount increases with time.

19. **C.**   The older a fossil is, the more fluorine would have been present. A modern jawbone would, on testing, yield a lesser amount of fluorine in comparison to an ancient cranium.

20. **D.**   Iron in this case was used to artificially color the mandible to match the cranium.

21. **C.**   The last fragment was quite thin; in reality it was chosen by the perpetrator of the hoax (Piltdown Hoax) to duplicate the thinnest part of the first skull.

22. **D.**   The passage points out that iron salts are oxidized.

23. **D.**   The chromium detected in the jawbone indicates that a dichromate solution was at first used by the forger in an attempt to assist the oxidation of iron salts used to stain the specimens.

24. **D.**   There were developments of several methods to study fossils in the 50 years it took to resolve this matter. Although one of the theories proposed was that the missing link was found, the investigation centered on solving the disparity of evidence between the cranium and the jaw. This was a brilliantly devised falsification and no one to date knows for sure who the culprit was.

25. **A.**   There is no evidence in the passage that Sara Murphy believed anything other than **A**, Zelda's inner complexity, caused her to appear different in the various photographs that were taken of her. Murphy's observation is cited in paragraph one.

26. **D.**   In paragraph four, the author characterizes Nancy Milford as Zelda's first major biographer. Sara Mayfield was Zelda's girlhood friend, and she wrote a biography after Milford had published hers. The passage does not provide that information, however. Arthur Mizener was Scott Fitzgerald's first major biographer, and Sara Murphy was a close friend of the Fitzgeralds. But again, the passage does not provide this information. **A**, **B**, and **C**, therefore, are incorrect answers.

27. **C.**   Paragraph two indicates that Fitzgerald was stationed at Fort Sheridan, near Zelda's hometown of Montgomery, and that he returned to New York after the war was over.

28. **A.**   In paragraph two, the author tells of Zelda's mother naming her after a gypsy queen in a novel she was reading, and goes on to add details that suggest Zelda's mother spoiled her daughter.

29. **B.**   Biographically there may be evidence to support the assertion that insanity ran in Zelda's family (**A**), but the passage does not supply such information. **C** and **D** present details that are not factual and do not appear in the passage. Milford's biography, according to paragraph four, presents a picture of Zelda as one who was exploited by her husband, but who also had conflicts not related to his treatment of her, the answer provided by **B**.

30. **B.**   While Zelda's friend, according to Scott, would have blamed her insanity on his drinking (**D**), and his friends would have blamed her insanity for his drinking (**C**), neither would have been correct: "liquor on my mouth is sweet to

her and I cherish her wildest hallucinations," he said, clearly characterizing their relationship to each other as mutually self-destructive. The correct answer, therefore, is **B**. Obviously he did not consider their friends as the best judges, the incorrect answer suggested in **A**. See paragraph five.

31.   **D.**   Paragraph three provides the works by Scott in which Zelda is the model for the heroine. The novel not listed in the passage is *The Last Tycoon* (**D**), which was in fact—though the passage does not say so—the only Fitzgerald novel for which Zelda was not the model for the main character.

32.   **C.**   Paragraph four in the passage notes the historical fact that Zelda died in 1948 while confined to a mental institution.

33.   **C.**   Paragraph one indicates that the fiftieth anniversary in the "Promised Land" was celebrated. Also found in paragraph one is the fact that the writer of *Leviticus* had God speak to Moses; there is no evidence in the passage that God ever spoke to Moses. The passage does point out that celebrating is an old practice of mankind, however; there is no comment anywhere to make the reader assume that most celebrations are joyous events.

34.   **C.**   Statements II and IV are supported by the passage. Paragraph two points out that even with birthdays we call special attention to the "big" years and, the quotation from John Adams leaves no doubt that our Independence Day celebration should be carried out "from this time forward for everyone."

35.   **D.**   Paragraph three mentions that the inauguration of a new enterprise is always an act of hope and when achievement is history a confident celebration is appropriate. Paragraph four mentions that a celebration is often viewed as the occasion for a new beginning.

36.   **D.**   Paragraph five indicates that nostalgia, although differently felt, is good for the human spirit. In paragraph four we are told that we usually think that the lives of pioneers are worth emulating and that anniversaries offer us an opportunity to reflect.

37.   **D.**   Paragraphs seven and eight mention the facts that human pride is a motor of an institutional machine, that we use anniversaries to emphasize legitimacy, and that one cannot ignore the commercial motivation behind celebrations.

38.   **B.**   The author did use the one hundred fiftieth anniversary of an institution to essentially write a treatise on why we need the act of regular celebrations.

39.   **C.**   The story cites universal experiences both in myth and in everyday life.

40.   **C.**   The passage focuses on choice, which, because it is human, is universal.

41.   **A.**   Because changing or not changing the sail was Theseus's choice, the death of his father resulting from that choice was clearly his responsibility.

42.   **A.**   The plot itself is a series of choices, one following the other.

43.   **B.**   The author shows how choices in a myth can be the same choices that anyone can face at any time.

44.   **B.**   The passage is concerned with the ways in which a character's actions determine his destiny and how major choices lead to other important choices. In Theseus's case, the primary problem is how he will kill the Minotaur.

45.   **D.**   All the other statements are supported by the passage. It is stated in the passage that caricatures must be based on *fact*.

46.   **C.**   Statements **A, B,** and **D** may be true, but they are not stated in the passage. Statement **C** is cited as a cause of laughter.

47.   **C.**   Although the author states **A** and **B,** they are not the main point. The passage is set up to lead toward statement **C.** Statement **D** is dismissed in the passage.

48.   **C.**   Statements I and III are stated in the passage to show how caricatures work. Statement II may be true, but it does not indicate *why* caricatures are effective.

49.   **A.**   The passage does not deal with the possible objections to caricatures stated in **B, C,** and **D**. However, **A** is cited as a danger.

50. **B.** The entire essay deals with the ways in which satirists use exaggeration as a means of communicating their ideas.

51. **B.** The first sentence of the passage identifies aggression as a neurochemical impulse. **A, C,** and **D** are contradicted in paragraph one.

52. **D.** **B** and **C** are not dealt with in the passage. Lorenz points out specifically that it is *not* the eating enemy, but competition within the species, that poses the greatest threat to an animal species.

53. **C.** According to the passage, there seems to be no other reason for this bickering among one's own, other than the need for stimulation. **A** and **B** are mentioned as the other two basic needs; **D,** structure, is not listed as a need.

54. **B.** The passage identifies the invention of weapons as important in throwing off the natural balance precisely because man possesses the killer instinct without the internal controls or safety devices to limit his use of this instinct.

55. **A.** Hunt's point that man is aggressive without having been programmed as to how he might channel the aggression is a major point on which the author of this passage relies in emphasizing the interdependence of instinct and culture in man's development.

56. **B.** The passage cites a number of ways, many of them perhaps surprising, in which activities of humans can be traced to innate aggression.

57. **D.** Although the essay addresses **A** and **B** specifically, the essay goes far beyond both of these. **D** incorporates both the cultural and the instinctual. The essay addresses the interdependence of the two.

58. **D.** Though one might think, the essay asserts, that people are congested in cities because they like to cooperate, it actually is due to aggressive needs.

59. **B.** The passage states this specifically, and adds that the Shield Soldiers to whom they submitted rendered only token punishment, thus acknowledging the appeasement gesture.

60. **B.** Indirect assessment scores are reliable, so **A** is incorrect. The tests may be biased, but

that issue is not addressed in the passage, so **C** is incorrect. **D** is not addressed.

61. **C.** Statement I is contradicted in the passage. Statement II is stated directly. Indirect assessments are an example of a reliable test that is not necessarily valid, so statement III is also correct. Statement IV cannot be true if statement II is true.

62. **B.** Statements **A, C,** and **D** are correct, but they do not deal with the idea in reader-response theory that readers bring their own experiences to the reading of a text.

63. **C.** It is the use of a scoring guide, not the particular kind of scoring guide (holistic, primary trait, analytic), that helps increase reliability.

64. **C.** Multiple readings increase the reliability of scores, so **A** is incorrect. **B** and **D** are not addressed in the passage.

65. **D.** The author points out problems with both kinds of testing and does not choose one type as better than the other. The author may agree with **C,** but that is not an evaluation.

PHYSICAL SCIENCES

66. **B.** In the absence of air resistance, both balls have the same vertical acceleration, $g = 9.8$ m/sec^2. Because they start from rest at the same height, they will fall equal distances in equal times as shown by the equation $y = \frac{1}{2} gt^2$.

67. **D.** The horizontal velocity of the second ball is $(10$ m/sec$)$ (COS $30°$) $= 8.7$ m/sec, so it takes it more than 1 s to reach the wall.

68. **A.** The easier way to solve this problem is to equate the work done against friction to the loss of kinetic energy of the masses, i.e.:
$F_f x = \frac{1}{2}$ mv^2, where $F_f = \mu$ N $= \mu$ mg where N is the "normal" force (equal to the weight in this case). Solving for $x = v^2/(2 \mu g) = 2$ m for *both* bodies. An alternative solution is to calculate the frictional force and the deceleration. One can then use the equations for uniformly accelerated motion to find the distance. The methods are completely equivalent.

69. **B.** It is possible to calculate the velocities exactly. The initial gravitational potential en-

ergy of the block and the ball are converted entirely into kinetic energy at the bottom of the incline. However, part of the kinetic energy of the ball is in the form of rotational kinetic energy about the ball's center of mass. Therefore, at the bottom of the incline, the velocity of the ball's center of mass is less than the linear velocity of the sliding block's center of mass. Understanding this concept, the question can be answered without calculating the velocities. One can do the actual calculations as follows:

Ball: $mgh = \frac{1}{2} mv^2 + \frac{1}{2} I \omega^2$

where I is the moment of inertia (of a sphere) and ω is the angular velocity. Substituting $I = \frac{2}{5} mr^2$ and $v = r\omega$, one can solve for v.

Ball: $v = \sqrt{(^{10}/_7)gh} = 2.646$ m/sec.

For the block,

Block: $mgh = \frac{1}{2} mv^2$ and $V = \sqrt{2gh} = 3.13$ m/sec.

70. **A.** At the terminal velocity (regardless of the actual terminal velocity), the upward frictional force of air resistance is equal to the weight. $F_f - mg = 0$, because the acceleration is zero. $F_f = 0.4 \times 9.8 = 3.92$ N.

71. **C.** This is a simple conversion problem. 205 lb $\times$ 1 kg/2.2 lb = 93.2 kg. $W = mg = 913$ N.

72. **B.** The gauge pressure in the foot is higher than the gauge pressure at the level of the aorta. (This is the reason blood pressures are taken with the cuff on the upper arm at the same approximate level as the aorta.) The height difference of 1.35 m creates a "pressure head" causing added pressure, $P_{add} = dgy$, where d is the density of the fluid (blood). Because the added pressure calculated will be in the standard SI units of N/m^2, the result must be converted to the units of mmHg, using the fact that 1 atmosphere = 1.01×10^5 N/m^2 = 760 mmHg. Then:

$P = 1050$ kg/m$^3 \times 9.8$ m/s$^2 \times 1.35$ m = 13900 N/m^2

= 13900 N/m$^2 \times (760$ mmHg/1.01 $\times 10^5$N/m^2) = 105 mmHg. and $P_{total} = 100 + 105 = 205$ mmHg.

73. **D.** This question is a straightforward conversion problem because all the data needed to answer the question is given. The excess intake is 1200 kcal/day or a total of 16,800 kcal in two weeks. Then the conversion of this excess

intake of energy to a corresponding mass of fat is given by: 16,800 kcal/9.5 kcal/g = 1,700 g.

74. **B.** This question deals with the concept of power as the "rate of doing work"; 1 watt = 1 joule/s. When the metabolic rate is 630 W the student is using 630 joules of energy each second. In 10 minutes (600 s.) the total energy expended is 378,000 joules. The number of liters of oxygen consumed is then obtained by a conversion: # liters = 378,000 joules $\times$ 1 L/20,000 joules = 19 L.

75. **B.** The object (the student) is in static equilibrium. The first law of equilibrium states that the vector sum of the forces acting on the body is zero. In this case, the sum of the upward vertical forces (the scale readings) equals the sum of the downward forces (the student's weight). 90 lb + 100 lb = 190 lb, which is the correct student weight. (The bathroom scales can be set to read zero even with a sturdy board on them.) The second law of equilibrium states that the sum of the counterclockwise torques equals the sum of the clockwise torques. If one takes the axis of rotation to be through the soles of the feet, there will be one counterclockwise torque caused by the force at the head (90 lb) with a lever arm of 1.83 m and one clockwise torque due to the total weight (190) acting down through the center-of-mass at an unknown lever arm, L, measured from the sole of the foot.

90 lb $\times$ 1.83 m $-$ 190 lb $\times L =$
$L = 0.87$m.

76. **B.** The energy of oxidation for fats and oils (9.5 kcal/gm) is given in question 73 above. The desired weight loss of 1 pound of fat corresponds to an energy expenditure of:

0.4545 kg $\times$ 1000 g/kg $\times$ 9.5 kcal/g $\times$ 4185 J/kcal = 1.8×10^7 joules.

500 Watt = 500 joules/sec. So the time required is $t = 1.8 \times 10^7$ joules/(500 joule/sec) = 3.615 $\times$ 10^4 sec = 10 hours.

77. **C.** The voltages of batteries connected in series add. The 6- and 12-volt batteries in series are equivalent to an 18-volt battery. Applying Ohm's law, $V = IR$, to the equivalent circuit; the current through the resistor is:

$I = V/R = 18$ volts/10 ohm = 1.8 A.

78. **B.** The expression for the equivalent resistance of resistors connected in series is: $R_s = R_1 + R_2 + \ldots = 4 + 8 = 12$ ohms. We can

find the current in this circuit using Ohm's law: $I = V/R_s = \frac{6}{12} = 0.5$ A. The power consumed in the *8-ohm resistor* is then found from $P = I^2R = (0.5)^2 \times 8 = 2$ watts. There is additional power consumed in the 4-ohm resistor, of course.

79. **D.** Although this question could be answered in the same manner as the preceding question, one would have to find the individual current through the 8-ohm resistor. It is easier and simpler to note that the full 12 volts is applied across the terminals of the 8-ohm resistor. The power consumed can be found using the expression: $P = IV = (V/R)V = V^2/R$ where we have applied Ohm's law, $V = IR$ to the 8-ohm resistor. Then: $P = 12^2/8 = 18$ watts.

80. **D.** We can find the power from the given information: $P = V^2/R = 18$ W. Power is the "time rate of doing work": (1 W = 1 J/s) $P = E/t$ so that $E = Pt$ where t is the time in seconds. Thus: $E = 18$ joules/s $\times 300$ s $= 5400$ joules.

81. **A.** $(t_i = 20°C)$ This heat is generated electrically in the resistor, $H = E = Pt = (V^2/R)t$. Then $m\, C_W\, (t_f - t_i) = (V^2/R)t$. We can solve this expression for t_f, the only unknown. $t_f = 22.6°C$.

82. **C.** In any standing wave, the antinodes and nodes always alternate and their separation is always exactly one-quarter wavelength. In this problem, the 25 cm tube length is equal to one-quarter wavelength because the fundamental frequency is the longest wavelength at which resonance can occur. (It is possible for higher frequency resonances to occur at shorter wavelengths so that the tube length will be some odd number of quarter wavelengths.) In this case the wavelength is equal to 4 tube lengths, that is; $\lambda = 1$ m. Then $v = 340$ Hz $\times 1$ m $= 340$ m/s.

83. **B.** Using the velocity expression: $v = f_1 \lambda_1 = 20,000$ Hz $\times 1.7 \times 510^{-2}$ m $= 340$ m/sec. The velocity is nearly the same for any frequency, so that $\lambda_2 = v/f_2 = 2.3 \times 10^{-2}$ m $= 2.3$ cm.

84. **A.** If one simply uses the given expression and takes the ratio of the energies, the constant K and the amplitude squared terms may be cancelled: $W_{20}/W_{15} = K(20000)^2A^2/K(15000)^2A^2 = (20)^2/(15)^2 = 1.8$.

85. **B.** Only transverse waves can be polarized. None of the other answers is true. Longitudinal waves can have either longer or shorter wavelengths and/or frequencies than transverse waves so that **A** and **D** are false. **C** is false because transverse waves, as their name implies, vibrate perpendicularly (transverse) to the direction the wave is traveling.

86. **A.** The quantum of energy for a photon is given, $E = hf$. By substituting for f from the velocity expression, $c = f\lambda$; E may be written as: $E = hc/\lambda$. Then the ratio of energies is $E_{400}/E_{750} = (hc/400)/(hc/750) = 750/400 = 1.88$. (The result illustrates the important fact that short wavelength electromagnetic radiation is more energetic than longer wavelength radiation, because the photon energies are *inversely* proportional to the wavelengths.) Notice that when taking the ratio, one does not have to convert nm to m because all the units cancel (as do the constants hc) leaving a pure number for the ratio.

87. **B.** The speed of sound does not depend on either the frequency or the wavelength. It depends on the properties of the air (pressure, temperature, and so on). Thus the speed of sound is the same for both frequencies and the ratio of the speeds is 1.

88. **A.** The total linear momentum, $P = m_c v_c + m_t v_t$, of the car-truck system is conserved (constant) during the collision. Take the East direction to be *positive* velocity. Momentum conservation yields:

$m_c v_c = (1000$ kg$)(+ 21$ m/sec$)$
$m_t v_t = (3000$ kg$)(- 21$ m/sec$)$, and
$(m_t + m_c)V = (4000$ kg$)V = (1000)(21) - (3000)(21)$
so that: $V = -(2000)(21)/4000 = -10.5$ m/sec.
    (The minus sign means the common velocity is West.)

89. **D.** The velocity of any wave is the product of its frequency and wavelength: $v = f\lambda$. Thus the ratio of the wavelengths is:
$\lambda_r \lambda_s = (c/f)/(v/f) = c/v = 300,000,000/340 = 882,353$.

90. **C.** The frequency of a simple harmonic oscillator is given by:
$f = (1/2\pi)\sqrt{k/m}$ where k is the spring constant. We will take the ratio of f_2 to f_1.

$$f_2 / f_1 = (4 \text{ Hz})/(2 \text{ Hz}) = \frac{(1/2\pi) \sqrt{k/m_2}}{(1/2\pi) \sqrt{k/m_1}}$$

Then, $2 = \sqrt{m_1/m_2} = \sqrt{4/m_2}$ or $4 = 4/m_2$ and $m_2 = 1$ kg.

91. **C.** The initial angular velocity is:

$\omega_0 = (60000 \text{ rev/min})(1 \text{ rev}/2\pi \text{ rad})(1 \text{ min}/60 \text{ sec})$

$= 2000\pi$ rad/sec.

Using $\omega = \omega_0 + \alpha t$, we know that $\omega = 0$ at $t = 100$ sec,

$\alpha = \omega_0/t = -2000\pi \text{ rad}/100 \text{ sec} = 20\pi \text{ rad/sec}^2$.

92. **B.** The magnetic force, evB, (on a charge $q = e$, moving with velocity v perpendicular to a magnetic field B) provides the required centripetal force for the circular path. The centripetal force, $F_c = mv^2/r$ where m is the mass and r the radius for a particle with velocity v. Equating these forces:

$mv^2/r = qvB$ and solving for r:

$r = mv/qB$. The ratio r_p/r_e is therefore:

$r_p/r_e = (m_p v/eB)/(m_e v/eB)$. Cancelling the common quantities v, e, and B:

$r_p/r_e = m_p/m_e = 1.007276 \text{ } u/0.0005486 \text{ } u = 1836$.

93. **B.** The thin lens formula can be used to find the image distance, q, when $f = +12$ cm and the object distance is $p = 6$ cm.

$1/f = 1/p + 1/q$

$1/q = 1/f - 1/p = 1/12 - 1/6 = 1/12 - 2/12$

$= -1/12$. Then:

$q = -12$ cm.

The linear magnification is given by:

$m = -(q/p) = +2 =$ image height/object height.

The object height is then:

$h_o = h_i/m = (8 \text{ cm})/2 = 4$ cm.

94. **C.** The initial kinetic energy of the sliding box is used up by the friction work done by the friction force, f, in stopping the box in the distance x.

The friction force, $f = \mu N$, where N is the "normal force" between the box and floor. In this case the normal force is the weight, $N = mg$, of the box. Equating the initial KE to the work, fx, done by f:

$1/2 \text{ } mv^2 = fx = \mu Nx = \mu mgx$.

$\mu_k = v^2/2gx = (3 \text{ m/sec})^2/(2)(9.8 \text{ m/sec}^2)(3.4\text{m}) = 0.14$.

95. **A.** Conservation of mechanical energy requires that the sum of the initial kinetic energy and potential energy equal the sum of the final kinetic energy and potential energy. In the problem the actual numerical values of m, v, h and the angles of projection are not important as long as $v_{initial}$, $h_{initial}$, (and h_{final}) are the *same* (as they are here). The angle of projection is not used since the problem does not involve vectors (the energies are scalar quantities). Then

(a) $1/2 \text{ } m_1 v^2 + m_1 gh = 1/2 \text{ } m_1 V^2$

(b) $1/2 \text{ } m_2 v^2 + m_2 gh = 1/2 \text{ } m_2 V'^2$

Cancelling mass m_1 in (a) and m_2 in (b) we find the final speeds V and V' are:

$V^2 = 1/2 \text{ } v^2 + gh$

$V'^2 = 1/2 \text{ } v^2 + gh$, so that $V = V'$.

96. **B.** f, p, and q are all positive because the light rays do travel from the object toward the lens and from the lens toward the image point.

$$1/f = 1/18 + 1/36; f = 12 \text{ cm}.$$

97. **A.** The linear magnification is the negative ratio of the image distance to the object distance. $M = -q/p = -36/18 = -2$. The minus sign indicates that the image is inverted and it is 2 times the size of the object. (If q were negative as it might be for a virtual image the magnification would be positive, $-(-q/p)$, which would indicate that the image was upright and not inverted with respect to the object.)

98. **A.** The object is placed inside the focal length (closer to the lens than the focal length). This is the way that one uses a magnifying glass. The image is virtual as shown by the negative image distance; is upright and it is magnified.

$$1/q = 1/f - 1/p = 1/24 - 1/6$$

and $q = -8$ cm. The image is on the same side of the lens as the object (in "front") and can only be seen by looking through the lens at the image.

99. **B.** The magnification of a simple refracting telescope is known as the angular magnification and is given by the ratio of the focal length of the objective to the focal length of the eyepiece:

$$M = f_o/f_e = 3 \text{ X}.$$

100. **C.** For a microscope, the magnification is the product of the magnification of the objective and the magnification of the eyepiece. $M = M_o M_e$

$$M_o = M/M_e = 400/10 = 40\times.$$

101. **D.** This problem is solved by two successive applications of the thin lens formula. One must calculate the object distance for lens #2. Lens #1: $1/q_1 = 1/f_1 - 1/p_1$; $q_1 = 24$ cm (behind #1). For lens #2, $p_2 = 72$ cm $- 24$ m $= 48$ cm (in front of #2). Then $1/q_2 = 1/f_2 - 1/p_2 = 1/24 - 1/48$, and thus $q_2 = +48$ cm (behind #2) The final image is real.

102. **D.** The magnification is the ratio of the image distance, q, to the object distance, p, for a thin lens. ($m = -q/p$). In order to find the image distance, q, we use the thin lens formula:

$1/f = 1/p + 1/q$, $1/q = 1/f - 1/p$ or
$1/q = 1/24 - 1/12 = -1/24$. Then $q = -24$ cm

and the magnification is: $m = -\left(\dfrac{-24}{12}\right) = +2$.

The image is twice as large as the object, or 10 cm tall. (The plus sign means that this viritual image is upright.)

103. **B.** This problem is done exactly as in the explanation for question 102. This time the focal length $f = -24$ cm so that the image distance is found to be: $1/q = -1/24 - 1/12$ or $q = -8$ cm. The magnification is then equal to: $m = -(-8)/12 = +0.67$ and the image is only 3.3 cm tall. (This image is upright as shown by the plus sign for the magnification. A diverging lens always produces an upright image.)

104. **C.** The very distant objects, such as stars, are effectively an infinite distance away. The thin lens formula, $1/f = 1/p + 1/q$, then yields the result that the image distance is the same as the focal length because $1/p$ is equal to zero for $p =$ infinity. The image must appear at the actual far-point of the eye, that is, at -80 cm (for the virtual image) and thus the required focal length is also -80 cm.

105. **D.** The power in diopters is equal to the reciprocal of the focal length in *meters*. Thus:

$P = 1/f$. Then $f = 1/P = -1/4$ meter $= -0.25$ m
or $f = -25$ cm.

106. **A.** The coolant is compressed to form a liquid and becomes warm. The heat is dissipated by a fan. Then the pressure is released from the liquid, allowing its conversion to a gas. This conversion requires heat, the heat of vaporization. It draws heat from surrounding materials.

107. **B.** The transition temperature from solid to liquid should be the same without regard to the direction from which it is approached.

108. **D.** Sublimation is the process of a solid becoming a gas without an intervening liquid.

109. **A.** Increased pressure increases the boiling point.

110. **B.** The critical temperature is the highest temperature at which a gas may be condensed by imposition of high pressure.

111. **B.** Velocity varies in linear fashion with variation of substrate in the area of point A. In this area, the reaction is first order with respect to substrate.

112. **A.** In the area where point B is located, there is no significant change in velocity with a change in substrate. This is zero order with respect to substrate.

113. **C.** At point C the reciprocal substrate concentration is zero, and the substrate concentration would be infinite. Obviously this point cannot be determined by laboratory measurement but must be extrapolated from other data.

114. **B.** The ordinate is reciprocal velocity, and the reciprocal of reciprocal velocity is velocity. Because this extrapolated point corresponds to the reciprocal of infinite substrate, it also will correspond to the reciprocal of maximum velocity.

115. **D.** Point B represents essentially maximum velocity and point C represents the reciprocal of maximum velocity. The zero order portion of the first graph (encompassing point B) does show some change, and it is somewhat difficult to ascertain at what point maximum velocity has been attained.

116. **B.** The three phases will exist together only at the triple point, point 2.

117. **B.** To raise the temperature without changing the pressure, one would proceed on a horizontal line to the right. Such a line intersects the phase transition line for liquid/gas at point 7.

118. **D.** Proceeding vertically toward the top of the diagram, no phase transition from the existing solid phase is indicated.

119. **A.** No liquid can exist above point 1, regardless of the pressure.

120. **C.** The transition from liquid to gas indicates the boiling temperature at the indicated pressure.

121. **A.** This is the definition of equilibrium constant. Note that the coefficients in the reaction equation become exponents in the equilibrium equation.

122. **B.** When the resultants on the right are written in the numerator, a small number such as this indicates that the reaction as written will be favored to go toward the left.

123. **A.** Five moles of gas are being converted to two moles of gas. Increased pressure will improve reaction toward the right, thus relieving the pressure (Principle of LeChatelier).

124. **C.** At STP, a mole of any gas occupies 22.4 liters. Three moles times 22.4 liters equals 67.2 liters.

125. **D.** Equilibrium constant indicates the concentrations at equilibrium. It does not deal with the rate in reaching equilibrium.

126. **A.** Knowing the atomic weight of hydrogen as 1.0 and oxygen at 16.0, the simplest proportions are one H and one O. Thus, the empirical formula is HO.

127. **B.** The empirical formula has only a molecular weight of 17.0. Because the true molecular weight is determined as 34.0, the molecular formula must be a multiple, in this case H_2O_2.

128. **B.** $H_2O_2 \rightleftharpoons H_2O + O_2$ (unbalanced)
Note that we have two hydrogen atoms on each side. However, we have two oxygen atoms on the left side and three on the right.

We may try to balance by multiplying H_2O and H_2O_2 by two. We now have
$$2 H_2O_2 \rightleftharpoons 2 H_2O + O_2$$
and find that this is balanced. As written, one mole of H_2O_2 will produce only 0.5 mole of O_2.

129. **C.** The balanced equation indicates two moles of H_2O_2 will produce two moles of H_2O or one mole of H_2O_2 will produce one mole of H_2O.

130. **C.** As noted above, one mole of H_2O_2 will produce 0.5 mole of O_2. Because one mole of any gas occupies a volume of 22.4 liters at S.T.P., 0.5 mole will occupy 11.2 liters.

131. **B.**
$$\overset{34}{2 H_2O_2} \rightleftharpoons \underset{68}{} 2 H_2O + \overset{x}{\underset{36}{O_2}}$$
$$\frac{34}{68} = \frac{x}{36}$$
$$x = \frac{(36)(34)}{68} = 18.$$

132. **C.** The LeChatelier principle indicates that if a system in equilibrium experiences a change in conditions, chemical reaction will occur to shift the equilibrium and reduce the effect of the changed conditions. Even if reactants and products are all in the gaseous state, there are two moles on the left side and three moles on the right side. Increased pressure would be expected to shift an equilibrium to the left.

133. **C.** If an equilibrium exists, there is an equilibrium constant. Addition of one or more products without changing conditions otherwise will not change the equilibrium constant, but the concentrations of reactants and other products must adjust to maintain the equilibrium constant.

134. **B.** See above. The equilibrium constant would not be affected.

135. **D.** Although it is expected that this would be a first order reaction (rate = k $[H_2O_2]$) it cannot be predicted with certainty. The order of the reaction must be determined on the basis of experimental evidence.

136.   **D.**   A catalyst is defined as a substance that increases the velocity of a chemical reaction. They are not consumed.

137.   **A.**   *Hypertonic:* the solution has a higher osmotic pressure than the solution with which it is compared. There is a higher concentration of solute and a lower concentration of solvent. *Hypotonic:* a lower concentration of solute and a higher concentration of solvent are present. *Isotonic:* both solutions have the same osmotic pressure.

138.   **C.**   One mole of any compound contains 6.02×10^{23} molecules. Two moles of carbon dioxide would contain one mole of molecules more than that contained by one mole of oxygen.

139.   **A.**   Acid salts are formed by di- and tribasic acids. For example, H_2CO_3 can form the acid salt ($NaHCO_3$) known as sodium hydrogen carbonate or sodium bicarbonate.

140.   **D.**   NaOH may be called a base because it produces OH^- ions, but it is more properly called a base because it consumes H^+ ions.

141.   **C.**   The thermal decomposition of $KClO_3$ to produce oxygen will occur if the temperature is sufficiently high. The addition of a catalyst MnO_2 will decrease the activation energy and increase the rate at a lower temperature.

142.   **B.**   See explanation for question 141.

WRITING SAMPLE

Part 1, Essay

The definition of a wise man generated by this quote hinges on the interpretation of the words "ought" and "can." These words, however, as well as "see," remain ambiguous out of context, thus permitting opposing definitions of a "wise man." If "ought" is taken as a limitation of "can," that is if the wise man sees only what he should or is obliged to see, then the quote takes on overtones of pragmatism. The wise man, or man who would be happy, does not see further than he ought. He sees less than he "can" or could. To see all he is capable of seeing would be unwise, perhaps because seeing all would be painful or would necessitate prying. He could find out more but sees only that which is his business. The wise man limits even his perception to avoid painful realities.

On first reading, the quote seems to imply some such limited wisdom, perhaps because the shades of meaning in "ought" and "can" have changed over time. Repulsed by the definition of wisdom generated by this interpretation, one might be driven to reverse the relative magnitude of the terms "ought" and "can." What a wise man ought to see is more than what he can see. He must go beyond what is obvious or visible. The implication here is that the wise man looks beyond or below the surface of perceptible reality. "See" begins to take on shades of meaning akin to "understand" or "infer" beyond superficial perception. The obligation implied by "ought" becomes an obligation to extend rather than an obligation to limit. This second wise man, to be wise, must either dig for more information (things he "ought" to see) or use intuition to understand more than he can see. Without further information on the context of the quote, two possible and opposing wise men remain.

Situations in which the pragmatic position does not apply can be found in psychology. If one believes that unconscious urges or forgotten traumas can have harmful effects on the individual, the wise man might be advised to "see" more than he "can." A man might, for example, have difficulty relating to authority figures who, judging by what he "can" see, restrict him unfairly. If he can "dig down" to or be made to see oedipal impulses underlying the perception of oppression, he may become better able to respond to authority in a prudent, less self-defeating manner. Seeing only what one ought may also have parallels in jurisprudence, where a judge sometimes suppresses information. A decision reached based on the visible, limited facts may then be different (not to mention wrong) from a conclusion based on what one ought to have seen beyond what could be seen. This analogy, if true, argues that if one only attends to what he can see he may be misled. The other wise man, the one who sees more than he "can," may have a less assailable position. Perhaps, the pragmatic wise man is the best example of a situation in which limited wisdom is advisable. It is arguable that seeing too much is painful and potentially harmful. A man might travel to study different cultures only to be more and more sickened by the pain and misery he finds everywhere. One could argue, I suppose, that he would have been wiser, that is happier, less potentially misanthropic, had he limited his vision.

In my mind there are no conditions under which vision or perception or understanding should be limited, if wisdom is the goal. According to the pragmatic reading of the quote, seeing all one can is a mistake, but I would argue limited wisdom is self-contradictory. The truly wise man is one who sees not only all he "can," but what he "ought" as well. In other words, his vision intuits or infers beyond the visible. The wise man and the happy man may inhabit mutually exclusive positions due to the potential pain involved in seeing too far into oneself or others. However, pleasure and the avoidance of pain should not be used as conditions for defining wisdom.

Part 1
Explanation of First Response: 5

The paper focuses on the statement and addresses the three writing tasks. The most difficult task in writing this essay is the first: explaining what Montaigne's quotation actually means. This essay confronts the difficulty squarely, making it clear that one's interpretation of the quotation depends very much on the meanings of the words "ought" and "can." The irony is that "ought" in one sense could be considered a weaker word than "can"; but in another it is stronger. The essay suggests that one must conclude that two entirely different wise men emerge from the quotation depending on the way in which "ought" is defined. Paragraph two, then, moves to the task of providing specific situations in which the two different wise men see as much as they ought and then as much as they should. The example taken from the psychology of unconscious motivation is appropriate and the analogy using judge and jury is particularly imaginative. Finally the essay confronts the ambiguities and paradoxes raised when one considers Montaigne's quotation by taking the stand that a wise man never limits his vision. And ultimately, the essay concludes, wisdom should not be defined in terms simply of pleasure or the avoidance of pain.

This essay provides a sensitive insight into a difficult quotation. The introduction is tightly reasoned; the writing is clear. Paragraph two brings the essay down into the realm of the concrete in its use of unconscious motives and of the judge-jury examples. Because the subject is so highly philosophical, this essay would be strengthened by the use of more concrete details, both in paragraphs one and two. The final paragraph, in which the essay winds down nicely, would especially benefit from a well-chosen concrete illustration. The addition of such specific details would elevate the rating of this essay rating from 5 to 6.

Part 2, Essay

History exists, according to Emerson, only as a document tracing the events of men. Without people, there can be no history. Therefore, history is not a recording of events, but of the men who participated in them. The history of the Cathedral at Chartres does not concern itself primarily with the building, not its stones, its ironworks, its bells. The history of the Cathedral at Chartres focuses on the men who designed and built it, who worshipped and died in it, who tended their flocks in its walls. It is their history, and the history of these men is biography.

If it is true that by definition history is necessarily biography, then the events must take second place to the individuals. After all, biography is typically a document showing how the events have shaped the individual. Is history about the individual? It is not. True, history without the human element is dead, but history enjoys a longer continuum than the life of those it influences, and those influenced by it. History is about eras, thoughts, and ages. The Age of Reason is neither a biography of Rousseau, nor a story with those who believed the tenets as the main characters. It is about the events that took place during the time. History encompasses wars, art, politics, science, and philosophy. No biography can encompass all this. History is a larger container than just the human beings. It must hold many men, many actions, both intended and accidental. History records mistakes, quirks, even coincidences and accidents. So, the history of the Cathedral at Chartres is not about Abbot Sugar or King Louis, it is larger than that. Like the stones, the cathedral's history is longer than the life of man, for the stones live longer than an abbot or king. The space is larger than the area taken up by the bodies it encompasses. It holds many ages of men, their thoughts, errors, treasons, and hopes. No, history cannot be biography, for biography is only a part of history. There are no biographies of stones and ideas, of errors and wars; there are only biographies of men.

But who shaped and stacked the stones? From whom do the errors, ideas, and reasons come? Though one man cannot live as long as a cathedral, the cathedral is nothing but a pile of stones and shards of glass without man and his God to give it meaning. Eras are eras of Man, and the Age of Reason reflects a change of thinking in the minds of man. For if we think of history as biography, we must think of Man as opposed to men. Emerson believed that Man and nature were inextricably entwined. Man and his consciousness were part stone, part God, part evil, part time. Though one man's story cannot be history, Man's story, Man's biography, certainly can, and this story is what we call history. History, then, redefines biography. This definition of biography is not about us as the limited creatures we are as individuals so much as it is about the limitless, encompassing Man as a unified whole. The stones are part of Man, and when labeled as Cathedral and joined to religion, the stones become more of Man. The history of the stones and of the space are then the history of Man, and that, true, is biography.

Part 2
Explanation of Second Response: 5

The essay focuses on the topic defined by Emerson's statement and addresses the three writing tasks. Paragraph one explains Emerson's idea that "there is properly no history; only biography" and illustrates the explanation with a concrete reference to the Cathedral at Chartres. The second paragraph explores in detail the other side of the issue, arguing through historical references that there is, indeed, history independent of biography. The final paragraph presents a balanced consideration of the relation between biography and history, concluding finally that the history of Man, not of men, is biography.

The first section of the essay uses an interesting rhetorical strategy: that of paraphrasing Emerson's statement in such a way that the paraphrases become premises leading to the conclusion that "Therefore, history is not a recording of events, but of the men who participated in them." Some will argue that Emerson's statement is not saying "without people, there can be no history" (the essay's second premise), and thus some will question the foundation of the essay from the beginning. A simple qualifier, such as "perhaps," would strengthen the logic. The second paragraph provides an eloquent defense of the idea that there is indeed history that includes more than biography. It does so by extending the example of the Cathedral at Chartres used in paragraph one and by citing various historical eras and ages. The essay's final paragraph brings the point back to Emerson's assertion and balances it by introducing the concept of the history of Man, a creative solution to the task of exploring the circumstances that determine the relationship between history and biography.

The writing in this essay is clear, and it flows nicely from sentence to sentence. The essay could use a clear transition leading into paragraph two. This is the paragraph that reverses the position explained in paragraph one, and the reader could use help in getting into that position. The essay is rich in concrete details. Especially effective is the extended reference to the Cathedral at Chartres. If this paper had led the reader more smoothly from one task to the next, and if the logic in the first several sentences were tightened, the paper would receive a rating of 6.

BIOLOGICAL SCIENCES

143–148.   (143-B) (144-A) (145-C) (146-D) (147-A) (148-B)   Let us identify the components of the neuron numbered: (2) nucleus with nucleolus, containing the genetic material of the cell and directing the synthetic activity of the cell; (3) Golgi apparatus (zone), the packaging and concentrating area of the cell's secretory activity; (4) dendrites; dendrites are the processes that pick up an impulse and carry it towards the cell body; (5) endoplasmic reticulum (rough in this case—ribosomes are attached), the synthetic machinery of the cell (proteins etc.,); (6) cell membrane, semipermeable and the protector of the cell from its environment; (7) cytoplasm (specifically the area here is called the axon hillock); (8) myelin sheath (Schwann cell covered by its neurilemma, the insulator of the axon); (1) direction of conduction of an impulse; axon (10a) and (10b) conducts impulses away from the dendrites to the function with the dendrites of another neuron. The junction point is known as the synaptic area; the impulse can cross the synapse only from the axon to the dendrite and no backflow is permitted; (11) terminal branches of the axon. In a lesion (cut) the process distal from the cell body would completely degenerate; retrograde degeneration would be detected in the proximal portion and the cell body, however, the proximal portion has the capacity and will regenerate.

149.   **C.**   Because glucose is absorbed at a faster rate than xylose, due to both passive and active transport, then as the glucose is absorbed, water follows. The transport system for glucose is working maximally as indicated by the initial concentration of glucose being 50 times the apparent Km of transport.

150.   **D.**   A 1.8% solution contains 1.8 g/100 ml of solution. This is 1,800 mg/100 ml, which is 18 mg/ml. For the recovery of 1.8 mg, this represents $(1.8/18 \times 100)$ a 10% recovery meaning that 90% has been metabolized or transported out of the lumen of the intestine.

151.   **D.**   Hemoglobin is a large (64,000 MW) molecule. Because the gut was ligated below the pancreas and proteolytic enzymes present were washed out, no digestion of the protein could occur. Large molecules are not readily transported across cell membranes. Due to the vast surface area of the small intestine with its many microvilli, some of the protein would be adsorbed on this surface and visible through the heme prosthetic group color.

152. **D.** All are correct. I. D-galactose is transported by the same carrier as glucose, therefore, by addition of galactose, a competition for transport between glucose and galactose occurs. II. The transport carrier is sodium ion selective. A larger cation, while having the appropriate charges, does not fit the selective carrier. III. The carrier is specific for the D-glucose; L-glucose would be transported by passive diffusion only. IV. Because the carrier is an energy requiring process, by limiting the supply of ATP, the transport is decreased.

153. **A.** A 25% solution of $MgSO_4$ is hypertonic. Neither Mg nor SO_4 ions are readily transported so the net effect is a water flow into the lumen becoming an isotonic solution.

154. **B.** Hemoglobin is not absorbed and an aqueous solution is not isotonic. Assuming that the hemoglobin is not ionized, a $0.3\ M$ solution would have to have $64,000 \times 0.3$ g/liter. This solution must be hypotonic, which can be only modified by water flow out of the lumen.

155–157. **(155-B) (156-C) (157-C)** The answers can be found in the flow diagram of the question. Thyroid hormones (T_3 and T_4) are iodothyronines. The union of iodine and tyrosine is called iodination, and the active thyroid principal is protein-bound during transport to the target organs.

158. **D.** Hyperthyriodism, hypothyroidism, and euthyroidism can be associated with goiter. In hyperthyroidism, thyroxin is released into the bloodstream at a rate exceeding needs. BMR accelerates resulting in rapid pulse and respiration, increased appetite with concomitant weight loss, nervousness, and protruding eyes. If not treated, goiter and thyroid exhaustion can occur; treatment involves antithyroid drugs or thyroidectomy. The opposite, hypothyroidism, exhibits a gland that cannot meet secretory demands; the body's metabolic rate is depressed and symptoms are the reverse of the above cited. When hypothyroidism occurs during childhood, a cretin is the result; mental retardation and stunted growth are features. Treatment requires administration of thyroid hormone. Goiter simply means enlargement of the gland and can be present in the normal (euthyroid) state.

159. **A.** Thyroid stimulating hormone produced by the basophils of the anterior pituitary is a glycoprotein made up of two peptide chains (alpha and beta). Certain regions of the hypothalamus have a neuroendocrine function because neurosecretory cells release hormones that affect anterior pituitary function. TRH secreted by the hypothalamus reaches the pituitary via the hypophyseal-portal circulation and elicits TSH production. Thyroxin binds to TBG. Exposure to cold would elicit a compensatory increase in BMR and, hence, thyroid activity.

160. **D.** Also see explanations for questions 158 and 159. Control of thyroid principal is via the pituitary. TSH stimulates the thyroid to produce thyroxin; its release is related to levels in the bloodstream. Low levels increase TSH and thyroxin release, but as levels rise to normal and above, further production and release of TSH is curtailed and thyroxin production falls. This feedback system maintains balance.

161. **C.** See explanations for questions 158–160.

162. **A.** The effect of repeated close-spaced stimuli is that a summation occurs: each contraction is somewhat larger than the preceding one.

163. **C.** ATP continues to be supplied in adequate amounts, even during the period of loss of contraction ability (fatigue). Some link between the stimulating event and the responding event (sliding of actins over myosins), however, gradually becomes less efficient.

164. **B.** During the summation period each new stimulus arrives before the preceding twitch can reach the relaxation period, and elastic elements in the muscle become stretched without rebounding to their original shape. The muscle eventually reaches a steady state of nearly full contraction (region 2), when all elastic elements are fully stretched.

165. **A.** When a volley of stimuli is applied to a muscle, each succeeding stimulus may arrive before the muscle can completely relax from the contraction caused by the preceding stimulus. The result is summation, an increased strength of contraction. If the frequency of stimulation is very fast, individual contractions fuse and the muscle smoothly and fully contracts. This is a tetanus.

166. **D.** The word contraction refers to those processes that are manifested externally by either a shortening of a muscle or by tension development in a muscle. If the muscle length is held constant, the contraction is referred to as an isometric contraction. In an isometric contraction, the passive tension remains constant with the active tension being added to it to produce the total tension of the muscle. If the muscle shortens during contraction, it is called an isotonic contraction and the total tension remains constant.

167. **C.** The drug most closely resembles PHT (phenytoin) in terms of its high efficacy in the electroshock model of tonic-clonic seizures and its adequate efficacy in the kindling model of partial complex seizures. **A**, though not completely incorrect, is not the best answer. PHT, the drug this experimental agent AntiEpp acts most like, is not effective in the audiogenic mouse model of myoclonic seizures, which is also a form of generalized convulsive seizures. **D** is also incorrect for this reason. The better answer is **C**.

168. **B.** Ethosuximide is the only drug that is exclusively effective against the animal model of absence seizures. **A** is incorrect because carbamazepine has highest efficacy in the kindling model and in partial complex seizures. **C** is incorrect because valproic acid shows some degree of efficacy in all seizure models and the corresponding clinical conditions. Again, Compound X, like ethosuximide, shows efficacy only against the GABA challenge model of absence seizures. Given the premise that investigational compounds are selected in part because of a chemical nature similar to presently used compounds, there is enough information to respond that this agent is "probably most similar" to ethosuximide. So **D** is also incorrect.

169. **C.** It is stated that 1 in 200 persons suffer from epilepsy in the United States and that there are 7 million persons in New York City. Thus, the correct answer can be derived as follows:

$$\frac{1}{200} = \frac{X}{7,000,000} \text{ or rearranging,}$$

$$X = \frac{(7,000,000)\ (1)}{200} \text{ or } X = 35,000$$

This can be calculated more rapidly in your head realizing that:

$$\frac{1}{200} = \frac{.5}{100} = \frac{5}{1,000} = \frac{50}{10,000} = \frac{500}{100,000} =$$

$$\frac{5,000}{1,000,000} \text{ or } \frac{35,000}{7,000,000}$$

A or **D** reflect a mathematical mistake. **B** is the probable number of yearly deaths from status epilepticus.

170. **C.** Status epilepticus is defined in the first paragraph of the passage as a seizure that persists for over 30 minutes. A partial seizure emanates from a restricted region. This woman's seizure is described as having lasted for "over an hour" and was observed on the electroencephalogram as "localized only to a restricted region." Thus, "partial status epilepticus" is the *best* answer. **A**, status epilepticus is correct but does not fully describe the patient's condition. Neither does partial complex seizure (**D**). Finally, generalized seizures, you are told, arise from the entire brain simultaneously. Again, this woman's seizure is restricted or partial. For this reason, **B** is incorrect.

171. **B.** The reading passage states that there are approximately 1.2 million persons with epilepsy in the United States. It also indicates that 25% of patients with epilepsy continue to have seizures at least once per month. So, the correct answer is generated by taking 25% of 1.2 million, or

$$0.25 \times 1,200,000 = 300,000$$

A, 30,000 represents a mathematical mistake. So does **D**, 250,000. **C**, ¼ million, is just another way of saying 250,000 and is also incorrect.

172. **B.** It is the purpose of this experiment to determine the sequence of events in cells stimulated to undergo mitosis, and to compare the data to those gathered from unstimulated cells.

173. **A.** Analysis of the graphs clearly shows that RNA synthesis precedes increased protein synthesis; at around 17 hours they are equal and RNA continues to drop, whereas protein synthesis increases.

174. **D.** It is safe to assume that unstimulated lymphocytes synthesize RNA, DNA, and protein at a low rate. One of the premier functions of DNA is the production of RNA; most RNA is

produced in the nucleus. DNA determines and acts as a template for RNA synthesis. With the help of a transcription enzyme (RNA polymerase), a complimentary RNA strand is produced; once produced it moves into the cytoplasm.

175. **B.** The cell is the basic unit of structure and function and the basis of all life; all cells come from preexisting cells.

176. **B.** A complete set of chromosomes ($2n$) is passed on to each daughter cell as a result of mitotic cell division. Cells that are produced mitotically are genetically alike.

177. **C.** Messenger RNA (mRNA) from the nucleus brings the coded message for protein synthesis to ribosomes in the cytoplasm.

178. **C.** Mitosis is divided into:
    (1) prophase—chromosomes become distinct and nucleoli disappear; centrioles, asters, and spindle appear; nuclear membrane disappears.
    (2) metaphase—chromosomes move to equator of cell.
    (3) anaphase—the two chromatids split apart and start migration toward the poles of the spindle, and the spindle loses its definition.
    (4) telophase—chromosomes lengthen and become less distinct and nucleoli reappear.
    (5) interphase—cell growth, protein + DNA synthesis, and chromosomes duplicate.

179. **B.** During metaphase of mitosis, the centrioles with asters are at the opposite poles; the chromosomes move to the equator of the cell. Also see explanation for question 178.

180. **D.** Nuclei have the highest DNA concentration among cellular organelles. The DNA in fraction 3 is in mitochondria.

181. **C.** Cytochrome oxidase is the enzyme complex that transfers electrons from the mitochondrial electron transport chain to oxygen and is therefore located in mitochondria.

182. **A.** Most of the RNA found in a mature cell is ribosomal RNA, and the cytoplasmic ribosomal RNA in a hepatocyte should occur in a mixture of free ribosomes and rough endoplasmic reticulum. Because only one peak of RNA occurred at the top of the gradient, fraction 1 must contain both free and membrane-bound ribosomes and therefore contains the rough endoplasmic reticulum. The RNA in fraction 3 probably represents ribosomes in mitochondria. The RNA in fraction 4 is probably partially assembled ribosomes in the nucleoli in the nuclei.

183. **B.** Acid phosphatase is a lysosomal enzyme and occurred only in fraction 2 among the choices.

184. **A.** Cytochrome P-450 is involved in detoxification reactions in smooth endoplasmic reticulum and only occurred in fraction 1 among the choices.

185. **C.** Krebs cycle enzymes are located in the mitochondria and should therefore occur in the same fractions that contain cytochrome oxidase activity.

186. **A.** Plasma proteins are secreted proteins and therefore should be made on the rough endoplasmic reticulum in fraction 1.

187. **A.** A cell that secretes large amounts of protein (such as a pancreatic exocrine cell) should contain large arrays of rough endoplasmic reticulum, which would increase fraction 1. Secretory granules could increase fraction 2 or fraction 3, but the assays used would not detect pancreatic enzymes or their contribution to a fraction.

188. **B.** Phagocytic cells, such as monocytes or macrophages, contain large numbers of lysosomes that would contribute to the acid phosphatase activity measured in fraction 2.

189. **C.** Proximal convoluted tubule lining cells contain large numbers of mitochondria that supply the large amounts of energy needed to support the active transport used for resorption of solutes from urine. High numbers of mitochondria should increase fraction 3.

190. **D.** Two moles of carbon dioxide formed and 12 ATP formed per mole of acetyl CoA. The reactions produce three moles of NADH

and one mole of $FADH_2$. Reoxidation of these coenzymes in the respiratory assembly will produce three ATP/NADH and two ATP/$FADH_2$. The remaining one ATP is a substrate level phosphorylation of GDP to GTP by succinyl CoA. GTP can phosphorylate ADP to ATP.

191. **B.** The reaction acetyl CoA to pyruvate does not occur. This is one of the reasons that we cannot make (net) glucose from acetyl CoA. Choice **D** shows two very similar reactions of oxidative decarboxylation. The same coenzymes, mechanism, and release of CO_2 occur. Choice **A** indicates both oxidations of a secondary alcohol. The product, oxalosuccinate, spontaneously decarboxylates due to the instability of the keto acid formed to yield alpha ketoglutarate. Choice **C** indicates both hydration reactions.

192. **A.** For the citric acid cycle to function, as acetyl CoA is catabolized it reacts with oxaloacetate to form citrate. In specific reactions, CO_2 is lost and oxaloacetate is regenerated. Oxaloacetate may be considered catalytic for the cycle. Oxaloacetate plus acetyl CoA forms $2 CO_2$ and oxaloacetate. **B** is a true statement in that the synthesis of fatty acids in the cytoplasm occurs through this step. **C** is also true because the first step in the synthesis of the porphyrin ring (heme) occurs from succinyl CoA. The last two choices are also true because transamination from these keto acids (using some other amino acids as the amino group donor) results in the formation of the specific amino shown.

193. **D.** Net synthesis of glucose does not take place because the reaction pyruvate to acetyl CoA is not reversible under physiological conditions and also because for every acetyl CoA condensing with oxaloacetate, $2 CO_2$ is formed. Choice **A** is true because specific enzymes of the pathway are inhibited by high levels of ATP (citrate synthase) or stimulated by low levels of ADP (isocitrate dehydrogenase). Choice **B** is correct. One control of the glycolytic pathway has citrate as a negative effector (phosphofructokinase). Choice **C** is a true statement. The citric acid cycle is the final metabolic pathway for many metabolites.

194. **A.** The red blood cell (mature RBC) does not contain mitochondria where the citric acid cycle takes place; see **B.** Choice **C** is true; for

every acetyl CoA (two per glucose mole) 12 ATP are formed. Substrate level phosphorylation (GTP + ADP to ATP + GDP) form one and reoxidation of reducing equivalents in oxidative phosphorylation forms 11 ATP. When acetyl CoA levels are high, several things can happen: (1) the citric acid cycle may be maximal (depends on ATP needs); (2) fatty acids may be synthesized; (3) ketone bodies may be formed; (4) gluconeogenesis is stimulated because the enzyme pyruvate carboxylase requires high levels to activate it for the synthesis of net oxaloacetate from pyruvate and CO_2. Eventually glucose may be formed anew from the pyruvate (gluconeogenesis).

195. **B.** L-amino acids are those coded for translation into proteins. D-amino acids are rare, although found in some bacteria. All of the amino acids with one exception, glycine, are optically active. This is a physical property that molecules may have when they are chiral.

196. **C.** In contrast to the amino acids, all of the main carbohydrates are of the D configuration. Notable exceptions are some L sugars found in blood group glycoproteins, such as L-fucose.

197. **B.** Diastereomers (diastereo-isomers) are not mirror images (enantiomers) and have different chemical, physical, and biological properties. If the question had asked D-glucose and D-galactose, the answer would be **D.** That is, they are both epimers and diastereomers.

198. **D.** D-galactose is an epimer at C4 of glucose, and D-mannose is an epimer at C2 of glucose. D-fructose is a keto hexose and has similar OH configuration to D-glucose at C atoms 3, 4, 5.

199. **D.** One may compare D-glyceraldehyde to D-glucose. It is as if the three carbon atom difference were by addition to the C-1 of glyceraldehyde.

200. **D.** Pyruvate is formed from the high energy compound phosphoenolpyruvate catalyzed by the enzyme pyruvate kinase. As NADH builds up from an earlier step, the keto acid pyruvate is reduced to the hydroxy-acid lactate. Choice **A** is the first product formed in all cells that metabolize glucose. Carbon dioxide (**B**) is not produced in the glycolytic pathway. Acetyl

CoA (**C**) is formed in mitochondria from pyruvate by the pyruvate dehydrogenase complex.

201. **D.** The glycolytic pathway takes place in the cytoplasm. The first step, glucose to glucose-6-phosphate, is catalyzed by a kinase and uses ATP to phosphorylate glucose.

202. **D.** Choice **A** requires ATP, whereas **B** and **C** are substrate level phosphorylations (ADP + high energy phosphate to give ATP).

203. **C.** The enzyme glucose-6-phosphate dehydrogenase, the first enzyme in the hexosemonophosphate shunt, catalyzes the oxidation to 6-phosphogluconate and the reduction of $NADP^+$ to NADPH. Red cell lysis occurs for a number of different reasons, including changes in hemoglobin, such as the oxidation of ferrous ion to ferric ion (which does not carry oxygen). Failure to maintain a reduced cell membrane results in a cell that does not fit through capillaries. Pyruvate is reduced to lactate by NADH.

204. **D.** After the formation of pentose phosphate, further catabolism produces common intermediates, such as glyceraldehyde-3-P, and fructose-6-phosphate provide an interchange between these two pathways. Only the hexose monophosphate shunt produces carbon dioxide in the red blood cell. This occurs by oxidation of 6-phosphogluconate to reduce $NADP^+$. The oxidized product is decarboxylated to a pentose phosphate and carbon dioxide. Another name for the hexose monophosphate shunt is the pentose pathway.

205. **C.** Except for statement **C**, all of the others are supported by the evidence. To infer that the experimenters should have paid closer attention to body weights is not supported because the greatest difference between the six groups (8 animals/group) was 8 grams, organ weights were corrected for body weight, and organ weights/g body weight do not appear to vary with body weight.

206. **B.** This study was designed to determine what vitamins were missing from diet A. The data indicated that diet A lacked the B vitamins. Thiamine (B_1) is essential for the proper functioning of the nervous system; deficiency will result in beriberi. Riboflavin (B_2) converts tryptophan to nicotinic acid; general problems

with vision, skin, coordination, and growth can occur. In the experiment, the difference between the percentage losing weight and percentage mortality within each group is best explained by individual variation among mice within each group.

207. **B.** Acidophils (alpha cells) of the pituitary secrete somatotropic hormone (STH, growth hormone), which stimulates generalized body growth. Hypersecretion before ossification is complete results in giantism, whereas thereafter, acromegaly is the consequence. Hyposecretion leads to dwarfism. Our assay had to be conducted on hypophysectomized rats because the pituitary produces growth hormone that might interfere with the assay.

208. **D.** The purpose of this experiment was to observe X ray effect on growth. X rays can be lethal; they are used in combination with chemotherapy to treat certain malignant growths. The table also shows that plants exposed to 24,000 r units exhibit a marked effect; growth from the cotyledon to the first node was greatly decreased. This was the part most affected; the midrib lengths were not affected.

209. **D.** Because the Y-chromosome always passes from father to son, all male offspring (half of the total, on average) have the father's Y-chromosome. If the gene is dominant, all males will exhibit the trait. Female offspring could not, because they get the father's X-chromosome, not the Y.

210. **D.** Melanoma is a malignancy. The data shows that an Ag A phenotype containing three seems to be related to higher antibody production. If one possesses a 1/3 Ag A phenotype, the mouse resulting from a cross of Strain 2 with one of Strain 3 would probably be a better antibody producer than a sibling having a 1/1 Ag A phenotype. Statements **A** and **C** are clearly contradicted by the data, whereas statement **B** is neither contradicted nor supported.

211. **D.** Statement **C** is neither supported nor contradicted by the data. Statement **D** is contradicted by the evidence because even after 90–100% resurfacing, an endothelial labeling index of 2.5% is exhibited. Statements **A** and **B** are supported by the information presented.

212. **D.** The actions of LH and FSH in the male on the testes are to promote androgen secretion

and spermatogenesis. Androgenic actions of testosterone are: (1) maintenance of secondary sex organs; (2) promotion of secondary sex characteristics (size of genitalia, voice, muscle development, and hair distribution); (3) normal development of body growth and psychological balance. The statement (**D**) that bilateral castration removes a major source of sex hormones is clearly the only one supported by the experiment; all others are contradicted.

213. **D.** Thyroid hormone controls the rate of metabolism, growth, maturation, and differentiation of the organism, and it influences nervous system activity. All the statements are consistent with the information and are true concerning thyroid activity. The quantity of heat liberated is decreased by deficiencies and elevated by excesses of thyroxin; after thyroidectomy the basal metabolic rate drops, and animals probably exhibit sluggishness and slight obesity.

214. **A.** It is obvious that because bacteria Z could grow following exposure to temperatures below 160°C, it cannot be destroyed in autoclave 1.

215. **A.** The testes of blinded hamsters weighed 1695 mg/100 g of body weight if no MTPH was given. Application of MTPH reduced the weight to 1419 mg/100 g, indicating increased atrophy.

216. **A.** Conversion of glycogen to glucose-1-phosphate is catalyzed by the enzyme, phosphorylase. Pancreatic amylase is usually not in contact with glycogen (except dietary glycogen); in any case it would not catalyze the formation of glucose-1-phosphate.

217. **C.** Production of glucose and fructose from sucrose and production of fatty acids and glycerol from triglycerides are both simple hydrolytic reactions in which essentially no energy is gained or lost. Production of steroids from acetate (as is true with most synthetic reactions) requires energy input. Production of CO_2 and water from fatty acids yields large amounts of energy.

218. **D.** A yellow precipitate of iodoform is produced in this reaction with methyl ketones, alcohols that may be oxidized to methyl ketones, or acetaldehyde.

219. **C.** We have described conditions for the formation of a diazonium salt and then replacement of the diazonium salt by Br to produce monobromobenzene. (The replacement is known as the Sandmeyer reaction.) The intermediate diazonium salt is often unstable at room temperature, so a lower temperature is used.

SCORING OF THE MCAT

A report of the results of your performance on the MCAT is sent to you, to the medical schools selected, and, with your agreement, to your Premedical Advisor, usually within six to eight weeks of taking the exam.

The score sheet will list the results of each of the four subtests. The score for the three multiple-choice subtests (but not the Writing Sample) is based on the number of correct answers. (Thus, guessing wrong will not induce a lowering of the score.)

The scores for three of the subtests—physical sciences, biological sciences, and verbal reasoning—are reported on a 1 to 15 scale. These *scaled scores* when reported are converted from *raw* scores (see chart on page 159). (The conversion factor varies with different exams and compensates for minor variations in difficulty between exams.)

The scaled scores earned are best interpreted in relation to the performance of other examinees by means of three data sheets, namely, means (and standard deviations) for each subtest, percentile rank ranges, and percentages of students receiving each scaled score, which are sent along with your scores.

SCORING YOUR MODEL MCAT PERFORMANCE _____

To obtain your score after you have completed the test, check your answers against those in the answer key (see page 140) and total up the number of correct answers in the verbal reasoning, physical sciences, and biological sciences subtests individually. Each of these totals is a *raw score* and has to be converted into a *scaled score*. Conversion is done by use of the table shown below.

Having completed the computation of your scaled scores for each of the three subtests, record them on the score card below.

Subtest	Maximum	Raw Score	Scaled Score
Physical Sciences	15		
Biological Sciences	15		
Verbal Reasoning	15		

A score of 11 or higher can be considered superior, 9 to 11 satisfactory, and 8 or less as deficient, requiring remediation in the relevant area tested. After assessing your performance, adjust your MCAT study plan and schedule appropriately.

The two writing samples will be scored independently by two readers, using a scale of 1 to 6. They will be evaluated on how well the challenge of addressing all three tasks has been met. The depth, clarity, coherence, and expository skill of the applicant will be assessed, and all four grades will be added to give a raw score. This score will be converted to an alphabetic scale whose range is J (lowest) to T (highest).

Verbal Reasoning		Physical Sciences		Biological Sciences	
Raw Score	Scaled Score	Raw Score	Scaled Score	Raw Score	Scaled Score
0–7	1	0–8	1	0–8	1
8–14	2	9–16	2	9–16	2
15–20	3	17–28	3	17–28	3
21–26	4	29–33	4	29–33	4
27–31	5	34–39	5	34–39	5
32–36	6	40–44	6	40–44	6
37–41	7	45–49	7	45–49	7
42–46	8	50–55	8	50–55	8
47–50	9	56–60	9	56–60	9
51–53	10	61–64	10	61–64	10
54–57	11	65–67	11	65–67	11
58–60	12	68–70	12	68–70	12
61–62	13	71–73	13	71–73	13
63–64	14	74–75	14	74–75	14
65	15	76–77	15	76–77	15

Source: *MCAT: How to Prepare for the Medical College Admission Test*, Hugo R. Seibel, Kenneth E. Guyer, et al. © 1997 by Barron's Educational Series. Reprinted with permission.

5 | Medical Schools

Basic data on medical schools

In this chapter you will find Table 5.1, Basic Data on the Medical Schools, which provides numerical data dealing with many school characteristics and serves as a quick source of information and a means for easily comparing features of schools you may be interested in.

BASIC DATA ON MEDICAL SCHOOLS

Table 5.1, Basic Data on the Medical Schools, contains the kind of information that will be useful in helping you decide which schools to apply to. At a glance you can see and compare application data, admissions statistics, academic statistics, and expenses.

Please note that while the information in this table is as up to date and accurate as possible, it is recommended that you check the individual medical school catalogs prior to applying.

For a very small number of schools, data for the 1996–97 year could not be secured. In such cases, which are identified by the symbol # after the school name, 1995–96 data is used. This fact should be borne in mind when using data for these schools.

How To Use This Table

This comprehensive table can help you formulate the initial and final list of medical schools to which you may wish to apply for admission. It will guide you at the outset to the schools located in your own and adjacent states where you may have a special priority (Column 1). It will also provide you with a ready means of identifying those schools that accept large numbers of out-of-state applicants (Column 8), which merit being placed on your list. If you are a woman or a minority group member, you can learn whether you should apply to a particular school by noting Columns 7 and 14, respectively. Assessing your potential academic suitability merely requires checking GPA (Column 11), and MCAT score averages (Column 15). Finally, affordability of a school will be indicated by Columns 17 and 18, which list tuition and other expenses, respectively.

After preparing your preliminary list based on geographical and residency considerations, you should then amend your list by taking into consideration such other factors as GPA, MCAT scores, and tuition. You should be cautioned not to automatically drop schools from the list merely because they are unsuitable in only one respect. In other words, if your GPA is 3.4 and the acceptance mean is 3.6, this by itself does not eliminate you from consideration since the 3.6 represents a mean, indicating that there probably was a range that included the 3.4 level. Similarly, the percentages of women and minorities accepted has to be taken in the context of total class size. Thus, 10% minorities accepted out of a class of 150 is 15, while 20% of a class of only 50 is 10. Finally, what you can afford to spend on the costly interview process needs to come into play when you are finalizing your list. It should prove very helpful when making up your list to refer to the profiles of the schools in Chapter 6.

Definitions

The following are explanations and definitions of the column headings in Table 5.1.

Application Fee

In most cases, this fee is required after your application has passed the initial screening by the medical school. This fee is sent at the time you submit your supplementary application. The preliminary application fee is usually the AMCAS application fee that is paid when submitting the form.

Earliest and Latest Filing Dates

These are usually firm dates.

Number of Applicants

This column gives an idea of how many applications were received for the 1996–97 class.

Applicants Enrolled

The columns indicate the men, women, and out-of-state students accepted for the 1996–97 class. The ratio of the total number of men and women accepted to the total number of applicants gives an indication of the competitive nature of admission at each school.

Class Size

The figures in this column refer to the 1996–97 class.

Percentage with Four Years of College

This shows the relative chances of a third-year student gaining admission.

Percent Interviewed

This indicates the relative importance of being granted an interview at a specific school.

Percent Residents

This indicates the desirability of a student to apply to a specific out-of-state school.

Percent Minorities

This column shows what percentage of the first-year class were members of a minority group.

Mean MCAT Scores

The mean MCAT scores for the three subtests for the 1996 entering class are listed in this column. The subtest abbreviations are P–physical sciences, B–biological sciences, and V–verbal reasoning.

Deposit

This column shows the amount of money that must be sent in to hold a place in the class. It may be applied toward eventual tuition cost and in some cases is refundable.

Tuition

1996–97 tuition costs (annual) for first-year students are given.

Other Expenses

This estimate covers the minimum room and board, fees, and other expenses, excluding microscope costs, for the first year.

Financial Aid

This column indicates the percentage of students receiving financial aid. This is awarded on the basis of demonstrated need in the form of grants, loans, and scholarships. Such financial support is usually available each year for the four-year study sequence. More information is available in Chapter 9.

Table 5.1. BASIC DATA ON THE MEDICAL SCHOOLS 1996–97

School	Fee	Application Data — Filing Dates — Earliest	Latest	Number of Applicants	Applicants Enrolled — Men	Women	Out-of-State	Class Profile — Class Size	% with 4 years College
ALABAMA									
*University of Alabama School of Medicine	$65	6/1**	11/1	2106	112	53	2	167	95
*University of South Alabama College of Medicine	$25	6/1**	11/15	1308	39	25	6	64	100
ARIZONA									
*University of Arizona College of Medicine	$ 0	6/15	11/1	531	49	51	0	100	100
ARKANSAS									
*University of Arkansas for Medical Sciences College of Medicine	$10	7/15	1/15	890	93	46	1	139	98
CALIFORNIA									
*Loma Linda University School of Medicine	$55	6/15**	11/1	4660	103	56	73	159	99
*Stanford University School of Medicine	$55	6/15**	11/1	6800	49	37	n/av	86	100
*University of California— Davis School of Medicine	$40	6/15	11/1	5491	59	34	3	93	93
*University of California— Irvine College of Medicine#	$40	6/1	11/1	5189	52	40	0	92	100
*University of California— Los Angeles—UCLA School of Medicine#	$40	6/1	11/1	6111	77	68	127	145	100
*University of California— San Diego School of Medicine	$40	6/1	11/1	5348	73	49	1	122	100
*University of California— San Francisco School of Medicine#	$40	6/1	11/1	5886	73	68	33	141	100
*University of Southern California School of Medicine	$70	6/1**	11/1	6509	81	69	25	150	100
COLORADO									
*University of Colorado School of Medicine	$70	6/1**	11/15	2700	67	62	24	129	100

```
*        AMCAS school
**       early decision available
#        1995–96 data
n/app    not applicable
n/av     data not available
```

| Mean GPA | Admission Statistics | | | Academic Statistics | Expenses | | | |
| | Class Profile | | | | | | | |
	% Interviewed	% Residents	% Minorities	Mean MCAT	Deposit	Tuition Res/Nonres	Other	% Financial Aid
3.55	26	84	9.7	P-9.7 B-9.9 V-9.8	$ 50	$ 5,780 $17,124	$15,940	75
3.60	17	92	13	P-9.6 B-9.9 V-9.8	$ 50	$ 7,000 $14,000	n/av	n/av
3.55	18	100	24	P-8.6 B-9.3 V-9.4	$ 0	$ 7,360 n/avpp	$ 1,613	85
3.52	50	99	10	P-8.9 B-9.1 V-9.5	$ 0	$ 7,712 $15,424	$ 9,848	75
3.54	10.2	54	7	P-9.6 B-9.8 V-9.5	$100	$23,944 $23,944	$ 7,900	n/av
3.60	7	n/av	11	P-11.4 B-11.7 V-10.3	$ 0	$25,350 $25,350	n/av	83
3.40	n/av	97	n/av	P-11.9 B-11.9 V-11.9	$ 0	$ n/av $ 8,394	$17,976	83
3.53	9	100	21	P-10.4 B-10.7 V-9.2	$ 0	$ 0 $ 7,699	$ 8,282	87
3.64	13	93	33	Required—scores not available	$ 0	$ 0 $ 7,699	$ 7,864	n/av
3.65	11	99	53	P-11.4 B-11.0 V-10.4	$ 0	$ 0 $ 8,394	$ 9,288	77
3.68	9	75	22	P-11.0 B-11.0 V-11.0	$ 0	$ 0 $ 7,699	$ 7,696	n/av
3.47	12	83	21	P-10.5 B-10.7 V-10.0	$100	$27,830 $27,830	$11,032	74
3.60	27	81	14	P-9.9 B-9.9 V-9.9	$200	$10,621 $49,849	$10,000	n/av

Table 5.1. BASIC DATA ON THE MEDICAL SCHOOLS 1996–97—CONTINUED

| School | Fee | Application Data | | Admission Statistics | | | | | |
| | | Filing Dates | | Number of Applicants | Applicants Enrolled | | | Class Profile | |
		Earliest	Latest		Men	Women	Out-of-State	Class Size	% with 4 years College
CONNECTICUT									
*University of Connecticut School of Medicine	$60	6/1	12/15**	3000	43	38	30	81	100
Yale University School of Medicine	$55	6/1**	10/15	3628	43	58	92	101	100
DISTRICT OF COLUMBIA									
*George Washington University School of Medicine and Health Sciences	$55	6/1**	12/1	7267	72	81	n/av	153	100
*Georgetown University School of Medicine#	$60	6/1**	11/1	12,248	96	69	2	165	100
*Howard University College of Medicine	$45	6/1	12/15	5989	53	58	107	111	94
FLORIDA									
*University of Florida College of Medicine#	$20	6/1	12/1	8612	48	37	4	85	100
*University of Miami School of Medicine	$50	6/1**	12/15	2873	71	68	4	139	70
*University of South Florida College of Medicine	$20	6/1**	12/1	1935	65	31	0	96	100
GEORGIA									
*Emory University School of Medicine	$50	6/1	10/15	8277	69	43	56	112	100
*Medical College of Georgia School of Medicine#	$0	6/1**	11/1	1911	115	65	4	180	99
*Mercer University School of Medicine#	$25	6/1**	12/1	1471	35	20	0	55	100
*Morehouse School of Medicine	$45	6/1**	12/1	2928	9	23	7	34	100
HAWAII									
*University of Hawaii John A. Burns School of Medicine#	$50	6/1**	12/1	1631	29	27	3	56	98

*	AMCAS school
**	early decision available
#	1995–96 data
n/app	not applicable
n/av	data not available

	Admission Statistics			Academic Statistics		Expenses		
	Class Profile							
Mean GPA	% Interviewed	% Residents	% Minorities	Mean MCAT	Deposit	Tuition Res/ Nonres	Other	% Financial Aid
3.50	10	90	11	P-10.0 B-10.0 V-10.0	$ 100	$ 8,400 $19,100	$15,390	81
3.60	23	9	17	P-11.2 B-11.5 V-10.7	$ 100	$24,700 $24,700	$13,075	n/av
3.40	14	n/av	16	P-10.0 B-10.0 V-10.0	$2,500	$30,200 $30,200	$ 2,370	n/av
3.58	12	0.8	6	P-10.0 B-10.0 V-10.0	$ 100	$23,625 $23,625	n/av	80
3.10	10	3.6	79	P-8.0 B-8.2 V-7.6	$ 250	$15,500 $15,500	$13,700	84
3.68	16	95	7	P-9.0 B-9.4 V-9.1	$ 0	$ 7,142 $19,522	$ 1,650	n/av
3.61	15	97	12	P-9.4 B-9.9 V-10.0	$ 75	$24,190 $24,190	$10,830	80
3.70	18	100	25	P-10.2 B-10.2 V-9.7	$ 0	$ 7,142 $20,141	$ 1,120	n/av
3.66	10	50	38	P-10.4 B-10.4 V-9.7	$ 0	$22,810 $22,810	$12,840	74
n/av	23	98	22	P-8.0 B-9.4 V-9.7	$ 50	$ 4,755 $14,976	$ 249	n/av
n/av	13	100	7	P-8.0 B-8.6 V-8.9	$ 100	$18,890 $18,890	n/av	80
n/av	8	71	91	P-6.8 B-7.2 V-6.9	$ 100	$16,500 $16,500	$ 1,986	86
3.55	15	96	2	P-8.5 B-9.0 V-8.8	$ 0	$5,996 $21,030	$ 8,700	61

Table 5.1. BASIC DATA ON THE MEDICAL SCHOOLS 1996–97—CONTINUED

School	Fee	Application Data — Filing Dates — Earliest	Latest	Number of Applicants	Admission Statistics — Applicants Enrolled — Men	Women	Out-of-State	Class Profile — Class Size	% with 4 years College
ILLINOIS									
*Chicago Medical School Finch University of Health Sciences	$65	6/1**	12/15	12,760	102	74	60	176	99
*Loyola University Chicago Stritch School of Medicine	$50	6/1**	11/15	10,106	74	56	65	130	100
*Northwestern University Medical School#	$50	6/1**	10/15	9522	85	89	93	174	100
*Rush Medical College of Rush University	$45	6/1**	11/15	5473	61	59	16	120	100
*Southern Illinois University School of Medicine	$50	6/1**	10/15	1965	42	30	0	72	100
*University of Chicago Pritzker School of Medicine	$55	6/1**	11/15	8709	54	50	58	104	99
*University of Illinois College of Medicine#	$30	6/1**	12/1	6655	225	92	19	317	100
INDIANA									
*Indiana University School of Medicine	$35	6/1**	12/15	2604	164	116	11	280	99
IOWA									
*University of Iowa College of Medicine#	$20	6/1**	11/1	3513	88	87	23	175	100
KANSAS									
*University of Kansas School of Medicine	$ 0	6/15**	10/15	1950	106	69	19	175	100
KENTUCKY									
*University of Kentucky College of Medicine	$ 0	6/1**	11/1	1866	56	39	10	95	100
*University of Louisville School of Medicine	$15	6/1**	11/1	1900	74	63	13	137	100
LOUISIANA									
*Louisiana State University School of Medicine in New Orleans#	$50	6/1**	11/15	1412	108	67	1	175	95

*   AMCAS school
**   early decision available
#   1995–96 data
n/app   not applicable
n/av   data not available

| | Admission Statistics | | | Academic Statistics | | Expenses | | | |
| | | Class Profile | | | | | | | |
Mean GPA	% Interviewed	% Residents	% Minorities	Mean MCAT	Deposit	Tuition Res/ Nonres	Other	% Financial Aid
3.30	6	40	12	P-9.0 B-9.0 V-9.0	$100	$29,980 $29,980	$16,966	76
3.50	6	50	3	P-9.4 B-9.8 V-9.4	$ 0	$27,150 $27,150	$14,104	91
3.51	5	47	4	P-9.6 B-9.8 V-9.7	$ 0	$25,446 $25,446	$ 0	61
3.51	8.3	13	10	P-9.0 B-9.0 V-9.0	$100	$23,868 $23,868	$13,400	81
3.45	13	100	0	P-9.0 B-10 V-10	$ 50	$10,920 $32,760	$ 7,520	85
3.55	6	44	15	P-10.3 B-10.5 V-10.0	$100	$21,660 $21,660	$12,400	83
3.41	n/av	96	27	P-9.2 B-9.3 V-9.3	$100	$ 9,520 $27,740	$ 1,218	n/av
3.68	38	96	6	P-9.7 B-9.7 V-9.7	$ 0	$11,040 $25,275	$ 3,885	n/av
3.60	n/av	86	13	P-9.3 B-9.7 V-9.5	$ 50	$ 8,428 $22,248	$ 172	n/av
3.60	19	89	10	P-9.4 B-9.7 V-9.6	$ 50	$ 8,830 $21,378	$11,500	88
3.61	19	85	n/av	P-9.2 B-9.3 V-9.01	$100	$ 8,643 $19,813	$13,016	86
3.60	53	91	n/av	P-8.7 B-8.7 V-8.9	$100	$ 8,480 $19,650	$12,392	89
3.40	27	99	31	P-8.4 B-8.6 V-8.9	$100	$ 6,776 $14,676	n/av	n/av

Table 5.1. BASIC DATA ON THE MEDICAL SCHOOLS 1996–97—CONTINUED

School	Fee	Application Data — Filing Dates — Earliest	Latest	Number of Applicants	Admission Statistics — Applicants Enrolled — Men	Women	Out-of-State	Class Profile — Class Size	% with 4 years College
*Louisiana State University School of Medicine in Shreveport	$50	6/1	11/15	1024	59	41	0	100	93
*Tulane University School of Medicine	$65	6/1	12/15	10,782	79	70	123	149	100
MARYLAND									
Johns Hopkins University School of Medicine#	$60	7/1**	11/1	3710	65	54	102	121	100
*Uniformed Services University of the Health Sciences F. Edward Hebert School of Medicine	$ 0	6/1	11/1	3380	119	46	n/av	165	100
*University of Maryland School of Medicine#	$40	6/1**	11/1	4645	74	72	25	14	100
MASSACHUSETTS									
*Boston University School of Medicine	$95	6/1**	11/15	11,586	84	54	87	138	75
Harvard Medical School#	$70	6/1	10/15	3914	82	85	152	165	100
*Tufts University School of Medicine#	$75	6/1**	11/1	11,534	92	84	124	176	100
*University of Massachusetts Medical School	$50	6/1**	11/15	1500	50	50	0	100	100
MICHIGAN									
*Michigan State University College of Human Medicine#	$50	6/1**	11/15	3719	51	53	25	104	100
*University of Michigan Medical School#	$50	6/1*	11/15	5873	96	69	65	165	100
*Wayne State University School of Medicine#	$30	6/1**	12/15	4409	161	86	17	247	100
MINNESOTA									
*Mayo Medical School	$60	6/1**	11/1	3791	19	23	34	42	100
*University of Minnesota—Duluth School of Medicine	$50	6/1**	11/15	1385	26	26	0	52	100

*   AMCAS school
**   early decision available
#   1995–96 data
n/av   data not available
n/app   not applicable

| Mean GPA | Admission Statistics | | | Academic Statistics | | Expenses | | | |
| | Class Profile | | | | | | | | |
	% Interviewed	% Residents	% Minorities	Mean MCAT	Deposit	Tuition Res/ Nonres	Other	% Financial Aid
3.45	20	100	7	P-9.0 B-9.2 V-9.0	$100	$ 6,776 $14,676	$ 3,063	82
3.50	13	17	7	P-9.8 B-10.0 V-9.9	$100	$26,610 $26,610	$12,341	81
n/av	19	15	13	Required—scores not available	$ 0	$21,800 $21,800	$ 1,828	80
3.47	18	n/av	7	P-10.4 B-10.2 V-9.9	$ 0	n/app n/app	n/app	n/av
3.50	19	82	16	P-9.8 B-10.1 V-9.6	$ 0	$10,751 $20,851	$ 1,833	71
n/av	10	37	11	P-9.6 B-9.8 V-9.3	$500	$31,520 $31,520	$10,790	89
3.80	27	7	14	P-11.0 B-11.0 V-10.0	$ 0	$23,200 $23,200	$ 1,519	n/av
3.54	8	30	8	P-9.6 B-9.8 V-9.1	$100	$28,800 $28,800	$ 330	74
3.50	33	100	6	P-10.0 B-10.0 V-10.0	$100	$ 8,700 n/app	$ 2,725	74
n/av	13	77	19	P-8.6 B-9.1 V-9.7	$ 50	$14,556 $31,038	$ 856	n/av
3.50	8	60	18	P-11.0 B-11.0 V-10.0	$100	$16,040 $25,140	$ 176	n/av
3.45	19	7	15	P-9.1 B-8.8 V-8.8	$ 50	$ 9,566 $19,061	$ 350	n/av
3.72	11	19	19	P-11.0 B-11.0 V-11.0	$100	$ 4,800 $ 9,900	n/av	n/av
3.55	13	0	7	P-8.7 B-9.0 V-9.0	$100	$15,672 $29,112	$ 7,834	90

Table 5.1. BASIC DATA ON THE MEDICAL SCHOOLS 1996–97—CONTINUED

School	Fee	Application Data — Filing Dates — Earliest	Latest	Number of Applicants	Men	Women	Out-of-State	Class Size	% with 4 years College
*University of Minnesota Medical School—Minneapolis	$ 50	6/1**	11/15	2330	86	89	13	175	100
MISSISSIPPI									
*University of Mississippi School of Medicine	$ 0	6/1**	11/1	313	70	30	0	100	100
MISSOURI									
*St. Louis University School of Medicine#	$100	6/1**	12/15	5307	90	62	110	152	100
*University of Missouri—Columbia School of Medicine	$ 0	6/1**	11/1	1123	54	38	1	92	100
University of Missouri—Kansas City School of Medicine	$ 25	8/1	11/15	871	38	61	72	99	n/app
*Washington University School of Medicine	$ 50	6/1	11/15	6500	62	60	110	122	100
NEBRASKA									
*Creighton University School of Medicine	$ 65	6/1**	12/1	7735	75	36	88	111	100
*University of Nebraska College of Medicine	$ 25	6/1	11/15	1236	67	56	2	123	100
NEVADA									
*University of Nevada School of Medicine	$ 45	6/1**	11/1	1222	31	21	5	52	100
NEW HAMPSHIRE									
*Darthmouth Medical School	$ 55	6/1**	11/1	7898	40	45	75	85	100
NEW JERSEY									
*New Jersey Medical School, University of Medicine and Dentistry of New Jersey	$125	6/1**	12/1	3957	113	57	13	170	82
*Robert Wood Johnson Medical School, University of Medicine and Dentistry of New Jersey	$125	6/1**	12/1	3973	87	52	18	139	100

*   AMCAS school
**   early decision available
\#   1995–96 data
n/av   data not available
n/app   not applicable

| Mean GPA | Admission Statistics | | | Academic Statistics | Expenses | | | |
| | Class Profile | | | | | | | |
	% Interviewed	% Residents	% Minorities	Mean MCAT	Deposit	Tuition Res/Nonres	Other	% Financial Aid
n/av	32	93	3	P-10.0 B-10.0 V-10.0	$ 0	$15,672 $29,112	$10,395	n/av
3.55	62	100	14	P-9.0 B-9.0 V-9.0	$100	$ 6,600 $12,600	$ 1,360	n/av
3.60	25	27	2	P-9.9 B-10.0 V-9.8	$100	$24,200 $24,200	$ 1,024	n/av
3.60	25	99	5	P-9.8 B-9.8 V-9.7	$100	$13,276 $26,580	$12,724	n/av
n/av	43	87	11	Not required	$100	$13,584 $27,968	$ 6,220	n/av
3.78	14	12	13	P-11.6 B-11.6 V-10.9	$100	$27,435 $27,435	$11,260	n/av
3.65	5	21	9	P-9.1 B-9.1 V-9.3	$100	$24,254 $24,254	$12,476	85
3.62	34	98	9	P-9.2 B-9.7 V-9.3	$100	$10,814 $20,908	$14,051	62
3.60	16	90	5	P-8.7 B-9.6 V-9.3	$ 0	$ 7,173 $10,458	$15,105	81
n/av	7	6	12	P-10.0 B-10.0 V-10.0	$ 0	$23,260 $23,260	$12,920	75
3.40	17	92	13	P-10.1 B-10.1 V-9.6	$100	$14,492 $22,679	n/app	75
3.45	19	13	19	P-10.0 B-10.0 V-9.1	$ 50	$14,492 $22,279	$19,120	78

Table 5.1. BASIC DATA ON THE MEDICAL SCHOOLS 1996–97—CONTINUED

School	Fee	Application Data Filing Dates Earliest	Latest	Number of Applicants	Admission Statistics Applicants Enrolled Men	Women	Out-of-State	Class Profile Class Size	% with 4 years College
NEW MEXICO									
*University of New Mexico School of Medicine	$25	6/15**	11/15	1165	33	40	3	73	92
NEW YORK									
*Albany Medical College	$60	6/1	11/15	9686	61	71	86	132	74
*Albert Einstein College of Medicine of Yeshiva University	$75	6/1**	11/1	9536	99	79	93	178	100
Columbia University College of Physicians and Surgeons	$65	6/15	10/15	4195	81	68	118	149	100
*Cornell University Medical College#	$65	6/1**	10/15	7429	51	50	40	101	100
*Mount Sinai School of Medicine of the City University of New York	$100	6/15**	11/1	5344	55	55	52	110	100
*New York Medical College#	$75	6/1**	12/1	12,289	115	73	146	188	100
New York University School of Medicine	$75	8/15	12/1	4840	105	57	87	162	100
*SUNY Health Sciences Center at Brooklyn College of Medicine	$65	6/1**	12/15	5000	108	77	1	185	99
*SUNY at Buffalo School of Medicine and Biomedical Sciences	$65	6/1**	11/1	3400	71	64	1	135	100
*SUNY at Stony Brook Health Sciences Center School of Medicine#	$65	6/1**	11/15	3982	57	43	8	100	100
*SUNY Health Sciences Center at Syracuse College of Medicine	$60	6/15**	12/1	3800	90	60	9	150	100
University of Rochester School of Medicine	$65	6/15	10/15	4088	59	41	65	100	100
NORTH CAROLINA									
*Bowman Gray School of Medicine of Wake Forest University	$55	6/1**	11/1	7884	71	37	49	108	100

*   AMCAS school
**   early decision available
#   1995–96 data
n/av   data not available
n/app   not applicable

| Mean GPA | Admission Statistics | | | Academic Statistics | Expenses | | | |
| | Class Profile | | | | | | | |
	% Interviewed	% Residents	% Minorities	Mean MCAT	Deposit	Tuition Res/ Nonres	Other	% Financial Aid
3.54	26	99	40	P-9.0 B-9.0 V-9.0	$ 0	$ 5,331 $15,318	$ 8,200	n/av
3.50	8	36	1	P-9.8 B-10.2 V-9.8	$100	$25,678 $26,613	$13,760	80
n/av	16	48	8	P-10.9 B-10.9 V-10.0	$100	$25,450 $25,450	$ 4,800	70
n/av	34	21	10	P-11.0 B-11.0 V-11.0	$ 0	$25,164 $25,164	$13,104	66
n/av	16	60	12	P-10.6 B-10.6 V-10.0	$100	$22,365 $22,365	$ 560	65
3.58	10	53	16	P-10.5 B-10.4 V-9.7	$ 0	$21,000 $21,000	$12,600	76
3.20	11	23	11	P-10.1 B-10.4 V-9.7	$100	$25,150 $25,150	$ 465	84
3.50	18	46	36	P-11.0 B-11.0 V-11.0	$100	$20,900 $20,900	$12,790	n/av
n/av	16	1	14	P-10.0 B-10.0 V-9.0	$100	$10,840 $21,940	$ 7,420	n/av
3.62	12	99	6	P-10.0 B-10.2 V-9.3	$100	$10,840 $21,940	$ 9,865	n/av
n/av	21	92	13	Required—scores not available	$ 0	$10,840 $21,940	$ 130	n/av
n/av	18	93	20	P-9.0 B-9.0 V-9.0	$ 0	$10,840 $33,225	$ 7,820	n/av
3.54	16	35	11	P-10.4 B-10.3 V-9.3	$ 0	$23,800 $23,800	$13,130	81
n/av	7	55	10	B-9.8 B-9.9 V-10.0	$100	$23,000 $23,000	$ 9,050	85

Table 5.1. BASIC DATA ON THE MEDICAL SCHOOLS 1996–97—CONTINUED

School	Fee	Application Data — Filing Dates — Earliest	Latest	Admission Statistics — Number of Applicants	Applicants Enrolled — Men	Women	Out-of-State	Class Profile — Class Size	% with 4 years College
*Duke University School of Medicine	$55	6/15	10/15	7181	61	38	61	99	100
*East Carolina University School of Medicine	$35	6/1**	11/15	1881	36	36	0	72	100
*University of North Carolina School of Medicine#	$55	6/1**	11/15	3420	91	69	17	160	100
NORTH DAKOTA									
University of North Dakota School of Medicine	$35	7/1	11/1	370	32	25	12	57	98
OHIO									
*Case Western Reserve University School of Medicine	$60	6/1**	10/15	7900	77	61	55	158	100
*Medical College of Ohio#	$30	6/1**	11/1	4800	84	51	19	135	100
*Northeastern Ohio Universities College of Medicine#	$30	6/1**	11/1	1378	14	11	1	25	100
*Ohio State University College of Medicine	$30	6/15**	11/15	4607	132	78	42	210	100
*University of Cincinnati College of Medicine	$25	6/1**	11/15	4787	88	63	25	151	100
*Wright State University School of Medicine	$30	6/1**	11/15	3582	41	49	15	90	100
OKLAHOMA									
*University of Oklahoma College of Medicine#	$50	6/1	10/15	1701	86	63	17	149	95
OREGON									
*Oregon Health Sciences University School of Medicine	$60	6/1	10/15	2100	48	48	30	96	100

*	AMCAS school
**	early decision available
#	1995–96 data
n/app	not applicable
n/av	data not available

| | Admission Statistics | | | Academic Statistics | | Expenses | | |
| | Class Profile | | | | | | | |
Mean GPA	% Interviewed	% Residents	% Minorities	Mean MCAT	Deposit	Tuition Res/ Nonres	Other	% Financial Aid
n/av	n/av	32	14	P-12.0 B-11.0 V-11.0	$100	$24,650 $24,650	$14,940	76
3.34	33	100	26	P-8.5 B-8.4 V-8.6	$100	$ 2,030 $21,386	$12,402	66
n/av	25	89	24	P-9.1 B-9.3 V-9.8	$100	$ 1,952 $20,466	$ 733	60
3.56	42	79	19	P-8.8 B-9.0 V-9.7	$ 75	$ 8,460 $22,588	$ 6,205	84
3.50	15	60	18	P-10.0 B-10.0 V-10.0	$ 0	$24,500 $24,500	$12,250	77
3.48	15	87	14	P-8.4 B-8.7 V-9.0	$ 0	$ 9,563 $12,963	$ 279	n/av
3.40	9	98	6	P-8.8 B-9.1 V-9.4	n/app	$ 9,717 $19,434	$ 699	75
3.50	14	80	8	P-10.3 B-10.3 V-10.0	$ 0	$ 10,155 $28,305	$ 9,124	n/av
3.45	13	83	15	P-9.7 B-9.9 V-9.4	$ 0	$11,478 $20,139	$12,713	78
n/av	12	87	21	Required—scores not available	$ 0	$ 9,642 $14,190	$ 2,388	85
3.57	22	91	17	P-8.8 B-9.0 V-9.6	$100	$ 7,550 $18,658	$ 325	90
3.60	8	30	8	P-10.0 B-10.0 V-10.0	$ 0	$14,118 $29,757	$12,139	92

Table 5.1. BASIC DATA ON THE MEDICAL SCHOOLS 1996–97—CONTINUED

School	Fee	Application Data — Filing Dates — Earliest	Latest	Number of Applicants	Applicants Enrolled — Men	Women	Out-of-State	Class Profile — Class Size	% with 4 years College
PENNSYLVANIA									
*Jefferson Medical College Thomas Jefferson University	$65	6/1**	11/15	11,600	152	71	124	223	75
*MCP/Hahnenann School of Medicine of Allegeheny University#	$55	6/1**	12/1	13,602	132	108	105	240	96
*Pennsylvania State University College of Medicine	$40	6/1**	11/15	7443	62	47	60	109	100
*Temple University School of Medicine#	$55	6/1**	12/1	8784	109	78	80	187	100
*University of Pennsylvania School of Medicine	$55	6/1	11/1	8552	72	78	43	150	100
*University of Pittsburgh School of Medicine	$50	6/1**	12/9	5904	85	61	55	146	100
RHODE ISLAND									
Brown University School of Medicine#	$60	8/15	3/1	2202	32	31	58	63	100
SOUTH CAROLINA									
*Medical University of South Carolina College of Medicine	$45	6/1**	1/1	3181	94	58	12	152	100
*University of South Carolina School of Medicine#	$45	6/1**	12/1	1878	41	31	8	72	100
SOUTH DAKOTA									
*University of South Dakota School of Medicine	$15	6/1	11/15	965	24	28	2	52	100
TENNESSEE									
*East Tennessee State University James H. Quillen College of Medicine	$25	6/15**	12/1	1826	39	21	6	60	100
*Meharry Medical College School of Medicine#	$25	6/1**	12/15	5548	42	38	71	80	95

*   AMCAS school
**   early decision available
#   1995–96 data
n/app   not applicable
n/av   data not available

	Admission Statistics			Academic Statistics		Expenses		
		Class Profile						
Mean GPA	% Interviewed	% Residents	% Minorities	Mean MCAT	Deposit	Tuition Res/ Nonres	Other	% Financial Aid
3.40	6	44	8	P-10.0 B-9.8 V-9.8	$100	$25,235 $25,235	$10,800	70
3.50	9	57	n/av	Required—scores not available	$100	$22,500 $22,500	$ 500	85
3.61	10	44	19	P-9.8 B-9.9 V-9.4	$100	$15,960 $22,981	$ 8,919	84
n/av	9	58	12	P-9.4 B-9.7 V-9.0	$100	$19,416 $24,555	$ 358	81
3.62	11	29	19	P-11.0 B-11.0 V-11.0	$100	$25,880 $25,880	$14,889	76
3.59	13	62	6	P-10.3 B-10.5 V-10.2	$100	$18,897 $25,271	$ 8,615	n/av
n/av	n/app	8	12	Not required	$ 0	$23,840 $23,840	$ 1,603	65
3.46	13	92	30	P-9.0 B-9.0 V-9.0	$132	$ 6,546 $18,620	$ 25	n/av
3.39	18	88	18	Required—scores not available	$100	$ 7,290 $18,620	$ 25	85
3.58	18	96	6	P-8.5 B-8.9 V-8.3	$100	$ 9,097 $21,479	$14,165	87
3.40	15	90	25	P-9.0 B-9.0 V-9.7	$100	$ 8,750 $16,424	$ 12,516	n/av
n/av	8	12	80	P-7.2 B-7.8 V-7.7	$100	$16,500 $16,500	$ 1,896	n/av

Table 5.1. BASIC DATA ON THE MEDICAL SCHOOLS 1996–97—CONTINUED

School	Fee	Filing Dates Earliest	Latest	Number of Applicants	Men	Women	Out-of-State	Class Size	% with 4 years College
*University of Tennessee College of Medicine	$25	6/1	11/15	1959	95	70	13	165	98
*Vanderbilt University School of Medicine	$50	6/1**	10/15	6436	67	37	90	104	100
TEXAS									
Baylor College of Medicine	$35	6/1**	11/1	3671	101	67	41	168	100
Texas A&M University College of Medicine#	$5	5/1	11/1	1519	40	24	1	64	97
Texas Tech University School of Medicine	$40	6/1**	11/1	1697	90	30	3	120	99
University of Texas Medical School at Galveston	$60	5/1	10/15	3335	128	72	45	200	95
University of Texas— Houston Medical School	$45	6/15	10/15	3471	106	94	55	200	99
University of Texas Medical School— San Antonio	$35	4/15	10/15	3400	111	89	15	200	96
University of Texas Southwestern Medical School at Dallas	$45	4/15	10/15	3418	120	81	32	201	99
UTAH									
*University of Utah School of Medicine#	$50	6/1**	10/15	1409	61	39	25	100	100
VERMONT									
*University of Vermont College of Medicine	$75	6/1**	11/1	8362	38	55	54	93	100
VIRGINIA									
*Eastern Virginia Medical School Medical College of Hampton Roads	$80	6/1**	11/15	7278	50	50	19	100	100
*Medical College of Virginia Virginia Commonwealth University	$75	6/15**	11/1	5302	101	71	50	172	100

The table has spanning headers: "Application Data" spans Fee and Filing Dates (Earliest, Latest); "Admission Statistics" spans Number of Applicants, Applicants Enrolled (Men, Women, Out-of-State), and Class Profile (Class Size, % with 4 years College).

*   AMCAS school
**   early decision available
#   1995–96 data
n/av   data not available
n/app   not applicable

| Mean GPA | Admission Statistics | | | Academic Statistics | Expenses | | | |
| | Class Profile | | | | | | | |
	% Interviewed	% Residents	% Minorities	Mean MCAT	Deposit	Tuition Res/ Nonres	Other	% Financial Aid
3.50	20	92	13	P-9.0 B-10.0 V-9.0	$100	$ 8,684 $16,858	$ 6,967	n/av
3.60	10	13	5	P-11.5 B-11.4 V-10.5	$ 0	$22,000 $22,000	$ 9,760	n/av
3.70	17	76	23	P-11.0 B-11.0 V-11.0	$300	$ 6,550 $19,650	$15,205	n/av
3.65	31	98	14	Required—scores not available	$ 0	$ 6,550 $19,650	$ 1,400	89
3.52	27	98	22	P-9.1 B-9.4 V-9.4	$100	$ 6,550 $19,550	$ 9,461	66
3.50	37	94	54	P-9.0 B-9.0 V-9.0	$ 0	$ 6,550 $19,650	$ 3,842	n/av
3.44	30	99	54	P-8.8 B-9.3 V-9.0	$ 0	$ 6,550 $19,650	$ 9,648	62
3.38	30	93	15	P-10.0 B-10.0 V-10.0	$ 0	$ 6,550 $19,650	$ 8,000	85
3.60	40	84	11	P-10.0 B-11.0 V-10.0	$ 0	$ 6,550 $19,650	$ 9,005	n/av
3.60	31	75	2	P-10.5 B-10.6 V-10.0	$100	$ 6,927 $14,760	$ 435	n/av
3.34	7	42	13	P-9.0 B-9.0 V-9.2	$100	$15,350 $27,850	$ 8,831	n/av
3.32	7.7	81	4	P-10.0 B-10.0 V-10.0	$200	$13,500 $24,000	$17,612	91
3.45	6	71	9	P-9.5 B-9.7 V-9.6	$100	$ 9,667 $24,278	$16,832	n/av

Table 5.1. BASIC DATA ON THE MEDICAL SCHOOLS 1996–97—CONTINUED

School	Fee	Application Data — Filing Dates — Earliest	Latest	Admission Statistics — Number of Applicants	Applicants Enrolled — Men	Women	Out-of-State[1]	Class Profile — Class Size	% with 4 years College
*University of Virginia School of Medicine	$50	6/1**	11/1	4879	73	66	48	139	100
WASHINGTON									
*University of Washington School of Medicine	$35	6/15	1/15	3603	82	84	75	166	100
WEST VIRGINIA									
*Marshall University School of Medicine	$30	6/1**	11/15	1156	31	17	3	48	94
*West Virginia University School of Medicine	$30	6/1**	11/15	1448	44	44	3	88	100
WISCONSIN									
*Medical College of Wisconsin#	$60	6/1**	11/15	7772	133	71	110	204	96
*University of Wisconsin Medical School#	$35	6/1**	11/1	3034	71	72	25	143	100
CANADA									
Dalhousie University Faculty of Medicine	$55	10/1	11/15	800	49	43	15	92	95
Laval University Faculty of Medicine	$55	1/1	2/1	1850	41	71	4	42	n/av
McGill University Faculty of Medicine	$60	9/1	11/15	1040	56	53	29	109	100
*McMaster University School of Medicine	$25	7/1	11/1	2900	27	73	n/av	100	77
Memorial University of Newfoundland Faculty of Medicine	$50	7/1	11/15	654	35	26	18	61	49
*Queen's University Faculty of Medicine	$75	7/1	11/1	1548	46	29	n/av	75	54
Université de Sherbrooke Faculté de Médicine	$30	11/1	3/1	1562	47	51	16	98	87
University of Alberta Faculty of Medicine	$60	7/1**	11/1	900	54	51	10	105	100

*	AMCAS school (U.S.) or OMSAS (Canadian)
**	early decision available
#	1995–96 data
n/app	not applicable
n/av	data not available
[1]	or Out-of-Province

| | Admission Statistics | | | Academic Statistics | | Expenses | | | |
| | Class Profile | | | | | | | | |
Mean GPA	% Interviewed	% Residents	% Minorities	Mean MCAT	Deposit	Tuition Res/ Nonres	Other	% Financial Aid
3.54	23	65	15	P-10.5 B-10.2 V-10.0	$ 0	$ 9,676 $22,006	n/av	81
3.58	23	92	11	P-10.0 B-10.4 V-10.0	$100	$ 8,172 $20,583	$11,403	80
3.40	25	94	19	P-8.7 B-8.8 V-9.6	$ 0	$ 8,550 $19,776	$ 1,325	80
3.61	20	97	8	P-9.0 B-9.3 V-9.1	$100	$ 8,380 $20,714	$ 2,075	n/av
n/av	8	54	4	P-9.6 B-9.6 V-9.5	$100	$12,894 $22,985	$ 35	n/av
3.51	7	18	15	P-9.5 B-9.7 V-9.4	$ 0	$13,041 $18,895	$ 0	n/av
n/av	100	90	98	P-10.0 B-10.0 V-10.0	$200	$ 5,515 $ 7,915	$ 2034	n/av
n/av	20	n/app	n/app	Not required	$ 0	$ 1,100 $10,000	$ 9,700	n/av
3.55	34	74	n/app	P-10.8 B-10.8 V-10.0	$500	$ 1,845 $ 7,634	$ 2,052	n/av
n/av	7	n/av	n/app	Not required	$ 0	$ 5,942 $27,395	$ 2,370	n/av
n/av	28	70	n/app	P-9.0 B-9.0 V-9.0	$100	$ 6,250 $30,000	$ 5,246	n/av
n/av	28	n/av	n/app	P-11.0 B-11.0 V-10.4	$ 0	$ 3,733	n/av	n/av
n/av	n/av	n/av	n/app	Not required	$200	$ 3,014 $11,697	$ 1,600	n/av
n/av	38	n/av	n/app	Required—scores not available	$200	$ 4,274 $ 8,548	$ 1,700	n/av

Table 5.1. BASIC DATA ON THE MEDICAL SCHOOLS 1996–97—CONTINUED

	Application Data			Admission Statistics					
		Filing Dates			Applicants Enrolled			Class Profile	
School	Fee	Earliest	Latest	Number of Applicants	Men	Women	Out-of-State[1]	Class Size	% with 4 years College
University of British Columbia Faculty of Medicine	$105	8/15	12/15	597	61	59	4	120	92
University of Calgary Faculty of Medicine	$60	7/15	11/30	1035	27	42	1	69	95
University of Manitoba Faculty of Medicine	$50	9/1	11/30	360	48	24	7	72	100
University of Montreal Faculty of Medicine#	$55	5/15	3/1	2202	65	96	10	161	52
*University of Ottawa Faculty of Medicine	$50	7/1	11/1	1903	39	45	9	84	41
University of Saskatchewan College of Medicine	$40	9/1	12/1	463	34	21	5	55	22
*University of Toronto Faculty of Medicine	$150	8/1	11/1	1759	105	72	27	177	55
*University of Western Ontario Faculty of Medicine	$50	7/1	11/1	1845	63	36	n/av	99	96

*	AMCAS school
**	early decision available
#	1995–96 data
n/app	not applicable
n/av	data not available
[1]	or Out-of-Province

	Admission Statistics			Academic Statistics		Expenses			
	Class Profile								
Mean GPA	% Interviewed	% Residents	% Minorities	Mean MCAT	Deposit	Tuition Res/ Nonres	Other	% Financial Aid
3.25	n/av	97	n/app	P-10.6 B-10.8 V-9.8	$300	$ 3,937	n/app	n/av
3.62	27	42	n/app	P-10.2 B-10.4 V-9.5	$100	$ 4,918 $ 9,836	$9,988	n/av
3.60	40	10	n/app	P-10.1 B-10.1 V-9.7	$100	$ 4,873 $ 4,873	$2,200	n/av
n/av	22	93	n/app	Not required	$ 0	$ 2,260 $ 7,450	$ 30	n/av
3.40	17	75	n/app	P-10.0 B-10.0 V-9.0	$100	$ 3,800 n/app	n/app	n/av
n/av	45	91	0.2	Not required	$100	$ 4,672 $ 4,672	n/av	n/av
3.70	20	85	n/app	P-10.3 B-10.3 V-10.0	$ 0	$ 4,037 $21,000	$ 563	n/av
n/av	21	n/av	n/app	P-8.0 B-8.0 V-9.0	$ 0	$ 4,700 n/av	$2,750	n/av

6 Medical School Profiles

In-depth medical school profiles

This chapter consists of in-depth medical school profiles that provide detailed information on various elements distinguishing individual schools.

IN-DEPTH MEDICAL SCHOOL PROFILES

The following profiles consist of in-depth descriptions of the 122 fully accredited U.S. medical schools and the 16 Canadian medical schools. Each school profile consists of three distinct components: (1) a box containing the school name, address, phone, fax, E-mail and World Wide Web numbers, (2) a data capsule containing a summary of vital statistics for the first year class (for more details, see Chapter 5), and (3) the school's specific descriptive characteristics, which are identified in the next paragraph and are defined below.

How To Use These Profiles

No two medical schools are the same. They differ in many ways, including their origins, admissions procedures and requirements, curriculum, grading policies, facilities, and special programs; each school is unique in what it has to offer.

After making a tentative list of schools to which you would consider applying (using the data in Table 5.1 in the preceding chapter), you should review each school's qualities in the profiles presented here to see if you qualify for admission and if the school will meet your personal needs.

The admissions requirements will let you know if you can meet the school's specific requirements beyond those mandated for all medical school applicants. If you cannot meet these requirements, applying is an exercise in futility. For instance, if a school limits its students exclusively to state residents, it is pointless to apply unless you meet this criterion. This section also suggests elective courses that may be advisable for you to take in your junior or senior years to make you more eligible for admission to specific schools.

Students should become familiar with the curriculum of the schools to which they are interested in applying. It is also recommended that, when visiting school campuses for an interview, you inquire from current students what their reaction is to the existing curriculum. Specific information on the performance under this curriculum on both parts of the USMLE can be of special value in assessing its impact. Also, the faculty's attitude toward the curriculum and any prospective modifications that will be introduced may be solicited from your interviewer (near the end of the session). You may wish to evaluate your findings with fellow premeds who have visited the same school, to determine how factual your data is. It may even prove worthwhile to secure information in advance of your visit about the curriculum from previous interviewees, so that you can then obtain specific information that you feel needs elaboration.

Familiarity with information regarding grading and promotion policies, facilities, and special programs will provide you with source material for making further inquires at the time of your interview and help make your visits more meaningful.

184

Definitions

Following are definitions of terms pertaining to the various features used in outlining each school's characteristics:

Introduction

A brief historical overview for the school is provided. It will usually also indicate other schools for the health professions that are affiliated with the university, as well as some geographical features that are of special importance.

Admissions

Though the minimum requirement for most schools is at least three years (90 credit hours) of undergraduate study at an accredited college, the percentage of those accepted with only this background is small. *The MCAT is required by almost all schools*, although in exceptional circumstances admission can be secured without having taken this exam, or it may be made contingent on securing satisfactory scores when taken at a later date. *Basic or minimum premedical science courses* means one year of biology, inorganic chemistry, organic chemistry, and physics plus appropriate laboratory work. Some schools have additional requirements such as English, mathematics, or certain advanced science courses. These are indicated along with any recommended courses. Since an interview is almost always by invitation, it is not indicated in each entry as a prerequisite for admission. *Transfer and advanced standing:* Transferring from one American medical school to another may present problems because of variations in curricula and length of programs. When these issues present no problem and space is available, transfer can be made at the end of the academic year. American citizens studying at foreign medical schools may be considered for admission to advanced standing, usually into the third-year class, at some schools. Generally, they must have completed their basic science courses and have taken the Medical Sciences Knowledge Profile examination.

Curriculum

Each curriculum is indicated as to length and type. The classifications used (except where a school preferred not to be identified in this manner) are: *traditional* (basic sciences are taught during first two years using a departmental or nonintegrated format. The last two years consist of clerkships in major and minor clinical specialties with little or no time allotted for electives); *semitraditional* (basic sciences are taught in traditional manner. The third year is devoted to clerkships in major specialties. The fourth year is mainly devoted to electives. Clinical correlation with basic sciences is usually provided); *semimodern* (one of the two years devoted to basic sciences is presented using a core or organ systems approach. The third year is devoted to clerkships in major specialties and the fourth year is mainly for electives. Clinical correlation with basic sciences is emphasized and the student is introduced to patients early in the preclinical program); *modern* (both basic science years are presented using core or organ systems approach. The third year is devoted to clerkships in major clinical specialties and the fourth year consists mainly of electives. Clinical correlation with basic sciences is strongly emphasized and the student is introduced to patients very early in the preclinical program). The following terms will be useful in understanding the various school curricula:

Introductory basic medical science courses
generally means anatomy, physiology, and biochemistry.

Advanced basic medical science courses
generally means microbiology, pharmacology, and pathology.

Clerkships
service on a hospital ward where the medical student works under direct supervision of a physician and becomes directly involved in the care of patients.

Major clinical specialties
usually medicine, surgery, pediatrics, obstetrics-gynecology, and psychiatry-neurology.

Minor clinical specialties
generally anesthesiology, dermatology, otolaryngology, ophthalmology, radiology, and public health-preventive medicine.

Subspecialty
specialized area of major specialty; for example, subspecialties of surgery are orthopedic surgery, neurosurgery, thoracic surgery, cardiac surgery, pediatric surgery, etc.

Preceptorship
service in a medical office or home situation where the student works under supervision of a family physician and becomes initiated into patient care in a nonhospital format.

Grading and Promotion Policies
The system used is not the same in all schools, so it is specifically identified for each school. Promotion usually is determined by a faculty committee and specific details concerning the policy of individual schools is outlined. Some schools require students to take only Steps 1 and 2 of the USMLE. Others may require a passing total score for promotion to the third year and graduation.

Facilities
Teaching
Facilities are of two kinds: those used for basic sciences and those used in clinical instruction. The former usually contain teaching and research laboratories, lecture rooms, and departmental and faculty offices. Clinical teaching occurs in hospitals with major facilities usually located on campus adjacent to the basic science building. Other hospitals in the city or area may be affiliated with the school (for example, have a contractual arrangement whereby the medical school faculty partly or completely staffs the hospital and uses its beds in teaching). Campus hospitals are frequently owned by the school and are then referred to as university hospitals. Major teaching and affiliated hospitals are noted in the description and the number of beds indicated. *Other:* Facilities concern the research and library facilities associated with the medical school. *Housing:* Facilities include information for single and married students. Off-campus accommodations are available near most schools and the Office of Student Affairs of the school may be able to assist students in securing such facilities. Details as to size, furnishings, and rental costs may be given in the school catalog.

Special Features
This section deals with two topics, *minority admissions* and *other degree programs*. In the former, the extent of a school's recruiting efforts of underrepresented students is identified and special summer programs are noted. Under the latter heading, combined programs (especially MD-PhD programs) are identified, and any unique areas of graduate training that are not part of the traditional basic sciences are mentioned.

ALABAMA

University of Alabama School of Medicine

University Station
A-100, Volker Hall
Birmingham, Alabama   35294

Phone: 205-934-2330   *Fax:* 205-934-8724
E-mail: ghand@uasom/,eos/uab.edu
WWW: http://www.lhl.uab.edu/vasom

Application Filing		Accreditation
Earliest:	June 1	LCME
Latest:	November 1	
Fee:	$65	**Degrees Granted**
AMCAS:	yes	MD, MD-PhD

Enrollment: 1996–97 First-Year Class

Men:	112	67%	Applied:	2106
Women:	53	32%	Interviewed:	548
Minorities:	16	10%	Enrolled:	167
Out of State:	2	1%		

1996–97 Class Profile

Mean MCAT Scores		*Mean GPA*
Physical Sciences:	9.7	3.55
Biological Sciences:	8.9	
Verbal Reasoning:	9.8	

Tuition and Fees

Resident	7920
Average (public)	9500
Average (private)	22,500
Nonresident	19,264
Average (public)	20,500
Average (private)	24,500

(in thousands of dollars)

Percentage receiving financial aid: 75%

Introduction

The School of Medicine began in Mobile in 1859. After several relocations, its main Medical Center campus was established in Birmingham in 1945. Branch campuses are also present in Huntsville and Tuscaloosa. The first 2 years of the educational program take place at the main campus, while clinical teaching occurs on all 3 campuses. The School of Medicine is one of the 6 health schools making up the University of Alabama Medical Center. The others are schools of Dentistry, Optometry, Nursing, Health-Related Professions, and Public Health.

Admissions (AMCAS)

Additional courses beyond the basic science requirements are recommended in the behavioral sciences. Only nonresidents of superior ability are accepted. The first 2 years of basic sciences are completed in Birmingham. The clinical rotations may be taken in either Birmingham, Huntsville, or Tuscaloosa.

Curriculum

4-year semitraditional. *First and second years:* Consist of education in the basic medical science as related to human biology and pathology. This is followed by an integrated study of organ system function and disorders. The humanities as related to medicine are also studied, and the skills necessary for physical diagnosis are developed. *Third and fourth years:* Consist of required rotations through clinical science disciplines, including participation in the cases of patients in both hospital and ambulatory settings (under faculty supervision). The clinical training curriculum requirements are similar at all 3 training centers.

Grading and Promotion Policies

A letter system is used for required courses and Pass/Fail for electives. All grades of D and F require remedial work satisfactory to the faculty. Obtaining a total passing score on Steps 1 and 2 of the USMLE is required for promotion to the third year and graduation after the fourth, respectively.

Facilities

Teaching: The school is part of the university's Medical Center. The Basic Science Building contains teaching facilities and administrative and faculty offices. The major clinical teaching facility is the University Hospital (817 beds) in Birmingham. Other facilities utilized are the VA Hospital (479 beds), the Children's Hospital, the Cooper Green Hospital, the Eye Foundation Hospital, and various community hospitals. *Other:* The Lyons-Harrison Research Building, Tinsley Harrison Tower, and basic science research and education buildings are the primary research facilities. Clinical facilities utilized in Tuscaloosa are the Druid City Hospital, the VA Medical Center, and the Capstone Medical Center. The Huntsville Hospital and the Ambulatory Care Center in Huntsville are also used. *Libraries:* The Lister Hill Library of the Health Sciences in Birmingham is a 4-story structure that contains more than 150,000 volumes. The Health Sciences Library at Tuscaloosa has about 10,000 volumes and subscribes to 475 journals. The library at Huntsville has about 9000 volumes. *Housing:* There are 178 modern apartment units in the Medical Center consisting of 28 efficiency, 84 one-bedroom, 62 two-bedroom, and 4 three-bedroom apartments. Preference is given to married students but consideration is given to single students for occupancy of the smaller units.

Special Features

Minority admissions: Minority Student Program to discover and encourage study of medicine among minority group members. The program awards summer fellowships to premedical and medical students. *Other degree programs:* Dual MD-PhD program; continuing education program for graduates.

University of South Alabama College of Medicine

Mobile, Alabama 36688

Phone: 334-460-7176   *Fax:* 334-460-2628
WWW: http://www.usouthal/edu/usa/deps-grd.html

Application Filing		Accreditation
Earliest:	June 1	LCME
Latest:	November 15	
Fee:	$25	**Degrees Granted**
AMCAS:	yes	MD, MD-PhD

Enrollment: 1996–97 First-Year Class

Men:	39	61%	Applied:	1308
Women:	25	39%	Interviewed:	222
Minorities:	8	13%	Enrolled:	64
Out of State:	6	9%		

1996–97 Class Profile

Mean MCAT Scores		*Mean GPA*
Physical Sciences:	9.6	3.6
Biological Sciences:	9.9	
Verbal Reasoning:	9.8	

Tuition and Fees

Resident	7567
Average (public)	9500
Average (private)	22,500
Nonresident	14,567
Average (public)	20,500
Average (private)	24,500

(in thousands of dollars)

Percentage receiving financial aid: n/av

Introduction

This public, state-sponsored medical school is located on the university's 1200 acre campus in the Springhill section of Mobile. It occupies 13 buildings, including a 400-bed Medical Center, which contains a Level I trauma center. The first class was admitted in 1973 and 64 applicants are enrolled annually. A 150-acre park containing recreational facilities lies adjacent to the campus. The first 2 years are taught in the main campus in the Medical Sciences Building; the last 2 clinical years are spent the University of South Alabama hospitals and clinics.

Admissions (AMCAS)

Required courses include the basic premedical sciences, English composition, 1 year of college mathematics, and 1 year of humanities. Recommended courses include quantitative analysis, comparative vertebrate anatomy, and vertebrate embryology. Nonresidents should have competitive MCAT and grade point averages to be considered for an interview. *Transfer and advanced standing:* None.

Curriculum

4-year semitraditional. *First and second years:* Consist largely of basic science courses that are intended to lay a foundation for the clinical understanding of medicine. In addition, courses such as medical ethics and medical practice and society are required in the first year, and behavioral science, genetics, and public health and epidemiology in the second. A weekly opportunity for clinical exposure occurs during the entire second year in the course introduction to clinical medicine. *Third and fourth years:* Provide the students with clinical involvement in almost every major aspect of medicine: internal medicine (12 weeks), psychiatry (6 weeks), obstetrics and gynecology (8 weeks), pediatrics (8 weeks), surgery (8 weeks), and family practice (6 weeks). Clerkships are primarily inpatient-oriented, and students are assigned as members of patient care teams with an intern, resident, and attending physician. Emphasis is on bedside teaching and students are expected to assume significant responsibility for their patients. The last year of medical school is elective. The 36-week year is planned by the student in conjunction with his/her own advisor. Each department offers a wide variety of clinical and research categories: surgical subspecialty, clinical neuroscience, primary care acting internship, subspecialty in medicine, pediatrics or ob/gyn, and ambulatory care.

Grading and Promotion Policies

An A, B, C, D, F system is used in the first 3 years; Honors, Pass, Fail is used in the senior year. Students must pass the Steps 1 and 2 of the USMLE. Step 1 is given at the end of the sophomore year and Step 2 during September of the senior year.

Facilities

Teaching: The basic sciences are housed in the Medical Sciences Building on the 1200-acre university campus in the western section of Mobile. Clinical teaching is conducted at the University of South Alabama Medical Center, USA Knollwood, and USA Doctors Children's and Women's Hospital. *Other:* Other facilities include the Moorer Clinical Sciences Building, University of South Alabama Cancer Center, Primate Research Laboratory, Laboratory of Molecular Biology, Family Practice Center, Mastin Building, Pediatric Outpatient Clinic, and Psychiatric Building. *Library:* The Biomedical Library contains more than 65,000 volumes and receives about 2500 periodicals. *Housing:* Furnished residence halls on campus are available for unmarried students. A university-owned subdivision immediately adjacent to campus offers housing for both married and single students.

Special Features

Minority admissions: An active recruitment program is coordinated by the Office of Student Affairs. *Other degree programs:* Combined MD-PhD degree programs are offered in the basic medical sciences.

ARIZONA

University of Arizona College of Medicine

P.O. Box 245075
Tucson, Arizona 85724

Phone: 520-626-6214 *Fax:* 520-626-4884
WWW: http://www.zax.radiology.arizona.edu/
introp.pic.html

Application Filing		Accreditation	
Earliest:	June 1	LCME	
Latest:	November 1		
Fee:	n/av	**Degrees Granted**	
AMCAS:	yes	MD, MD-PhD	

Enrollment: 1996–97 First-Year Class

Men:	49	49%	Applied:	531
Women:	51	51%	Interviewed:	96
Minorities:	24	24%	Enrolled:	100
Out of State:	0	0%		

1996–97 Class Profile

Mean MCAT Scores		*Mean GPA*
Physical Sciences:	n/av	3.55
Biological Sciences:	n/av	
Verbal Reasoning:	n/av	

Tuition and Fees

Resident	7426
Average (public)	9500
Average (private)	22,500
Nonresident	n/app

0   10   20   30   40   50
(in thousands of dollars)

Percentage receiving financial aid: 85%

Introduction

Authorization for establishment of the College of Medicine was granted in 1962 and the first class was initiated in 1967. The University Medical Center, completed in 1971, was expanded in 1994. The new Arizona Health Sciences Library and Learning Resource Center was completed in 1992.

Admissions (AMCAS)

Basic premedical science courses plus 2 semesters of English are required for admission. Applicants for both entering and transfer openings will be considered only from Arizona residents and certified and funded WICHE applicants. *Transfer and advanced standing:* Applicants must be matriculated in WHO-listed foreign medical schools, 2-year or 4-year U.S. LCME-accredited medical schools, or accredited schools of osteopathy and must have completed the basic sciences. All applicants must take the USMLE.

Curriculum

4-year semimodern. *First year:* A 40-week period when the basic sciences are presented. Patient contact is provided and behavioral sciences are emphasized. *Second year:* A 36-week period consisting of advanced basic science courses, behavioral sciences, and a continuation of the introduction to clinical sciences. *Third year:* A 48-week period when the clinical sciences are presented with at least 6 weeks of clerkships in each of the principal departments. *Fourth year:* A 33-week period for electives in the student's career path.

Biologic, cultural, psychosocial, economic, and sociologic concepts and data are provided in the core curriculum. Increasing emphasis is placed on problem-solving ability, beginning with initial instruction and carried through to graduation. Excellence in performance is encouraged and facilitated. Awareness of the milieu in which medicine is practiced is also encouraged. The learning environment encompasses lectures, small-group instruction, independent study, clinical clerkships, practice in physical diagnosis, computer-based instruction, and a variety of other modes for the learner. The Patient Instructor Program in the second year uses a unique method of clinical instruction. Real patients are trained to help students fine-tune their physical examination and history-taking skills. Students receive immediate feedback on their performance from the patient instructors, which helps to develop and improve the skills needed during the clinical years. Students learn in the classroom, conference room, laboratory, clinic, and physician's office, bed units of hospitals, special sites for diagnostic and therapeutic maneuvers, University Medical Center, and a variety of community inpatient and outpatient settings.

Grading and Promotion Policies

An Honors/Pass/Fail system is in operation. A written evaluation that characterizes specific student performance is also recorded with the Office of Student Affairs. The major criterion for promotion is that the student passes all required courses in the curriculum during each academic year. The student may repeat a course only once. A passing score must be recorded for both Steps 1 and 2 of the USMLE in order to graduate.

Facilities

Teaching: The Health Sciences Center complex is located adjacent to the university campus and consists of several interconnected buildings: Basic Science, Clinical Sciences, Outpatient Clinic, University Medical Center, Children's Research Center, the Health Sciences Library, and Cancer Center. *Other:* Additional facilities used are the Tucson VA Hospital and Tucson and Phoenix hospitals. *Library:* The Health Sciences Center Library houses 176,000 volumes and 3600 medical journals. It is the only major biomedical library in the area. *Housing:* Some rooms are available for single students in the residence halls and for married students at the Family Housing Project.

Special Features

Minority admissions: Disadvantaged, rural, and minority residents of Arizona are urged to apply for admission. *Other degree programs:* A combined MD-PhD program of study is also offered.

ARKANSAS

University of Arkansas for Medical Sciences

College of Medicine
4301 West Markham Street
Little Rock, Arkansas   72205

Phone: 501-686-5354   *Fax:* 501-686-5873
E-mail: tsouth @ comdean I.uams.edu.
WWW: http://www.amanda.uams.edu:80/uams.html

Application Filing	Accreditation
Earliest: July 15	LCME
Latest: January 15	
Fee: $10	**Degrees Granted**
AMCAS: yes	MD, MD-PhD, MD-MS

Enrollment: 1996–97 First-Year Class

Men:	93	67%	Applied:	890
Women:	46	33%	Interviewed:	445
Minorities:	14	10%	Enrolled:	139
Out of State:	1			

1996–97 Class Profile

Mean MCAT Scores		*Mean GPA*
Physical Sciences:	8.9	3.52
Biological Sciences:	9.1	
Verbal Reasoning:	9.5	

Tuition and Fees

Resident	8495
Average (public)	9500
Average (private)	22,500
Nonresident	16,207
Average (public)	20,500
Average (private)	24,500

0   10   20   30   40   50
(in thousands of dollars)

Percentage receiving financial aid: 75%

Introduction

In 1897 the Arkansas Industrial University established a medical department. This component became part of the University of Arkansas for Medical Sciences in 1975. The latter incorporates 5 colleges, training physicians, nurses, pharmacists, health-related professionals, and graduate students.

Admissions (AMCAS)

Prerequisites include the minimum premedical science courses plus 3 semesters of English and 2 semesters of mathematics. Recommended courses include genetics, embryology, quantitative analysis, statistics, cell biology, psychology, anthropology, world history, and literature. Nonresidents should have a GPA above 3.5 and an MCAT score of 9 or higher in each subtest. *Transfer*

and advanced standing: For upperclassmen only, with very limited places available. Applicants are considered on a case-by-case basis and must demonstrate strong ties to the state of Arkansas.

Curriculum

4-year semitraditional. *First year:* (36 weeks) Introductory basic sciences as well as opportunity for patient contact by means of the introduction to the medical profession course. *Second year:* (32 weeks) Consists of the advanced basic sciences and courses in behavioral science, physical diagnosis, and mechanism of disease. *Third year:* (48 weeks) Consists of clerkship rotations through the major clinical specialties. *Fourth year:* (from 36 to 48 weeks) Open to more than 200 electives selected with advice of a faculty advisor. Research may be carried out as part of elective. Off-campus study locally or elsewhere in U.S. or abroad may be selected.

Grading and Promotion Policies

A letter grading system is used in basic sciences and required clinical rotations; a Pass/Fail system is used in electives. Subjective assessments are used by a Promotions Committee in determining a student's eligibility for promotion. A passing grade must be recorded on Step 1 of the USMLE for promotion to the third year.

Facilities

Teaching: Medical Center includes a 9-story Educational Building that provides basic science facilities. University Hospital (400 beds) is the principal site for clinical training. This facility is augmented by the Ambulatory Care Center and the Arkansas Cancer Research Center. The school is affiliated with the Arkansas Children's Hospital and VA Hospitals in Little Rock and North Little Rock. It cooperates with other Little Rock hospitals in its training programs. *Other:* T. H. Barton Institute of Medical Research, Arkansas State Hospital for Nervous Diseases, Arkansas Rehabilitation Institute, Biomedical Research Center, Jones Eye Institute, and the Central Arkansas Radiation Therapy Institute. *Housing:* All single freshman and sophomore students are required to live in the residence hall unless special exemption is received. Approximately 35 one-bedroom furnished apartments are available for married students.

Special Features

Minority admissions: The college's Office of Minority Student Affairs conducts programs designed to identify and assist prospective admission candidates among minority and disadvantaged students in the state. *Other degree programs:* Dual MD-PhD and MS-MD programs available, offered in conjunction with the Graduate School of the university. Medical Student Research Program enables students to work in selected areas of research. Work done under this program may be applied toward a PhD degree.

CALIFORNIA

Loma Linda University School of Medicine
Loma Linda, California   92350

Phone: 909-824-4467   *Fax:* 909-824-4146
E-mail: jbuchanan@ccmail.llu.edu
WWW: http://www.llu.edu/sml. html

Application Filing		Accreditation	
Earliest:	June 1	LCME	
Latest:	November 1		
Fee:	$55	**Degrees Granted**	
AMCAS:	yes	MD, MD-PhD, MD-MS	

Enrollment: 1996–97 First-Year Class

Men:	103	65%	Applied:	4660
Women:	56	35%	Interviewed:	475
Minorities:	11	7%	Enrolled:	159
Out of State:	73	46%		

1996–97 Class Profile

Mean MCAT Scores		*Mean GPA*
Physical Sciences:	9.6	3.54
Biological Sciences:	9.8	
Verbal Reasoning:	9.5	

Tuition and Fees

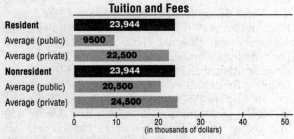

Resident	23,944
Average (public)	9500
Average (private)	22,500
Nonresident	23,944
Average (public)	20,500
Average (private)	24,500

(in thousands of dollars)

Percentage receiving financial aid: n/av

Introduction
This medical school, like its parent body, Loma Linda University, is owned and operated by the Seventh-Day Adventist Church. It was founded in 1909. The campus includes basic science facilities and a Medical Center. The school is located inland not far from Los Angeles. The curriculum of the university is approved by LCME.

Admissions (AMCAS)
Required courses include minimum science courses plus English. The MCAT also is required. Preference is shown to members of the Seventh-Day Adventist Church, but it is a firm policy of the admissions committee to admit each year a number of non-church-related applicants who have demonstrated a strong commitment to Christian principles.

Curriculum
4-year traditional. The freshman year is devoted to the basic sciences as well as behavioral science, community medicine, and physical diagnosis. The sophomore year includes the standard advanced basic science courses as well as continued work in community medicine and physical diagnosis. The last 2 are clinical years with the didactic work integrated with ward and clinic assignments. Five months are set aside for an elective experience.

Grading and Promotion Policies
Students are evaluated on a Pass/Fail basis; however, class ranks are determined on a percentile system. Passing Step 1 of the USMLE is required for promotion to clinical clerkships. Obtaining a total passing score on Steps 1 and 2 of the USMLE is required for promotion to the third year and graduation after the fourth year, respectively.

Facilities
Teaching: School is located on the university campus. Clinical teaching takes place at University Hospital (500 beds) and several affiliated hospitals. *Other:* A medium-scale, general-purpose computer facility serves the students and faculty of the university in instructional and research functions. *Library:* Medical and related fields make up more than half of the holdings of the Vernier Radcliff Memorial Library located on campus.

Special Features
Minority admissions: The school does not discriminate on the basis of race, age, sex, or handicap. *Other degree programs:* MD-MS and MD-PhD programs are available.

Stanford University School of Medicine

851 Welch Road
Palo Alto, California   94304

Phone: 415-723-6861   *Fax:* 415-725-4599
WWW: http://www.stanford.edu

Application Filing		Accreditation	
Earliest:	June 1	LCME	
Latest:	November 1		
Fee:	$55	**Degrees Granted**	
AMCAS:	yes	MD, MD-PhD	

Enrollment: 1996–97 First-Year Class

Men:	49	57%	Applied:	6800
Women:	37	43%	Interviewed:	476
Minorities:	9	11%	Enrolled:	86
Out of State:	n/av	n/av		

1996–97 Class Profile

Mean MCAT Scores		*Mean GPA*
Physical Sciences:	11.4	3.6
Biological Sciences:	11.7	
Verbal Reasoning:	10.3	

Tuition and Fees

Resident	25,957
Average (public)	9500
Average (private)	22,500
Nonresident	25,957
Average (public)	20,500
Average (private)	24,500

(in thousands of dollars)
0   10   20   30   40   50

Percentage receiving financial aid: 83%

Introduction

The School of Medicine was founded in 1858 as the medical department of the College of the Pacific. It later became affiliated with the University City College, and subsequently, in 1882, was given the name Cooper Medical College in honor of the original founder. In 1908 it was adopted by Leland Stanford Junior University and relocated to outside San Francisco. Stanford University School of Medicine was established in 1958. A new Medical Center was opened in 1959 and is located on an 8800-acre campus.

Admissions (AMCAS)

The standard premedical courses are required. Strongly recommended, but not required, are knowledge of a modern foreign language. Spanish is especially useful. Courses in calculus, biochemistry, physical chemistry, and behavioral sciences are strongly encouraged. No preference is shown to California residents. Foreign applicants must have completed a minimum of 1 year of study in a U.S., Canadian, or United Kingdom accredited college or university. *Transfer and advanced standing:* Transfer students are not accepted.

Curriculum

4-year modern. The goals of the curriculum are to develop outstanding clinical skills and the capacity for leadership in the practice of scientific medicine, and to prepare as many students as possible for careers in research and teaching. Stanford's flexible curriculum is its major innovative approach to medical education. It was designed to create an environment that encourages intellectual diversity and to provide opportunities for students to develop as individuals. While traditional courses and clerkships are required for graduation, the duration of study leading to the MD degree may vary from 4 to 6 years. Students have flexibility in sequencing courses by demonstrating competency through examination. This curriculum stimulates self-directed learning, and provides students time to pursue an investigative project, obtain teaching experience, perform community service, explore special interests, or obtain advanced degrees.

Grading and Promotion Policies

The grading system is Pass/Fail/Marginal Performance in the basic sciences and clinical clerkships. Narrative evaluations are used in the clerkships. Step 1 and Step 2 of the USMLE must be passed in order to graduate.

Facilities

Teaching: The school is part of the Stanford University Medical Center and consists of 26 departments. The major clinical teaching facilities are Stanford University Hospital (663 beds), Lucile Packard Children's Hospital (152 beds), Santa Clara Valley Medical Center (791 beds), and the Palo Alto Veterans Administration Hospital (1000 beds). *Library:* The Lane Medical Library contains more than 280,000 volumes and more than 3000 periodicals. The Fleischmann Learning Resource Center is an independent study center offering media and computer-based programs. SUMMIT (Stanford University Medical Media and Information Technologies) produces faculty- and student-authored programs. *Housing:* Apartments are available for single and married students.

Special Features

Minority admissions: The school believes that a student body that is both highly qualified and diverse in terms of culture, class, gender, race, ethnicity, background, work and life experiences, skills, and interests is essential to the education of physicians. Because of its strongly belief in the value of diversity, the school especially encourages applications from African Americans, Mexican Americans, Native Americans, and mainland Puerto Ricans, as well as from others whose backgrounds and experience provide additional dimensions that will enhance the school's program. An early matriculation program, which includes preclinical coursework and research opportunities, has been developed for students from disadvantaged backgrounds. *Other degree programs:* Combined MD-PhD programs are offered in most basic medical sciences as well as in cancer biology, epidemiology, immunology, neurobiology, and medical information sciences.

University of California—Davis School of Medicine

Davis, California 95616

Phone: 916-752-2717
WWW: http://www.ucdavis.edu

Application Filing		Accreditation	
Earliest:	June 1	LCME	
Latest:	November 1		
Fee:	$40	**Degrees Granted**	
AMCAS:	yes	MD, MD-PhD, MD-MPH	

Enrollment: 1996–97 First-Year Class

Men:	59	63%	Applied:	5491
Women:	34	37%	Interviewed:	5491
Minorities:	93	n/av	Enrolled:	93
Out of State:	3	3%		

1996–97 Class Profile

Mean MCAT Scores		*Mean GPA*
Physical Sciences:	n/av	3.4
Biological Sciences:	n/av	
Verbal Reasoning:	n/av	

Tuition and Fees

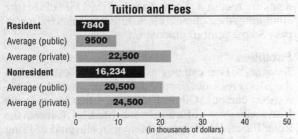

Resident	7840
Average (public)	9500
Average (private)	22,500
Nonresident	16,234
Average (public)	20,500
Average (private)	24,500

0   10   20   30   40   50
(in thousands of dollars)

Percentage receiving financial aid: n/av

Introduction

This medical school admitted its first class in 1968. Its educational goal is to provide students with a medical knowledge base that enables them to choose to pursue a career in primary care, specialty practice, public health, research, or administration. While most of the facilities necessary for earning the medical degree are located on the University of California Davis campus, most of the school's clinical space is at the UC Davis Medical Center in Sacramento.

Admissions (AMCAS)

Requirements include the basic premedical science courses plus 1 year each of English and mathematics that includes integral calculus. First preference goes to residents and next to WICHE applicants. *Transfer and advanced standing:* Currently enrolled students in good standing at U.S. or Canadian medical schools may apply for admission to the third year of study. Applications are considered on a space available basis.

Curriculum

4-year semimodern. The curriculum seeks to provide a balanced blend of basic and clinical sciences. *First year:* Consists of the introductory basic medical sciences, immunology, and general pathology. These are combined with social sciences, an introduction to the art of communicating with patients, and emergency medicine. *Second year:* Provides for a transition between basic and clinical sciences with the presentation of pathology, nutrition, pharmacology, microbiology, human sexuality, pathological basis of disease, and physical diagnosis, as well as laboratory diagnostic techniques and community health. *Third year:* Consists of clerkship rotations in the major specialties, maternal and child health, and psychiatry. *Fourth year:* Electives and elective clerkships, with required courses in medical ethics, medical economics, and medical jurisprudence.

Grading and Promotion Policies

Letter grades are given in required courses and letter grades or Satisfactory/Unsatisfactory in elective courses. At the end of each year, the medical school's Promotion Board evaluates each student's record. Students must record a passing total score on Step 1 of the USMLE for promotion to the third year and record a score on Step 2 to graduate.

Facilities

Teaching: The basic sciences are taught at the Medical Sciences I complex in Davis. Clinical facilities are provided by the University Medical Center (486 beds), which has over 100 specialty clinics. *Other:* Clinical instruction also takes place at the UCD Medical Center in Sacramento, Kaiser Foundation Hospitals in Sacramento, and other affiliated hospitals and family practice centers. *Library:* The Health Sciences Library is located adjacent to the School of Medicine and has more than 142,000 volumes and 3700 periodicals. The library has terminal access to MEDLINE, an on-line retrieval system for medical periodical information. A branch library is operated at the Sacramento Medical Center. *Housing:* Some on-campus housing is available at residence halls for unmarried students; a number of 1- and 2-bedroom units are available for married students.

Special Features

Minority admissions: An active recruitment program is coordinated by the Director of the Office of Research and Education for Medically Underserved. A 6-week summer prematriculation program is offered. *Other degree programs:* Combined MD-PhD programs are offered in a wide variety of disciplines including biomedical engineering, biophysics, endocrinology, genetics, nutrition, and psychology. MD-MBA and MD-MPH degree programs are offered through the University of California, Berkley School of Public Health and are given at the medical school.

University of California—Irvine College of Medicine

Irvine, California   92717

Phone: 714-824-5388   *Fax:* 714-824-2485
E-mail: reschrei @uci-edu
WWW: http://www.meded.com.uci.edu:80

Application Filing		Accreditation
Earliest:	June 1	LCME
Latest:	November 1	
Fee:	$40	**Degrees Granted**
AMCAS:	yes	MD, MD-PhD

Enrollment: 1996–97 First-Year Class

Men:	52	40%	Applied:	5189
Women:	40	43%	Interviewed:	467
Minorities:	19	21%	Enrolled:	92
Out of State:	0	0%		

1996–97 Class Profile

Mean MCAT Scores		*Mean GPA*
Physical Sciences:	10.4	3.56
Biological Sciences:	10.7	
Verbal Reasoning:	9.2	

Tuition and Fees

	(in thousands of dollars)
Resident	8280
Average (public)	9500
Average (private)	22,500
Nonresident	15,979
Average (public)	20,500
Average (private)	24,500

Percentage receiving financial aid: 87%

Above data applies to 1995–96 academic year.

Introduction

This school began as a private institution in 1896 and was incorporated into the University of California in 1965. Its location is on the 122-acre Irvine Campus. Its park-like setting and the year-round mild climate of Southern California provides a conducive environment for both study and relaxation.

Admissions (AMCAS)

Prerequisites for admission include the required pre-medical science courses plus 1 advanced biology course and 1 course in calculus. Preference is given to applicants with 4 years of undergraduate work. Nonresidents may apply, but preference is given to California residents.

Curriculum

4-year modern. The Doctor of Medicine curriculum entails 4 years of academic and clinical study—a period that, under special circumstances, may be lengthened. The current instructional year consists of 16 periods spread over 4 years, including a 10-week vacation period between the first and second years, and up to 12 weeks of vacation in the senior year. *First two years:* Basic science and preclinical instruction are scheduled on a modified quarter system. Each quarter in the first 2 years spans 9 to 15 weeks and consists of 8 to 14 weeks of instruction as well as 1 week of final and/or midcourse examinations. Basic science instruction includes gross anatomy and embryology, biochemistry, histology, neuroanatomy, physiology, microbiology, behavioral sciences, and nutrition. Preclinical instruction involves pathology, clinical pathology, behavioral science II, preventive medicine, examination of the patient, mechanisms of disease, and introductory courses to the clinical clerkships. *Third and fourth years:* Devoted to clinical rotations, which are scheduled according to 10-week quintiles. The 2-year clinical sciences component is spent in clerkships in medicine, pediatrics, obstetrics and gynecology, surgery, anesthesiology, ophthalmology, psychiatry, physical medicine and rehabilitation, neurosciences, primary care, and radiological sciences. Students are also provided ample opportunity to participate in clinical and research elective courses of their choosing.

Grading and Promotion Policies

An Honors/Pass/Fail grading system was adopted in the fall of 1994. After the second year, all medical students are required to pass Step 1 of the USMLE before continuing their clinical clerkships. Students must also pass Step 2 prior to graduation.

Facilities

Teaching: The campus is 40 miles south of Los Angeles. Preclinical instructions are conducted in facilities on campus. Clinical teaching takes place at the University of California Irvine Medical Center, the Long Beach VA Hospital, Memorial Hospital of Long Beach, and Children's Hospital of Orange County. Laboratories are organized on a multidisciplinary basis. *Other:* Other facilities include advanced equipment in medical imaging and laser medicine, electron microscope, analytical ultracentrifuge, amino acid analyzer, biometrics, medical illustration, medical vivarium, and research and development shop. *Library:* The Medical Sciences Library is located in the medical sciences facilities. *Housing:* An adequate number of apartments are available for single and married students.

Special Features

Minority admissions: Applications are encouraged from minority students and the school utilizes the Med-MAR list. A 6-week summer premedical program and a 7-week summer preentry program are offered for disadvantaged students to facilitate their admission and retention. *Other degree programs:* Interdisciplinary courses include those in community environmental medicine, mechanisms of disease, examination of patients, and a variety of elective courses. Students may take a leave of absence to pursue special research. A continuing education program is provided; a combined MD-PhD program is available in conjunction with the UCI School of Biological Sciences.

University of California— Los Angeles
UCLA School of Medicine

Los Angeles, California   90095

Phone: 310-825-6081
WWW: http://www.medctr.ucla.edu/

Application Filing		Accreditation	
Earliest:	June 1	LCME	
Latest:	November 1		
Fee:	$40	**Degrees Granted**	
AMCAS:	yes	MD, MD-PhD, MD-MPH	

Enrollment: 1996–97 First-Year Class

Men:	77	53%	Applied:		6111
Women:	68	47%	Interviewed:		794
Minorities:	22	15%	Enrolled:		145
Out of State:	127	88%			

1996–97 Class Profile

Mean MCAT Scores		*Mean GPA*
Physical Sciences:	n/av	3.64
Biological Sciences:	n/av	
Verbal Reasoning:	n/av	

Tuition and Fees

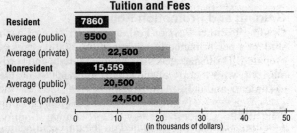

Resident	7860
Average (public)	9500
Average (private)	22,500
Nonresident	15,559
Average (public)	20,500
Average (private)	24,500

(in thousands of dollars)

Percentage receiving financial aid: n/av

Above data applies to 1995–96 academic year.

Introduction

This was the first University of California Medical School in Southern California, enrolling its charter class in 1951. The school is located on the UCLA campus and is closely connected with the University Medical Center. Both the School of Medicine and Medical Center have expanded along with the growth of Los Angeles into a major metropolitan urban center.

Admissions (AMCAS)

Prerequisites for admission include the required premedical science courses plus quantitative analysis (as part of inorganic chemistry), 1 year of advanced biology (including molecular, cellular, developmental, and genetic biology), and 1 year of mathematics (including college algebra). Introductory calculus is recommended. *Transfer and advanced standing:* Those who have completed 2 years in an approved U.S. medical school will be considered for the third-year class only.

Curriculum

4-year semitraditional. Stress is on the holistic approach in medicine. *First year:* Introductory basic sciences and patient contact and experience in history and physical examination as well as an elective program and a preceptorship program. *Second year:* Study of the process of disease through advanced basic science courses using an organ-system approach; diagnosis and treatment through courses in clinical surgery, clinical neurology, outpatient psychiatry, radiology, and obstetrics. *Third year:* Clerkships in clinical sciences and work in wards and outpatient clinics. *Fourth year:* Consists of electives—advanced elective clinical clerkships with primary patient responsibility, and indepth elective courses that can be centered on major area of clinical interest or a combination of related or diverse disciplines.

Grading and Promotion Policies

Letter grading in basic sciences, clinical sciences, and electives. Promotion is contingent upon satisfactory completion of required work each year. Completion of Steps 1 and 2 of the USMLE is required.

Facilities

Teaching: The School of Medicine is located in the Center for Health Sciences, which is the largest building in California. The University Hospital (517 beds) is the major clinical training center. Many other hospitals, including Harbor General (800 beds), are affiliated with the medical school. *Other:* The Brain Research Institute is a 10-story wing, connected to the Neuropsychiatric Institute and also houses the Los Angeles County Cardiovascular Research Laboratory. The Reed Neurological Research Center is an 8-story unit devoted to clinical research in neuromuscular disease. *Library:* The Biomedical Library is an 8-level facility in the northeast corner of the campus. *Housing:* Living accommodations are available in the university's residence halls or married students' housing.

Special Features

Minority admissions: The school has an active recruitment program and offers a 4-week summer prologue to medicine program for accepted students. *Other degree programs:* Combined MD-PhD degree programs are offered in a variety of disciplines including medical physics, biomathematics, engineering, and experimental pathology. An MD-MPH program is also offered.

University of California— San Diego School of Medicine

La Jolla, California   92093

Phone: 619-534-3880   *Fax:* 619-534-5282
E-mail: mlofftus@ucsd.edu
WWW: http://www.medicine.ucsd.edu

Application Filing		Accreditation	
Earliest:	June 1	LCME	
Latest:	November 1		
Fee:	$40	**Degrees Granted**	
AMCAS:	yes	MD, MD-PhD, MD-MPH	

Enrollment: 1996–97 First-Year Class

Men:	73	60%	Applied:	5348
Women:	49	40%	Interviewed:	588
Minorities:	65	53%	Enrolled:	122
Out of State:	1	1%		

1996–97 Class Profile

Mean MCAT Scores		*Mean GPA*
Physical Sciences:	11.4	3.65
Biological Sciences:	11	
Verbal Reasoning:	10.4	

Tuition and Fees

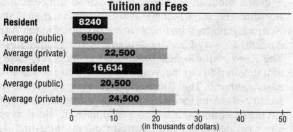

Resident	8240
Average (public)	9500
Average (private)	22,500
Nonresident	16,634
Average (public)	20,500
Average (private)	24,500

0   10   20   30   40   50
(in thousands of dollars)

Percentage receiving financial aid: 77%

Introduction

This school is located on the main campus of the University at La Jolla, making it accessible to a wide variety of educational opportunities. Its scenic location is unique, affording students special opportunities for both educational and cultural advancement.

Admissions (AMCAS)

It is recommended that students enter medical school after 4 years of undergraduate study; the absolute minimum requirement is attendance for 3 academic years at an approved college of arts and sciences. Students who have attended a foreign school must have completed at least 1 year of undergraduate study at an accredited 4-year college or university in the United States prior to application. Applicants are required to have completed the minimum premedical science courses and 1 year of mathematics (only calculus, statistics, or computer science is considered). The ability to express oneself clearly in both oral and written English is essential. A broad base of knowledge is advantageous in preparing for the many roles of a physician and may include courses in behavioral sciences, the biology of cells and development, genetics, biochemistry, English, social sciences, or conversational Spanish. Only permanent residents or U.S. citizens will be considered for admission and preference is given to California state residents. *Transfer and advanced standing:* Transfer students from either foreign or domestic medical schools are not accepted.

Curriculum

4-year modern. Program places emphasis upon human disease with aim of expanding scientific knowledge and in the context of social applicability. The curriculum is divided into 2 major components: the core curriculum and the elective programs. Both are pursued concurrently, with the core predominating in the early years and the elective in the latter. Elective programs offer students a set of choices suited to their unique background, ability, and career objectives. *Preclinical phase:* The first year includes social and behavioral sciences, biostatistics, and an introduction to clinical medicine as well as some introductory and advanced basic science courses. The second year includes anatomy as well as advanced electives. *Clinical phase:* An extended continuum consisting of rotation through the major clinical specialties and electives (which take up about half of the total time of these 2 years).

Grading and Promotion Policies

Grading is either Pass or Fail, and a narrative of each student's performance in his/her individual courses is prepared. These narratives are collated yearly and summarized, with a copy of the summary made available to students and their main advisor.

Facilities

Teaching: The school is located on the university campus in La Jolla. The primary teaching hospitals include the Veterans Administration Medical Center, UCSD Medical Center, and Balboa Naval Hospital. *Other:* Clinical teaching is also done at Mercy Hospital, Sharp Hospital, Children's Health Center, and the Kaiser Permanente Health Maintenance Organization as well as a wide spectrum of front-line, outpatient clinics, ranging from tiny Indian reservation facilities in North San Diego County, to the Clinica de Campesinos to the west, and the Northern California Rural Health Project some 500 miles to the north. *Library:* The Biomedical Library is located on the UCSD medical school campus and houses a large collection of books and journals. *Housing:* Limited on-campus housing is available.

Special Features

Minority admissions: The school conducts an active recruitment program and offers a summer preparatory program for disadvantaged students who have been accepted. *Other degree programs:* Combined MD-PhD programs available in a variety of disciplines, including biology, bioengineering, and chemistry. Also available is an MD-MPH program in conjunction with San Diego State University.

University of California— San Francisco School of Medicine

San Francisco, California   94143

Phone: 415-476-4044
WWW: http://www.ucsf.edu

Application Filing		Accreditation	
Earliest:	June 1	LCME	
Latest:	November 1		
Fee:	$40	**Degrees Granted**	
AMCAS:	yes	MD, MD-PhD	

Enrollment: 1996–97 First-Year Class

Men:	73	52%	Applied:	5886
Women:	68	48%	Interviewed:	530
Minorities:	31	22%	Enrolled:	141
Out of State:	33	23%		

1996–97 Class Profile

Mean MCAT Scores		*Mean GPA*
Physical Sciences:	11	3.68
Biological Sciences:	11	
Verbal Reasoning:	11	

Tuition and Fees

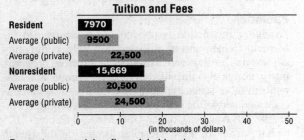

Resident	7970
Average (public)	9500
Average (private)	22,500
Nonresident	15,669
Average (public)	20,500
Average (private)	24,500

(in thousands of dollars)

Percentage receiving financial aid: n/av

Above data applies to 1995–96 academic year.

Introduction

The University of California—San Francisco School of Medicine can trace its roots back to Toland Medical College, founded in 1864. UCSF became affiliated with the state university system in 1873. It represents the only 1 of 9 campuses of the University of California that is devoted exclusively to the health professions. In addition to the School of Medicine, it has 3 other professional schools for Dentistry, Nursing, and Pharmacy.

Admissions (AMCAS)

Minimum premedical science courses are required; biology should include vertebrate zoology. Mathematics, upper-division biological sciences, and humanities courses are recommended. *Transfer and advanced standing:* No students are accepted at any level.

Curriculum

4-year program that allows flexibility in course sequence, in choice of third and fourth year clinical electives. *First year:* Devoted to anatomy (including clinical anatomy), cell, molecular, and tissue biology, human metabolism, genetics, endocrinology, physiology, psychiatry, epidemiology, and introduction to clinical medicine. *Second year:* Devoted to pharmacology, parasitology, pathology, immunology, infectious diseases, psychiatry, and radiology. Other courses are human sexuality; and reproduction, growth and development. *Third year:* Devoted to completion of the 52 weeks of clinical clerkships in the major specialties. *Fourth year:* Spent completing the required clerkships and clinical electives, including a month-long selective in clinical problem-solving and a year-end course in mechanism of disease and advanced cardiac life support. A career advising program allows students to devise a fourth year schedule to enhance clinical skills and prepare them for postgraduate training programs.

Grading and Promotion Policies

The grading system used is Honors/Pass/Not pass. Honors are not awarded in the first-year courses. The Student Screening Committee on Student Promotions assesses the performance of all students at the end of each quarter and recommends one of the following: promotion to the next quarter; promotion to the next quarter, subject to certain conditions; formal repetition of one or more quarters of work; or consideration of dismissal from the school. A passing total score must be recorded in Step 1 of the USMLE for promotion to the third year; Step 2 must be taken only to record a score.

Facilities

Teaching: Preclinical courses are offered at the Medical Sciences Building and the Health Sciences Instruction and Research Building. Core clinical instruction utilizes the Herbert C. Moffitt/Joseph M. Long Hospitals (540 beds), San Francisco General Hospital (520 beds), UCSF/Mount Zion Medical Center (439 beds), Veterans Administration Medical Center (252 beds), and Langley Porter Psychiatric Institute (44 beds), as well as other area hospitals. *Other:* There are 8 research facilities affiliated with the school: the Cancer Research Institute, Cardiovascular Research Institute, George Williams Hooper Foundation, Hormone Research Laboratory, Institute for Health Policy Studies, Laboratory of Radiobiology and Environmental Health, Metabolic Unit, and Reproductive Endocrinology Center. *Library:* The major portions of the library are housed in the Medical Sciences Building; there are more than 500,000 volumes and 8000 periodicals. *Housing:* The university operates Millberry Residence Hall for single students and Aldea San Miguel for married students.

Special Features

Minority admissions: With the exception of Howard and Meharry, this medical school has the highest minority enrollment of continental U.S. schools. Its multifaceted program seeks to identify, recruit, and prepare disadvantaged students for careers in the health sciences. Included in these efforts are academic support services and counseling opportunities. *Other degree programs:* Students are encouraged to engage in research and other scholarly activities. Dual-degree programs offering MS, MPH, and PhD degrees are offered for this purpose, along with many opportunities not linked to dual-degree programs. MD-PhD programs are offered in a variety of disciplines.

University of Southern California School of Medicine

1975 Zonal Avenue
Los Angeles, California   90033

Phone: 213-342-2552
E-mail: medadmit@ hsc.usc.edu
WWW: http://www.usc.edu/hsc/med-sch/med-home.html

Application Filing		Accreditation
Earliest:	June 1	LCME
Latest:	November 1	
Fee:	$70	**Degrees Granted**
AMCAS:	yes	MD, MD-PhD, BS-MD

Enrollment: 1996–97 First-Year Class

Men:	81	54%	Applied:	6509
Women:	69	46%	Interviewed:	781
Minorities:	32	21%	Enrolled:	150
Out of State:	25	17%		

1996–97 Class Profile

Mean MCAT Scores		*Mean GPA*
Physical Sciences:	10.5	3.47
Biological Sciences:	10.7	
Verbal Reasoning:	10	

Tuition and Fees

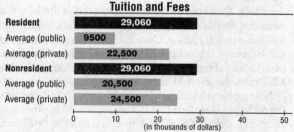

Resident	29,060
Average (public)	9500
Average (private)	22,500
Nonresident	29,060
Average (public)	20,500
Average (private)	24,500

(in thousands of dollars)

Percentage receiving financial aid: 74%

Introduction

This medical school was founded in 1885 and is part of a privately supported, nondenominational university. Its 31-acre campus is located in northeast Los Angeles, directly across from its major teaching hospital, which is one of the largest in the country. It is located 7 miles from the University Park campus and 3 miles from the Los Angeles Civic Center. It is the second largest of the university's 19 colleges and professional schools.

Admissions (AMCAS)

Minimum premedical science courses are required. A 1-semester course in molecular biology is also required. Developmental biology, cell physiology, genetics, biochemistry, and statistics are strongly recommended. The student body comes from all parts of the United States, as well as from several foreign countries. *Transfer and advanced standing:* Only second-year students enrolled and in good standing at LCME-approved medical schools may be considered for admission for the third year. Such students must pass Step 1 of the USMLE.

Curriculum

4-year modern. Students are progressively involved in patient care beginning with the first semester of the first year. An introduction to clinical medicine course begins in the freshman year and runs through the sophomore year. Doctor-patient relationships and interviewing are presented during the first year, and physical diagnosis and history-taking are discussed in the second. Groups of approximately 6 to 7 students are led by a faculty member who serves as a clinical tutor for their first 2 years. Basic sciences are taught largely in an organ system approach. Appropriate material in the basic sciences is presented during the study of these systems; patients are observed and examined for clinical illustration of the subject under discussion. In the second year, the student studies the pathologic aspects of medicine, also predominantly in organ system approach. In addition, a student may begin an investigative project. In the third year, student participation is required in the clinical clerkships, such as internal medicine and general surgery. Elective study is provided in the third and fourth years. The senior year consists almost entirely of work chosen by the student. In addition, students have an opportunity to engage in clinical or basic research through voluntary participation in a summer fellowship program between the freshman and sophomore years.

Grading and Promotion Policies

Grading basis is Honors, Satisfactory, Unsatisfactory.

Facilities

Teaching: Instruction is conducted on campus, in the Medical Center, and in affiliated hospitals, community clinics, and institutions. Through the elective program, instruction is also provided at medical schools and hospitals in other states and countries. The 30-acre campus is located across the street from its chief teaching hospital, the Los Angeles County-USC Medical Center (2105 beds). A 284-bed USC Hospital located on the Health Sciences Campus opened in 1991. *Other:* Additional clinical facilities include Norris Cancer Hospital and Research Institute, Doheny Eye Institute, Hospital of the Good Samaritan, Eisenhower Medical Center, and Barlow, California Huntington Memorial, and Presbyterian Inter-Community Hospitals. *Library:* The library can house 300,000 volumes and seat 250 readers. *Housing:* Information is not available.

Special Features

Other degree programs: Several components of the school provide direct support to students, including the Student Health Service, the Offices of Curriculum, Minority Affairs, Student Affairs, and the Office for Women. Services include tutorial assistance, health and counseling services, extensive extracurricular academic and nonacademic programs, school and university student government, services for students with disabilities, sophisticated library and electronic resources, and various other services. *Other degree programs:* The school sponsors an MD-PhD and a Research Scholar program. Apply during the first or second year of medical school. An 8-year Baccalaureate-MD program is offered to high school seniors.

COLORADO

University of Colorado School of Medicine

4200 East Ninth Avenue
Denver, Colorado   80262

Phone: 303-315-7361   *Fax:* 303-315-8494
E-mail: joey.seamans@uchsc.edu
WWW: http://www.uchsc. edu/

Application Filing		Accreditation	
Earliest:	June 1	LCME	
Latest:	November 15		
Fee:	$70	**Degrees Granted**	
AMCAS:	yes	MD, MD-PhD, MD-MPA	

Enrollment: 1996–97 First-Year Class

Men:	67	52%	Applied:	2700	
Women:	62	48%	Interviewed:	729	
Minorities:	18	14%	Enrolled:	129	
Out of State:	24	19%			

1996–97 Class Profile

Mean MCAT Scores		*Mean GPA*
Physical Sciences:	9.9	n/av
Biological Sciences:	9.9	
Verbal Reasoning:	9.9	

Tuition and Fees

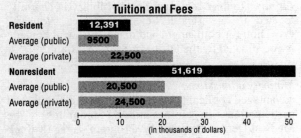

Resident	12,391
Average (public)	9500
Average (private)	22,500
Nonresident	51,619
Average (public)	20,500
Average (private)	24,500

0   10   20   30   40   50
(in thousands of dollars)

Percentage receiving financial aid: n/av

Introduction

The School of Medicine is one of the 4 components of the University of Colorado Health Sciences Center. The others are the schools of Dentistry and Nursing, and their Graduate School. The School of Medicine began in 1883 in Boulder. The first University Hospital was a 30-bed facility contracted in 1885, then relocated in 1911 to Denver, a city that offers many cultural and recreational facilities.

Admissions (AMCAS)

Required courses include the minimum premedical science courses plus 1 year of college-level mathematics and English literature, and 1 semester of English composition. About 85% of the approximately 125 first-year openings are awarded to residents. *Transfer and advanced standing:* Applicants in good standing from approved U.S. medical schools will be considered, when openings occur, for admission to sophomore classes. Preference is given to Colorado residents. Colorado residents who have completed their basic sciences at nonaccredited medical schools must have successfully passed Step 1 of the USMLE before being considered for openings in the sophomore class.

Curriculum

4-year semimodern. *First year:* Introductory basic sciences and courses in genetics and biometrics, as well as the first of a 3-year longitudinal course in primary care. *Second year:* Advanced basic sciences and courses in physical examination and preclerkship, pathophysiology of disease, clinical neurosciences, basic cardiac life support and primary care. *Third and fourth years:* Clerkship rotations through the major clinical specialties, electives, and free time. Seminars in minor clinical specialties are held throughout the school year. A large number of clinical and basic science opportunities are offered for the elective quarters. This allows students to major in certain specialties or subspecialties or to have experience in programs in community medicine, family medicine, or rural practice. It also provides for additional work in basic sciences or in laboratory research. An elective rural preceptorship is available, and participation in independent research during vacation is strongly encouraged. Among electives offered are courses in alcoholism, drug abuse, community medicine, ethical problems in medicine, geriatrics, health care delivery systems, human sexuality, occupational medicine, and environmental health hazards.

Grading and Promotion Policies

System used is Honors/Pass/Fail. The performance of each student is considered by curriculum and promotion committees, which determine when students have satisfactorily completed appropriate coursework.

Facilities

Teaching: Basic sciences are taught in the School of Medicine Building, which also has space for faculty offices and research laboratories. Clinical teaching takes place at the University Hospital (386 beds), at Colorado General Hospital (450 beds), at the VA Hospital (500 beds), and at Denver General Hospital (340 beds). *Other:* The Sabin Building for Cellular Research, the Webb-Waring Institute for Medical Research, the Clinical Research Wing of the Colorado General Hospital. *Library:* Denison Memorial Library is located in a building bearing the same name. The collection includes more than 150,000 volumes, and 2000 periodicals are received regularly. *Housing:* No residence halls available.

Special Features

Minority admissions: A minority-group students program gives special consideration to the applicants, provides advisory and tutoring services, and grants financial aid for eligible students. The school also offers an 8-week summer course, introduction to medical science, for some students. *Other degree programs:* Combined MD-PhD programs are offered in the basic medical sciences and in biometrics, biophysics, and genetics; there is a combined MD-MBA program.

CONNECTICUT

University of Connecticut School of Medicine

263 Farmington Avenue
Farmington, Connecticut   06030

Phone: 860-679-3874   *Fax:* 860-679-1282
E-mail: sanford@nso1.uchc.edu
WWW: http://www.uchc.edu/

Application Filing		Accreditation
Earliest:	June 1	LCME
Latest:	December 15	
Fee:	$60	**Degrees Granted**
AMCAS:	yes	MD, MD-PhD

Enrollment: 1996–97 First-Year Class

Men:	43	53%	Applied:	3000
Women:	38	47%	Interviewed:	300
Minorities:	9	11%	Enrolled:	81
Out of State:	30	37%		

1996–97 Class Profile

Mean MCAT Scores		*Mean GPA*
Physical Sciences:	10	3.6
Biological Sciences:	10	
Verbal Reasoning:	10	

Tuition and Fees

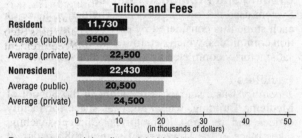

Resident	11,730
Average (public)	9500
Average (private)	22,500
Nonresident	22,430
Average (public)	20,500
Average (private)	24,500

0   10   20   30   40   50
(in thousands of dollars)

Percentage receiving financial aid: 81%

Introduction

The University of Connecticut has been in existence since 1881. The School of Medicine was activated in 1968 and together with the School of Dental Medicine and the University Hospital and Ambulatory Unit forms the University of Connecticut Health Center. The campus is located on 162 wooded acres, 7 miles west of Hartford in scenic Farmington. Boston and New York are each about 2 hours away.

Admissions (AMCAS)

Required courses include the basic premedical sciences. Applicants must demonstrate facility in quantitative and communicative skills. The faculty believes a broad liberal arts education provides the best preparation for those entering the medical profession. Strong preference is given to residents. *Transfer and advanced standing:* Third-year U.S. medical school transfers only.

Curriculum

4-year modern. It consists of 3 phases: *Phase 1:* Extends for 2 years. The didactic portion requires 20 hours per week devoted to the basic concepts and facts of medicine. It will involve lectures, laboratories, and seminars. Problem-based learning sessions will lead to an understanding of the material in a clinical context. Areas to be covered include: human system, human development in its environment, mechanism of disease, student practice, introduction to clinical medicine, Elective 1, and practical clinical experiences. *Phase 2:* Extends over 1 year. It is divided into 3 months of required experiences, 2 months of selectives, and 6 months of electives. A student practice preceptorship extends over the entire 4 years.

Grading and Promotions Policies

A Pass/Fail system is used. Students must take Steps 1 and 2 of the USMLE and record a score.

Facilities

Teaching: Students obtain most of their clinical experience in hospitals in the greater Hartford area and at the John Dempsey Hospital at the Health Center. The Health Center is a member of a consortium of hospitals that seeks to strengthen health education programs and improve patient care. Ten health care institutions are affiliated, and 11 are allied with the Health Center. *Library:* Lyman Maynard Stowe Library is centrally located in the Health Sciences Center. *Housing:* Provision for both single and married student housing is coordinated by the Office of Student Affairs.

Special Features

Minority admissions: The school actively recruits disadvantaged applicants by visits to area institutions and participation in informational programs. The Medical/Dental Preparatory Program is an 8-week summer program that simulates the first year of basic medical sciences. *Other degree programs:* MD-PhD programs are offered in a variety of disciplines including molecular biology and immunology.

Yale University
School of Medicine

333 Cedar Street
New Haven, Connecticut   06510

Phone: 203-785-2644   *Fax:* 203-785-3234
E-mail: medicalschool.admissions@quickmale.
          Yale.edu.
WWW: http://www.info.med.Yale.edu/medadmit

Application Filing   **Accreditation**
Earliest: June 1   LCME
Latest: October 15
Fee: $55   **Degrees Granted**
AMCAS: no   MD, MD-PhD, MD-MPH

Enrollment: 1996–97 First-Year Class

Men:	43	43%	Applied:	3628
Women:	58	57%	Interviewed:	834
Minorities:	17	17%	Enrolled:	101
Out of State:	92	91%		

1996–97 Class Profile

Mean MCAT Scores		*Mean GPA*
Physical Sciences:	11.2	3.6
Biological Sciences:	11.5	
Verbal Reasoning:	10.7	

Tuition and Fees

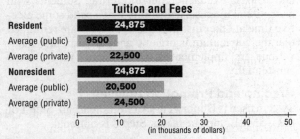

Resident	24,875
Average (public)	9500
Average (private)	22,500
Nonresident	24,875
Average (public)	20,500
Average (private)	24,500

0   10   20   30   40   50
(in thousands of dollars)

Percentage receiving financial aid: n/av

Introduction

This medical school was established by a state charter granted to Yale College in 1810. Subsequently, faculty members, local physicians, and other citizens raised funds that resulted in the New Haven Hospital, which served as a place to train medical students. In 1965 the hospital and the university became affiliated. The School of Medicine is a component of the Yale-New Haven Medical Center that also contains the School of Nursing and Yale-New Haven Hospital.

Admissions

Courses in the basic premedical sciences are required and courses in mathematics (calculus and statistics) and physical chemistry are recommended. *Transfer and advanced standing:* Students studying at other medical schools, domestic or foreign, are not encouraged to apply. In a few cases, students are accepted into second or third year.

Curriculum

First year: Four-year semimodern. The curriculum emphasizes normal biological form and function, and has been designed to coordinate information from various disciplines. It features a development approach to human behavior as related to health and illness. Anatomy and physiology are taught intensively two-thirds of the academic year. The first year includes a medicine, society, and public health series. Students are introduced to the principles and skills in medical interviewing and physical examination. *Second year:* The emphasis is on the disease process. A special feature is a series of all-day colloquia investigating diseases in an in-depth format. Basic principles of diagnostic radiology and laboratory medicine are included during the first 14 weeks. There are opportunities to enhance skills in history-taking and physical examination. The remaining 18 weeks feature modules in cardiovascular, clinical neuroscience and psychiatry, endocrine, female reproductive, GI/liver, lung/respiratory, musculoskeletal, renal/urinary tract, general oncology, and hematology. The medicine, society, and public health series continues. *Third and fourth years:* The clinical experience consists of direct patient care. Rotations include internal medicine and 3 subspecialties of surgery. There are clerkships in obstetrics and gynecology, psychiatry, pediatrics, clinical neuroscience, and primary care.

Grading and Promotion Policies

It is not the policy of this school to grade its students, and numerical standings are not determined. The performance of the students is carefully evaluated and reported by the faculty. All students must also pass Step 1 and Step 2 of the USMLE as a threshold requirement for graduation.

Facilities

Teaching: The school occupies several city blocks about one-half mile southwest of the University Center. Basic sciences are taught at the Jane Ellen Hope Building, Lander Hall, and Brady Memorial Laboratory. Clinical instruction takes place primarily at Yale-New Haven Hospital (900 beds) and the VA Hospital (513 beds) in West Haven. *Library:* Yale Medical Library is located in Sterling Hall and contains more than 380,000 volumes, receives 2600 journals, and has more than 90,000 other books of the last 2 centuries. The library is one of the country's largest medical libraries. *Housing:* Edward S. Harkness Memorial Hall provides living accommodations for single men and women and married students.

Special Features

Minority admissions: The school receives a substantial number of minority group applications even though it does not have a special recruitment program. *Other degree programs:* Combined degree programs are available for an MD-PhD in a variety of disciplines including anthropology, biology, chemistry, economics, engineering, genetics, biophysics, and psychology. MD-MDIV, MD-MPH, and MD-JD programs are also offered.

DISTRICT OF COLUMBIA

George Washington University School of Medicine and Health Sciences

2300 Eye Street, N.W.
Washington, D.C.   20037

Phone: 202-994-8749   *Fax:* 202-994-1753
E–mail: u.gwumc@gwis.circ.gwu.edu
WWW: http://www.gwu.edu/-gwu.edu/-gwumc/
medschool.html

Application Filing	Accreditation
Earliest: June 1	LCME
Latest: December 1	
Fee: $55	**Degrees Granted**
AMCAS: yes	MD, MD-PhD, MD-MPH

Enrollment: 1996–97 First-Year Class

Men:	72	47%	Applied:	7267
Women:	81	53%	Interviewed:	1017
Minorities:	24	16%	Enrolled:	153
Out of State:	n/av	n/av		

1996–97 Class Profile

Mean MCAT Scores		*Mean GPA*
Physical Sciences:	10	3.4
Biological Sciences:	10	
Verbal Reasoning:	10	

Tuition and Fees

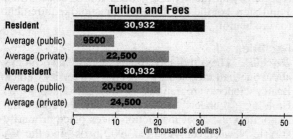

Resident	30,932
Average (public)	9500
Average (private)	22,500
Nonresident	30,932
Average (public)	20,500
Average (private)	24,500

0   10   20   30   40   50
(in thousands of dollars)

Percentage receiving financial aid: n/av

Introduction

The university began in 1821 as Columbian College and changed its name in honor of the first president in 1904. The School of Medicine was established in 1825. In 1844 Congress granted it the use of the Washington Infirmary, thereby establishing one of the earliest general teaching hospitals in the country. The School of Medicine is now one of the components of the George Washington Medical Center, which includes the University Hospital, a Health Sciences Library, and several other buildings.

Admissions (AMCAS)

Courses in English composition and literature are required in addition to the standard premedical science courses. School accepts many students from out of state. An early selection program for second-year Columbian (G.W.U.) College students is available. *Transfer and advanced standing:* Transfer students are accepted into the second- and third-year classes.

Curriculum

Practice of Medicine (POM) was recently incorporated into the first year. POM introduces students to the clinical setting in the first 2 years while teaching the basic sciences. In the final 2 years, POM reinforces and reintegrates the basic sciences as students' clinical experience progresses. *First year:* Introduction to normal human biology and function, including anatomy, biochemistry, physiology, neurobiology. *Second year:* Focus on abnormal human biology with the introduction of pharmacology, pathology, microbiology, psychopathology taught initially in a core curriculum and then progressing to an interdisciplinary, organ-system-organized discussion of the pathology, pharmacology, and the natural history of disease. *Third year:* Eight-week clerkships through the 5 major clinical disciplines and a 6-week primary care clerkship. *Fourth year:* Includes 37 weeks of course work and must include a 4-week "acting internship" in medicine, pediatrics, or family practice; three 2-week courses in anesthesiology, emergency medicine, and neuroscience; two selected 2-week courses to be selected from urology, orthopedics, otolaryngology, pediatric surgery, and ophthalmology; a course in medical decision making; and at least 1 didactic course offering. Students with exceptional interests and ability may spend some elective time at other institutions. Applicants are reminded that the curriculum is organic and, as curricular innovations are implemented, some details may change substantially.

Grading and Promotion Policies

System used is Honors/Pass/Conditional/Fail. Step 1 of the USMLE must be taken. Step 2 is optional.

Facilities

Teaching: Walter G. Ross Hall is the basic science building. Clinical instruction takes place at the 550-bed University Hospital and University Clinic, as well as at numerous affiliated hospitals. *Library:* The Himmelfarb Health Sciences Library is expanding, with a capacity for 80,000 volumes. *Housing:* Most students live off campus.

Special Features

Minority admissions: Admission Committee members visit selected schools to discuss the school's program with minority students. *Other degree programs:* Combined MD-PhD degree programs are offered in all the basic sciences as well as an MD-MPH program. In addition, there are BA-MD and integrated engineering programs.

Georgetown University School of Medicine

3900 Reservoir Road, N.W.
Washington, D.C.   20007

Phone: 202-687-1154
WWW: http://www.dml.georgetown.edu/schmed/

Application Filing		Accreditation
Earliest:	June 1	LCME
Latest:	November 1	
Fee:	$60	**Degrees Granted**
AMCAS:	yes	MD, MD-PhD

Enrollment: 1996–97 First-Year Class

Men:	96	58%	Applied:	12,448
Women:	69	42%	Interviewed:	1494
Minorities:	10	6%	Enrolled:	165
Out of State:	2	1%		

1996–97 Class Profile

Mean MCAT Scores		*Mean GPA*
Physical Sciences:	10	3.58
Biological Sciences:	10	
Verbal Reasoning:	10	

Tuition and Fees

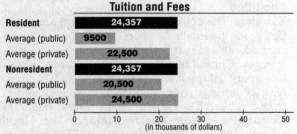

Resident	24,357
Average (public)	9500
Average (private)	22,500
Nonresident	24,357
Average (public)	20,500
Average (private)	24,500

(in thousands of dollars)

Percentage receiving financial aid: 80%

Above data applies to 1995–96 academic year.

Introduction

Founded in 1851, this is the oldest Catholic and Jesuit-sponsored medical school in the United States. It is named according to its location, the Georgetown section of Washington, D.C. The school is a component of Georgetown University Hospital and a Concentrated Care Center containing 12 modern surgical suites. The curriculum of the School of Medicine was approved by the LCME.

Admissions (AMCAS)

Required courses include the basic premedical sciences as well as 1 year each of English and mathematics. Courses considered useful preparation are biochemistry, computer science, cellular physiology, genetics, embryology, biostatistics, quantitative analysis. Some preference is given to District residents and Georgetown University undergraduates. *Transfer and advanced standing:* Students from foreign or domestic medical schools may apply to transfer to the second or third year. Transfers must take and pass Step 1 of the USMLE and must have taken the MCAT.

Curriculum

Georgetown's 4-year curriculum combines departmentally based basic science courses and laboratory work, prescribed clinical clerkships, multidisciplinary courses and conferences, and electives. Courses in the first 2 years focus on the development of fundamental knowledge concerning the body's normal and altered structure and functions. Small-group teaching and problem-based presentations have replaced a portion of the large class lectures.

In the third year, clinical clerkships stress the skills required to acquire and interpret patient-based data, while the fourth year further develops skills in patient management, including rotations in ambulatory care settings. Twenty-four weeks of electives are available during this final year, 4 of which may be used for vacation.

Faculty-student review of the curriculum is an important continuing endeavor of the School of Medicine.

Grading and Promotion Policies

At Georgetown the grading system consists of Honors, High Pass, Pass, and Fail. Students who receive an F in any course will be considered to be in a position of jeopardy, and their case will be referred to the Committee on Students for Review. A failure could lead to dismissal, repeating a year, or doing additional work in a specific course. Passing Step 1 of the USMLE is required prior to entering the third year.

Facilities

Teaching: Basic sciences are taught in the School of Medicine Building, the Preclinical Science Building, and the Basic Science Building. Clinical teaching takes place at University Hospital (535 beds), and a complex in close proximity to institutions providing access to approximately 7000 beds. *Other:* The District location provides students with opportunities such as federal laboratories, libraries, and museums. The National Library of Medicine and the laboratories of the Department of Agriculture and Bureau of Standards are affiliated with the university. *Library:* Dahlgren Memorial Library houses about 160,000 volumes and subscribes to 1650 periodicals. Also available for students' use are the Library of Congress, the National Library of Medicine, the National Institutes of Health Library, Agriculture Department Library, and the Public Library of District of Columbia. *Housing:* none.

Special Features

Minority admissions: Special admissions programs for underrepresented minority students include a prematriculation year of study supplemented with academic enrichment and advising. *Other degree programs:* A research track for medical students and a combined MD-PhD program are also available; the PhD may be taken in a basic medical science department, the neurosciences, or in philosophy-bioethics.

Howard University College of Medicine

520 W Street, N.W.
Washington, D.C.   20059

Phone: 202-806-6270   *Fax:* 202-806-7934
E–mail: bhlogan@access.howard.edu
WWW: http://www.cldc.howard.edu/-bhlogan/
                    hucm-cat.html

Application Filing		Accreditation	
Earliest:	June 1	LCME	
Latest:	December 15		
Fee:	$45	**Degrees Granted**	
AMCAS:	yes	MD, MD-PhD, BS-MD	

Enrollment: 1996–97 First-Year Class

Men:	53	48%	Applied:	5989
Women:	58	52%	Interviewed:	599
Minorities:	88	79%	Enrolled:	111
Out of State:	107	96%		

1996–97 Class Profile

Mean MCAT Scores		*Mean GPA*
Physical Sciences:	8	3.1
Biological Sciences:	8.2	
Verbal Reasoning:	7.6	

Tuition and Fees

Resident	16,288
Average (public)	9500
Average (private)	22,500
Nonresident	16,288
Average (public)	20,500
Average (private)	24,500

(in thousands of dollars) 0 10 20 30 40 50

Percentage receiving financial aid: 84%

Introduction

This is the oldest and largest African-American medical school in the country. It began in 1868 as the university's medical department, with the goal of training physicians in medically underserved areas. Its students come from all over the world and its alumni make up a significant segment of the nation's minority physicians.

Admissions (AMCAS)

Requirements include a minimum of 62 credits (2 years) of undergraduate work, plus minimum premedical science courses and 1 year of English. There are no residence restrictions; 70% of the students are African-American; about 50% are women. Selection is based not only on academic achievements and personal qualities, but also on the likelihood of practice in commu-

nities or facilities needing physician services. *Transfer and advanced standing:* Placement is infrequent, and usually at the end of the second year. Foreign transfers are not accepted.

Curriculum

4-year modern. Program is flexible in order to produce the physician-scientist. *First year:* Core concept presentation of introductory basic sciences and interdisciplinary courses, plus optional electives. *Second year:* Continued core concept presentation of advanced basic sciences plus interdisciplinary courses in pathophysiology of organ systems, infectious diseases, and physical diagnosis. Elective courses are offered. *Third year:* A series of clerkships through the major clinical specialties. Possibility for involvement in community health care is also provided. *Fourth year:* A 9-month program similar to junior year, except that periods of specialization are increased by allotment of 24 weeks of elective time (4 of which can be used for vacation).

Grading and Promotion Policies

System used is the Honors/Satisfactory/Unsatisfactory. Students must take Step 1 of the USMLE and obtain a passing total score for promotion to the third year. To graduate, students must record a passing total score on Step 2.

Facilities

Teaching: The college is part of Howard University Center for the Health Sciences. It is housed in a modern building and is the site for teaching basic medical sciences. Clinical teaching is at the 300-bed Howard University Hospital. Several other hospitals in the District area provide additional training facilities. *Other:* Research is carried out in several buildings, including a Cancer Center. *Library:* The Health Sciences Library contains more than 265,000 volumes, and 1750 periodicals. National Institutes of Health and National Library of Medicine are available to students. *Housing:* Professional students are not usually allocated accommodations on campus, but a university-owned apartment complex is nearby.

Special Features

Minority admissions: The college is dedicated to training minority applicants and has a strong recruitment program that includes early admission and academic reinforcement for admitted students. *Other degree programs:* A dual-degree program is available for the MD-PhD in most of the basic sciences; a BS-MD program is also offered. Continuing education is available for graduates.

FLORIDA

University of Florida College of Medicine

Gainesville, Florida   32610

Phone: 352-392-4569   *Fax:* 352-846-0622
WWW: http://www.med.ufl.edu/

Application Filing	Accreditation
Earliest: June 1	LCME
Latest: December 1	
Fee: $20	**Degrees Granted**
AMCAS: yes	MD, MD-PhD

Enrollment: 1996–97 First-Year Class

Men:	48	56%	Applied:	8612
Women:	37	44%	Interviewed:	1378
Minorities:	6	7%	Enrolled:	85
Out of State:	4	5%		

1996–97 Class Profile

Mean MCAT Scores		*Mean GPA*
Physical Sciences:	9	3.68
Biological Sciences:	9.4	
Verbal Reasoning:	9.1	

Tuition and Fees

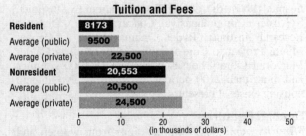

Resident	8173
Average (public)	9500
Average (private)	22,500
Nonresident	20,553
Average (public)	20,500
Average (private)	24,500

(in thousands of dollars)

Percentage receiving financial aid: n/av

Above data applies to 1995–96 academic year.

Introduction

This medical school began in 1956 and occupies the southeast corner of the 2000-acre University of Florida campus. It is a component of the University of Florida Health Sciences Center, which also consists of colleges of Dentistry, Veterinary Medicine, Nursing, Pharmacy, and Health-Related Professionals.

Admissions (AMCAS)

Only the minimum premedical science courses are required. The college gives strong preference to those who have completed the requirements for a bachelor's degree and who are state residents. Very few of the class are nonresidents; out-of-state applicants should have a 3.5 or better GPA. *Transfer and advanced standing:* Transfer students are rarely considered. The state's program in medical sciences provides for the easy transfer of students only from Florida State University, Florida

A & M, and the University of West Florida.

Curriculum

4-year semitraditional. *First year:* In addition to the basic sciences, courses in medical ethics, human behavior, and molecular genetics are presented. *Second year:* Aside from the advanced basic sciences, courses in ophthalmology, radiology, and physical diagnosis are offered. *Third year:* Eight clinical clerkships extending over 52 weeks. *Fourth year:* Surgical and medical clerkships, coursework, and electives in selected categorical areas related to medicine within the medical school or at 2 nonuniversity settings.

Grading and Promotion Policies

The system used is letter/number. At the end of each quarter the Committee on Academic Status reviews each student's performance on the basis of grades and comments by faculty and recommends suitable action to the dean. Students who receive Fs in 2 major courses in one semester will be dropped automatically. In order to graduate, the student must take Steps 1 and 2 of the USMLE.

Facilities

Teaching: Basic sciences are taught in J. Hillis Miller Health Center, which includes the Shands Teaching Hospital (405 beds). Clinical teaching also takes place at the nearby VA Hospital (450 beds). *Other:* Research facilities are present in the Health Center, VA Hospital, and an animal research farm. *Library:* The Health Center Library has a collection of more than 193,000 books and periodicals. Computer-based retrieval services are available. *Housing:* Accommodations are available for single students in Beaty Towers and Schucht Village, and for married students in Cory, University, Maguire, and Diamond Memorial Villages. The latter contain 1-, 2-, and some 3-bedroom apartments.

Special Features

Minority admissions: The college encourages well-qualified students from minority groups and women students to apply. A summer workshop for new minority matriculants is sponsored annually. It is an orientation and academic preparation program. *Other degree programs:* The Medical Sciences Program allows students at Florida State University and Florida A & M to combine baccalaureate study with first year of medical study for combination degree. The college also offers a dual MD-PhD program for Medical Scientist Training Program. Continuing education is available for graduates.

University of Miami School of Medicine

P.O. Box 016159
Miami, Florida 33101

Phone: 305-243-6791 *Fax:* 305-243-6548
E-mail: rhinkley@mednet.med.miami.edu
WWW: http://www.miami.edu

Application Filing	Accreditation
Earliest: June 15	LCME
Latest: December 1	
Fee: $50	**Degrees Granted**
AMCAS: yes	MD, MD-PhD

Enrollment: 1996–97 First-Year Class
Men:	71	51%	Applied:	2873
Women:	68	49%	Interviewed:	431
Minorities:	17	12%	Enrolled:	139
Out of State:	4	3%		

1996–97 Class Profile
Mean MCAT Scores		*Mean GPA*
Physical Sciences:	9.4	3.61
Biological Sciences:	9.9	
Verbal Reasoning:	10	

Tuition and Fees

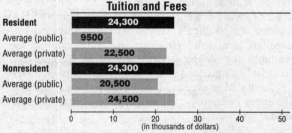

Resident	24,300
Average (public)	9500
Average (private)	22,500
Nonresident	24,300
Average (public)	20,500
Average (private)	24,500

(in thousands of dollars)

Percentage receiving financial aid: 80%

Introduction
This is the oldest and largest medical school in Florida and was established in 1952. The School of Medicine is located next to Jackson Memorial Hospital in the Civic Center area of Miami. The school has undergone considerable growth and is especially noted for its extensive research.

Admissions
Required courses include minimum premedical science courses plus 2 semesters of English. School gives strong preference to residents. *Transfer and advanced standing:* Transfer applicants must be Florida residents and currently enrolled in another medical school. Students are accepted into second- and third-year classes only. All applicants must be U.S. citizens or permanent residents of the United States.

Curriculum
4-year modern. *First year:* Designed to provide the student with a background of normal structure, function, and behavior. Basic sciences are integrated into study of organ systems. These courses include gross anatomy, cell biophysics, neuroscience, biochemistry, and systemic physiology. The latter is an interdisciplinary course dealing with structure and function of organ systems. The Community Clinical Experience runs throughout the first and second years. It provides a setting in which students acquire clinical skills through direct patient contact from the beginning of the freshman year. *Second year:* Initial weeks are devoted to general concepts of advanced basic sciences. A major course in mechanisms of disease emphasizes the disease processes that affect various organ systems. The transition to third-year work is prepared for by physical diagnosis. *Third year:* Consists of clerkship rotations through the major clinical specialties. *Fourth year:* Consists of electives. Students may select from a number of programs at the school and at other institutions, if approved. Students may choose from clinical (direct patient care and consultative care), academic, and research electives.

Facilities
Teaching: Basic sciences are taught in the Rosenstiel Medical Sciences Building. Clinical teaching takes place at Jackson Memorial Hospital (1500 beds) and the VA hospital (900 beds). *Other:* Bascom Palmer Eye Institute, Sylvester Comprehensive Cancer Center, Diabetes Research Institute, Ryder Trauma (Level 1) Center, Miami Project to Cure Paralysis. *Library:* The Calder Memorial Library houses more than 180,000 volumes and more than 2100 periodicals. *Housing:* No student housing exists at present.

Special Features
Minority admissions: Applications from women and socioeconomically disadvantaged candidates are encouraged, as are those from older applicants. *Other degree programs:* MD-PhD program for qualified applicants with extensive prior research experience.

University of South Florida College of Medicine
12901 Bruce B. Downs Boulevard
Tampa, Florida   33612

Phone: 813-974-2229   *Fax:* 813-974-4990
WWW: http://www.coml.med.usf.edu/

Application Filing
Earliest: June 1
Latest: December 15
Fee: $20
AMCAS: yes

Accreditation
LCME

Degrees Granted
MD, MD-PhD, MD-MPH

Enrollment: 1996–97 First-Year Class
Men:	65	68%	Applied:	1935
Women:	31	32%	Interviewed:	348
Minorities:	24	25%	Enrolled:	96
Out of State:	0	0%		

1996–97 Class Profile
Mean MCAT Scores		*Mean GPA*
Physical Sciences:	10.2	3.7
Biological Sciences:	10.2	
Verbal Reasoning:	9.7	

Tuition and Fees
Resident	8262
Average (public)	9500
Average (private)	22,500
Nonresident	21,261
Average (public)	20,500
Average (private)	24,500

(in thousands of dollars)

Percentage receiving financial aid: n/av

Introduction
This school, established in 1971, is one of the 3 colleges of the University of South Florida Health Sciences Center. Its location on a 1600-acre site of the northeast section of Tampa, which is an expanding metropolitan area of over 2 million people, has enhanced the rapid growth of the institution.

Admissions (AMCAS)
Required courses include the minimum premedical science courses plus 2 semesters of English and mathematics. Recommended courses include physical chemistry or biochemistry, embryology, cell biology, comparative anatomy, genetics, statistics, logic, and rhetoric. Coursework in communication, arts, humanities, and natural sciences is encouraged. Applicants who present a bachelor's degree from a liberal arts college are preferred. A 3-year applicant must present a superior academic record and demonstrated maturity. To be competitive, Florida residents should have a GPA of 3.0 or better on a 4.0 scale and score at least 8 in each category of the MCAT. *Transfer and advanced standing:* Information is not available.

Curriculum
4-year semitraditional. The 4-year curriculum is designed to permit the student to learn the fundamental principles of medicine, to acquire skills of critical judgment based on evidence and experience, and to develop an ability to use principles and skills wisely in solving problems in health and disease. It includes the sciences basic to medicine, the major clinical disciplines, and other significant elements such as behavioral science, medical ethics, and human values. The intent is to foster in students the ability to learn through self-directed, independent study throughout their professional lives. Using both ambulatory and hospital settings, students are given increasing responsibility for patient care in preparation to enter graduate medical education residencies.

Grading and Promotion Policies
Students' performance in academic coursework will be evaluated by assignment of grades of Honors (H), Pass with Commendation (PC), Pass (P), Requires Remediation (D), Fail (F), or Incomplete (I). Passing grades are H, PC, and P in order of excellence. Deficient grades are D, F, or I. The D, F, or I grade may be given to a student who fails to complete course requirements or who fails to attend or participate in required course activities.

Facilities
The USF Health Sciences Center offers hospital educational opportunities at facilities with more than 3500 patient beds. The primary teaching facilities are H.L. Moffitt Cancer Center and Research Institute, James A. Haley Veterans' Hospital, and Tampa General Hospital. The university's 538 College of Medicine faculty members work both on and off campus. Health Sciences Center affiliates for clinical education also include the following: USF Medical Clinic, University Diagnostic Clinic, University Psychiatry Center, All Childrens' Hospital, Bayfront Medical Center, Bay Pines Veterans' Hospital, and the Shriner Hospital for Crippled Children.

Special Features
Minority admissions: Special efforts are made to encourage qualified minority students to apply. *Other degree programs:* The school has an MD-PhD program for a select few students interested in a research career. Likewise, students interested in public health, preventive medicine or related areas can secure an MD-MPH degree. This degree requires minimal additional time and is awarded by The College of Public Health.

GEORGIA

Emory University School of Medicine

Atlanta, Georgia 30322

Phone: 404-727-5660 *Fax:* 404-727-0045
E-mail: medschadmiss@medadm.emory.edu
WWW: http://www.emory.edu/whsc/

Application Filing		Accreditation
Earliest:	June 1	LCME
Latest:	October 15	
Fee:	$50	**Degrees Granted**
AMCAS:	yes	MD, MD-PhD

Enrollment: 1996–97 First-Year Class

Men:	69	62%	Applied:	8277
Women:	43	38%	Interviewed:	828
Minorities:	43	38%	Enrolled:	112
Out of State:	56	50%		

1996–97 Class Profile

Mean MCAT Scores		*Mean GPA*
Physical Sciences:	10.4	3.66
Biological Sciences:	10.4	
Verbal Reasoning:	10	

Tuition and Fees

Resident	23,240
Average (public)	9500
Average (private)	22,500
Nonresident	23,240
Average (public)	20,500
Average (private)	24,500

(in thousands of dollars) 0 10 20 30 40 50

Percentage receiving financial aid: 74%

Introduction

Emory is a privately controlled university affiliated with the Methodist Church. The Emory University School of Medicine was established in 1915. The forerunner of this school was the Atlanta Medical College, which was established in 1856. This school was merged with Southern Medical College to form the Atlantic College of Physicians and Surgeons, and a subsequent merger took place with the Atlanta School of Medicine in 1905. In 1919 the name was changed to Emory University School of Medicine. It is located on 620 acres in the Druid Hills section of Atlanta.

Admissions (AMCAS)

Required courses, aside from the standard premedical sciences, include 1 year of English and 18 semester hours of humanities and/or social and behavioral sciences. Biochemistry is highly recommended. Applications from well-qualified students are seriously

considered regardless of geographic origin; however, 50% of the positions are given to state residents. Foreign students on visas must document ability to fund their medical education. *Transfer and advanced standing:* Properly qualified students from LCME-accredited schools will be considered for the second- or third-year classes.

Curriculum

4-year semitraditional. Years 1 and 2 utilize a continuum course in medical problem solving to assist students in their approach to patients and their problems. Along with traditional lectures and laboratories, the problem-based learning format allows students to integrate and apply basic science and psychosocial knowledge in solving clinical problems. *First year:* Interdepartmental course in cellular biology and biochemistry and in neurobiology; physiology, human anatomy, and genetics; introduction to the doctor-patient relationship, patient interviewing, and biostatistics. *Second year:* Advanced basic sciences and courses in behavioral science, nutrition, human values, and clinical methods. *Third year:* 12-week clerkship in internal medicine, 12-month interdisciplinary ethics clerkship, 8-week clerkship in other major clinical specialties, and a family medicine clerkship of 4 weeks duration. *Fourth year:* 4-week clerkships in medicine, neurology, and 4 weeks on a surgical selection, 2 weeks in dermatology, anesthesiology, and radiology, and 12 weeks of elective work in any area.

Grading and Promotion Policies

Grades of A through F are used in required courses and grades of Satisfactory/ Unsatisfactory are used in electives. At the end of the year, the promotion committees for each class review the records of all students to determine whether they should be unconditionally promoted to the next year's program, whether they need remedial work, whether they must repeat work deemed unsatisfactory, or whether they are to be asked to withdraw. For promotion to the third year, a passing total score must be recorded in Step 1 of the USMLE; Step 2 must be taken only to record a score.

Facilities

Teaching: Basic sciences are taught primarily on the Emory campus. Clinical instruction takes place primarily at University Hospital (600 beds), Grady Memorial Hospital (1000 beds), the VA Hospital (604 beds), Crawford Long Hospital (583 beds), and at many other ambulatory primary care sites. *Library:* The Health Sciences Library has more than 200,000 volumes and 3000 periodicals. Other clinical libraries are located in Emory University, Crawford Long, and Grady hospitals. *Housing:* A variety of on-campus and off-campus housing is available for graduate-level students.

Special Features

MD-PhD programs are offered in a variety of disciplines. An MD-MPH program is also available. There is a continuing education program for graduates.

Medical College of Georgia School of Medicine

1120 15th Street
Augusta, Georgia   30912

Phone: 706-721-3186   *Fax:* 706-721-0959
WWW: http://www.mcg.edu/

Application Filing		Accreditation	
Earliest:	June 1	LCME	
Latest:	November 1		
Fee:	n/av	**Degrees Granted**	
AMCAS:	yes	MD, MD-PhD	

Enrollment: 1996–97 First-Year Class

Men:	115	64%	Applied:	1911	
Women:	65	36%	Interviewed:	440	
Minorities:	40	22%	Enrolled:	180	
Out of State:	4	2%			

1996–97 Class Profile

Mean MCAT Scores		*Mean GPA*
Physical Sciences:	9.2	n/av
Biological Sciences:	9.4	
Verbal Reasoning:	9.7	

Tuition and Fees

Resident	5004
Average (public)	9500
Average (private)	22,500
Nonresident	15,225
Average (public)	20,500
Average (private)	24,500

(in thousands of dollars)

Percentage receiving financial aid: n/av

Above data applies to 1995–96 academic year.

Introduction

The University System of Georgia includes all state-operated institutions of higher education. The Medical College of Georgia is one of the 4 universities of this system. It consists of 5 schools: Medicine, Dentistry, Nursing, Allied Health, and Graduate Studies. The medical school, founded in 1828, is located in Augusta, which is on the south bank of the Savannah River, midway between the Great Smoky Mountains and the Atlantic Coast.

Admissions (AMCAS)

The basic premedical science courses are required as well as courses in English sufficient to satisfy baccalaureate degree requirements. Very strong preference is given to state residents, as well as to candidates with 4 years of undergraduate work. *Transfer and advanced standing:* Applicants from other MD programs are considered on a space-available basis.

Curriculum

4-year modern. *Year 1:* A 36-week core with elective time available in the third quarter. The core period is concerned with molecular, cellular, and human biology. Structure and function of the healthy body are approached by classical methods. The elective courses, which can be chosen from a wide variety of offerings, are aimed at strengthening skills and increasing knowledge. In addition, students begin their first contact with patients in the first year with courses such as physical diagnosis and the physician and patient. *Year 2:* A 35-week program coordinating the advanced basic sciences that are concerned with the study of the biology of diseases. Physical diagnosis is taught in relation to the study of pathophysiology. Additional contributions are made by various clinical departments. *Year 3:* A 48-week period of rotating clerkships in the major clinical specialties. Up to 8 weeks of electives can be taken. *Year 4:* 24 weeks of electives, which can be advanced clinical clerkships, basic science electives, or research electives. Some of the electives may be taken in other institutions and community hospitals.

Grading and Promotion Policies

Letter grades are used. Steps 1 and 2 of the USMLE are required of all students.

Facilities

Teaching: Basic sciences are taught primarily in the Research and Education Building that was opened in 1971. Clinical teaching takes place at the Medical College of Georgia Hospital and Clinics (540 beds) and 4 affiliated hospitals. *Other:* A 9-floor Clinical Research Annex at the teaching hospital contains special laboratories for research. *Library:* The library houses more than 150,000 volumes and 1650 periodicals. *Housing:* Accommodations are available in 3 residence halls for single students. One- and 2-bedroom apartments are available for married students.

Special Features

Minority admissions: The college conducts an intensive recruitment program and is committed to increasing minority representation in the student body. The college also conducts an 8-week summer program for high school and college students to strengthen their academic backgrounds and introduce them to the practical aspects of the health careers. *Other degree programs:* MD-PhD programs are offered in a variety of disciplines including endocrinology.

Mercer University School of Medicine

Macon, Georgia   31207

Phone: 912-752-2542
E-mail: kothanek.j@gain.mercer.edu

Application Filing		Accreditation	
Earliest:	June 1	LCME	
Latest:	December 1		
Fee:	$25	**Degrees Granted**	
AMCAS:	yes	MD	

Enrollment: 1996–97 First-Year Class

Men:	35	64%	Applied:	1471
Women:	25	45%	Interviewed:	191
Minorities:	4	7%	Enrolled:	55
Out of State:	0	0%		

1996–97 Class Profile

Mean MCAT Scores		*Mean GPA*
Physical Sciences:	8	n/av
Biological Sciences:	8.6	
Verbal Reasoning:	8.9	

Tuition and Fees

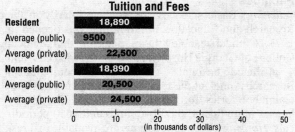

Resident	18,890
Average (public)	9500
Average (private)	22,500
Nonresident	18,890
Average (public)	20,500
Average (private)	24,500

(in thousands of dollars)

Percentage receiving financial aid: 80%

Above data applies to 1995–96 academic year.

Introduction

This school, founded in 1982, has the special mission of training physicians whose service will help meet the health care needs of rural and other underserved areas of Georgia. Located in Macon, in the heart of central Georgia, it is within driving distance of both Atlanta and Savannah.

Admissions (AMCAS)

The basic premedical science courses are required. Applicants with rural backgrounds are encouraged to apply. To date, only legal residents of Georgia have been accepted. *Transfer and advanced standing:* Transfer students from LCME-accredited medical schools are considered for admission into the junior year. Applicants must be legal residents of Georgia.

Curriculum

4-year problem-based. A 4-program educational scheme is used to train physicians for service in rural and/or medically underserved areas of Georgia. *Program 1 (Biomedical Problems):* During this 74-week program groups of 6 to 7 students work with faculty in a tutorial setting to study the basic medical and behavioral science concepts that underlie medical problems. The array and the sequence of problems are chosen to ensure that students acquire the basic medical and behavioral science knowledge requisite to medical practice. *Program 2 (Clinical Skills and Community Office Practice):* This occurs throughout the first 2 years during which students learn the skills basic for interaction with patients. Students interview and examine actual and standardized patients and have opportunities to practice their skills in the offices of supervising community physicians. *Program 3 (Community Science):* This program spans 4 years. Initially, students attend seminars and group discussions on biostatistics, epidemiology, and public health. Each student is assigned to a rural community and makes site visits to learn about medical practice and the health care needs of the area. In the fourth year this culminates in a 4-week community-based primary care clerkship during which the student lives in the community and participates in the practice of the supervising physician. *Program 4 (Clerkships-Electives):* The third year contains rotations in internal medicine, surgery, ambulatory family medicine, pediatrics, obstetrics/gynecology, and psychiatry. During year 4, critical care, substance abuse, and surgery rotations, in addition to 20 weeks of electives, are required.

Grading and Promotion Policies

A Pass/Fail system is used. Students must pass Steps 1 and 2 of the USMLE for promotion to year 3 and graduation, respectively.

Facilities

Teaching: The basic sciences are taught at the Education Building, and clinical training is offered at the Medical Center of Central Georgia and regional hospitals. A 40-room ambulatory care unit is also utilized. *Library:* A comprehensive medical library is available for student and faculty use. *Housing:* Apartments are available on campus and within a 15-minute drive of the school.

Special Features

Minority admissions: There is a program that involves strong recruiting efforts directed toward traditionally black colleges in Georgia. *Other degree programs:* Combined programs are not currently available.

Morehouse School of Medicine

720 Westview Drive, S.W.
Atlanta, Georgia   30310

Phone: 404-752-1650   *Fax:* 404-752-1512
E-mail: Karen@link.nism.edu
WWW: http://www.msm.edu/

Application Filing		Accreditation	
Earliest:	June 1	LCME	
Latest:	December 1		
Fee:	$45	**Degrees Granted**	
AMCAS:	yes	MD, MD-PhD, MD-MPH	

Enrollment: 1996–97 First-Year Class

Men:	11	32%	Applied:		2928
Women:	23	68%	Interviewed:		234
Minorities:	6	17%	Enrolled:		34
Out of State:	7	26%			

1996–97 Class Profile

Mean MCAT Scores		*Mean GPA*
Physical Sciences:	n/av	n/av
Biological Sciences:	n/av	
Verbal Reasoning:	n/av	

Tuition and Fees

Resident	18,433
Average (public)	9500
Average (private)	22,500
Nonresident	18,433
Average (public)	20,500
Average (private)	24,500

(in thousands of dollars)

Percentage receiving financial aid: n/av

Introduction

Morehouse School of Medicine is independent of its parent school Morehouse College. Morehouse School of Medicine is the most recent member of the Atlanta University Center, which is an organization of 6 independent institutions making up the largest predominantly African-American private educational structure in the world. It is one of 3 medical schools in the nation founded by historically African-American institutions. It began as a 2-year school in 1978 and was later transformed into a 4-year institution, graduating its first class in 1985.

Admissions (AMCAS)

The basic premedical science courses plus mathematics and English are required. Courses in biochemistry, embryology, and genetics are recommended. *Transfer and advanced standing:* Into second year only, provided space is available.

Curriculum

4-year traditional. *First and second years:* Devoted to the basic medical sciences as well as courses in human behavior and psychopathology, nutrition, community medicine, and biostatistics, along with human values in medicine and introduction to clinical medicine courses. *Third and fourth years:* These 2 years involve rotation through the clinical specialties plus 20 weeks of electives.

Grading and Promotion Policies

Letter grades are used. Students must obtain passing total scores on Steps 1 and 2 of the USMLE for promotion to the third year and graduation, respectively.

Facilities

Teaching: The first 2 years are taught at the Basic Medical Sciences Building. Clinical training is available at a number of affiliated hospitals in Atlanta and surrounding areas. *Library:* The medical library collection meets both student and faculty needs. *Housing:* Not available on campus.

Special Features

Minority admissions: The school's recruitment officer is actively involved in identifying, informing, and encouraging potential applicants. *Other degree programs:* An MD-PhD program is available in the biomedical sciences.

HAWAII

University of Hawaii
John A. Burns School of Medicine

1960 East-West Road
Honolulu, Hawaii   96822

Phone: 808-956-8300   *Fax:* 808-956-9547
E-mail: nishikim@jabsom.biomed.hawaii.edu
WWW: http://www.petersons.com/sites/775800 si.html

Application Filing		Accreditation	
Earliest:	June 1	LCME	
Latest:	December 1		
Fee:	$50	**Degrees Granted**	
AMCAS:	yes	MD, MD-PhD, MD-MS	

Enrollment: 1996–97 First-Year Class

Men:	29	52%	Applied:		1631
Women:	27	48%	Interviewed:		245
Minorities:	1	2%	Enrolled:		56
Out of State:	3	5%			

1996–97 Class Profile

Mean MCAT Scores		*Mean GPA*
Physical Sciences:	8.5	3.55
Biological Sciences:	9	
Verbal Reasoning:	8.8	

Tuition and Fees

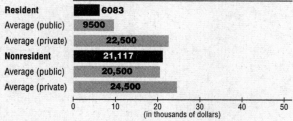

Resident	6083
Average (public)	9500
Average (private)	22,500
Nonresident	21,117
Average (public)	20,500
Average (private)	24,500

0   10   20   30   40   50
(in thousands of dollars)

Percentage receiving financial aid: 61%

Above data applies to 1995–96 academic year.

Introduction

The University of Hawaii is located in Honolulu. In 1961 the John A. Burns School of Medicine was founded as a 2-year program and expanded in 1973 to 4 years. The medical school is one of the components of the College of Health Science and Social Welfare, which includes schools of Nursing, Public Health, and Social Work.

Admissions (AMCAS)

Specific work required for entrance consists of the minimum premedical science courses. Courses should be of the type acceptable for students majoring in these areas and must include laboratory experience. Other science courses are not required, and breadth of education in the liberal arts is stressed. Residents of Hawaii and the Pacific Islands are given preference.

Curriculum

4-year. *First and second years:* The basic medical sciences are taught during the first 2 years of problem-based curriculum. *Third year:* 46 weeks of required clerkships (family practice, medicine, surgery, obstetrics-gynecology, pediatrics, and psychiatry). *Fourth year:* 35 weeks of clerkships and electives.

Grading and Promotion Policies

Grading system is Credit/No Credit/Honors. The student must obtain passing total scores on Steps 1 and 2 of the USMLE for graduation.

Facilities

Teaching: The Biomedical Sciences Building on the University of Hawaii Manoa campus houses the basic science departments. The clinical departments are based in affiliated community hospitals, where clinical teaching takes place. *Library:* The principal library resources are the Hawaii Medical Library adjacent to the Queen's Medical Center and Hamilton Library on the University of Hawaii at Manoa campus. Several hospital libraries are also available. *Housing:* Students are expected to make their own living arrangements.

Special Features

Minority admissions: A special program provides students from socioeconomically and academically underprivileged areas with the opportunity to study medicine. *Other degree programs:* Dual MD-MS and MD-PhD programs are offered in a variety of disciplines.

ILLINOIS

Chicago Medical School

Finch University of Health Sciences
3333 Green Bay Road
North Chicago, Illinois   60064

Phone: 847-578-3206   *Fax:* 847-578-3284
E-mail: foxd@mid.finchc.ms.edu
WWW: http://www.uchicago.edu/u.acadunits/bsd.html

Application Filing		Accreditation	
Earliest:	June 1	LCME	
Latest:	December 15		
Fee:	$65	**Degrees Granted**	
AMCAS:	yes	MD, MD-PhD	

Enrollment: 1996–97 First-Year Class

Men:	102	58%	Applied:		1276
Women:	74	42%	Interviewed:		1
Minorities:	21	12%	Enrolled:		176
Out of State:	12	7%			

1996–97 Class Profile

Mean MCAT Scores		*Mean GPA*
Physical Sciences:	9	3.6
Biological Sciences:	9	
Verbal Reasoning:	9	

Tuition and Fees

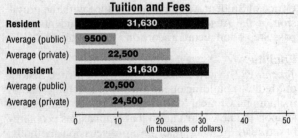

Resident	31,630
Average (public)	9500
Average (private)	22,500
Nonresident	31,630
Average (public)	20,500
Average (private)	24,500

(in thousands of dollars)

Percentage receiving financial aid: 76%

Introduction

This school was established in 1912 with the goal of enabling men and women to study medicine at night, a common practice at that time. It attracted a staff of excellent teachers and practitioners in 1917 when an older medical school in Chicago closed and its faculty transferred to the Chicago Medical School. In 1930 the school moved to a complex located west of downtown Chicago, and in 1967 the University of Health Sciences was established. The university consists of the Chicago Medical School, the School of Related Health Sciences, and the School of Graduate and Postdoctoral Studies.

Admissions (AMCAS)

Only minimum premedical science courses are required. Completion of a minimum of 90 semester hours is required and a baccalaureate degree is preferred. The school does not impose geographical restrictions. *Transfer and advanced standing:* None.

Curriculum

4-year semitraditional. Students may be permitted to finish requirements in 5 years, if they choose. *Year 1:* 30 weeks of class time in the basic sciences. *Year 2:* A clinically oriented introduction to medicine begins in the first quarter and increases progressively. Interdepartmental cooperation between clinical and basic science departments is emphasized. Overall, 30 weeks devoted to the advanced basic sciences. *Year 3:* 48 weeks devoted to clerkships in major specialties. Correlation of clinical instruction with basic sciences in conferences and seminars. *Year 4:* 36 weeks devoted to electives and selectives in affiliated hospitals and extramural institutions, along with a medical subinternship and neurology clerkship.

Grading and Promotion Policies

Letter grades are used in required courses and Pass/Fail in electives. There is a monthly review of performance by departments and a quarterly review by an evaluation committee. Students must record passing scores on Steps 1 and 2 of the USMLE in order to graduate.

Facilities

Teaching: The basic science instruction takes place in the classroom and administration building in North Chicago. Primary clinical teaching occurs in affiliated hospitals: Cook County Hospital, Edward Hines Veterans Affairs Medical Center, North Chicago Veterans Medical Center, Illinois Masonic Center, Lutheran General Hospital, Resurrection Hospital, and Mount Sinai Hospital Medical Center. *Library:* The library contains 75,000 volumes and subscribes to 1200 periodicals. *Housing:* None available on campus.

Special Features

Minority admissions: The school is actively involved in the recruitment of disadvantaged students and participates in the Chicago Area Health and Medical Careers Program. *Other degree programs:* MD-PhD programs are offered in a variety of basic science disciplines. A 7-year honors program in engineering and medicine is offered in conjunction with the Illinois Institute of Technology.

Loyola University Chicago Stritch School of Medicine

2160 South First Avenue
Maywood, Illinois   60153

Phone: 708-216-3229
WWW: http://www.meddean,iuc.edu/

Application Filing		Accreditation	
Earliest:	June 1	LCME	
Latest:	November 15		
Fee:	$50	**Degrees Granted**	
AMCAS:	yes	MD, MD-PhD	

Enrollment: 1996–97 First-Year Class

Men:	74	57%	Applied:	10,106
Women:	56	43%	Interviewed:	1
Minorities:	4	3%	Enrolled:	130
Out of State:	65	50%		

1996–97 Class Profile

Mean MCAT Scores		*Mean GPA*
Physical Sciences:	9.4	3.5
Biological Sciences:	9.8	
Verbal Reasoning:	9.4	

Tuition and Fees

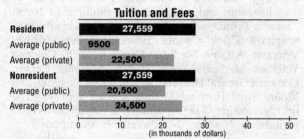

Resident	27,559
Average (public)	9500
Average (private)	22,500
Nonresident	27,559
Average (public)	20,500
Average (private)	24,500

0   10   20   30   40   50
(in thousands of dollars)

Percentage receiving financial aid: 91%

Introduction

Loyola is an autonomous school with a Jesuit/Roman Catholic connection. The Medical Center of Loyola works closely with several renowned hospitals in Chicago. The School of Medicine was founded in 1870; by 1920 it underwent a major reorganization. In 1969 the Loyola University Medical School was built in Maywood, a suburban community located about 12 miles west of Chicago.

Admissions (AMCAS)

This school requires satisfactory completion of the basic premedical science courses, all with laboratory. A semester or quarter of biochemistry can be substituted for part of the organic chemistry requirements. About half of the first-year openings are reserved for residents. A GPA of 3.0 and MCAT scores above 8 are considered competitive. *Transfer and advanced standing:* Space for transfers from domestic schools are based upon attrition.

Curriculum

4-year traditional. *First and second years:* The first year familiarizes the students with the science basic to normal structure and function of the body from cell to organ. The Introduction to Medicine I course provides students with skills and experience crucial in the patient-doctor relationship. The second year familiarizes students with the mechanisms of human disease and the therapeutic approach. The Introduction to the Practice of Medicine II course expands the clinical skills and reasoning to allow transition to the third year. It is devoted to developing an understanding of the sciences basic to the practice of medicine. During the early clinical experience course, students are provided training in clinical skills and experiences in ambulatory medicine settings. *Third and fourth years:* Organized into clinical clerkships. The core curriculum includes medicine (12 weeks), surgery (12 weeks), pediatrics (6 weeks), psychiatry (6 weeks), family medicine (6 weeks), neurology (4 weeks), obstetrics and gynecology (6 weeks), and subinternship experiences in medicine or pediatrics including critical care experience (8 weeks). Students also take between 32 and 40 weeks of electives during these 2 years. Through these electives, they anticipate their residency training and prepare for careers in medicine suited to their particular interests and talents.

Grading and Promotion Policies

The system used is Honors/High Pass/Pass/Fail. Student performance is regularly reviewed by the Office of Student Affairs in accordance with the provision of the Academic Policy Manual. Students must pass Step 1 and record a score on Step 2 of the USMLE.

Facilities

Teaching: The new 200,000 square foot Stritch School of Medicine building opened in 1997. Teaching spaces, including a Clinical Skills Laboratory, are designed to support the new curriculum that emphasizes problem-based learning and small group discussion methods. Clinical teaching takes place at the University Hospital and Ambulatory Center, the Hines VA Hospital, and affiliated hospitals. *Other:* Research facilities are available at the Medical Center. *Library:* The Medical Center Library has a collection of 172,803 volumes (62,714 books; 109,152 journals). *Housing:* There is no on-campus housing.

Special Features

Minority admissions: The school has joined other medical schools in the area to offer a Minority Medical Education Program sponsored by the AAMC and Robert Wood Johnson Foundation. Applications from minority group members from Illinois are encouraged. *Other degree programs:* An MD-PhD dual degree program is available.

Northwestern University Medical School

303 East Chicago Avenue
Chicago, Illinois   60611

Phone: 312-503-8206
WWW: http://www.ghsl.nwu.edu/healthweb/

Application Filing		Accreditation	
Earliest:	June 1	LCME	
Latest:	October 15		
Fee:	$50	**Degrees Granted**	
AMCAS:	yes	MD, MD-PhD, MD-MS	

Enrollment: 1996–97 First-Year Class

Men:	85	49%	Applied:	9522	
Women:	89	51%	Interviewed:	476	
Minorities:	7	4%	Enrolled:	174	
Out of State:	93	53%			

1996–97 Class Profile

Mean MCAT Scores		*Mean GPA*
Physical Sciences:	9.6	3.51
Biological Sciences:	9.8	
Verbal Reasoning:	9.7	

Tuition and Fees

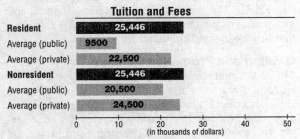

Resident	25,446
Average (public)	9500
Average (private)	22,500
Nonresident	25,446
Average (public)	20,500
Average (private)	24,500

0   10   20   30   40   50
(in thousands of dollars)

Percentage receiving financial aid: 61%

Above data applies to 1995–96 academic year.

Introduction
Northwestern University, established in 1851, is a private university. The medical school was opened in 1859 and the university became one of the first to provide an expanded medical education. The school is located on the university's lakefront Chicago campus. Among the school's major contributions to medicine involves the production of a whooping cough vaccine and innovation in the area of microscopy and laser surgery.

Admissions (AMCAS)
One year of English is required in addition to the minimum premedical science courses. About 50 openings are available to out-of-state students. *Transfer and advanced standing:* Applications to the second and third years are considered.

Curriculum
4-year semitraditional. *Basic sciences:* Work related to fundamental principles of molecular, cellular, tissue and gross architecture and function, followed by study of alteration in functions and structure by disease. Some degree of patient contact occurs throughout the first 2 years through courses such as introduction to clinical medicine and physical diagnoses. *Clinical sciences:* One year of clerkships in major clinical areas, ward rounds, teaching conferences, seminars, and increasing responsibility for patient care. Senior year is devoted exclusively to a program of electives. There is the option of spending 1 academic quarter at another school in the United States or abroad.

Grading and Promotion Policies
The system used is Honors/Pass/Fail. A Committee on Promotion reviews student records at the end of each year and determines those qualified for promotion. Taking Step 1 of the USMLE and recording a score is required. Taking Step 2 is optional.

Facilities
Teaching: Basic science teaching takes place in the Montgomery Ward and Searle Buildings. Clinical facilities are provided by 5 area hospitals that, together with the medical and dental schools, make up the Northwestern-McGraw Medical Center. *Other:* The Northwestern Health Sciences Building houses the NU Cancer Center and NU Memorial Hospital's acute care services. Morton Building contains research laboratories. *Library:* The Archibald Church Medical Library, located in the Searle Building, houses 228,000 volumes and more than 2500 periodicals. In addition, other libraries of Northwestern University are open to the students. *Housing:* Rooms are available for single men and women in Abbott Hall and 2 high-rise residence halls located on campus. A limited number of apartments for married students without children is also available in the facility.

Special Features
Minority admissions: Recruitment is conducted on the high school and college levels. The school participates in the summer program of the Chicago Area Health Careers Opportunity Program. *Other degree programs:* A combined MD-PhD program is available for students interested in research in a variety of disciplines including molecular biology, tumor cell biology, and clinical psychology. MD-MS and MD-MPH combined programs are also offered.

Rush Medical College of Rush University

600 S. Paulina Street
Chicago, Illinois   60612

Phone: 312-942-6913   *Fax:* 312-942-2333
E-mail: webadm@rpslmc.edu
WWW: http://www.rpslmc.edu/

Application Filing		Accreditation	
Earliest:	June 1	LCME	
Latest:	November 15		
Fee:	$45	**Degrees Granted**	
AMCAS:	yes	MD, MD-PhD	

Enrollment: 1996–97 First-Year Class

Men:	61	51%	Applied:	5473
Women:	59	49%	Interviewed:	454
Minorities:	12	10%	Enrolled:	120
Out of State:	16	13%		

1996–97 Class Profile

Mean MCAT Scores		*Mean GPA*
Physical Sciences:	9	3.51
Biological Sciences:	9	
Verbal Reasoning:	9	

Tuition and Fees

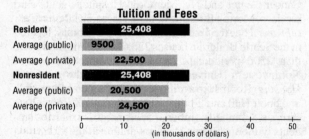

Resident	25,408
Average (public)	9500
Average (private)	22,500
Nonresident	25,408
Average (public)	20,500
Average (private)	24,500

(in thousands of dollars)

Percentage receiving financial aid: 81%

Introduction

Rush University began as 1 college and now consists of 4 colleges. They include Rush Medical College, the College of Nursing, the College of Health Sciences, and the Graduate College. The medical school was originally founded in 1837, remained in existence till 1943, and reopened in 1971. It is located on the west side of Chicago near the Loop.

Admissions (AMCAS)

The standard premedical courses are required. Consideration is given primarily to state residents, although competitive out-of-state residents are encouraged to apply. Rush Medical College students come from a wide variety of educational and social backgrounds. The Committee on Admissions considers both the academic and nonacademic qualifications of applicants in making its decisions.

Curriculum

4-year semitraditional. *First year:* Provides students with exposure to the vocabulary and fundamental concepts upon which the clinical sciences are based. The first year is made up of 3 quarters of basic science material organized by disciplines and emphasizing the structure, function, and behavior of the normal person. Students participate in a 2-year longitudinal generalist curriculum. Courses include interviewing and communications, physical diagnosis, and a primary care preceptorship. *Second year:* Students study the causes and effects of disease and therapeutics and initiate their work with patients in programs that emphasize interviewing, history-taking, and the physical examination. *Third and fourth years:* Provide students with training in clinical skills, diagnosis, and patient management in a variety of patient care settings. The clinical curriculum includes required core clerkships in family medicine, internal medicine, neurology, pediatrics, psychiatry, obstetrics/gynecology, and surgery for a total of 60 weeks. A total of 18 weeks of elective study in areas of special interest to each student is also required. *Alternative curriculum:* Rush has established an innovative preclinical curriculum for 24 students in each entering class. The Alternative Curriculum strives to give beginning medical students more experience with clinical problems, emphasizes personal responsibility for learning, and fosters the development of interpersonal skills. The new program involves individual and group assignments and uses elements of new information processing and computer technology.

Grading and Promotion Policies

The final evaluation in coursework is recorded as Honors, Pass, or Fail. The Committee on Student Evaluation and Promotion receives evaluations of each clinical period and determines when students are eligible for promotion. A total passing score must be obtained on Step 1 of the USMLE and a score recorded on Step 2.

Facilities

Teaching: Rush Medical College is located on the campus of Rush University at Rush-Presbyterian-St. Luke's Medical Center on Chicago's near west side. The Academic Facility houses the physical facilities for classroom instruction, laboratory research and private study. Clinical teaching takes place at Rush-Presbyterian-St. Luke's Hospital (903 beds) and other affiliated institutions. *Library:* The library of Rush University is located in the Academic Facility, has more than 93,000 volumes, and subscribes to more than 2050 journals.

Special Features

Minority admissions: The college encourages applications from disadvantaged minority group members who are underrepresented in the medical profession. *Other degree programs:* MD-PhD programs are offered in a variety of disciplines including immunology and psychology.

Southern Illinois University School of Medicine

P.O. Box 19230
Springfield, Illinois   62794

Phone: 217-782-2860   *Fax:* 217-785-5538
WWW: http://www.c-som.siu.edu/

Application Filing		Accreditation	
Earliest:	June 1	LCME	
Latest:	October 15		
Fee:	$50	**Degrees Granted**	
AMCAS:	yes	MD, MD-JD	

Enrollment: 1996–97 First-Year Class

Men:	42	58%	Applied:	1965
Women:	30	42%	Interviewed:	255
Minorities:	0	0%	Enrolled:	72
Out of State:	0	0%		

1996–97 Class Profile

Mean MCAT Scores		*Mean GPA*
Physical Sciences:	9	3.45
Biological Sciences:	10	
Verbal Reasoning:	10	

Tuition and Fees

Resident	12,180
Average (public)	9500
Average (private)	22,500
Nonresident	34,020
Average (public)	20,500
Average (private)	24,500

(in thousands of dollars) — scale 0 to 50

Percentage receiving financial aid: 85%

Introduction

The Southern Illinois University School of Medicine at Springfield is one of 5 campuses in the Southern Illinois University system. Southern Illinois University began as a teachers' college in the late 1800s, and the School of Medicine was opened in 1969. The first year of medical school is spent on the Carbondale campus; the remaining 3 years are spent on the Springfield campus. The Carbondale campus is located in a rustic setting; the Springfield campus is located in the state capital.

Admissions (AMCAS)

The minimum premedical science courses are recommended. *Transfer and advanced standing:* School will consider applications from students in good standing at other LCME-accredited medical colleges. For requirements for consideration for advanced standing, contact the Office of Student and Alumni Affairs.

Curriculum

4-year modern. Academic year begins in August. *First year:* Designed to develop competence in several disciplines basic to medicine, such as physiology, biochemistry, anatomy, behavioral sciences, and clinical medicine, the curriculum is organized around organ systems rather than traditional disciplines, focuses on the normal organism, and is taught in Carbondale. *Second year:* Presented in Springfield, instruction is integrated and organized around organ systems, but the focus is on abnormalities associated with disease. The major academic disciplines include pathology, pharmacology, microbiology, immunology, radiology, and clinical medicine. A problem-based learning curriculum is optional for the first 2 years. *Third year:* Clinical clerkships are provided in the following major specialties: internal medicine, surgery, obstetrics/gynecology, pediatrics, family practice, psychiatry, and anesthesiology. *Fourth year:* There are 32 weeks of elective study that may include advanced clinical clerkships, basic science research, and medical application of ancillary disciplines. Third and fourth year clerkships in medical humanities is mandatory.

Grading and Promotion Policies

An Honors/Pass/Fail system is used. Students must pass Step 1 of the USMLE before graduation.

Facilities

Teaching: The educational program is conducted at both the medical education facilities in Carbondale and the medical center in Springfield. The split campus allows the School of Medicine to maximize the existing resources of a major university and the long-established clinical facilities in Springfield: Memorial Medical Center and St. John's Hospital. *Libraries:* One library is located within Carbondale's Morris Library Science Division, consists of more than 100,000 bound volumes, and subscribes to 1000 periodicals. In Springfield, the library is located in the Medical Instruction Facility, contains 113,000 bound volumes and subscribes to 1600 periodicals. *Housing:* Married housing units are available in Carbondale. In Springfield, only off-campus housing is available.

Special Features

Minority admissions: The school sponsors a non-degree-granting Medical-Dental Education Preparatory Program (MED-PREP) for disadvantaged students who are underrepresented. *Other degree programs:* 6-year MD-JD program.

University of Chicago
Pritzker School of Medicine

Chicago, Illinois   60637

Phone: 312-702-1939   *Fax:* 312-702-2598
WWW: http://www.uchicago.edu/u.acadunits/
bsd.html &I

Application Filing		Accreditation	
Earliest:	June 1	LCME	
Latest:	November 15		
Fee:	$55	**Degrees Granted**	
AMCAS:	yes	MD, MD-PhD	

Enrollment: 1996–97 First-Year Class

Men:	54	52%	Applied:	8709
Women:	50	48%	Interviewed:	523
Minorities:	6	6%	Enrolled:	104
Out of State:	58	56%		

1996–97 Class Profile

Mean MCAT Scores		*Mean GPA*
Physical Sciences:	10.3	3.55
Biological Sciences:	10.5	
Verbal Reasoning:	10	

Tuition and Fees

Resident	23,310
Average (public)	9500
Average (private)	22,500
Nonresident	23,310
Average (public)	20,500
Average (private)	24,500

0   10   20   30   40   50
(in thousands of dollars)

Percentage receiving financial aid: 83%

Above data applies to 1995–96 academic year.

Introduction

The University of Chicago is located approximately 7 miles from downtown Chicago in the Hyde Park section. The Pritzker School of Medicine, established in 1927, is part of the Division of Biological Sciences of the University of Chicago.

Admissions (AMCAS)

The minimum premedical science courses are required, but 1 semester of biochemistry may be substituted for the second semester of organic chemistry. Studies in the social sciences, humanities, English composition, and mathematics are recommended but not required. When appropriate, reasonable accommodation is made to otherwise qualified handicapped students. *Transfer and advanced standing:* If space is available, students from LCME-accredited institutions may be considered for transfer into second- or third-year openings on the basis of compelling personal reasons, including pursuit of a specified research area not available at the home institution.

Curriculum

4-year semimodern. *First year:* Consists of courses in the basic sciences. A 2-quarter clinical medicine course introduces students to patients with diseases illustrating the medical correlates of the subjects taught concurrently. The summer is available for research or other activities. *Second year:* Consists of advanced courses. Clinical medicine, including physical diagnosis, continues through the second year. *Third year:* Consists of 5 major clinical clerkships (internal medicine, surgery, pediatrics, psychiatry, and obstetrics and gynecology) with 1 month of the pediatrics rotation and 1 month of the surgery rotation offering opportunities to experience subspecialties. Students also attend departmental seminars and conferences. *Fourth year:* The fourth year is entirely elective and normally consists of consult electives, research, basic science coursework, reading courses, subinternships, ambulatory experiences, and away rotations in other countries.

Grading and Promotion Policies

Courses in the first 2 years and most electives and research are graded on the Pass/Fail basis. Clinical clerkships use internal designators of Honors/High Pass/Pass/Low Pass/Fail. Research is required to graduate with honors. Promotion and continuance of students is in accordance with published guidelines and recommendations made by the Committee on Promotions. Students are not required to take the USMLE Steps 1 and 2 to progress through the medical school.

Facilities

Teaching: Basic sciences are taught in the Biological Sciences Learning Center. Clinical teaching takes place in the university hospitals and predominates in 2 other major off-site community-based hospitals. *Other:* Research laboratories are located throughout the medical center and in other nearby facilities that are part of the University of Chicago campus. Most are grouped by general area of research. A new center for molecular medicine, Knapp Institute, adjoining the new Biological Sciences Learning Center was completed in 1993 as well. *Library:* The Crerar Library houses more than 996,000 volumes and 7000 periodicals, constituting one of the largest science holdings in the United States. *Housing:* 1100 apartments are available.

Special Features

The Division of Biological Sciences permits special curricular opportunities for medical students. *Minority admissions:* The medical school actively seeks minority students through city-wide and national recruitment efforts. MCAT preparation, study skills, and a test-taking skills development course in conjunction with other Chicago area medical schools are offered. *Other degree programs:* A special Medical Scientist Training Program (MSTP) is offered for a combined MD-PhD degree in a 7-year period. This program is limited to 6 students yearly.

University of Illinois College of Medicine

808 South Wood Street m/c 783
Chicago, Illinois   60612

Phone: 312-996-5635   *Fax:* 312-996-6693
WWW: http://www.vic.edu/depts/mcam/

Application Filing		Accreditation	
Earliest:	June 1	LCME	
Latest:	December 1		
Fee:	$30	**Degrees Granted**	
AMCAS:	yes	MD, MD-PhD, MD-MS	

Enrollment: 1996–97 First-Year Class

Men:	225	71%	Applied:	6655
Women:	92	29%	Interviewed:	n/av
Minorities:	86	27%	Enrolled:	317
Out of State:	19	6%		

1996–97 Class Profile

Mean MCAT Scores		*Mean GPA*
Physical Sciences:	9.2	3.41
Biological Sciences:	9.3	
Verbal Reasoning:	9.3	

Tuition and Fees

Resident	10,740
Average (public)	9500
Average (private)	22,500
Nonresident	28,960
Average (public)	20,500
Average (private)	24,500

(in thousands of dollars) 0 10 20 30 40 50

Percentage receiving financial aid: n/av

Above data applies to 1995–96 academic year.

Introduction

In 1867 the University of Illinois was chartered as a land grant institution. The medical school was founded in 1881 as the College of Physicians and Surgeons of Chicago. The College of Medicine has 4 campuses: Chicago, Urbana-Champaign, Peoria, and Rockford. The University of Illinois College of Medicine at Chicago is located in the west side medical center district.

Admissions (AMCAS)

The minimum premedical science courses as well as mathematics and behavioral science are recommended. Strong preference is given to state residents. The College of Medicine consists of 4 geographic sites, located in Chicago, Peoria, Rockford, and Urbana-Champaign, and 2 educational tracks. Students enrolled on the Chicago Track attend there all 4 years.

Students enrolled on the Urbana, Peoria, or Rockford (UPR) Track spend the first year at Urbana-Champaign for basic science study and will remain there (mainly students enrolled in the combined degree Medical Scholars Program [MSP]) or move to Peoria or Rockford for the next 3 years. *Transfer and advanced standing:* A limited number of students who pass the school's qualifying exam may be admitted to the second year on a space-available basis. Third-year transfers are considered only from among students currently enrolled in the second year of an out-of-state U.S. or Canadian allopathic medical school, with preference given to state residents with compelling reasons to return to Illinois.

College of Medicine at Chicago

This site is located about 2 miles west of downtown Chicago and is the largest of the 4 geographic sites. The College of Medicine at Chicago offers a 4-year program providing a solid foundation in the basic and clinical sciences leading to the MD degree. The curriculum consists of 2 years of basic and preclinical sciences followed by 2 years of clinical work. *First year:* This covers the introductory basic sciences. Clinical conferences are offered to reinforce basic science principles relevant to the practice of medicine. *Second year:* In addition to the advanced basic sciences, LPC courses are offered in medical ethics and human sexuality as well as physical diagnosis and problem solving. *Third year:* Rotation through 6 major clinical specialties. *Fourth year:* Involves rotations. The balance of the time is devoted to electives.

College of Medicine at Peoria

The college is located a few blocks west of downtown Peoria. This site includes basic science facilities and is affiliated with the Methodist Medical Center of Illinois and St. Francis Medical Center, allowing access to 1100 beds. Only the upper 3 years are taught, including advanced basic sciences and clinical studies. *Second year:* This serves as an introduction to clinical medicine, using a systemic pathophysiological teaching approach. *Third year:* The basic required clerkship rotations are taught, with the emphasis on the clinical practice of medicine and the delivery of health care. *Fourth year:* Consists of at least 36 weeks of instruction.

College of Medicine at Rockford

Located near the northeast side of the city, the college consists of a teaching center and 3 associated hospitals—Rockford Memorial, St. Anthony Medical Center, and Swedish-American Hospital. The program at Rockford includes a unique experience in primary health care delivery at one of 3 Community Health Centers (CHC). This experience continues for 2 half days per week during the M-3 and M-4 years. *Second year:* This consists of pathology, pharmacology, issues in contemporary medicine, and clinical medicine skills, as well as a systemic-oriented introduction to clinical medicine. *Third year:* This consists of the required core clerkships in the CHC experience. *Fourth year:* This consists of a 4-week clerkship in neurology, and additional work in the CHC experience.

College of Medicine at Urbana-Champaign

Located on the university campus, the college has, in addition to its basic science facilities, affiliations for clinical training with almost all the hospitals in the east-central region of Illinois. The college offers a complete 4-year medical education program leading to an MD degree. The first-year basic medical science program at Urbana-Champaign also serves those students who complete the last 3 years of medical school in Peoria or Rockford. *First year:* All the basic sciences except pharmacology, pathology, and epidemiology are taught and are organized into learning units distributed among 8 clinical problem themes directly relating basic medical science to human disease. First-year students have an option to participate in the Medical Doctor Adviser (MDA) Program, which enables them to meet with practicing physicians for advisement and instruction. *Second year:* The remaining basic sciences are offered as well as introduction to clinical medicine in the second semester of the sophomore year, which includes direct student contact with hospitalized patients. *Third and fourth years:* The core clinical clerkships, medical electives, and in-depth individual study experiences comprise the last 2 years.

Grading and Promotion Policies

A Pass/Fail system is used for the first year with a 5-item grading system for the clinical portion of the curriculum. Students must record passing total grades on Step 1 and Step 2 of the USMLE for graduation.

Special Features

Minority admissions: Recruitment is conducted through the Urban Health Program, and a 6-week summer prematriculation program is offered for accepted students. *Other degree programs:* Combined MD-MS and MD-PhD programs are offered by the College of Medicine at Chicago in the basic sciences and public health and at Urbana-Champaign in over 40 disciplines including the basic sciences. A special decompressed first-year program is available. An opportunity to engage in an Independent Study Program is available at the Chicago, Rockford, and Peoria sites for students interested in this type of curriculum.

INDIANA

Indiana University School of Medicine

1120 South Drive, Fesler Hall 213
Indianapolis, Indiana   46202

Phone: 317-274-3772   *Fax:* 317-278-0211
WWW: http://www.iupui.edu/it/medschl/home.html

Application Filing		Accreditation	
Earliest:	June 1	LCME	
Latest:	December 15		
Fee:	$35	**Degrees Granted**	
AMCAS:	yes	MD, MD-PhD, MD-MS	

Enrollment: 1996–97 First-Year Class

Men:	164	59%	Applied:	2604
Women:	116	41%	Interviewed:	990
Minorities:	17	6%	Enrolled:	280
Out of State:	11	4%		

1996–97 Class Profile

Mean MCAT Scores		*Mean GPA*
Physical Sciences:	9.7	3.68
Biological Sciences:	9.7	
Verbal Reasoning:	9.7	

Tuition and Fees

Resident	11,040
Average (public)	9500
Average (private)	22,500
Nonresident	25,275
Average (public)	20,500
Average (private)	24,500

(in thousands of dollars) 0 10 20 30 40 50

Percentage receiving financial aid: n/av

Introduction

The Indiana University School of Medicine began in 1907 on the Bloomington campus. In 1908 Indiana University became responsible for all medical education in the state of Indiana, and in 1971 the Indiana Statewide Medical Education System was put into effect. It has teaching centers in all major cities in Indiana. The Indiana University Medical Center includes schools of Medicine, Dentistry, Nursing, and Allied Health Sciences, as well as university hospitals, and research laboratories.

Admissions (AMCAS)

Only minimum premedical science courses are required. Preference is given to residents; a few out-of-state residents are accepted yearly. *Transfer and advanced standing:* Only transfers of Indiana residents from American or foreign medical schools are considered.

Curriculum

4-year semimodern. The major objectives of the curriculum are the concentration of core material in both preclinical and clinical years, early exposure to patients, and extensive elective time. The *first year* is devoted to core basic science courses and introduction to clinical medicine. *Second year* to core basic science courses and continuing patient contact through the introduction to medicine courses. *Third year* (12 months) is devoted to clinical experience in pediatrics, obstetrics, gynecology, psychiatry, medicine, and surgery. *Fourth year* (9 months). Experience in a variety of clinical specialties and the remainder is reserved exclusively for electives.

Grading and Promotion Policies

System used is Honors/High Pass/Pass/Fail. Students must pass Steps 1 and 2 of the USMLE to graduate.

Facilities

The Medical Center is located in Indianapolis; the School of Medicine has students on 8 other campuses. *Teaching:* In Indianapolis, preclinical teaching takes place in the Medical Sciences Building. Clinical facilities are provided by the University Hospital, Robert W. Long Hospital, William H. Coleman Hospital for Women, and James Whitcomb Riley Hospital for Children. *Other:* Emerson Hall accommodates clinical departments; Fesler Hall houses clinical laboratories and offices. Riley Hospital has connecting wings for pediatric and cancer research. A psychiatric research unit is also located at the center. Combined hospitals of the medical center contain 2000 beds. Neighboring hospitals provide some additional experience. *Library:* The medical library and nursing library combined house more than 125,000 volumes and subscribe to 2500 periodicals. *Housing:* Very limited on-campus housing.

Special Features

Minority admissions: The school has an active program to identify, advise, and recruit disadvantaged students. *Other degree programs:* Students interested in medical science can work to combine an MD degree with either an MS or a PhD in biomedical disciplines. The combined MD-PhD may also be earned in other sciences, and law, social and behavioral sciences, and the humanities on the Bloomington campus.

IOWA

University of Iowa College of Medicine

CMAB
Iowa City, Iowa 52242-1101

Phone: 319-335-8052 *Fax:* 319-335-8052
E-mail: medical-admission@uiowa.edu
WWW: http://www.medadmin.uiowa.edu/osac/
admiss.htm

Application Filing		Accreditation	
Earliest:	June 1	LCME	
Latest:	November 1		
Fee:	$20	**Degrees Granted**	
AMCAS:	yes	MD, MD-PhD	

Enrollment: 1996–97 First-Year Class

Men:	88	50%	Applied:	3513
Women:	87	50%	Interviewed:	3513
Minorities:	23	13%	Enrolled:	175
Out of State:	23	13%		

1996–97 Class Profile

Mean MCAT Scores		*Mean GPA*
Physical Sciences:	9.3	3.6
Biological Sciences:	9.7	
Verbal Reasoning:	9.5	

Tuition and Fees

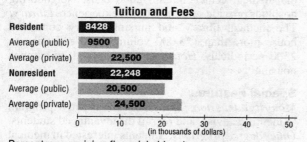

Resident	8428
Average (public)	9500
Average (private)	22,500
Nonresident	22,248
Average (public)	20,500
Average (private)	24,500

0 10 20 30 40 50
(in thousands of dollars)

Percentage receiving financial aid: n/av

Above data applies to 1995–96 academic year.

Introduction

The University of Iowa is located in Iowa City, and includes the College of Medicine, which was founded in 1850. This school has evolved into the state's major health center. It includes a large University Hospital and clinics. The Health Science Center also contains schools of Nursing, Dentistry, and Pharmacy, and is located on a 900-acre campus.

Admissions (AMCAS)

College requires minimum premedical science courses plus 1 advanced biology course and college algebra and trigonometry. Iowa residents are given strong preference, but some nonresidents are admitted. *Transfer and advanced standing:* Not available.

Curriculum

4-year semitraditional. *First and second years:* The 2-year introductory phase comprises the basic medical sciences as well as some electives in each year. One semester of the second year is devoted to an introduction to clinical medicine. *Third year:* Comprises summer session and 2 semesters of rotating clinical clerkships in major specialties, in which student participates in patient care. *Fourth year:* Devoted to 32–47 weeks of electives in which the student focuses on whatever facet of medical education best relates to his/her professional interests. Elective courses are offered in alcoholism, biomedical engineering, community medicine, drug abuse, emergency medicine, medical ethics, medical jurisprudence, and nutrition.

Grading and Promotion Policies

System used is Honors/Pass/Fail in basic and clinical sciences and Pass/Fail in the electives. Promotions committees consisting of faculty members review the accomplishments of their students and determine their eligibility for advancement at the close of the academic year.

Facilities

Teaching: Preclinical sciences are taught at the Medical Laboratories Building and the Basic Science Building. Clinical teaching takes place at the University Hospital (1100 beds), and VA Hospital (440 beds). *Other:* The major research facility is the Medical Research Center. *Library:* The Health Sciences Library houses 111,000 volumes and more than 125,000 periodicals. *Housing:* Information not available.

Special Features

Minority admissions: Recruitment is coordinated by means of the college's Educational Opportunities Program, which sponsors a summer program for accepted students. *Other degree programs:* Combined MD-PhD programs are offered in a variety of disciplines including radiation biology and community medicine.

KANSAS

University of Kansas School of Medicine

3901 Rainbow Boulevard
Kansas City, Kansas   66160

Phone: 913-588-5283   *Fax:* 913-588-5259
WWW: http://www.kumc.edu/instruction/medicine/
som.html

Application Filing		Accreditation	
Earliest:	June 15	LCME	
Latest:	October 15		
Fee:	n/av	**Degrees Granted**	
AMCAS:	yes	MD, MD-PhD	

Enrollment: 1996–97 First-Year Class

Men:	106	61%	Applied:	1950
Women:	69	39%	Interviewed:	371
Minorities:	18	10%	Enrolled:	175
Out of State:	19	11%		

1996–97 Class Profile

Mean MCAT Scores		*Mean GPA*
Physical Sciences:	9.4	3.6
Biological Sciences:	9.7	
Verbal Reasoning:	9.6	

Tuition and Fees

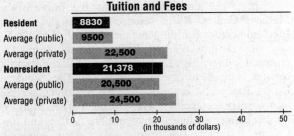

Resident	8830
Average (public)	9500
Average (private)	22,500
Nonresident	21,378
Average (public)	20,500
Average (private)	24,500

0   10   20   30   40   50
(in thousands of dollars)

Percentage receiving financial aid: 88%

Introduction

The University of Kansas opened in 1866. In 1899 a 1-year preparatory course for medical school was initiated. Students who completed the year then transferred to other medical schools. The curriculum was lengthened to 2 years in 1899. In 1905 clinical training began at Bell Memorial Hospital and graduating with a medical degree became possible. In 1924 the medical school and hospital expanded and moved to its present location. The Medical Center now consists of schools of Medicine, Nursing, and Allied Health, and Office of Graduate Studies.

Admissions (AMCAS)

The school requires a bachelor's degree and minimum premedical science courses. Statistics is recommended.

Preference is given to residents, but nonresidents are accepted. *Transfer and advanced standing:* If vacancies exist, candidates for the third-year class are considered from other U.S. medical schools.

Curriculum

4-year semitraditional. *First and second years:* Basic medical sciences are taught in structured course format of traditional curriculum. Courses in medical jurisprudence and introductory clinical medicine are included in preclinical years. Clinical correlation of various aspects of basic sciences is emphasized. *Third year:* Clerkship rotations and a preceptorship extending over 56 weeks. *Fourth year:* Five 4-week electives.

Grading and Promotion Policies

Grading is by letter. A passing total score is required on Step 1 of the USMLE for promotion to the third year and on Step 2 for graduation.

Facilities

Teaching: The school is part of the university's Medical Center. Orr-Major Hall provides classrooms and labs for teaching basic science courses as well as space for individual research and departmental offices. The University Hospital provides facilities used in clinical training. *Library:* Dykes Medical Library contains more than 110,000 volumes. *Housing:* Information not available.

Special Features

Combined MD-PhD programs are offered in a variety of disciplines.

KENTUCKY

University of Kentucky College of Medicine

800 Rose Street
Lexington, Kentucky   40536

Phone: 606-323-6161   *Fax:* 606-323-2076
E-mail: mathew@pop.uky.edu
WWW: http://www.uky.edu/medicine

Application Filing		Accreditation	
Earliest:	June 1	LCME	
Latest:	November 1		
Fee:	n/av	**Degrees Granted**	
AMCAS:	yes	MD, MD-PhD, MD-MS	

Enrollment: 1996–97 First-Year Class

Men:	56	59%	Applied:	1866
Women:	39	41%	Interviewed:	355
Minorities:	95	n/av	Enrolled:	95
Out of State:	10	11%		

1996–97 Class Profile

Mean MCAT Scores		*Mean GPA*
Physical Sciences:	9.2	3.61
Biological Sciences:	9.3	
Verbal Reasoning:	9	

Tuition and Fees

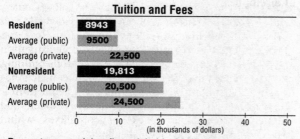

Resident	8943
Average (public)	9500
Average (private)	22,500
Nonresident	19,813
Average (public)	20,500
Average (private)	24,500

(in thousands of dollars)

Percentage receiving financial aid: 86%

Introduction

In 1956 the University of Kentucky Medical Center was established. The College of Medicine is one of the programs offered at the University of Kentucky Medical Center campus in Lexington. The College of Medicine is part of the University of Kentucky Chandler Medical Center, which also contains schools of Dentistry, Nursing, Pharmacy, and Allied Health profession, as well as the University Hospital and Ambulatory Care Center.

Admissions (AMCAS)

In addition to the basic premedical science courses, 1 year of English is required. Courses in mathematics and in the psychological and social sciences are recommended. Preference is given to residents, but a number of nonresidents who have a clear interest in pursuing their medical education in Kentucky are accepted each year.

Curriculum

4-year semimodern. *First and second years:* Consist of 48 and 36 weeks, respectively, of scheduled class work in the basic sciences. Each week has about 23 hours of scheduled activities. *Third year:* Clerkship rotations through the major clinical specialties and primary care are required. *Fourth year:* Selection of specialty and electives. One rotation is required in a surgery and medical active internship, one emergency medicine rotation, one advanced clinical pharmacology and anesthesiology course, one gerontology elective, a dean's colloquium, a selective in primary care or rural medicine, and 2 elective rotations.

Grading and Promotion Policies

Grades are A, B, C, E (Failure), P (Pass), W (Withdrawal), U (Unsatisfactory), and I (Incomplete). A student who is doing unsatisfactorily in 2 or more classes in one academic year may be dropped. At regular intervals the Student Progress and Promotions Committee for each class reviews the record of each student and makes recommendations relative to promotion, adjustment of academic load, remediation, or dismissal. Students must record total passing scores on Step 1 of the USMLE for promotion to the third year and on Step 2 for graduation.

Facilities

Teaching: The college is part of the university's Medical Center. Basic sciences are taught at the Medical Science Building and the major clinical teaching site is the 473-bed University of Kentucky Hospital. *Other:* The Kentucky Clinic offers comprehensive outpatient medical services. The Sander-Brown Research Center on Aging is a national gerontology resource facility. The Lucille Parker Markey Cancer Center includes a patient care facility and the Combs Research Building. *Library:* The Medical Center Library houses more than 160,000 volumes and 2000 periodicals. *Housing:* University housing is available.

Special Features

Minority admissions: The college has an active recruitment program and offers a summer prematriculation program for accepted students. *Other degree programs:* Combined MD-PhD degree programs are offered in the basic medical sciences.

University of Louisville School of Medicine

Health Sciences Center
Louisville, Kentucky   40292

Phone: 502-852-5193
E-mail: mesklaoi@ulkyum.louisville.edu
WWW: http://www.medical.informatics.louisvillesch/
medschool/

Application Filing		Accreditation	
Earliest:	June 1	LCME	
Latest:	November 1		
Fee:	$15	**Degrees Granted**	
AMCAS:	yes	MD, MD-PhD	

Enrollment: 1996–97 First-Year Class

Men:	74	54%	Applied:	1900	
Women:	63	46%	Interviewed:	1007	
Minorities:	n/av	n/av	Enrolled:	137	
Out of State:	13	9%			

1996–97 Class Profile

Mean MCAT Scores		*Mean GPA*
Physical Sciences:	8.7	3.6
Biological Sciences:	8.7	
Verbal Reasoning:	8.9	

Tuition and Fees

Resident	8480
Average (public)	9500
Average (private)	22,500
Nonresident	19,650
Average (public)	20,500
Average (private)	24,500

0   10   20   30   40   50
(in thousands of dollars)

Percentage receiving financial aid: 89%

Introduction

The University of Louisville School of Medicine was originally part of the Louisville Medical Institute when it was established in 1833. In 1846 it became part of the University of Louisville, which is part of the state university system. In 1908 the school merged with 4 others and adopted its present name. In the late 1980s the school embarked on a comprehensive building program, which included the construction of the University of Louisville Hospital. The Health Science Center consists of the schools of Medicine, Dentistry, and Nursing, and the Division of Allied Health.

Admissions (AMCAS)

Requirements include minimum premedical science courses plus 1 semester of calculus (or 2 semesters of other college mathematics courses) and 2 semesters of English. Preference is given to state residents. *Transfer and advanced standing:* Applicants from LCME-accredited schools with documented circumstances necessitating the need to return to Kentucky will be considered on a limited basis.

Curriculum

4-year semitraditional with an introduction to clinical medicine. *First and second years:* Consist of basic science courses; 2 hours of elective time per semester is required. *Third year:* Devoted to required clerkships. *Fourth year:* Five required clinical rotations and health policy and management courses, an ACLS, and 12 weeks of electives.

Grading and Promotion Policies

A grade of Pass or Fail is submitted at the completion of each course. The Committee on Student Promotions approves the scholastic activities of the individual or may recommend one of several courses of action if work is unsatisfactory. A passing total score on Step 1 of the USMLE is needed for promotion to the third year. Taking Step 2 is required.

Facilities

Teaching: Basic sciences are taught in the Instructional Building at the Health Science Center near downtown Louisville. Primary clinical facilities are University of Louisville, Kosair-Children's Hospital, and Veterans Administration Medical Center. Other clinical affiliates are the Bingham Child Guidance Clinic, Inc., Audubon Hospital, Frazier Rehabilitation Center, Jewish Hospital, James Graham Brown Cancer Center, Allient Norton Hospital, St. Anthony Hospital, and Trover Clinic (Madisonville). *Other:* The Research Building is devoted entirely to scientific investigation by all departments of the school. A commons building houses the Health Sciences library, auditorium, cafeteria, and bookstore. *Housing:* Medical-Dental dormitory located near the Health Sciences Center, and numerous affordable apartment complexes within 10–15 minutes of the medical school.

Special Features

Minority admissions: The Office of Professional and Graduate Minority Affairs aids in recruitment and retention of minorities. *Other degree programs:* A combined MD-PhD program is available in a variety of disciplines including biophysics, immunology, and toxicology.

LOUISIANA

Louisiana State University School of Medicine in New Orleans

1901 Perdido Street
New Orleans, Louisiana 70112

Phone: 504-568-6262
E-mail: shuadm@isumc.edu
WWW: http://www.lib-sh.lsumc.edu

Application Filing		Accreditation
Earliest:	June 1	LCME
Latest:	November 15	
Fee:	$50	**Degrees Granted**
AMCAS:	yes	MD, MD-PhD

Enrollment: 1996–97 First-Year Class

Men:	108	62%	Applied:	1412
Women:	67	38%	Interviewed:	381
Minorities:	54	31%	Enrolled:	175
Out of State:	1	1%		

1996–97 Class Profile

Mean MCAT Scores		*Mean GPA*
Physical Sciences:	8.4	3.4
Biological Sciences:	8.6	
Verbal Reasoning:	8.9	

Tuition and Fees

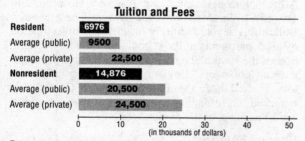

Resident	6976
Average (public)	9500
Average (private)	22,500
Nonresident	14,876
Average (public)	20,500
Average (private)	24,500

0 10 20 30 40 50
(in thousands of dollars)

Percentage receiving financial aid: n/av
Above data applies to 1995–96 academic year.

Introduction

The Louisiana State University School of Medicine in New Orleans was founded in 1931. The School of Medicine is located next to Charity Hospital, adjacent to the city's central business district. It is a major component of the Louisiana State University Medical Center, which includes schools of Dentistry, Nursing, Allied Health Sciences, and Graduate Studies.

Admissions (AMCAS)

Recommended courses include English composition and public speaking. Only state residents are accepted into the first-year class.

Curriculum

4-year semitraditional. First and second years: Combination of basic sciences and clinical medicine. Introduction to patient care and contact is provided at the beginning of the second year in the introduction to clinical medicine course. *Third and fourth-years:* Teaching is on a pure block system and is basically small-group instruction (on a conference and seminar basis) in hospitals, clinics, and private practice facilities. All third-year students are required to take a 4-week clerkship in family medicine, which is given in a community physician's office. During the final year, blocks in ambulatory care, general medicine, neurosciences, special topics, and an acting internship are required. The special-topics block includes nutrition, geriatrics, drug and alcohol abuse, office management, and financial planning. The other 5 months may be scheduled as electives.

Grading and Promotion Policies

Grades are Honors, High Pass, Pass, Fail, Withdrew Passing, and Withdrew Failing. Periodic reviews are made of student performance by means of exams, staff reports, and other forms of appraisal. Eligibility for promotion rests on completion of all coursework and requirements and approval by the Promotions Committee. A passing score must be recorded for Step 1 of the USMLE prior to entering the third year. Step 2 must be passed prior to graduation.

Facilities

Teaching: The Medical Education Building is the site for basic science instruction. The school is located near the center of the New Orleans business district. The two main teaching hospitals are the Medical Center of Louisiana at New Orleans and University Hospital. Ten other hospitals are affiliated with LSU. An auditorium equipped with the most up-to-date audiovisual facilities provides space for medical meetings and faculty/student assemblies and lectures. *Library:* The library is located in the Resource Center. It services all professional schools in the Medical Center with more than 176,000 volumes and current periodicals in excess of 1500 titles. *Housing:* University-controlled housing is provided for 300 married and single students. Located 3 blocks from the school, the residence hall provides 1-, 2-, or 3-bedroom apartments for married students and double rooms for single men and women. Recreational facilities are located in the dormitory.

Special Features

Minority admissions: The Office of Minority Affairs coordinates recruitment. The school offers a Minority Summer Prematriculation Program for accepted first-year students to facilitate adjustment to medical school. *Other degree programs:* Combined MD-PhD programs are offered in a variety of disciplines.

Louisiana State University School of Medicine in Shreveport

1501 Kings Highway, P.O. Box 33932
Shreveport, Louisiana 71130

Phone: 318-675-5190 *Fax:* 318-675-5244

Application Filing			Accreditation
Earliest:	June 1		LCME
Latest:	November 15		
Fee:	$50		**Degrees Granted**
AMCAS:	yes		MD, MD-PhD

Enrollment: 1996–97 First-Year Class

Men:	59	59%	Applied:	1024
Women:	41	41%	Interviewed:	n/av
Minorities:	7	7%	Enrolled:	100
Out of State:	0	0%		

1996–97 Class Profile

Mean MCAT Scores		*Mean GPA*
Physical Sciences:	9	3.45
Biological Sciences:	9.2	
Verbal Reasoning:	9	

Tuition and Fees

Resident	6976
Average (public)	9500
Average (private)	22,500
Nonresident	14,876
Average (public)	20,500
Average (private)	24,500

0 10 20 30 40 50
(in thousands of dollars)

Percentage receiving financial aid: 82%

Introduction

The Louisiana State University School of Medicine in Shreveport was founded in 1966. The medical school facilities are located next to the Louisiana State University Hospital. The permanent medical facilities were occupied in 1975, 2 years after the first MD degrees were awarded by the school.

Admissions (AMCAS)

Required courses, in addition to the minimum premedical sciences, include English (6 semester hours). MCAT scores within 3 years are also required.

Curriculum

4-year semitraditional. *First year:* Courses include introductory basic sciences plus introductory classes in comprehensive health care, genetics, radiology, psychiatry, and biometry. *Second year:* Advanced basic sciences with a major course in clinical diagnosis to prepare students for clinical years and neurology, perspectives in medicine II and comprehensive care are also offered. *Third and fourth years:* Emphasis on supervised experience in patient care, especially in the development of clinical skills. All of the fourth year is electives with opportunities for extramural and intramural work in family practice, other clinical specialties, basic sciences, and research.

Grading and Promotion Policies

A letter system is used for coursework and Pass/Fail for electives.

Facilities

Teaching: Louisiana State University Hospital (675 beds) is the principal teaching facility. The ten-story medical school adjoining the University Hospital houses lecture halls and laboratories used for most didactic teaching and basic science research. A separate ambulatory care facility is used for a multi-year course in ambulatory and family medicine. *Other:* Shreveport VA Hospital (450 beds) and E. A. Conway Hospital in nearby Monroe are affiliated with the school. *Library:* A fully modern library houses more than 90,000 volumes and subscribes to more than 1300 periodicals. A local network of terminals accesses several national data bases for study and research. *Housing:* None.

Special Features

Minority admissions: Recruitment of disadvantaged students is facilitated by visits to Louisiana colleges and communications with other educational institutions. *Other degree programs:* Combined MD-PhD programs are offered in a variety of disciplines.

Tulane University School of Medicine

1430 Tulane Avenue
New Orleans, Louisiana   70112

Phone: 504-588-5187   *Fax:* 504-585-6462
E-mail: jpisano@tmcpop.tmc.tulane.edu
WWW: http://www.mcl.tulane.edu/departments/admiss

Application Filing		Accreditation	
Earliest:	June 1	LCME	
Latest:	December 15		
Fee:	$65	**Degrees Granted**	
AMCAS:	yes	MD, MD-PhD, MD-MS	

Enrollment: 1996–97 First-Year Class

Men:	79	53%	Applied:	10,782
Women:	70	47%	Interviewed:	1
Minorities:	10	7%	Enrolled:	149
Out of State:	123	83%		

1996–97 Class Profile

Mean MCAT Scores		*Mean GPA*
Physical Sciences:	9.8	3.5
Biological Sciences:	10	
Verbal Reasoning:	9.9	

Tuition and Fees

	(in thousands of dollars)
Resident	23,310
Average (public)	9500
Average (private)	22,500
Nonresident	23,310
Average (public)	20,500
Average (private)	24,500

Percentage receiving financial aid: 81%

Introduction

The Tulane University School of Medicine was established in 1834 as the Medical College of Louisiana. In 1845 the school became the Medical Department of the University of Louisiana. The school was closed during the Civil War. It later reopened and struggled financially for its survival until 1884, when a local merchant, Paul Tulane, provided funds for what became Tulane University. A major multidisciplinary Medical Center was later established incorporating the School of Medicine, School of Public Health and Tropical Medicine, and Medical Center Hospital and Clinic.

Admissions (AMCAS)

Only the minimum premedical science courses are required. Large numbers of out-of-state students and a few 3-year students are accepted. Half the students will be drawn each year from the South. *Transfer and advanced standing:* A few students are accepted annually as transfers to second- and third-year classes. Premedical sciences required.

Curriculum

4-year semimodern. The aim of the first 2 years is to have students develop clinical problem-solving skills. *First year:* Core courses in the introductory basic sciences. Students begin clinical medical training and study human behavior, community medicine, epidemiology, and biostatistics. *Second year:* Consists of core courses in the advanced basic sciences and preparation for clinical studies such as physical diagnosis and introduction to clinical medicine. There are opportunities for elective and independent study time. *Third year:* Consists of 48 weeks devoted to basic core clerkships in the major clinical areas, with direct responsibility for diagnosis and management of clinical problems presented by patients in the hospital. *Fourth year:* Consists of 2 components: required clerkships and electives. Electives in all clinical departments include ethics, jurisprudence, engineering, and health delivery systems. Clerkships include outpatient medicine or pediatrics and a subinternship in major clinical areas and in community medicine.

Grading and Promotion Policies

Grades are Honors, High Pass/Pass/Conditional/Fail. Any grade of below Pass constitutes an academic deficiency that must be removed by remedial work and/or examination, in order to advance to the succeeding year. Steps 1 and 2 of the USMLE are optional.

Facilities

Teaching: Located in downtown New Orleans, the school occupies a full city block and consists of 4 units: the Hutchinson Memorial Building, the Libby Memorial Building, the Burthe-Cottam Memorial Building, and the Environmental Medicine Building. Clinical teaching takes place at the Tulane Medical Center Hospital (300 beds) and Charity Hospital (1877 beds). Six other hospitals in New Orleans provide supplementary teaching facilities and others located elsewhere in the area are available. *Other:* The Leon M. Wolf Graphic Arts Laboratories houses facilities for medical photography and illustration. A television network is utilized for instructional purposes; Souchon Museum of Anatomy is an award-winning collection of over 400 specimens; the Computer Center provides services to the medical center; the Delta Regional Primate Research Center is involved in work in communicable diseases, genetics, developmental disorders, and other medical problems. *Library:* The Rudolph Matas Library houses more than 130,000 volumes, and 1200 periodicals are received. *Housing:* Accommodations for single and married students are available.

Special Features

Minority admissions: The school has an active recruitment program targeted at the southeastern and southwestern parts of the country. A Summer Reinforcement and Enrichment Program is available for minority undergraduate premedical students. *Other degree programs:* Combined MD-PhD programs are offered in a variety of disciplines. MD-MS and MD-MPH programs are also available.

MARYLAND

Johns Hopkins University School of Medicine

720 Rutland Avenue
Baltimore, Maryland   21205

Phone: 410-955-3182
WWW: http://www.infonet.welch.jhu.edu/education/
prospectives.html

Application Filing		Accreditation	
Earliest:	July 1	LCME	
Latest:	November 1		
Fee:	$60	**Degrees Granted**	
AMCAS:	yes	MD, MD-PhD, MD-MPH	

Enrollment: 1996–97 First-Year Class

Men:	65	55%	Applied:	3710
Women:	54	45%	Interviewed:	3710
Minorities:	15	13%	Enrolled:	119
Out of State:	102	86%		

1996–97 Class Profile

Mean MCAT Scores		*Mean GPA*
Physical Sciences:	n/av	n/av
Biological Sciences:	n/av	
Verbal Reasoning:	n/av	

Tuition and Fees

Resident	22,628
Average (public)	9500
Average (private)	22,500
Nonresident	22,628
Average (public)	20,500
Average (private)	24,500

0   10   20   30   40   50
(in thousands of dollars)

Percentage receiving financial aid: 80%

Above data applies to 1995–96 academic year.

Introduction

Johns Hopkins University was established in 1876 after Johns Hopkins provided 7 million dollars to establish a university, hospital, and teaching center. The School of Medicine opened in 1893. The main School of Medicine campus is located in eastern Baltimore.

Admissions

Bachelor's degree or its equivalent required, minimum premedical science course requirements plus 1 semester of calculus and 24 semester hours of social and behavioral sciences and humanities. Courses in biochemistry and advanced biology are recommended. There are no residence requirements and no preference is shown in selection of applicants. Aside from the regular program, the school has a multiple-option Flexible Medical Admissions Program (FlexMed) that assures admission to juniors after college graduation or delayed matriculation for seniors. This enables students to pursue alternative educational pathways, work experiences, and humanitarian service in keeping with their interests and career goals. *Transfer and advanced standing:* Transfer applications are considered for the second- or third-year class, and are accepted only into the standard 4-year curriculum, if places are available.

Curriculum

4-year semimodern. The program includes the integration of basic sciences and clinical experiences and the expanded use of case-based, small group learning sessions. Students have early contact with clinical medicine by working with community-based physicians. The physician and society course spans the 4-year program and covers a wide range of topics. *First year:* Integrated coverage of introductory basic sciences, neuroscience, and epidemiology. *Second year:* Devoted to advanced basic sciences, clinical skills, and start of clerkships. *Third and fourth years:* Required clerkships in major clinical areas and electives.

Grading and Promotion Policies

Letter grades are used in required courses and clerkships and Honors/Pass/Fail are used for electives. Grades are based on the composite judgment of responsible instructors, and not solely upon results of examinations. At the end of each academic year, the Committee on Student Promotions decides what actions will be taken regarding student status. The USMLE is not used to evaluate students for promotion or graduation.

Facilities

Teaching: Most of the preclinical departments are situated in the W. Barry Wood Basic Science Building. The Johns Hopkins Hospital (1100 beds) occupies 14 acres of land adjacent to buildings that house the preclinical departments. Separate buildings contain specialty clinics such as the new outpatient center. The school is also affiliated with Bayview Medical Center (665 beds), Good Samaritan Hospital (277 beds), and Sinai Hospital of Baltimore (516 beds), and is associated with other institutions. *Other:* Research facilities for the preclinical sciences and clinical investigation are located in the Basic Science and Traylor Research Buildings. The Ross Research Building contains 240 modern laboratory suites. *Library:* The Welch Medical Library is located in a separate building adjacent to the other buildings of the School of Medicine and houses more than 354,000 volumes and 3600 periodicals. *Housing:* Reed Residence Hall is available for single students. A housing office assists other students in finding off-campus housing.

Special Features

Minority admissions: The school has an active admissions program. *Other degree programs:* Combined MD-PhD programs are available in all the basic sciences as well as in biomedical engineering, biophysics, medical history, human genetics, and molecular biology. The school also offers combined MD-MPH and MD-DSc in Public Health programs.

Uniformed Services University of the Health Sciences F. Edward Hebert School of Medicine

4301 Jones Bridge Road
Bethesda, Maryland   20814

Phone: 301-295-3102   *Fax:* 301-295-3545
E-mail: dreston@uduhd.mil
WWW: http://www.usuhs.mil

Application Filing		Accreditation	
Earliest:	June 1	LCME	
Latest:	November 1		
Fee:	n/av	**Degrees Granted**	
AMCAS:	yes	MD	

Enrollment: 1996–97 First-Year Class

Men:	119	72%	Applied:	3380	
Women:	46	28%	Interviewed:	608	
Minorities:	12	7%	Enrolled:	165	
Out of State:	n/av	n/av			

1996–97 Class Profile

Mean MCAT Scores		*Mean GPA*
Physical Sciences:	10.4	3.47
Biological Sciences:	10.2	
Verbal Reasoning:	9.9	

Tuition and Fees

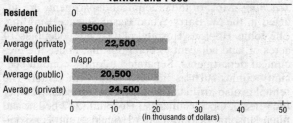

Resident	0
Average (public)	9500
Average (private)	22,500
Nonresident	n/app
Average (public)	20,500
Average (private)	24,500

(in thousands of dollars)

Percentage receiving financial aid: n/app

Introduction

The Uniformed Services University of the Health Sciences is located at the National Naval Medical Center. The university was created by the Department of Defense in 1972 to train career medical officers. The establishment of the school was sponsored by the late congressman F. Edward Hebert, whose initiative secured congressional approval for the creation of the Uniformed Services University. This is a tuition-free school, whose graduates provide medical services to the military.

Admissions (AMCAS)

The basic premedical science courses plus 1 semester of calculus and 1 of college English are required. *Transfer and advanced standing:* None.

Curriculum

4-year semitraditional. *First year:* After a 4-week officer orientation program, the introductory basic sciences are taught. In addition, courses are offered in epidemiology and biometrics, human context in health care, military studies and medical history, diagnostic parisitology and medical zoology, medical psychology, and introduction to Clinical Medicine I. *Second year:* In addition to the advanced basic sciences, courses presented include clinical concepts, preventive medicine, radiographic interpretation, and introduction to Clinical Medicine II. *Third year:* A 48-week period of rotations through the major clinical specialties including family practice. *Fourth year:* Consists of medical, surgical, and psychiatric selective blocks, neurology, military preventive medicine, contingency and emergency medicine, subinternships, and elective clerkships.

Grading and Promotion Policies

Letter grades are used for courses and clerkships and Pass/Fail for electives. Both steps of the USMLE must be taken and passed.

Facilities

Teaching: The school is located on the grounds of the Naval Hospital. Four buildings contain faculty offices, classrooms, student multidisciplinary and other laboratories and various support units. Thirteen affiliated hospitals provide clinical teaching facilities. *Library:* The Learning Resources Center possesses about 75,000 volumes and receives about 1500 medical periodicals. *Housing:* None available on campus.

Special Features

Minority admissions: Recruitment is sponsored by the Minority Affairs Program, which can be contacted through the Office of Admissions. *Other degree programs:* PhD programs are offered.

University of Maryland School of Medicine

655 West Baltimore Street
Baltimore, Maryland 21201

Phone: 410-706-7478
WWW: http://www.som./ab.umd.edu/som.html

Application Filing		Accreditation	
Earliest:	June 1	LCME	
Latest:	November 1		
Fee:	$40	**Degrees Granted**	
AMCAS:	yes	MD, MD-PhD	

Enrollment: 1996–97 First-Year Class

Men:	74	51%	Applied:	4645
Women:	72	49%	Interviewed:	883
Minorities:	23	16%	Enrolled:	146
Out of State:	25	17%		

1996–97 Class Profile

Mean MCAT Scores		*Mean GPA*
Physical Sciences:	9.8	3.5
Biological Sciences:	10.1	
Verbal Reasoning:	9.6	

Tuition and Fees

Resident	12,584
Average (public)	9500
Average (private)	22,500
Nonresident	22,684
Average (public)	20,500
Average (private)	24,500

0   10   20   30   40   50
(in thousands of dollars)

Percentage receiving financial aid: 71%
Above data applies to 1995–96 academic year.

Introduction

The University of Maryland School of Medicine is located on the Baltimore City Campus, and is the fifth oldest medical school in the United States. The first class graduated in 1810. It was one of the first colleges to build its own hospital for clinical instruction. The school is part of the 11 campuses of the University of Maryland system. The School of Medicine at the Baltimore Campus is the central component of a large academic Health Center that provides for medical education, patient care, biomedical research, and community service.

Admissions (AMCAS)

In addition to the minimum premedical science courses, requirements include 1 year of English. Applicants must also have completed a minimum of 90 semester hours at an accredited college or university. Strong preference is given to residents.

Curriculum

First and second years: The basic sciences are integrated and taught as systems, using interdisciplinary teaching with both basic and clinical science faculty. Contact hours have been reduced, with an emphasis on independent study. A half-day course in introduction to clinical practice is dedicated to the instruction of interviewing, physical examination, intimate human behavior, ethics, and the dynamics of ambulatory care. *Third year:* Clerkships through major medical specialties. A mandatory rotation in family medicine is included. There is emphasis on ambulatory teaching in all other disciplines and a longitudinal half-day experience in a clinical setting in which the student will have continuity of care for patients and families. *Fourth year:* Devoted to ambulatory care, student subinternships, and electives.

Grading and Promotion Policies

A letter grade system is used. Step 1 of the USMLE is required, and promotion to the third year is dependent on passing.

Facilities

Teaching: The school is located a short distance from the newly developed downtown Charles Center. University Hospital and affiliated hospitals around Baltimore have more than 1400 beds for teaching purposes. *Other:* The school also is affiliated with the Shock Trauma Center, Cancer Center, Institute of Psychiatric and Human Behavior, and the Sudden Infant Death Syndrome Institute. *Library:* The Health Sciences Library houses more than 240,000 volumes and subscribes to 3100 periodicals. It also provides access to a wide range of data bases. *Housing:* Dormitory rooms are available in the Baltimore Student Union; apartments are available a short distance from the campus.

Special Features

Minority admissions: The school has an active recruitment program that involves visits to colleges, seminars, and workshops. A 10-week preprofessional summer program is sponsored for undergraduates interested in health science careers, and a prematriculation summer program is available for those accepted into the first year. *Other degree programs:* Combined MD-PhD programs are available in all the basic sciences and in epidemiology, human genetics, and preventive medicine.

MASSACHUSETTS

Boston University School of Medicine

80 East Concord Street
Boston, Massachusetts   02118

Phone: 617-638-5300   *Fax:* 617-638-5258
E-mail: preich@bu.edu
WWW: http://www.med-amsa.bu.edu/

Application Filing		Accreditation
Earliest:	June 1	LCME
Latest:	November 15	
Fee:	$95	**Degrees Granted**
AMCAS:	yes	MD, MD-PhD, MD-MPH

Enrollment: 1996–97 First-Year Class

Men:	84	61%	Applied:	11,586
Women:	54	39%	Interviewed:	1159
Minorities:	15	11%	Enrolled:	138
Out of State:	87	63%		

1996–97 Class Profile

Mean MCAT Scores		*Mean GPA*
Physical Sciences:	9.6	n/av
Biological Sciences:	9.8	
Verbal Reasoning:	9.3	

Tuition and Fees

Resident	31,895
Average (public)	9500
Average (private)	22,500
Nonresident	31,895
Average (public)	20,500
Average (private)	24,500

(in thousands of dollars)

Percentage receiving financial aid: 89%

Introduction

The Boston University system includes 15 different schools and was founded in 1839. Boston University opened the School of Medicine when it joined in 1873 with the New England Female Medical College, which was the first medical school for women in the world. The School of Medicine became a component of the Boston University Medical Center in 1962. It is located in the south end of Boston, between Boston City Hospital and Boston University Medical Center Hospital.

Admissions (AMCAS)

The school is known for offering more pathways leading to the MD degree than any other medical school in the country. Students are accepted after high school, or after 2 years of college, in addition to being able to complete the first year of medical school over 2 academic years. For the traditional applicant who plans to enter after completing college, 1 year of English (composition or literature) and humanities is required in addition to the minimum premedical science courses. It is recommended that the student have a knowledge of calculus and of quantitation in chemistry. *Transfer and advanced standing:* Applicants considered for second- and third-year places must have appropriate basic science preparation. Transfer students must pass Step 1 of the USMLE.

Curriculum

4-year semimodern. *First year:* The first-year curriculum presents a study of man in a biopsychosocial model. Courses are offered in the traditional biologic disciplines that lead to an understanding of normal structure and function of the human body. Gross anatomy and histology emphasize the structure. Biochemistry, physiology, and endocrinology emphasize the mechanisms of normal function. Neurosciences and immunology utilize the resources of several departments to present material in an integrated format. A first semester course in psychiatry and second semester courses in sociomedical sciences, biostatistics, and epidemiology present, respectively, the spectrum of human development and social organizations in which people participate as professionals, patients, and citizens. *Second year:* The first semester of this year is composed of the traditional courses in microbiology and infectious diseases, pharmacology, and pathology. The second semester is devoted to an interdisciplinary course, Biology of Disease, a systems-based pathophysiology course in which emphasis on the clinical sciences is closely integrated with the basic sciences. Two courses, integrated problems and introduction to clinical medicine, are given throughout the first 2 years of the curriculum. They serve as a means of relating the basic sciences to each other and of making the transition to the clinical years. Integrated Problems is conducted through both the first and second years in a problem-based learning format. It is a student-centered course in which student participation, cooperative group learning, problem solving, and integration of information from concurrent courses are primary features. Introduction to Clinical Medicine is based predominantly in clinical settings where student-to-faculty ratios are as little as 1:1. In the first year, the course explores the various aspects of the doctor-patient relationship, with a major emphasis on effective communication, and the relationship of medicine to some of the broader social issues such as substance abuse, children at risk, and the effects of cultural diversity. In the second year of introduction to clinical medicine, communication skills are reinforced and techniques of physical examination are introduced so that students are appropriately prepared for their third year clerkships. *Third year:* The principal clinical clerkship year is composed of clerkships in medicine, surgery, obstetrics and gynecology, pediatrics and psychiatry. *Fourth year:* The fourth year is composed of required, 4-week courses on the home medical service (geriatrics), neurology, radiology, ambulatory medicine (primary care), and a subinternship. The remaining 20 weeks of electives may be scheduled at each student's discretion. The elective period permits considerable flexibility in developing a program fitted to the individual needs and interests of each medical student. Diversification is thus possible during the fourth year and may include courses in other schools and colleges of Boston University, other approved educational institutions in the Boston area, and clinical and research electives in other medical schools or medical-school-affiliated hospitals in this country and abroad.

Grading and Promotion Policies
The student's record contains for each course the appropriate Honors/Pass/Fail designation and a detailed written narrative. If the student is unable to pass any given course, the Promotion Committee determines the action to be taken. Passing Step 1 of the USMLE is required for graduation. Taking Step 2 is optional.

Facilities
Teaching: The 14-story Instructional Building includes space for student activities, administrative offices, two 130-seat auditoriums, teaching laboratories, faculty offices, research laboratories, and a 3-floor library. The first floor of an adjacent research building houses 13 seminar, conference, and computer rooms. Several small seminar rooms are open for evening use by students. The principal teaching hospitals are Boston Medical Center and affiliated Veterans Administration hospitals. *Other:* The school is affiliated with a network of at least 12 community hospitals, neighborhood health centers and other private practice settings, all of which provide clinical settings for all years. *Library:* The library contains more than 80,000 volumes and receives approximately 1500 periodicals. Fifty-five PCs are available 7 days a week and until 10:30 P.M. on week nights in the library's full service computer lab.

Special Features
Minority admissions: The school is committed to the recruitment, admission, and retention of disadvantaged students. It conducts a 6-week summer enrichment Pre-entrance Program for accepted students and maintains articulation agreements with a consortium of historic African-American colleges and universities to allow early acceptance to medical school. *Other degree programs:* Combined MD-PhD programs in all basic sciences are offered as is an MD-MPH program. As an alternative curriculum, students may schedule the requirements of the first 3 semesters over a 5-semester period.

Harvard Medical School

25 Shattuck Street
Boston, Massachusetts   02115

Phone: 617-432-1550   *Fax:* 617-432-3307
E-mail: hmsadm@warren.med.harvard.edu
WWW: http://www.med.harvard.edu/

Application Filing		Accreditation	
Earliest:	June 1	LCME	
Latest:	October 15		
Fee:	$70	**Degrees Granted**	
AMCAS:	yes	MD, MD-PhD	

Enrollment: 1996–97 First-Year Class

Men:	82	50%	Applied:		3914
Women:	83	50%	Interviewed:		1057
Minorities:	23	14%	Enrolled:		165
Out of State:	152	92%			

1996–97 Class Profile

Mean MCAT Scores		*Mean GPA*
Physical Sciences:	11	3.82
Biological Sciences:	11	
Verbal Reasoning:	10	

Tuition and Fees

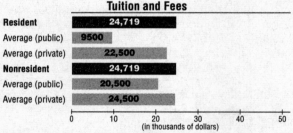

Resident	24,719
Average (public)	9500
Average (private)	22,500
Nonresident	24,719
Average (public)	20,500
Average (private)	24,500

(in thousands of dollars)

Percentage receiving financial aid: n/av

Above data applies to 1995–96 academic year.

Introduction

The Harvard Medical School was founded in 1782. It has been located on the Longwood Avenue Quadrangle since 1906. In 1987 the Medical Education Center was opened next to the Medical School. It is a diverse academic medical center and has cooperative links to 18 independent medical institutions.

Admissions

Minimum science courses are required in addition to 1 year of calculus and 1 year of expository writing. Recommended courses include 16 hours in these areas: literature, languages, the arts, humanities, and social sciences. Selection is not based on residence. *Transfer and advanced standing:* Limited number of students are admitted to third-year class.

Curriculum

4-year modern. Two programs are offered. The New Pathway Program is designed to accommodate the vari-ety of interests, educational backgrounds, and career goals that characterize the student body. Basic science and clinical content are interwoven throughout the 4 years. *First and second years:* Uses a problem-based approach that emphasizes small-group tutorials and self-directed learning, complemented by laboratories, conferences, and lectures. Students are expected to analyze problems, locate relevant material in library and computer-based resources, and develop habits of life-long learning and independent study. *Third and fourth years:* Core clinical clerkships; advance science or independent project; patient-doctor III; and electives. The second MD Pathway is the Harvard-MIT Division of Health Sciences and Technology Program (HST). The curriculum of this program is designed for the student with a strong interest and background in quantitative science. The curriculum is in a semester format. HST students join students of the New Pathway Program for their clinical rotation. Thirty students are admitted each year.

Grading and Promotion Policies

System used is Honors/Pass/Fail. Promotion Boards for each of the first 3 years determine those qualified to be promoted. Students must record total passing scores on Steps 1 and 2 of the USMLE for promotion and graduation, respectively.

Facilities

Teaching: Preclinical courses are taught in the buildings that compose Longwood Avenue Quadrangle. Clinical instruction takes place in Beth Israel Hospital (368 beds), Brigham and Women's Hospital (650 beds), Massachusetts General Hospital (1060 beds) and others. *Other:* Research facilities available in most of the medical school buildings. *Library:* The Countway Library of Medicine is one of the largest in the country. *Housing:* Dormitory housing is available for men and women; apartments for married students are nearby.

Special Features

Minority admissions: A full-time administrator coordinates the active minority recruitment program, which is geared to enroll students having academic strength, community commitment, and leadership ability. An 8-week prematriculation summer program is offered for a limited number of disadvantaged students to enhance their academic preparation and provide exposure to research. *Other degree programs:* The MD-PhD program exists for qualified applicants who wish to integrate medical school and intensive scientific training.

Tufts University School of Medicine

136 Harrison Avenue
Boston, Massachusetts   02111

Phone: 617-636-6571
E-mail: sgp@cor.cdm.nemc.org
WWW: http://www.nemc.org/tusu/about

Application Filing		Accreditation	
Earliest:	June 1	LCME	
Latest:	November 1		
Fee:	$75	**Degrees Granted**	
AMCAS:	yes	MD, MD-PhD, MD-MPH	

Enrollment: 1996–97 First-Year Class

Men:	92	52%	Applied:	11,534	
Women:	84	48%	Interviewed:	923	
Minorities:	14	8%	Enrolled:	176	
Out of State:	124	70%			

1996–97 Class Profile

Mean MCAT Scores		*Mean GPA*
Physical Sciences:	9.6	3.54
Biological Sciences:	9.8	
Verbal Reasoning:	9.1	

Tuition and Fees

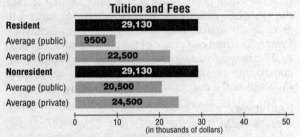

Resident	29,130
Average (public)	9500
Average (private)	22,500
Nonresident	29,130
Average (public)	20,500
Average (private)	24,500

(in thousands of dollars)

Percentage receiving financial aid: 74%

Above data applies to 1995–96 academic year.

Introduction

Tufts University was established in 1850 as the Tufts Institute of Learning. In 1872 the name was changed to Tufts College, and in 1953 it became Tufts University. This reflects transition from the small liberal arts college to a complex multi-campus university. The School of Medicine was established in 1893. Because of the diverse hospitals affiliated with the school, students are provided with clinical experiences that range from inner-city tertiary-level hospitals to rural-based individual preceptorships.

Admissions (AMCAS)

Minimum premedical science courses are required, as is proficiency in written and spoken English. Courses in calculus, statistics, and computers are desirable. There is no preference for state residents. *Transfer and advanced standing:* Acceptance into the second or third year is possible as places become available.

Curriculum

4-year modern. *First year:* Major themes during this year include fundamental principles applicable to the normal human, the biopsychosocial determinants of human behavior, the impact of health care systems and society on the individual patient and physician, an introduction to the doctor-patient relationship, and an introduction to human nutrition. *Second year:* This year involves a progressive introduction to human abnormal biology and therapeutics through a series of interdisciplinary courses organized by organ system. A course in psychopathology is also offered, as is one in physical diagnosis. *Third year:* Consists of rotations through the major clinical specialties and rotations in neurology, rehabilitative medicine, ophthalmology, otolaryngology, and therapeutic radiology. *Fourth year:* Involves eight 4-week rotations, two of which are ward service. The remainder of the time is free for electives.

Grading and Promotion Policies

The system used is Honors/High Pass/Pass/Low Pass/Fail. Passing Steps 1 and 2 of the USMLE is required for graduation.

Facilities

Teaching: The major school structure is the Sackler Center. Clinical teaching facilities are provided by the New England Center Hospital (452 beds) and off campus by St. Elizabeth's Hospital (385 beds), Bayside Medical Center (950 beds), VA Hospital (769 beds), Lemuel Shattick Hospital (250 beds), and others. *Other:* Clinical research is carried out in the Ziskind Research Building of New England Medical Center Hospital. *Library:* The Health Sciences Library houses 92,000 volumes and subscribes to 1400 periodicals. *Housing:* A residence hall for men and women is located 1 block from the main building.

Special Features

Minority admissions: Recruitment of minority applicants is directed primarily to the Boston, New England, and New York areas. A preadmission summer program is offered for accepted applicants. *Other degree programs:* Combined MD-PhD programs are offered in a variety of disciplines including immunology and molecular biology. A combined MD-MPH program is also offered.

University of Massachusetts Medical School

55 Lake Avenue, North
Worcester, Massachusetts   01655

Phone: 508-856-2323
E-mail: admissions@banyan.ummed.edu
WWW: http://www.ummed.edu:800/

Application Filing		Accreditation	
Earliest:	June 1	LCME	
Latest:	November 1		
Fee:	$50	**Degrees Granted**	
AMCAS:	yes	MD, MD-PhD	

Enrollment: 1996–97 First-Year Class

Men:	50	50%	Applied:	1500	
Women:	50	50%	Interviewed:	495	
Minorities:	6	6%	Enrolled:	100	
Out of State:	0	0%			

1996–97 Class Profile

Mean MCAT Scores		*Mean GPA*
Physical Sciences:	10	3.5
Biological Sciences:	10	
Verbal Reasoning:	10	

Tuition and Fees

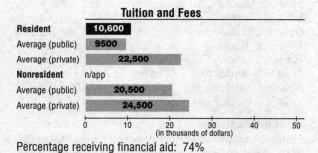

Resident	10,600
Average (public)	9500
Average (private)	22,500
Nonresident	n/app
Average (public)	20,500
Average (private)	24,500

(in thousands of dollars)

Percentage receiving financial aid: 74%

Introduction

The University of Massachusetts Medical School opened in 1970 and is located in Worchester. The school seeks to train residents of Massachusetts for service in the state, especially underserved areas. The school is affiliated with the University of Massachusetts Medical Center, which encompasses a regional trauma center as well as an air ambulance reception area. The school is located on the banks of Lake Quinsigamond.

Admissions (AMCAS)

The standard premedical science courses and 1 year of English are required. Courses in calculus, psychology, sociology, and statistics are recommended. *Transfer and advanced standing:* Applicants will be accepted, provided there are vacancies in the class.

Curriculum

4-year semimodern. *First and second years:* The curriculum in the preclinical sciences emphasizes thoughtful coordination across disciplines and interdiscipli-

nary courses. Throughout the first 2 years, students also participate in twice-weekly sessions consisting of The Patient, Physician, and Society (PPS) and the Longitudinal Preceptorship Program (LPP). Both courses are tightly integrated and coordinated with concurrent basic science disciplines. *Third and fourth years:* The clerkship years comprise the third and fourth years of study. Required clerkships consist of clinical rotations in internal medicine, family practice, pediatrics, obstetrics and gynecology, psychiatry, neurology, and surgery. The medicine clerkship includes 4 weeks in an internist's office. The surgery clerkship consists of a hospital-based, 8-week component and a 4-week ambulatory component. The fourth year consists of a required 4-week clerkship in neurology and a 4-week subinternship in medicine plus a minimum of an additional 24 weeks of electives. With the guidance and counsel of faculty members, students plan a balanced program of study appropriate to their field of interest, combining work in both basic science and clinical medicine. The Senior Scholars Program also exists for selected students who desire intensive study in a field of special interest or research. Under the guidance of a faculty mentor, a unique program of at least 3 months combining both basic science and clinical experience in a given discipline is arranged.

Grading and Promotion Policies

System used is Honors/Satisfactory/Marginal/Unsatisfactory/ Incomplete. Students are not required to take the USMLE, although it is anticipated that most will elect to do so for purposes of subsequent licensure. Promotion from one phase of the curriculum to the next will be determined by the Committee on Promotions, consisting of instructors from each department involved in the curriculum of a given period of study.

Facilities

Teaching: A 10-story Basic and Clinical Sciences Building was completed in 1973. A 400-bed teaching hospital that adjoins the Sciences Building opened in 1976. The Medical Center is the designated regional trauma center for Central Massachusetts as well as the base of operation for New England Life Flight. *Other:* Among the affiliated hospitals for clinical teaching are the St. Vincent Hospital (600 beds), Worcester City Hospital (250 beds), Worcester Memorial Hospital (379 beds), and Berkshire Medical Center (365 beds). *Library:* The Medical School Library is housed in the Sciences Building and includes the capacity for more than 100,000 volumes. *Housing:* The school has limited on-campus facilities for housing single students, reserved for first-year students. Most find housing in the community.

Special Features

Minority admissions: Minority students who are legal residents of Massachusetts are invited to apply for admission. A 4-week Summer Enrichment Program (SEP) is available for sophomore and higher level college students. *Other degree programs:* Combined MD-PhD programs are offered in all the basic medical sciences and in immunology and molecular genetics.

MICHIGAN

Michigan State University College of Human Medicine

East Lansing, Michigan   48824

Phone: 517-353-9620   *Fax:* 517-432-0021
E-mail: mdadmissions@ msu.edu
WWW: http://www.msu.edu/academics/
             academics2.html

Application Filing		Accreditation	
Earliest:	June 1	LCME	
Latest:	November 15		
Fee:	$50	**Degrees Granted**	
AMCAS:	yes	MD, MD-PhD, MD-MA	

Enrollment: 1996–97 First-Year Class

Men:	51	49%	Applied:	3719
Women:	53	51%	Interviewed:	3719
Minorities:	20	19%	Enrolled:	104
Out of State:	25	24%		

1996–97 Class Profile

Mean MCAT Scores		*Mean GPA*
Physical Sciences:	8.6	n/av
Biological Sciences:	9.1	
Verbal Reasoning:	9.7	

Tuition and Fees

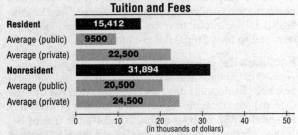

Resident	15,412
Average (public)	9500
Average (private)	22,500
Nonresident	31,894
Average (public)	20,500
Average (private)	24,500

0   10   20   30   40   50
(in thousands of dollars)

Percentage receiving financial aid: n/av

Above data applies to 1995–96 academic year.

Introduction

The aim of the College of Human Medicine at Michigan State University is to train primary care physicians in order to provide superior health care for everyone. It is essentially a large university operating in a small college setting. The university's health care educational complex incorporates, in addition, an Allopathic Medical School, a College of Osteopathic Medicine, and a College of Veterinary Medicine.

Admissions (AMCAS)

Requirements include the basic premedical science courses, 1 year of English, and psychology and/or sociology. Preference is given to applicants from Michigan. *Transfer and advanced standing:* Applicants are considered when vacancies exist.

Curriculum

The curriculum is divided into 3 blocks integrating the basic biological and behavioral sciences with clinical training and problem-solving skills. *Block I:* A 1-year discipline-based experience that provides an introduction to the fundamentals of the basic biological and psychological/social sciences, along with mentor group and early clinical skills training that includes patient contact. *Block II:* A 1-year experience in the second year that is problem-based and learner-centered with the majority of learning occurring in the small group setting. An extended curricular option for both Blocks I and II is offered at no extra cost. *Block III:* An 84-week experience that includes the traditional clinical clerkships plus core competency and primary care experiences. This period is spent in 1 of the 6 communities affiliated with the university. Students live in their assigned community for the total period of required clinical training. Electives may be taken elsewhere. The community physicians work closely with community-based faculty members of the college to provide a unique and highly relevant learning environment.

Grading and Promotion Policies

All grading in the school is Honors/Pass/Fail. A total passing score on Steps 1 and 2 of the USMLE is required for promotion to the third year and graduation, respectively.

Facilities

Teaching: The primary facilities utilized in basic science instruction are Life Sciences Building, Fee Hall, and Giltner Hall. The Clinical Center is an ambulatory care facility where students are trained in clinical sciences during the first 2 years of the curriculum. Students receive their formal clinical training during the last 2 years in community settings in 18 hospitals in 6 Michigan communities. *Library:* Information not available. *Housing:* On-campus dormitory rooms and apartments for both single and married students. There is also a large selection of off-campus housing.

Special Features

Minority admissions: A major effort is made to include applicants from inadequately represented geographic, economic, and ethnic groups. *Other degree programs:* Combined MA-MD and MD-PhD programs available in basic and behavioral science departments by individual arrangement.

University of Michigan Medical School

1301 Catherine Street
Ann Arbor, Michigan   48109-0010

Phone: 313-764-6317   *Fax:* 313-764-4542
WWW: http://www.med.umich.edu/

Application Filing		Accreditation	
Earliest:	June 1	LCME	
Latest:	November 15		
Fee:	$50	**Degrees Granted**	
AMCAS:	yes	MD, MD-PhD, BA-MD	

Enrollment: 1996–97 First-Year Class

Men:	96	58%	Applied:	5873
Women:	69	42%	Interviewed:	470
Minorities:	99	60%	Enrolled:	165
Out of State:	65	39%		

1996–97 Class Profile

Mean MCAT Scores		*Mean GPA*
Physical Sciences:	11	3.5
Biological Sciences:	11	
Verbal Reasoning:	10	

Tuition and Fees

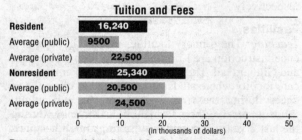

Resident	16,240
Average (public)	9500
Average (private)	22,500
Nonresident	25,340
Average (public)	20,500
Average (private)	24,500

(in thousands of dollars) 0 10 20 30 40 50

Percentage receiving financial aid: n/av

Above data applies to 1995–96 academic year.

Introduction

The University of Michigan Medical School is located in the University of Michigan Medical Center in Ann Arbor along with the University of Michigan hospitals. Its origin can be traced back to the establishment of the university in 1817. The first class graduated in 1851. The beginning of the modern Medical School came in 1869 when it replaced the proprietary school. The quality of the new school was already praised in the famous Flexner Report. The University Hospital, the most modern in the world at that time, was opened up in 1925. The school is located on an 84-acre campus and provides large city facilities with a small city atmosphere.

Admissions (AMCAS)

In addition to the basic premedical science courses, 6 credits of English and 18 credits of nonscience subjects are required. A biochemistry course is also required. Advanced courses in biology and/or chemistry are recommended. Preference is given to residents, but a significant number of nonresidents are admitted. Thirty-five highly qualified high school graduates who have been accepted by the University of Michigan College of Literature, Science and the Arts will be admitted to the 8-year Integrated Premedical-Medical Program. They earn their BA degree after the fourth year. *Transfer and advanced standing:* None.

Curriculum

4-year semimodern. *First year:* Basic science fundamentals courses, 1 interdisciplinary course (molecular and cellular biology), and introduction to the patient, a clinical interviewing and clinical skills course. *Second year:* A series of organ-based sequences designed to provide advanced basic science material in a clinical context, and a continuation of the introduction to the patient course. *Third year:* Clerkship rotation through the major clinical specialties, with some opportunity for career electives, and weekly clinical conferences; a primary care clerkship experience is required of all students; it may be completed in the third or fourth year. *Fourth year:* An 8-week subinternship is required of all students (students may choose department and specialty), and also an advanced basic science experience (students may choose from a list of experiences). There is also ample opportunity for varied experiences on campus and at other institutions.

Grading and Promotion Policies

The first year is Pass/Fail only; in the second, third, and fourth years, a modified system comprised of Honors, High Pass, and Pass. Clinical clerkship grades are usually accompanied by a narrative description of student performance. Students are required to pass Step 1 of the USMLE for promotion to the third year, and are required to pass Step 2 for graduation.

Facilities

Teaching: Basic sciences are taught in Medical Sciences Buildings Unit I and II in the Medical Center. Clinical instruction takes place at the University Hospitals (888 beds) supplemented by the use of St. Joseph Mercy Hospital (522 beds) and the VA Hospital (486 beds). The University Hospital was opened in 1986. *Other:* Medical Center includes: Simpson Memorial Institute devoted to cancer research and diseases of the blood; 3 Kresge buildings for clinical research; and the Buhl Research Center for Human Genetics. Two new Medical Sciences Research Buildings were opened in 1986 and 1988 and a third in 1994. *Library:* The A. Alfred Taubman Medical Library houses more than 200,000 volumes and 3000 periodicals; the Learning Resource Center is housed in the library building and includes computers, laser printers, and an extensive audiovisual collection for student use. *Housing:* Some facilities available.

Special Features

Minority admissions: The school has an active minority-student recruitment program. Some scholarships for underrepresented minority students are available. *Other degree programs:* School offers combination MD-PhD programs in a variety of disciplines including human genetics.

Wayne State University School of Medicine

540 East Canfield Avenue
Detroit, Michigan   48201

Phone: 313-577-1466   *Fax:* 313-577-1330
WWW: http://www.phypc.med.wayne.edu/

Application Filing		Accreditation	
Earliest:	June 1	LCME	
Latest:	December 15		
Fee:	$30	**Degrees Granted**	
AMCAS:	yes	MD, MD-PhD	

Enrollment: 1996–97 First-Year Class

Men:	161	65%	Applied:	4409
Women:	86	35%	Interviewed:	838
Minorities:	37	15%	Enrolled:	247
Out of State:	17	7%		

1996–97 Class Profile

Mean MCAT Scores		*Mean GPA*
Physical Sciences:	9.1	3.45
Biological Sciences:	8.8	
Verbal Reasoning:	8.8	

Tuition and Fees

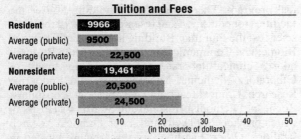

Resident	9966
Average (public)	9500
Average (private)	22,500
Nonresident	19,461
Average (public)	20,500
Average (private)	24,500

(in thousands of dollars)

Percentage receiving financial aid: n/av

Above data applies to 1995–96 academic year.

Introduction

The Wayne State University School of Medicine was established in 1868. It is associated with the Detroit Medical Center, which contains 6 health care institutions. It is located in the northcentral area of Detroit. The facilities of the School of Medicine are relatively modern, having been completed in the last 25 years.

Admissions (AMCAS)

Applicants should have taken the basic premedical courses plus 1 year of English. School does consider nonresidents for admission. *Transfer and advanced standing:* Applicants from U.S. or Canadian allopathic and osteopathic schools will be considered for second- and third-year classes.

Curriculum

4-year modern. Curriculum consists of a core program, early correlation of clinical medicine, coordinated clin-ical experience, and expanded elective studies. *First year:* Consists of study of structure and function of the normal human through a disciplinary approach. Social and behavioral sciences as related to community health problems are also considered. *Second year:* Consists of a study of abnormalities in structure and function. Behavior is also considered. Time is allotted for an intensive course in interviewing techniques, taking medical histories, and physical examination. *Third year:* Consists of rotating clerkships through major specialties and family medicine. *Fourth year:* A broad program of 32 weeks of structured electives. Time can be spent at another university.

Grading and Promotion Policies

System used is Honors/Pass/Fail. In order to qualify for promotion to the next class, a student must demonstrate competency on all subject examinations. All students will be required to pass Step 1 of the USMLE in order to be promoted into the third year.

Facilities

Teaching: The School of Medicine is located in the heart of the 236-acre Detroit Medical Center. Gordon Scott Hall houses the school's basic science departments, as well as administrative and service offices. Clinical teaching takes place at the Harper Hospital (557 beds), Children's Hospital (320 beds), Grace Hospital (957 beds), Hutzel Hospital (360 beds). *Other:* Clinical teaching also takes place off campus at the Detroit Receiving Hospital (700 beds) and VA Hospital (890 beds). *Library:* Shiffman Medical Library houses more than 150,000 volumes. *Housing:* Available in the campus area.

Special Features

Minority admissions: The school's Office of Recruitment is actively engaged in furthering minority-student enrollment. Entering students can participate in a summer program designed to facilitate the transition to medical school. *Other degree programs:* Combined MD-PhD degree programs are offered in a variety of basic science disciplines.

MINNESOTA

Mayo Medical School

200 First Street, S.W.
Rochester, Minnesota 55901

Phone: 507-284-3671 *Fax:* 507-284-2634
WWW: http://www.mayo.edu/education/mms

Application Filing		Accreditation	
Earliest:	June 1	LCME	
Latest:	November 1		
Fee:	$60	**Degrees Granted**	
AMCAS:	yes	MD, MD-PhD	

Enrollment: 1996–97 First-Year Class

Men:	19	45%	Applied:	3791
Women:	23	55%	Interviewed:	417
Minorities:	8	19%	Enrolled:	42
Out of State:	34	81%		

1996–97 Class Profile

Mean MCAT Scores		*Mean GPA*
Physical Sciences:	11	3.72
Biological Sciences:	11	
Verbal Reasoning:	11	

Tuition and Fees

Resident	4800
Average (public)	$9500
Average (private)	$22,500
Nonresident	$9900
Average (public)	$20,500
Average (private)	$24,500

(in thousands of dollars)

Percentage receiving financial aid: n/av

Introduction

As part of the Mayo Clinic, the Mayo Medical School is managed by the Mayo Foundation. Its origin goes back to 1863, when Dr. William Worrall Mayo settled in Rochester. He was joined 20 years later by his two physician sons who set up a private integrated group practice in which they were joined by other respected physicians. This led to the formation of the renowned Mayo Clinic. The faculty of the Medical School is associated with the Clinic and several hospitals.

Admissions (AMCAS)

Only the minimum premedical science courses are required. A course in biochemistry is also required. Forty-two students comprise each class.

Curriculum

4-year modern. The small class size facilitates a personalized course of instruction characterized by extensive clinical interaction and the integration of basic and clinical sciences throughout all segments of the curriculum. Patient contact begins early in the first year and increases commensurate with student progress. The integration of basic and clinical sciences occurs in a manner that strengthens basic science concepts, stresses the patient orientation appropriate for an undergraduate medical school, and utilizes a variety of active, problem-oriented, faculty-guided and self-learning techniques to aid student comprehension. Integration of the various components of the curriculum is promoted by organization of course material into broad functional units that span several curricular years. The curricular units are: the cell; the organ; the patient, physician, and society; the scientific foundations of medical practice; clinical experiences; and the research trimester. This type of curricular organization enables content integration of the basic and clinical sciences and between basic and clinical science.

Grading and Promotion Policies

An Honors/Pass/Fail system is used. Students are required to take Steps 1 and 2 of the USMLE. Promotion will be based on evidence of behavior and maturation, consonant with the student's talents and defined professional goals.

Facilities

Teaching: Located in Rochester, the school makes use of the facilities of the Mayo Foundation in its preclinical program. The Guggenheim Building houses the facilities for education and research in most of the basic sciences; the Plummer Building houses the library and Biomedical Communications; and the Hilton Building houses clinical laboratories of the Department of Laboratory Medicine, Microbiology, and Endocrine Research. Clinical teaching takes place at 2 hospitals: Rochester Methodist Hospital and St. Mary's Hospital, which provide 2000 beds and several clinical research facilities. *Other:* Facilities for research are located in the Medical Sciences Building, Guggenheim Building, and Rochester Methodist and St. Mary's Hospitals. *Library:* Information not available. *Housing:* Students are responsible for finding their own housing in the area.

Special Features

Minority admissions: The school actively seeks minority students and welcomes their application for admission. *Other degree programs:* Combined MD-PhD programs are offered in several disciplines including immunology and pathology. A combined MD-Oral Maxillofacial Surgery program is also offered to candidates who have completed the DDS degree.

University of Minnesota—Duluth School of Medicine

10 University Drive
Duluth, Minnesota   55812

Phone: 218-726-8511   *Fax:* 218-726-6235
E-mail: jcarls 10@l.umn.edu
WWW: http://www.d.umn.edu/medweb/

Application Filing	Accreditation
Earliest: June 1	LCME
Latest: November 15	
Fee: $50	**Degrees Granted**
AMCAS: yes	None

Enrollment: 1996–97 First-Year Class

Men:	26	50%	Applied:	1385
Women:	26	50%	Interviewed:	180
Minorities:	4	7%	Enrolled:	52
Out of State:	0	0%		

1996–97 Class Profile

Mean MCAT Scores		*Mean GPA*
Physical Sciences:	8.7	3.55
Biological Sciences:	9	
Verbal Reasoning:	9	

Tuition and Fees

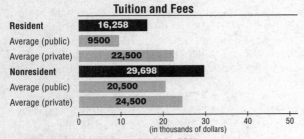

Resident	16,258
Average (public)	9500
Average (private)	22,500
Nonresident	29,698
Average (public)	20,500
Average (private)	24,500

(in thousands of dollars)

Percentage receiving financial aid: 90%

Introduction

In 1947 the University of Minnesota—Duluth became an associate campus of the University of Minnesota. The University of Minnesota—Duluth School of Medicine was founded in 1969. This school provides the first 2 years of medical education, after which students automatically transfer to the partent school in Minneapolis for the completion of their training. The school seeks to provide practitioners for northern Minnesota and Wisconsin.

Admissions (AMCAS)

Requirements include the minimum premedical science courses and 1 year of English composition, mathematics through calculus, humanities, and behavioral science. Only residents of Minnesota, Ashland, Bayfield, Burnett Douglas, Iron, Price, Sawyer and Washburn counties of Wisconsin, and the Canadian province of Manitoba are considered. The school offers a 2-year program that prepares students for transfer to a clinical program at a degree-granting institution. A mechanism has also been established for transfer to the University of Minnesota Medical School in Minneapolis on a noncompetitive basis for completion of MD requirements.

Curriculum

2-year traditional. *First year:* The basic medical sciences are covered in a course-oriented curriculum. About 10 hours of a 40-hour week remain as unprogrammed time. A preceptorship, during which students spend periods each week with a physician engaged in family practice, will be initiated during the first year. *Second year:* The curriculum is course-oriented with a heavier emphasis on clinical science.

Grading and Promotion Policies

An Honors/Pass/Fail system is used, and Step 1 of the USMLE must be taken and passed for promotion to the third year of the medical curriculum in Minneapolis.

Facilities

Teaching: A basic medical sciences building was constructed on the main Duluth campus. Clinical teaching takes place at St. Mary's, St. Luke's, and Miller-Dawn Hospitals of Duluth. *Other:* The original facilities are for research purposes. *Library:* The Health Science Library is part of the Duluth campus library system and presently includes 60,000 volumes; more than 500 periodicals are received regularly. *Housing:* Housing is available on the main Duluth campus and in the surrounding community.

Special Features

Minority admissions: Applicants from minority groups underrepresented in the health professions, particularly Native Americans, are encouraged to apply.

University of Minnesota Medical School—Minneapolis

420 Delaware Street, S.E.
Minneapolis, Minnesota 55455

Phone: 612-624-1122 *Fax:* 612-626-6800
E-mail: reilloo2@maroon.tc.umn.edu
WWW: http://www.med.umn.edu/

Application Filing		Accreditation	
Earliest:	June 1	LCME	
Latest:	November 15		
Fee:	$50	**Degrees Granted**	
AMCAS:	yes	MD, MD-PhD	

Enrollment: 1996–97 First-Year Class

Men:	86	49%	Applied:	2330
Women:	89	51%	Interviewed:	746
Minorities:	5	3%	Enrolled:	175
Out of State:	13	7%		

1996–97 Class Profile

Mean MCAT Scores		*Mean GPA*
Physical Sciences:	10	n/av
Biological Sciences:	10	
Verbal Reasoning:	10	

Tuition and Fees

Resident	16,258
Average (public)	9500
Average (private)	22,500
Nonresident	29,698
Average (public)	20,500
Average (private)	24,500

(in thousands of dollars) 0 10 20 30 40 50

Percentage receiving financial aid: n/av

Introduction

The University of Minnesota Medical School was established in 1888 when 3 of the 4 proprietary medical schools in the area joined together; a fourth joined later. By 1911 the first unit of the University Hospital was dedicated. The school has a long tradition of research and clinical achievement and is characterized by strong departments in the basic medical sciences.

Admissions (AMCAS)

Requirements include a bachelor's degree, the basic premedical science courses, English (3 quarters), liberal arts courses (27 quarters), and calculus. Courses in genetics and psychology are recommended. Preference for admission is given to legal residents of Minnesota. *Transfer and advanced standing:* Transfer students are accepted into the third year and usually only from the 2-year medical school of the University of Minnesota-Duluth.

Curriculum

4-year semitraditional. *First year:* Consists of the basic science courses and clinical correlations. During the summer, topics in clinical medicine, human behavior, genetics, and clinical diagnostic skills are presented. *Second year:* Consists of the advanced basic sciences and pathophysiology of organ systems. Clinical exposure to internal medicine, pediatrics, neurology, and family practice is provided. *Third and fourth years:* Very flexible; consists of externships (4 quarters), electives (2 quarters). Research activities are encouraged.

Grading and Promotion Policies

Information not available.

Facilities

Teaching: The University Hospital and most of the major hospitals in the Minneapolis-St. Paul area are affiliated with the medical school and provide clinical training facilities. *Other:* Facilities for research are located in the Health Sciences Center. *Library:* A comprehensive medical library that contains many books and subscribes to numerous periodicals is available for student use. *Housing:* Information is not available.

Special Features

Minority admissions: Minority applicants are encouraged to apply. *Other degree programs:* A 7-year MD-PhD program is available for superior students planning academic medicine careers.

MISSISSIPPI

University of Mississippi School of Medicine

2500 North State Street
Jackson, Mississippi   39216

Phone: 601-984-1080   *Fax:* 601-984-1079
E-mail: bmb@fiona.umsmed
WWW: http://www.fiona.umsmed.edu/

Application Filing		Accreditation
Earliest:	June 1	LCME
Latest:	November 1	
Fee:	n/av	**Degrees Granted**
AMCAS:	yes	MD

Enrollment: 1996–97 First-Year Class

Men:	70	70%	Applied:	313
Women:	30	30%	Interviewed:	194
Minorities:	14	14%	Enrolled:	100
Out of State:	0	0%		

1996–97 Class Profile

Mean MCAT Scores		*Mean GPA*
Physical Sciences:	9	3.55
Biological Sciences:	9	
Verbal Reasoning:	9	

Tuition and Fees

Resident	6715
Average (public)	9500
Average (private)	22,500
Nonresident	12,715
Average (public)	20,500
Average (private)	24,500

0   10   20   30   40   50
(in thousands of dollars)

Percentage receiving financial aid: n/av

Introduction

The University of Mississippi School of Medicine, located in Jackson, is part of the University of Mississippi Medical Center. The Medical Center also includes Schools of Dentistry, Nursing, Health-Related Professions, Graduate Studies in the Medical Sciences, and the University Hospital. The School of Medicine opened in 1903 and operated as a 2-year institution until 1955 when it expanded to a 4-year program and relocated to the 158-acre campus in Jackson.

Admissions (AMCAS)

In addition to the basic premedical sciences, required courses include 1 year of mathematics, 1 year of English, and 1 of advanced science. High priority is given to state residents. *Transfers and advanced stand-*

ing: Applications are considered from those who are in good standing at their previous school.

Curriculum

4-year traditional. *First year:* Introductory basic sciences plus psychiatry and cardiopulmonary resuscitation. *Second year:* Advanced basic sciences as well as courses in parasitology, genetics, psychiatry, epidemiology, and biostatistics, all of which are covered in the first 2 quarters. The third quarter is devoted to multidepartmental introduction to clinical medicine which provides classroom instruction in history taking and physical examination. This is supplemented by weekly tutorial sessions conducted by members of the faculty and is correlated with instruction in clinical laboratory diagnosis. *Third year:* Rotating clerkships in major clinical specialties as well as in family medicine and radiology. *Fourth year:* Consists of 9 required calendar-month blocks of clinical subjects. One block must come from 2 of the 3 major clinical specialties. Two courses must be taken in an ambulatory setting and 1 block in neuroscience, medicine, and surgery is required.

Grading and Promotion Policies

A numerical grading system is used. Students must achieve not less than 70 in each course and a weighted average of not less than 75 each year. Students must record scores in specific individual exams of Steps 1 and 2 of the USMLE.

Facilities

Teaching: The school is part of the University of Mississippi Medical Center located on the 158-acre campus in the heart of the city. It consists of an 8-story complex whose north wing is occupied by the medical school. The east, west, and south wings house the University Hospital (552 beds) that serves as the principal clinical teaching facility. Three other hospitals in the Jackson area cooperate in the teaching program. *Library:* The Rowland Medical Library houses more than 161,000 volumes and 2500 periodicals and is located in the Holmes Learning Resource Center. *Housing:* A dormitory for women students and efficiency, 2-, and 3-bedroom apartments are available.

Special Features

Minority admissions: The school has a strong commitment to enrolling and retaining minority and/or disadvantaged students. Its efforts are coordinated by its Office of Minority Affairs. It offers a 9-week preparatory reinforcement and enrichment program and a preentry summer program for accepted minority students. *Other degree programs:* Combined MD-PhD programs are offered in the basic sciences and preventive medicine.

MISSOURI

St. Louis University Health Sciences Center

1402 South Grand Boulevard
St. Louis, Missouri 63104

Phone: 314-577-8205 *Fax:* 314-577-8214
E-mail: galofrea@sluvca.slu.edu
WWW: http://www.slu.edu/colleges/med/

Application Filing		Accreditation
Earliest:	June 15	LCME
Latest:	December 15	
Fee:	$100	**Degrees Granted**
AMCAS:	yes	MD, MD-PhD

Enrollment: 1996–97 First-Year Class

Men:	90	59%	Applied:	5307
Women:	62	41%	Interviewed:	1327
Minorities:	3	2%	Enrolled:	152
Out of State:	110	72%		

1996–97 Class Profile

Mean MCAT Scores		*Mean GPA*
Physical Sciences:	9.9	3.6
Biological Sciences:	10	
Verbal Reasoning:	9.8	

Tuition and Fees

Resident	25,200
Average (public)	9500
Average (private)	22,500
Nonresident	25,200
Average (public)	20,500
Average (private)	24,500

(in thousands of dollars)

Percentage receiving financial aid: n/av

Above data applies to 1995–96 academic year.

Introduction

St. Louis University, established by the Jesuits in 1818, was the first university chartered west of the Mississippi. The School of Medicine was opened in 1836. It is one of the university's 4 professional schools, the others being Business, Law, and Social Service. During the last half of the nineteenth century political developments forced the separation of the medical school from the university. Reintegration took place in 1963. It was at that time that many distinguished physicians also joined the faculty.

Admissions (AMCAS)

In addition to the basic premedical science courses, requirements include 1 year of English and 12 credits of humanities and behavioral science courses. Recommended courses include calculus, biochemistry, and physical chemistry. More than half of each class are nonresidents. *Transfer and advanced standing:* Applicants from accredited U.S. medical schools are considered for the second- and third-year classes.

Curriculum

4-year semitraditional. *Basic sciences:* First 2 years include the introductory and advanced basic sciences, with appropriate exposure to the clinical sciences. Elective time is available each year, as are correlative conferences. Courses are offered on human sexuality, nutrition, bioethics and medical communication skills, and death and dying. A multidisciplinary course is offered for neural sciences. *Clinical sciences:* Third year consists of clerkships in major clinical areas. Senior year is divided into required programs in clinical neuroscience and clinical floor service, ambulatory care, and 18 weeks of electives.

Grading and Promotion Policies

The system used is Honors/Pass/Fail. Overall achievement and the promise of students is taken into consideration in deciding promotion. Students must record a passing total score on Step 1 of the USMLE for promotion to the third year and on Step 2 for graduation.

Facilities

Teaching: The school occupies a full block and consists of a medical sciences building (Schwitalla Hall) from which E-shaped wings project. Clinical facilities consist of 4 hospitals: Firmin Desloge Hospital (367 beds), Cardinal Glennon Memorial Hospital for Children (190 beds), Saint Mary's Health Center (568 beds), the Anheuser Busch Eye Institute, and the Wohl Memorial Mental Health Institute (40 beds). Several other hospitals are affiliated with the school. *Other:* Laboratory facilities are available at the University Hospital and School of Medicine. *Library:* The Medical Center Library has a collection of 107,000 volumes and receives 1728 periodicals. *Housing:* A medical fraternity offers housing; other housing is available at Fusz Hall, the university's graduate residence facility.

Special Features

Minority admissions: The school offers a 1-year enrichment program in the medical morphological sciences. *Other degree programs:* Combined MD-PhD programs are available in the basic medical sciences and in molecular virology. A student may also receive the MD degree with distinction in research or distinction in community service.

University of Missouri—Columbia School of Medicine

One Hospital Drive
Columbia, Missouri   65212

Phone: 573-882-2923   *Fax:* 573-884-4808
E-mail: shari-I-swindella@muccmail.missouri.edu
WWW: http://www.miaims.missouri.edu/index.html

Application Filing		Accreditation
Earliest:	June 1	LCME
Latest:	November 1	
Fee:	n/av	**Degrees Granted**
AMCAS:	yes	MD, MD-PhD, MD-MS

Enrollment: 1996–97 First-Year Class

Men:	54	59%	Applied:	1123
Women:	38	41%	Interviewed:	281
Minorities:	5	5%	Enrolled:	92
Out of State:	1	1%		

1996–97 Class Profile

Mean MCAT Scores		*Mean GPA*
Physical Sciences:	9.8	3.6
Biological Sciences:	9.8	
Verbal Reasoning:	9.7	

Tuition and Fees

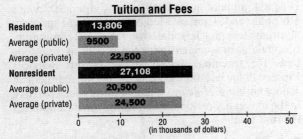

Resident	13,806
Average (public)	9500
Average (private)	22,500
Nonresident	27,108
Average (public)	20,500
Average (private)	24,500

(in thousands of dollars) 0 10 20 30 40 50

Percentage receiving financial aid: n/av

Introduction

The University of Missouri has 4 campuses: Columbia, Kansas City, Rolla, and St. Louis. The Columbia campus, the oldest and largest, is the site of the university's Columbia School of Medicine. This institution, established in 1872 as a 2-year medical school, expanded in 1956 into its present 4-year program. The University of Missouri Health Sciences Center includes the School of Medicine, University Hospital, VA Hospital, and other facilities.

Admissions (AMCAS)

In addition to the basic premedical science courses, mathematics and English composition are required. State residents are given very strong preference, especially those from small cities, towns, and rural areas. *Transfer and advanced standing:* Limited number admitted into third year. Applicants to the third year must post passing USMLE scores. Missouri residency is required for advanced standing positions.

Curriculum

4-year semimodern. *First and second years:* Preclinical training is in eight 10-week blocks, each block consisting of 8 weeks of instruction followed by a week of evaluation and a week of vacation. A 10-week summer vacation falls between blocks 4 and 5. Each learning block is comprised of 2 components—the Basic Science Backbone/Problem-based Learning (PBL) component and the Introduction to Patient Care (IPC) component. Using a clinical case format, the PBL component integrates the traditional basic sciences. Students work together to gather and organize information and then to generate and test hypotheses. In the IPC component, students explore a variety of content and skill-building experiences, including the physical exam skills, interviewing, health care/health policy, epidemiology, use of diagnostic tests and psychosocial aspects of medicine. Beginning in their first semester, students work with physician mentors and with standardized patients. Students also are assigned to a weekly clinic for an ambulatory care experience. *Third and fourth years:* The third year features six 8-week required clerkships in child health, family medicine, internal medicine, obstetrics and gynecology, psychiatry/neurology, and surgery. The fourth year has three 8-week required advanced clinical selectives from a medical area, a surgical area, and one other selective. Also required in the fourth year are 8-weeks of advanced biomedical sciences and 12 weeks of general electives.

Grading and Promotion Policies

The School of Medicine uses a multilevel grading system with Satisfactory/Unsatisfactory in the first year, Honors/Satisfactory/Unsatisfactory in the second year, and Honors/Letter of Commendation/Satisfactory/Unsatisfactory in the third and fourth years. Students must pass USMLE Step 1 prior to their fourth year and Step 2 to graduate.

Facilities

Teaching: The School of Medicine is located on the main, or Columbia, campus of the university and is part of the University Hospital and Clinics. Basic sciences are taught in the Medical Sciences Building; newly renovated student "labs" are rooms designed for PBL sessions, small-group discussions, and home-basic study rooms. Clinical teaching takes place at the University Hospital (495 beds), Mid-Missouri Mental Health Center (87 beds), the VA Hospital (480 beds), and other affiliated off-campus hospitals. *Other:* The Rusk Rehabilitation Center is part of the Health Sciences Center complex. *Library:* The Medical Library is located in the new Medical Annex and has more than 196,000 volumes. About 2000 periodicals are received regularly.

Special Features

Minority admissions: The school has an active program and offers special summer programs for high school and undergraduate minority students. *Other degree programs:* Combined MD-MS program, as well as MD-PhD in the basic sciences, is offered.

University of Missouri— Kansas City School of Medicine

2411 Holmes
Kansas City, Missouri 64108

Phone: 816-235-1870 *Fax:* 816-235-5277
WWW: http://www.hsc.missouri.edu/som/docs/
somadd.html

Application Filing		Accreditation	
Earliest:	August 1	LCME	
Latest:	November 15		
Fee:	$25	**Degrees Granted**	
AMCAS:	no	BA-MD, MD	

Enrollment: 1996–97 First-Year Class

Men:	38	38%	Applied:	871
Women:	61	62%	Interviewed:	375
Minorities:	11	11%	Enrolled:	99
Out of State:	72	73%		

1996–97 Class Profile

Mean MCAT Scores		*Mean GPA*
Physical Sciences:	n/av	n/av
Biological Sciences:	n/av	
Verbal Reasoning:	n/av	

Tuition and Fees

Resident	14,064
Average (public)	9500
Average (private)	22,500
Nonresident	28,448
Average (public)	20,500
Average (private)	24,500

0 10 20 30 40 50
(in thousands of dollars)

Percentage receiving financial aid: n/av

Introduction

In 1971 a combined 6-year undergraduate and graduate program of study was offered at the University of Missouri Kansas City School of Medicine for the first time; thus, rather than being patterned after the traditional program of 4 years of undergraduate study followed by 4 years of medical school, the program at this school is designed to accept high school graduates, who will spend 6 years and receive combined baccalaureate-medical degrees at the completion of their studies. The school is located on a 135-acre campus.

Admissions

Major emphasis of school is the combined 6-year BA-MD program for graduating high school seniors. Only limited number of places will be open for Missouri residents completing the usual premedical college pro-

gram. *For year 1:* High school students should have strong science background and take other courses that will prepare them for a medical school education that is community oriented. *For year 3:* Minimum of a baccalaureate degree is required. *Transfer and advanced standing:* Not applicable.

Curriculum

6-year modern. Program operates on a 48-week year and has the objective of preparing physicians committed to comprehensive health care. *Years 1 and 2:* These years comprise liberal arts and introductory medical courses. Emphasis is on team approach and courses integrate patient interviews and examinations with basic medical sciences, psychology, and sociology. *Years 3 through 6:* A clinical scholar is assigned for each small group of students and will act as their guide during the balance of study. Clinical sciences are taught in the affiliate hospitals, with a problem-centered approach. Student attains a specific set of clinical competencies as a precondition to attaining degree.

Grading and Promotion Policies

A Pass/Fail system is used, and obtaining a total passing score on Steps 1 and 2 of the USMLE is required for promotion and graduation, respectively.

Facilities

Teaching: A new medical school building has been completed. Clinical facilities include Children's Mercy Hospital, a major acute Psychiatric Center, St. Luke's Hospital, and Truman Medical Center, the primary adult care teaching hospital. *Other:* Several community hospitals are associated with the school and provide beds for teaching. *Library:* The Health Sciences Library is located on the second floor of the medical school building. *Housing:* Students are expected to live in the university residence hall on the main campus for the first year.

Special Features

Minority admissions: A Minority Recruitment Committee works to identify and recruit health science students early in their secondary schooling. *Other degree programs:* None.

Washington University School of Medicine

660 South Euclid Avenue
St. Louis, Missouri   63110

Phone: 314-362-6857   *Fax:* 314-362-4658
E-mail: wumscag@molly.wustl.edu
WWW: http://www.med.school.wutl.edu/admissions/

Application Filing		Accreditation	
Earliest:	June 1	LCME	
Latest:	November 15		
Fee:	$50	**Degrees Granted**	
AMCAS:	yes	MD, MD-PhD, MD-MA	

Enrollment: 1996–97 First-Year Class

Men:	62	51%	Applied:		6500
Women:	60	49%	Interviewed:		910
Minorities:	16	13%	Enrolled:		122
Out of State:	110	90%			

1996–97 Class Profile

Mean MCAT Scores		*Mean GPA*
Physical Sciences:	11.6	3.78
Biological Sciences:	11.6	
Verbal Reasoning:	10.9	

Tuition and Fees

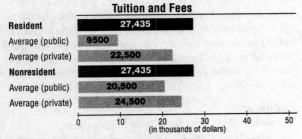

Resident	27,435
Average (public)	9500
Average (private)	22,500
Nonresident	27,435
Average (public)	20,500
Average (private)	24,500

0   10   20   30   40   50
(in thousands of dollars)

Percentage receiving financial aid: n/av

Introduction

The St. Louis Medical College was established as an independent school in 1842 and became the medical division of Washington University in 1891. In 1899 the Missouri Medical College became part of Washington University as well. The Medical Center is located on the eastern edge of Forrest Park in St. Louis and includes the School of Medicine and a number of teaching hospitals.

Admissions (AMCAS)

Required courses include the basic premedical sciences and differential and integral calculus. *Transfer and advanced standing:* Third-year class positions are available to well-qualified individuals enrolled in U.S. medical schools who have compelling personal reasons for transfer.

Curriculum

4-year modern. *First and second years:* (38 and 36 weeks, respectively) Devoted to basic medical sciences with preparatory courses for the clinical sciences included. *Third year:* (48 weeks) Clinical clerkships. *Fourth year:* (48 weeks) Students must complete 36 weeks of clinical electives or research.

Grading and Promotion Policies

A Pass/Fail grading system is used for the first year. Thereafter, the grades are Honors, High Pass, Pass, and Fail. In the third and fourth years, grades are accompanied by comments characterizing each student's performance. Promotions are made by committees on academic evaluation of students. Taking Steps 1 and 2 of the USMLE is recommended.

Facilities

Teaching: The 9-story McDonnell Medical Sciences Building contains lecture halls, teaching laboratories, research laboratories, and animal quarters. Local affiliated teaching hospitals were incorporated in 1962 to form the Washington University Medical Center, Barnes-Jewish, Children's, Barnard Hospitals and the Central Institute for the Deaf. Through a series of mergers that began in 1993, this system expanded to form the BJC Health System. It includes 39 hospital sites with 5262 beds and 6010 medical personnel, and is the first system in the nation to integrate an academic medical center with rural, suburban, and metropolitan-based health care facilities. The 10-story Clinical Sciences Research Building provides research facilities for 7 clinical departments. *Library:* The Library and Biomedical Communication Center is an 8-level structure that houses more than 450,000 volumes and subscribes to 3200 journals. The facility includes a computer teaching laboratory that links students to a large health information network. *Housing:* The Spencer T. Olin Residence Hall accommodates approximately 250 single men and women.

Special Features

Recruitment of underrepresented minority students is facilitated by the school's Associate Dean for Diversity Programs. *Other degree programs:* 5-year MA-MD program offering a year of research training, and 6-year combined MD-PhD program in various basic sciences including biology, biophysics, and genetics.

NEBRASKA

Creighton University School of Medicine

2500 California Plaza
Omaha, Nebraska 68178

Phone: 402-280-2798   *Fax:* 402-280-1241
E-mail: medschadm@creighton.edu
WWW: http://www.creighton.edu

Application Filing		Accreditation
Earliest:	June 1	LCME
Latest:	December 1	
Fee:	$65	**Degrees Granted**
AMCAS:	yes	MD, MD-PhD, MD-MS

Enrollment: 1996–97 First-Year Class

Men:	75	68%	Applied:	7735
Women:	36	32%	Interviewed:	387
Minorities:	10	9%	Enrolled:	111
Out of State:	88	79%		

1996–97 Class Profile

Mean MCAT Scores		*Mean GPA*
Physical Sciences:	9.1	3.65
Biological Sciences:	9.1	
Verbal Reasoning:	9.3	

Tuition and Fees

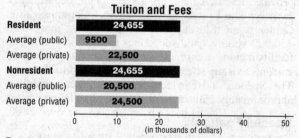

Resident	24,655
Average (public)	9500
Average (private)	22,500
Nonresident	24,655
Average (public)	20,500
Average (private)	24,500

0   10   20   30   40   50
(in thousands of dollars)

Percentage receiving financial aid: 85%

Introduction

Creighton University, a Jesuit institution, has 4 health science schools. The School of Medicine was established in 1892. Clinical instruction is carried out in several institutions.

Admissions (AMCAS)

The basic premedical science courses and 1 year of English are required. There are no restrictions on residence. *Transfer and advanced standing:* Possible to the second or third year for qualified applicants when spaces are available. Admission restricted to those who have either a Creighton University affiliation or a compelling reason to seek admission.

Curriculum

4-year semimodern. A new curriculum has been introduced, divided into 4 components. *Component one:*

The biomedical fundamentals serves as the foundation of the educational program. *Component two:* Comprised of more complex basic science information presented in a clinically relevant context consisting of a series of organ-based and disease-based courses. *Component three:* Consists of redesigned, required core clerkships emphasizing basic medical principles, primary care, and preventive medicine. *Component four:* Provides additional responsibilities for patient care. A 12-week block of critical care medicine and the 24 weeks of electives provide subinternship experience. At least 4 weeks of an implied, in-depth basic science experience is also part of this component. Clinical experience is a prominent part of the curriculum in all components, beginning with the physical diagnosis instruction in the first year and with students assigned to longitudinal clinics throughout the curriculum. The curriculum also integrates ethical and societal issues into all 4 components. Instructional methodology utilizes case-based small-group sessions and computer-assisted instruction in all components.

Grading and Promotion Policies

This school uses a Satisfactory/Unsatisfactory/Honors Evaluation system. Students are evaluated individually against curriculum standards and are not ranked among their peers. An Unsatisfactory grade will not be accepted for graduation credit. Promotion to the next higher class depends upon a record of acceptable conduct and satisfactory completion of the entire year's work with a minimum of Satisfactory in each course. All students are required to pass Step 1 of the USMLE before promotion into the clinical years of the curriculum and to take Step 2 of the USMLE in their senior year. Successful completion is not required for promotion but is necessary for licensure to practice.

Facilities

Teaching: Basic medical sciences are taught in the Criss Medical Center. This 3-unit center houses the School of Medicine offices, research facilities, laboratories, lecture halls, extensive television teaching classrooms, and other facilities for Medicine. Saint Joseph Hospital is the principal site for Creighton medical instruction. Creighton students also participate in clinical instruction at Saint Joseph Center for Mental Health, Children's Hospital, Omaha Veterans Medical Center, Bergan Mercy Medical Center, and some clinical services at other area hospitals. *Library:* The library is part of the Creighton University Bioinformation Center. Over 200,000 volumes of print and nonprint material are available. Access is provided to many bibliographic databases such as MEDLINE, Micromedex, etc. *Housing:* Creighton University has limited space in the apartment-style Towers residence hall for families. The Department of Residence Life, 104 Swanson Hall, posts information on rentals in the area of campus. Arrangements are left to individual students.

Special Features

Minority admissions: The Office of Minority Affairs coordinates an active recruitment program.

University of Nebraska College of Medicine

600 South 42 Street
Omaha, Nebraska 68198

Phone: 402-559-6468   *Fax:* 402-559-6796
E-mail: jwagner@unme.edu
WWW: http://www.unmc.edu/

Application Filing		Accreditation	
Earliest:	June 1	LCME	
Latest:	November 15		
Fee:	$25	**Degrees Granted**	
AMCAS:	yes	MD, MD-PhD	

Enrollment: 1996–97 First-Year Class

Men:	67	54%	Applied:	1236	
Women:	56	46%	Interviewed:	420	
Minorities:	11	9%	Enrolled:	123	
Out of State:	2	2%			

1996–97 Class Profile

Mean MCAT Scores		*Mean GPA*
Physical Sciences:	9.2	3.62
Biological Sciences:	9.7	
Verbal Reasoning:	9.3	

Tuition and Fees

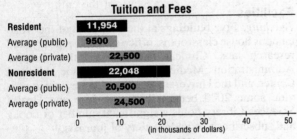

Resident	11,954
Average (public)	9500
Average (private)	22,500
Nonresident	22,048
Average (public)	20,500
Average (private)	24,500

(in thousands of dollars)

Percentage receiving financial aid: 62%

Introduction

The University of Nebraska College of Medicine was established in 1902 when Omaha Medical College joined the University of Nebraska. The latter was established in 1880. Currently, the University of Nebraska Medical Center includes the colleges of Medicine, Nursing, and Pharmacy, School of Allied Health Professions, University Hospital, and several other facilities. Omaha is located in the western part of the state and is its largest city.

Admissions (AMCAS)

The basic premedical science courses, introductory calculus or statistics, 4 courses in social sciences and humanities, and a course in writing are required. Few out-of-state residents are accepted. *Transfer and advanced standing:* No transfers from non-LCME-approved schools or from non-medical professional schools are accepted.

Curriculum

4-year semitraditional. *First year:* Introductory cores that present traditional basic sciences in an integrated manner emphasizing the "normal" state. An Integrated Clinical Experience introduces students to ethics, history and physical examination techniques, patient care in a longitudinal clinic, and the biopsychosocial model of health and disease. *Second year:* An introduction to "disease" processes through a systems approach to traditional basic sciences. The Integrated Clinical Experience continues to present issues involved in the doctor-patient relationship. *Third year:* Required clerkships in all major areas including a 2-month community preceptorship. Students participate in an outpatient specialty clinic in a continuation of the Integrated Clinical Experience. *Fourth year:* A 1-month required experience in surgery and 1 month required basic science elective provide advanced training. Basic science-clinical correlations are offered as part of the Integrated Clinical Experience. Seven months of clinical serves are required.

Grading and Promotion Policies

For class of 1997 and class of 1998, system used is letter grades and narrative comments from clerkship and elective directors. A student must obtain a C average in each of the first 2 years of medical curriculum and a C+ average in each of the clinical years to advance and/or graduate. For the class of 1999 and class of 2000, system used is Honors/High Pass/Pass/Marginal, and Fail. Students are limited to 5 years of enrollment to complete the medical curriculum. Passage of USMLE Step 1 is required for the class of 1998 and beyond for promotion to the senior year. Taking Step 2 of the USMLE is optional.

Facilities

Teaching: Basic sciences are taught in 2 buildings—Wittson Hall and Eppley Institute. Clinical teaching takes place at University Hospital (364 beds). Nine other affiliated hospitals provide access to over 2800 additional beds for teaching purposes. *Library:* The McGoogan Library of Medicine is situated in Wittson Hall and houses more than 234,000 volumes and 2200 periodicals. *Housing:* Student Services has a listing of private off-campus housing available to students.

Special Features

Minority admissions: The school has an active recruitment program for disadvantaged and rural students. It also offers summer enrichment programs for college juniors and seniors, depending on availability of grant funds. *Other degree programs:* Combined MD-PhD programs available in all the basic sciences.

NEVADA

University of Nevada School of Medicine

Reno, Nevada 89557

Phone: 702-784-6063 *Fax:* 702-784-6194
E-mail: dagmar@scs.unr.edu
WWW: http://www.med.unt.edu/homepage/one/

Application Filing		Accreditation
Earliest:	June 1	LCME
Latest:	November 1	
Fee:	$45	**Degrees Granted**
AMCAS:	yes	MD, MD-PhD

Enrollment: 1996–97 First-Year Class

Men:	31	60%	Applied:	1222
Women:	21	40%	Interviewed:	196
Minorities:	3	5%	Enrolled:	52
Out of State:	5	10%		

1996–97 Class Profile

Mean MCAT Scores		*Mean GPA*
Physical Sciences:	8.7	3.6
Biological Sciences:	9.6	
Verbal Reasoning:	9.3	

Tuition and Fees

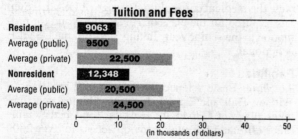

Resident	9063
Average (public)	9500
Average (private)	22,500
Nonresident	12,348
Average (public)	20,500
Average (private)	24,500

0 10 20 30 40 50
(in thousands of dollars)

Percentage receiving financial aid: 81%

Introduction

The University of Nevada School of Medicine is a community-oriented medical school that was founded in 1969. Supplementing university-based faculty, community physicians serve as teachers. The goal is to train physicians in primary care to be able to provide both rural health care delivery and treatment in an office or hospital setting. This school is one of a small group of community-based institutions.

Admissions (AMCAS)

In addition to the basic premedical science courses, 1 additional year of biology, and 2 behavioral science courses are required. There is no quota for out-of-state residents, but few are accepted into the second and third years. *Transfer and advanced standing:* Possible from U.S. schools only.

Curriculum

4-year semimodern. *First and second years:* The program is concentrated in the classroom and laboratories on the Reno campus. The curriculum emphasizes biomedical and behavioral sciences basic to medicine. Basic science disciplines are often integrated with each other and with clinical problems to facilitate meaningful understanding of major organ systems of the body. Students are encouraged to use this basic information to solve clinical problems. In addition to courses in anatomy, behavioral science, biochemistry, microbiology, pharmacology, physiology, pathology, and community health, students learn the basic physician skills of interviewing, obtaining a medical history, and performing a physical examination on patients. *Third and fourth years:* The curricula include experiences in community hospitals and physicians' offices in family medicine, internal medicine, obstetrics and gynecology, pediatrics, psychiatry, and surgery. These last 2 years concentrate on the common problems encountered by primary care physicians and are spent in Reno, Las Vegas, and rural Nevada; graduates will have a realistic understanding and interest in health problems of Nevada and will know what it is like to be a physician caring for Nevadans.

Grading and Promotion Policies

Letters and numbers are used in addition to a Pass/Fail system. Both steps of the USMLE must be taken.

Facilities

Teaching: Five buildings at the north end of the Reno campus house classrooms, office space, the library, and research labs. Clinical facilities are the Veterans Administration Medical Center, Washoe Medical Center, and the University Medical Center, which provide some 2000 beds. *Library:* A Life and Health Sciences Library holds a significant number of books and subscribes to a wide variety of journals.

Special Features

Minority admissions: Recruitment of minorities is coordinated by the Minority Student Affairs Office. *Other degree programs:* A combined MD-PhD program can be arranged in some disciplines.

NEW HAMPSHIRE

Dartmouth Medical School

7020 Remsen, RM 3006
Hanover, New Hampshire   03755

Phone: 603-650-1505   *Fax:* 603-650-1614
WWW: http://www.dartmouth.edu/ims/

Application Filing		Accreditation	
Earliest:	June 1	LCME	
Latest:	November 1		
Fee:	$55	**Degrees Granted**	
AMCAS:	yes	MD, MD-PhD, MD-MBA	

Enrollment: 1996–97 First-Year Class

Men:	40	47%	Applied:	7898
Women:	45	53%	Interviewed:	553
Minorities:	10	12%	Enrolled:	85
Out of State:	75	88%		

1996–97 Class Profile

Mean MCAT Scores		*Mean GPA*
Physical Sciences:	10	n/av
Biological Sciences:	10	
Verbal Reasoning:	10	

Tuition and Fees

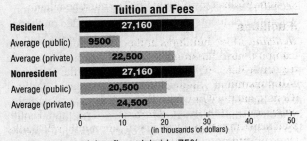

Resident	27,160
Average (public)	9500
Average (private)	22,500
Nonresident	27,160
Average (public)	20,500
Average (private)	24,500

(in thousands of dollars)

Percentage receiving financial aid: 75%

Introduction

Dartmouth Medical School, located in Hanover, New Hampshire, is the fourth oldest medical school in the United States. Founded in 1797, the school is a component of the Dartmouth Hitchcock Medical Center. The school is located on a 250-acre wooded site in a major winter resort area.

Admissions (AMCAS)

The basic premedical science courses and a course in calculus are required. There are no residence restrictions, but special consideration is given to applicants from New Hampshire and Maine. In addition to the 64 students accepted each year for the 4-year Dartmouth MD track, up to 20 students are accepted for a joint program with Brown, in which the first 2 years are spent at DMS and the last 2 at Brown. For this program, the MD is awarded by Brown. *Transfer and advanced standing:* Transfers are considered only when places are available; preference is given to students from other U.S. schools with compelling needs to be in Hanover.

Curriculum

4-year semimodern. The New Directions curriculum is designed to integrate the study of basic and clinical sciences throughout medical school while supporting close working relationships between students and the faculty. *First and second years:* The first and second years include the Longitudinal Clinical Experience, a course that pairs students with faculty practitioners in local communities and alternates with biweekly, small group tutorials on campus. The first year also emphasizes basic science courses. *Third year:* Clerkships in many disciplines are scheduled in three 16-week blocks of the third year. *Fourth year:* Fourth year students take advanced courses to complete a neurology clerkship, a subinternship, and an elective.

Grading and Promotion Policies

System used is Honors/ High Pass/Pass/Fail. Promotion is by vote of the faculty and no student will be promoted who has not passed all courses. Taking Steps 1 and 2 of the USMLE is optional.

Facilities

Teaching: Dartmouth Medical School, located on the campus of Dartmouth College, is a component of the Dartmouth-Hitchcock Medical Center (DHMC), a 429-bed facility dedicated to serving a patient population of over 1.5 million people. DHMC is home to one of the nation's 5 largest multi-specialty group practices. The Norris Cotton Cancer Center, one of only 28 comprehensive cancer centers designated by the National Cancer Institute; the Children's Hospital at Dartmouth, which includes a 30-bed intensive care nursery; the Community Health Center, a primary care facility that emphasizes preventive care; and the Borwell Research Building; home to Dartmouth's $55 million sponsored research program are prominent facilities of DHMC. The White River Junction (Vermont) Veterans Administration Hospital is a component of DHMC and a major teaching hospital. *Other:* The C. Everett Koop Institute at Dartmouth was founded in 1992 to facilitate reforms in medical education. Dr. Koop serves as the Institute's Senior Scholar. *Libraries:* Two libraries, containing 225,000 volumes in medicine and the life sciences and receiving 3000 current journals, offer a full range of traditional and electronic information services, including MEDLINE, CD-ROM databases, audiovisual resources, networked Macintosh and MS-DOS computers and peripherals, laser disc systems, and advanced workstations. *Housing:* College-owned apartments are available for married students. Most students live in off-campus housing.

Special Features

Minority admissions: The school actively encourages applications from qualified minority students. *Other degree programs:* Combined MD-PhD programs are offered in several disciplines. An MD-MBA program is offered in conjunction with Dartmouth's Amos Tuck School.

NEW JERSEY

New Jersey Medical School University of Medicine and Dentistry of New Jersey

185 South Orange Avenue
Newark, New Jersey   07103

Phone: 201-982-4631   *Fax:* 201-982-7986
WWW: http://www.njmsa.umdnj.edu/

Application Filing		Accreditation	
Earliest:	June 1	LCME	
Latest:	December 1		
Fee:	$125	**Degrees Granted**	
AMCAS:	yes	MD, MD-PhD, BA-MD	

Enrollment: 1996–97 First-Year Class

Men:	113	13%	Applied:	3957
Women:	57	34%	Interviewed:	673
Minorities:	22	13%	Enrolled:	170
Out of State:	13	8%		

1996–97 Class Profile

Mean MCAT Scores		*Mean GPA*
Physical Sciences:	10.1	3.4
Biological Sciences:	10.1	
Verbal Reasoning:	9.6	

Tuition and Fees

Resident	15,592
Average (public)	9500
Average (private)	22,500
Nonresident	23,779
Average (public)	20,500
Average (private)	24,500

(in thousands of dollars)

Percentage receiving financial aid: 75%

Introduction

As part of the University of Medicine and Dentistry of New Jersey, the New Jersey Medical School is located in Newark and was established in 1977. The University of Medicine and Dentistry of New Jersey also includes a second Medical School in Piscataway, a School of Osteopathic Medicine in Stratford, a Dental School in Newark, Graduate School for Biomedical Sciences in Newark, as well as a Health-Related Professional School and School of Nursing.

Admissions (AMCAS)

Minimum premedical science courses plus 1 elective in biology (excluding botany or invertebrate zoology) plus 1 year of English are required. A course in mathematics is recommended. *Transfer and advanced*

standing: Applications to the second and third-year classes from those in other medical schools will be considered.

Curriculum

4-year semitraditional. *First and second years:* Consists of basic science courses correlated with problem-based learning and clinical experiences. Part of the second year is devoted to an introduction to the clinical sciences, during which student receives instruction in history-taking and physical diagnosis. In addition, courses in preventive medicine and community health, psychiatry, and mental health are offered. *Third year:* The year is spent in rotations through all of the clinical departments. This is a closely supervised, hands-on, comprehensive endeavor through which the student acquires the basic knowledge and techniques of clinical medicine. Instruction is mainly in small groups and individual instruction. *Fourth year:* Senior is an active member of a group of individuals responsible for study and care of patients. This method provides the advantages of the apprentice system in scientifically supervised atmosphere. Twenty weeks of electives are available.

Grading and Promotion Policies

An Honors/High Pass/Pass/Fail system is used. Decisions on promotion are made by executive faculty on recommendation of a Promotions Committee. Decisions are based upon a comprehensive evaluation of accomplishments. A score must be recorded on Steps 1 and 2 of the USMLE and a passing grade on Step 1 is needed for graduation.

Facilities

Teaching: A new campus on a 58-acre site in Newark is the hub of a major medical educational complex, including the Biomedical Science Building, the University Hospital, and a library. *Other:* Clinical teaching facilities include University Hospital, East Orange; VA Hospital, Hackensack; University Medical Center; Morristown Memorial Hospital; Children's Hospital of New Jersey; Kessler Institute; and Bergen Pines Hospital. *Library:* Library of Medicine houses 70,000 volumes and 2000 periodicals. *Housing:* No facilities available on campus, but there are many rooms or apartments in the local area.

Special Features

Minority admissions: The school conducts an extensive recruitment program. Accepted minority students attend an 8-week summer pre-enrollment enrichment program. *Other degree programs:* Combined MD-PhD programs are offered in all the basic sciences and a 7-year BA-MD program with 7 undergraduate colleges.

Robert Wood Johnson Medical School
University of Medicine and Dentistry of New Jersey

675 Hoes Lane
Piscataway, New Jersey   08854

Phone: 908-235-4576   *Fax:* 908-235-5078
WWW: http://www2.umdnj.edu/rwjms.html

Application Filing		Accreditation	
Earliest:	June 1	LCME	
Latest:	December 1		
Fee:	$125	**Degrees Granted**	
AMCAS:	yes	MD, MD-PhD	

Enrollment: 1996–97 First-Year Class

Men:	87	63%	Applied:		3973
Women:	52	37%	Interviewed:		755
Minorities:	26	19%	Enrolled:		139
Out of State:	18	13%			

1996–97 Class Profile

Mean MCAT Scores		*Mean GPA*
Physical Sciences:	10	3.45
Biological Sciences:	10	
Verbal Reasoning:	9.1	

Tuition and Fees

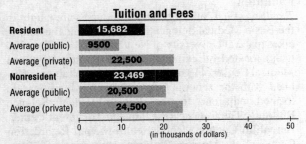

Resident	15,682
Average (public)	9500
Average (private)	22,500
Nonresident	23,469
Average (public)	20,500
Average (private)	24,500

(in thousands of dollars)

Percentage receiving financial aid: 78%

Introduction

Robert Wood Johnson Medical School has 2 campuses located in Camden and Piscataway. All students get their basic science education at the Piscataway campus. The school originally was known as Rutgers Medical School when it began in 1961 as a 2-year medical school. It became part of the University of Medicine and Dentistry in 1970. A major financial source of support was the president of the Johnson & Johnson Company, in whose honor the school was named.

Admissions (AMCAS)

The basic premedical science courses as well as 1 semester of mathematics and 1 year of English are required. Some nonresidents are accepted. In addition to the campus in Piscataway, the school has a division in Camden.

Separate applications are not required. Students who matriculate into this program receive their clinical education in Camden. *Transfer and advance standing:* Applicants to the third-year class are considered.

Curriculum

4-year. *Basic sciences:* Most basic science instruction is carried out in multidisciplinary teaching laboratories where a high degree of individualized attention is possible. Students are exposed to clinical problems from the outset and take some clinically oriented courses in the first 2 years. *Clinical years:* The third year consists of an 8-week rotation through the major specialties and family medicine and psychiatry. The fourth year consists of 12 weeks of electives as well as advanced clerkships in medicine, surgery, and neurology, and a 2-week course in clinical community and professional correlates and a subinternship in medicine, surgery, pediatrics, or family medicine. At the Camden campus the third- and fourth-year curriculum is identical to the one in central New Jersey.

Grading and Promotion Policies

System used is Honors/High Pass/Pass/Low Pass/Fail. A passing score on the USMLE Step 1 is required for promotion into the third year, and passage of Step 2 is required for graduation.

Facilities

Teaching: The Medical Science Complex in Piscataway includes the Medical Sciences Tower, Kessler Teaching Laboratories, Institute of Mental Health Sciences, Library of Science and Medicine, Center for Advanced Biotechnology and Medicine, and Environmental and Occupational Health Sciences Institute. Clinical teaching takes place at the Robert Wood Johnson University Hospital and other affiliated hospitals in central New Jersey. In Camden, clinical teaching takes place principally at the Cooper Hospital/University Medical Center. *Library:* The Rutgers University Library of Science and Medicine adjoins the Medical Science Complex in Piscataway, and clinical libraries are available in Camden and New Brunswick. *Housing:* Students are assisted in finding nearby housing.

Special Features

Minority admissions: The school has an active recruitment program and offers a 10-week summer enrichment program for incoming minority students. *Other degree programs:* Combined MD-PhD programs are offered in the basic medical sciences.

NEW MEXICO

University of New Mexico School of Medicine

Albuquerque, New Mexico   87131

Phone: 505-277-4766   *Fax:* 505-277-2755

Application Filing	Accreditation
Earliest: June 15	LCME
Latest: November 15	
Fee: $25	**Degrees Granted**
AMCAS: yes	MD, MD-PhD

Enrollment: 1996–97 First-Year Class

Men:	33	45%	Applied:	1165
Women:	40	55%	Interviewed:	303
Minorities:	29	40%	Enrolled:	73
Out of State:	3	4%		

1996–97 Class Profile

Mean MCAT Scores		*Mean GPA*
Physical Sciences:	9	3.54
Biological Sciences:	9	
Verbal Reasoning:	9	

Tuition and Fees

Resident	5363
Average (public)	$9500
Average (private)	$22,500
Nonresident	$15,350
Average (public)	$20,500
Average (private)	$24,500

0   10   20   30   40   50
(in thousands of dollars)

Percentage receiving financial aid: n/av

Introduction

In 1961 the School of Medicine at the University of New Mexico was established, and by 1966, it had become a 4-year program. The school is located on the north campus of the university and provides an opportunity for both professional and graduate education.

Admissions (AMCAS)

The basic premedical science courses are required. Recommended courses include calculus, biochemistry, and Spanish. Residents of New Mexico are given primary consideration for admission. Secondary consideration is given to residents of Alaska, Montana, and Wyoming. *Transfer and advanced standing:* Transfer is occasionally possible if places are available.

Curriculum

4-year modern. The current curriculum incorporates problem-based and student-centered learning, early mastery of clinical skills, peer teaching, and computer-assisted instruction. *Phase I:* In the first year and a half, the curriculum is organized around organ systems, each incorporating 3 perspectives—biologic, behavioral, and population. Hands-on medical skills are gained through weekly clinical skills and laboratory sessions. Students can utilize learning resources appropriate for individual needs, and participate in a 3-month, in-depth experience in a professional setting, in either a rural or urban community or a research laboratory. They also work on a research or creative project. *Phase II:* In the next year and a half, students will continue problem-based tutorial learning in both inpatient and ambulatory settings and reinforcement of basic and clinical science integration of basic science learning resources. Time will be spent with patients with and without prior diagnoses and on various inpatient services (pediatrics, family medicine, general surgery, internal medicine, neuropsychiatry, and obstetrics) in small group tutorials. *Phase III:* The fourth year will feature more hospital-based clinical experiences with progressive responsibility for patient care. Students will also be able to select clinical experiences that will assist them in making future specialty decisions. One month will be spent in a community preceptorship.

Grading and Promotion Policies

The school uses grades of Outstanding, Good, Satisfactory, Marginal, and Unsatisfactory. Step 1 of the USMLE must be passed for promotion into the third year and Step 2 must be taken to record a score.

Facilities

Teaching: First- and second-year courses are taught in the Basic Medical Science Building. Clinical teaching takes place at University of New Mexico Hospital (300 beds) located on campus, and the Regional Federal Medical Center (413 beds). Six other hospitals are affiliated with the school. *Other:* Research facilities are located adjacent to the Basic Medical Science Building. The Cancer Research and Treatment Center, Bernalillo County Mental Health-Mental Retardation Center, New Mexico Children's Psychiatric Center, Family Practice Center, and a variety of other institutions. Library: Students have use of the Medical Center Library as well as University Library. *Housing:* None is available on campus.

Special Features

Minority admissions: The school has active minority admissions program that encourages applications from Hispanic, Native American, and African-American residents of New Mexico. *Other degree programs:* A combined MD-PhD program is available.

Albany Medical College

47 New Scotland Avenue
Albany, New York   12208

Phone: 518-262-5521
WWW: http://www.albanyanesth.com/index.html

Application Filing		Accreditation	
Earliest:	June 1	LCME	
Latest:	November 15		
Fee:	$70	**Degrees Granted**	
AMCAS:	yes	MD, MD-PhD, BS-MD	

Enrollment: 1996–97 First-Year Class

Men:	61	46%	Applied:	9686	
Women:	71	54%	Interviewed:	775	
Minorities:	1	1%	Enrolled:	132	
Out of State:	86	65%			

1996–97 Class Profile

Mean MCAT Scores		*Mean GPA*
Physical Sciences:	9.8	3.5
Biological Sciences:	10.2	
Verbal Reasoning:	9.8	

Tuition and Fees

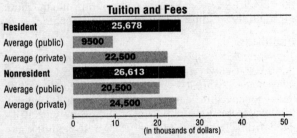

Resident	25,678
Average (public)	9500
Average (private)	22,500
Nonresident	26,613
Average (public)	20,500
Average (private)	24,500

(in thousands of dollars)

Percentage receiving financial aid: 80%

Introduction

This private medical school has been in existence since 1839. It is a coeducational and nondenominational school. In 1873 Albany Medical College joined with Union College and Albany Law School to form Union University. The Medical School is administratively linked with the Albany Medical Center Hospital. Albany, the state capital of New York, is readily accessible to New York City and Boston.

Admissions (AMCAS)

Applicants must have completed a minimum of 3 years of college work in an accredited college or university. Required courses include 1 year of general biology or zoology, inorganic chemistry, organic chemistry, and general physics. Applicants for first-year admission are also required to take the Medical College Admission Test and submit official scores. *Advanced standing:* Opportunities may exist for advanced standing admission to the second and third years.

Curriculum

4-year. The curriculum focuses students on the principles of comprehensive care, considering all aspects of patients' needs, including medical, preventive, palliative, and social support. The curriculum also emphasizes the pivotal role of the primary care physician while stressing the collaborative relationship between primary care physicians and specialists. The medical education process is seen as a 4-year continuum. The basic sciences are integrated within clinical medicine to emphasize the relevance of a scientific knowledge base to understanding, treating, and explaining symptoms and diseases. This effectively alters the process of medical education from memorization to that of reasoning and problem solving. *First year:* Basic science instruction is combined with clinical cases to focus on normal function. *Second year:* Focuses primarily on abnormal function and the disease state. *Third year:* Clinical clerkships offered emphasize ambulatory care in varied settings: rural, urban, managed care, and private practice. *Fourth year:* Required experiences are hospital based, preparing students for residency and practice. Additional elective time allows students to round out their education and further explore specific areas of interest. During both the third and fourth years, basic science material is revisited within the context of a student's clinical experience. Several other modules span the entire 4-year experience. Health Care and Society introduces students to the psychosocial, humanistic, ethical, and legal aspects of care. Comprehensive Care Case Study emphasizes primary care, systems of care, comparisons of care in different settings, issues related to the epidemiology of disease, prevention and wellness, geriatrics, AIDS, and substance abuse. This module focuses students' attention on the concept of health care delivered by a team rather than an individual. Clinical Skills Laboratory teaches interviewing and physical diagnostic skills, procedural skills, and laboratory medicine. All 4-year-long modules are correlated with the clinical and basic science issues that the students are learning concurrently.

Grading and Promotion Policies

Students are graded on a modified Pass/Fail system. Grades assigned are Excellent, Good, Marginal, and Unsatisfactory. Distinguished performance is recognized by the grade of Excellent with Honors. Academic performance is reviewed periodically by a promotions committee, and students with an accumulation of Marginal or Unsatisfactory grades will be required to remedy their deficiencies before they are eligible for promotion. Students must take Steps 1 and 2 of the USMLE as candidates and record scores.

Facilities

Teaching: The Albany Medical College is located in the state's capital among private, federal, and state-operated health care and research facilities. The school consists of a 7-floor Medical Education Building and a 5-story Medical Research Building, which together provide teaching facilities, research laboratories, faculty and administrative offices, clinic areas, a bookstore, student lounge, and library. The Albany Medical College and the Albany Medical Center Hospital are physically joined in 1 large complex. The hospital provides comprehensive diagnostic procedures and medical care for nearly 2,000,000 inhabitants of 24 counties of eastern New York and western New England. The 1674-bed Albany Medical Center Hospital, the nearby 1489-bed Veterans Administration Medical Center, and other affiliated hospitals in the Capital District and surrounding area provide excellent facilities for clinical instruction. *Library:* The library possesses about 111,300 volumes, 1500 audiovisual programs (including computer programs), and receives 1250 medical periodicals on a regular basis. *Housing:* A residence hall accommodating 168 single students is located within easy walking distance.

Special Features

Minority admissions: The school conducts an active minority recruitment program. A Minority Affairs Office provides academic, social, and cultural support services for enrolled students. *Other degree programs:* Joint programs with 3 undergraduate schools at Rensselaer Polytechnic Institute and Union College enable qualified students to earn both BS and MD degrees in 7 calendar years. It is also possible for individuals desiring to be trained as medical scientists, making research and academic medicine a career, to develop individualized programs leading to both MD and PhD degrees. A program of this type usually takes 6 years to complete.

Albert Einstein College of Medicine of Yeshiva University

1300 Morris Park Avenue
Bronx, New York   10461

Phone: 718-430-2106   *Fax:* 718-430-8825
E-mail: admissions@aecom.yu.edu
WWW: http://www.aecom.yu.edu/

Application Filing		**Accreditation**
Earliest:	June 1	LCME
Latest:	November 1	
Fee:	$75	**Degrees Granted**
AMCAS:	yes	MD, MD-PhD

Enrollment: 1996–97 First-Year Class

Men:	99	56%	Applied:	9536
Women:	79	44%	Interviewed:	1526
Minorities:	14	8%	Enrolled:	178
Out of State:	93	52%		

1996–97 Class Profile

Mean MCAT Scores		*Mean GPA*
Physical Sciences:	10.9	3.4
Biological Sciences:	10.9	
Verbal Reasoning:	10	

Tuition and Fees

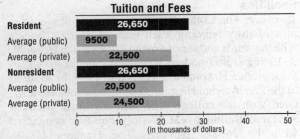

Resident	26,650
Average (public)	9500
Average (private)	22,500
Nonresident	26,650
Average (public)	20,500
Average (private)	24,500

(in thousands of dollars)

Percentage receiving financial aid: 70%

Introduction

A part of Yeshiva University, Albert Einstein College of Medicine was established in 1955. It is a privately endowed coeducational institution. Affiliated with the school are 2 postgraduate divisions, the Sue Goldberg Graduate Division of Medical Sciences and the Belfer Institute for Advance Biomedical Studies, making the school a major center for medical education, clinical care (through its affiliated hospitals), and biomedical research.

Admissions (AMCAS)

Required courses include the basic premedical sciences and 1 year of mathematics and English. Recommended courses are quantitative analysis, calculus, and biochemistry. *Transfer and advanced standing:* None.

Curriculum

4-year semimodern. *First year:* In addition to courses dealing with normal biological structures and function, there is an extensive introduction to clinical medicine course on early patient-centered experiences in clinical and small group settings. *Second year:* There is a major organ-system-based integrated course in pathophysiology and pathology, plus courses dealing with drug action and infectious diseases. The introduction to clinical medicine course continues, with increasing emphasis on the physical examination and physical diagnosis. *Third year:* There are clerkship rotations in all major disciplines, including family medicine and geriatrics and increasing emphasis on ambulatory care in non-hospital settings. *Fourth year:* This includes a subinternship and a rotation through ambulatory care. There is also a 6-month elective period. Many students opt to study abroad for all or part of their elective time, much of which is funded by international fellowships.

Grading and Promotion Policies

Grades are Honors, Pass, and Fail. Narrative evaluations do not appear on transcripts but are part of the permanent record of the student and are used in preparation of school recommendations. In order that students be promoted to clerkships, they must have passed all courses in the Preclinical Core Program. Passing total test scores on Steps 1 and 2 of the USMLE must be recorded prior to graduation.

Facilities

Teaching: The school is located in the Westchester Heights section of the Bronx. Facilities for teaching include computer workstations and laboratories equipped with audiovisual hardware. Clinical teaching is carried out at the Beth Israel Medical Center, Bronx Municipal Hospital Center, Montefiore Medical Center, Bronx-Lebanon Hospital Center, North Central Bronx Hospital, and Long Island Jewish Medical Center. In all, Einstein cares for 2 million people. *Other:* Ullmann Research Center is a 12-story building that houses research in the basic biological sciences. *Library:* Gottesman Library houses more than 180,000 volumes and 2400 periodicals. *Housing:* The college operates 2 apartment complexes that provide apartments for single as well as married students. A modern, fully equipped athletic center with a swimming pool is located on campus.

Special Features

Minority admissions: The college's director of the Office of Minority Student Affairs is in charge of minority student recruitment. A 2-week prematriculation summer preparatory course is offered to students with relatively weak science backgrounds. *Other degree programs:* For those interested in the combined MD-PhD, there is a Medical Scientist Training Program, which is available in all the basic science disciplines.

Columbia University College of Physicians and Surgeons

630 West 168th Street
New York, New York   10032

Phone: 212-305-3595
E-mail: pt8@columbia.edu
WWW: http://www.cpmchet.columbia.edu/dept/ps

Application Filing		Accreditation
Earliest:	June 15	LCME
Latest:	October 15	
Fee:	$65	**Degrees Granted**
AMCAS:	yes	MD, MD-PhD, MD-MPH

Enrollment: 1996–97 First-Year Class

Men:	81	54%	Applied:	4195
Women:	68	46%	Interviewed:	1426
Minorities:	15	10%	Enrolled:	149
Out of State:	118	79%		

1996–97 Class Profile

Mean MCAT Scores		*Mean GPA*
Physical Sciences:	11	3.5
Biological Sciences:	11	
Verbal Reasoning:	11	

Tuition and Fees

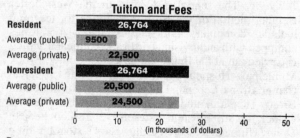

Resident	26,764
Average (public)	9500
Average (private)	22,500
Nonresident	26,764
Average (public)	20,500
Average (private)	24,500

(in thousands of dollars)

Percentage receiving financial aid: 66%

Introduction

Columbia University was established in 1754 and by 1767 it had its own medical instructors. Originally known as King's College, the school's name was changed to Columbia University in the City of New York in 1912. In 1814 the medical faculty of Columbia College merged with the College of Physicians and Surgeons. The Columbia-Presbyterian Medical Center was opened in 1928. Seven years later a permanent alliance was established with the university, and the college is now part of the Columbia-Presbyterian Medical Center, incorporating the Medical School, a Dental School, Presbyterian Hospital, and its subdivisions.

Admissions

Requirements include the basic premedical science courses plus 1 other course in chemistry and 1 year of English. The college welcomes applications from candidates in all geographical areas. *Transfer and advanced standing:* Transfer students from colleges in the United States or Canada are considered. Relatively few candidates whose previous education was not obtained in this country or in Canada are admitted to an entering class or with advanced standing.

Curriculum

4-year semitraditional. *First year:* Basic science courses with frequent correlation clinics through which basic science material may be related to medical problems. An introduction to medical practice course is also offered. *Second year:* One semester of advanced basic science course with the addition of interdepartmental courses in abnormal human biology and an introduction to the evaluation of patients and their problems. *Third year:* Consists of a rotation in or clerkships in the clinical discipline. *Fourth year:* Clinical and basic science electives. An elective in medicine in the tropics is available to fourth-year students who serve for 3 months in hospitals in South America, Africa, or Asia. An elective in the ambulatory care area is required.

Grading and Promotion Policies

The system used is Honors/Pass/Fail. Students may be advanced to the next academic year or be allowed to repeat a year only upon the recommendation of the faculty members under whom they studied during the previous year.

Facilities

Teaching: The College of Physicians and Surgeons is in a 17-story building, each floor of which connects with the wards and service of the Presbyterian Hospital. A 10-story ultramodern hospital located adjacent to Presbyterian Hospital was opened in 1989. In addition to the Presbyterian Hospital, 7 other hospitals are affiliated with the college. The William Black Medical Research Building is a 20-story building connected with the college building. The Hammer Health Sciences Center contains multidisciplinary teaching laboratories, classrooms, and research laboratories and the Psychiatric Institute is housed in a new research building. Other facilities include a Clinical Cancer Center and a General Clinical Research Center. *Library:* The medical library occupies the first 4 floors of the Hammer Health Sciences Center. In addition to its large collection of books and periodicals, the library contains extensive and comfortable areas for study. *Housing:* Bard Hall is the residence for men and women, and there are a limited number of apartments for married students available at Bard Haven.

Special Features

Minority admissions: The school has designated its Office of Special Projects to coordinate its minority recruitment program. This office offers a 6-week summer MCAT preparation course. *Other degree programs:* Hospital residencies for the training of specialists and continuing education courses offer medical training beyond the MD degree. Combined MD-PhD programs are available in a variety of disciplines. An MD-MPH program is also available.

Cornell University Medical College

445 East 69th Street
New York, New York 10021

Phone: 212-746-1067
WWW: http://www.med.cornell.edu/

Application Filing		Accreditation	
Earliest:	June 1	LCME	
Latest:	October 15		
Fee:	$65	**Degrees Granted**	
AMCAS:	yes	MD, MD-PhD	

Enrollment: 1996–97 First-Year Class

Men:	51	50%	Applied:	7429	
Women:	50	50%	Interviewed:	1189	
Minorities:	12	12%	Enrolled:	101	
Out of State:	40	40%			

1996–97 Class Profile

Mean MCAT Scores		*Mean GPA*
Physical Sciences:	10.6	3.55
Biological Sciences:	10.6	
Verbal Reasoning:	10	

Tuition and Fees

Resident	22,925
Average (public)	9500
Average (private)	22,500
Nonresident	22,925
Average (public)	20,500
Average (private)	24,500

(in thousands of dollars) 0 10 20 30 40 50

Percentage receiving financial aid: 65%

Above data applies to 1995–96 academic year.

Introduction

The Cornell University Medical College was established in 1898 and is situated on the upper east side of New York City. Although the university is located in Ithaca, New York, the medical school was established in New York City to provide students with clinical experience and laboratory-oriented instruction. An academic medical center was established that affiliated Cornell Medical School with New York Hospital. With the relocation, both these components became part of a common campus—the New York Hospital-Cornell Medical Center.

Admissions (AMCAS)

A solid background in science is important. Required courses include the basic premedical science courses and 1 year of English. Calculus is strongly recommended. *Transfer and advanced standing:* When vacancies occur, students are considered for admission to the second or third year. Candidates must furnish evidence of satisfactorily completed work and must present a letter of current good standing from their U.S.-accredited school.

Curriculum

4-year. Instruction is conducted in small groups whenever possible, using seminars, clinical tutorials, and special projects; interdisciplinary teaching is emphasized. Electives begin in the first year. *First year:* Introductory basic sciences and introductory medicine, which includes basic elements of interviewing technique, and sociological and emotional aspects of disease. Clinical conferences are presented to illustrate application of basic sciences to clinical medicine. *Second year:* Advanced basic sciences and physical diagnosis, psychiatry, ethics, and public health. Attendance in a weekly clinicopathologic conference is required for second-year students. *Third year:* Initial 4 weeks devoted to an introductory course to the clinical year and radiology, 48 weeks devoted to clerkship rotations through major clinical specialties as well as neurology and public health. *Fourth year:* 32 weeks made up of four 4-week selectives and four 4-week electives. The program for each individual is decided on in consultation with an advisor. However, it must include a required advanced clinical clerkship and ambulatory care experience. Three other short courses must be selected from a variety of offerings. Each student has a faculty advisor, who throughout the 4 years provides counseling and guidance.

Grading and Promotion Policies

Performance is graded by an Honors/Pass/Fail system, supplemented by detailed faculty evaluations. Taking the USMLE is optional.

Facilities

Teaching: Basic sciences are taught in a series of joined buildings. Clinical instruction is carried on in New York Hospital; Memorial Sloan-Kettering Cancer Center; the Hospital for Special Surgery; Lenox Hill Hospital; New York Hospital—Queens Medical Center, and Burke Rehabilitation Center in White Plains, New York. *Library:* The library for the school houses more than 125,000 volumes and 1700 periodicals. *Housing:* Housing owned by Cornell is available for both single and married students in the immediate vicinity of the Medical Center.

Special Features

Minority admissions: The school makes a nationwide effort to enroll qualified minority group students. It conducts a research fellowship program for minority college premedical students who have completed their junior year. *Other degree programs:* The school offers a fully funded combined MD-PhD program, which is coordinated with the Rockefeller University, Memorial Sloan-Kettering Cancer Center, and the Cornell University Graduate School of Medical Sciences.

Mount Sinai School of Medicine of the City University of New York

One Gustave L. Levy Place
New York, New York   10029

Phone: 212-241-6696   *Fax:* 212-369-6013
WWW: http://www.mssm.edu/

Application Filing		Accreditation
Earliest:	June 15	LCME
Latest:	November 1	
Fee:	$100	**Degrees Granted**
AMCAS:	yes	MD, MD-PhD

Enrollment: 1996–97 First-Year Class

Men:	55	50%	Applied:	5344
Women:	55	50%	Interviewed:	534
Minorities:	18	16%	Enrolled:	110
Out of State:	52	47%		

1996–97 Class Profile

Mean MCAT Scores		*Mean GPA*
Physical Sciences:	10.5	3.58
Biological Sciences:	10.4	
Verbal Reasoning:	9.7	

Tuition and Fees

Resident	21,825
Average (public)	9500
Average (private)	22,500
Nonresident	21,825
Average (public)	20,500
Average (private)	24,500

(in thousands of dollars)

Percentage receiving financial aid: 76%

Introduction

The Mount Sinai School of Medicine is an integral part of the Mount Sinai Medical Center, which was established in 1852. It is a privately endowed coeducational institution. The Medical Center is a 22-building complex containing a major teaching hospital, numerous laboratories, and a Postgraduate School of Medicine and Biological Sciences.

Admissions (AMCAS)

Requirements include the basic premedical science courses and 1 year each of English and mathematics. Recommended courses are psychology, embryology, comparative anatomy and/or physical chemistry, and advanced organic chemistry. *Transfer and advanced standing:* Students from domestic and foreign schools are considered for second- and third-year classes when vacancies occur.

Curriculum

4-year semimodern. *First year:* Basic sciences are scheduled in block times and take up the first two-thirds of the year. Remainder of time is devoted to integrated study of 2 organ systems—the neurosciences and the musculoskeletal. Some time is allotted to biostatistics; a total of 300 hours of elective and free time are included. *Second year:* Greater portion of year is devoted to continued integrated study of organ systems. Courses include human ecology, growth and development, and disease processes. In this period, 300 hours of elective and free time are provided for study at all institutions affiliated with school as well as off-campus study. Up to 200 hours are devoted to the interdepartmental course introduction to medicine, which is begun in the first year and carries through the second year. *Third and fourth years:* Devoted primarily to rotation through series of required clerkships in clinical specialties. Student is given 23 weeks of elective time during which he/she may continue with additional clinical studies or engage in lab work.

Grading and Promotion Policies

During the first 2 years, grades of Pass or Fail are given. In the clinical years, students receive Honors, Pass, or Fail grades. Students are evaluated for promotion by a promotions committee. Passing Steps 1 and 2 of the USMLE is required.

Facilities

Teaching: The school is part of Mount Sinai Medical Center in upper Manhattan. The basic science departments and nearly all clinical departments have teaching and office facilities in the 31-story Annenberg Building. Clinical teaching is done at Mount Sinai Hospital (1200 beds) and at 4 off-campus hospitals. *Other:* Nathan Cummings Science Building provides facilities for a variety of educational programs. *Library:* The Levy Library occupies one and a half floors of the Annenberg Building. *Housing:* Apartments in buildings owned by the Medical Center are available for married students; single students are housed in a separate residence hall.

Special Features

Minority admissions: The school has an active recruitment program and offers a 2-month summer enrichment program for accepted students. *Other degree programs:* The school offers a 6-year Medical Scientist Training Program for combined MD-PhD degrees in a variety of disciplines including cellular and molecular pathology and human genetics.

New York Medical College

Valhalla, New York   10595

Phone: 914-993-4507   *Fax:* 914-993-4976
E-mail: webmaster@nymc.edu
WWW: http://www.nymc.edu/nymc.htm

Application Filing		Accreditation
Earliest:	June 1	LCME
Latest:	December 1	
Fee:	$75	**Degrees Granted**
AMCAS:	yes	MD, MD-PhD

Enrollment: 1996–97 First-Year Class

Men:	115	61%	Applied:	12,289
Women:	73	39%	Interviewed:	1352
Minorities:	21	11%	Enrolled:	188
Out of State:	146	78%		

1996–97 Class Profile

Mean MCAT Scores		*Mean GPA*
Physical Sciences:	10.1	3.2
Biological Sciences:	10.4	
Verbal Reasoning:	9.7	

Tuition and Fees

	(in thousands of dollars)
Resident	25,615
Average (public)	9500
Average (private)	22,500
Nonresident	25,615
Average (public)	20,500
Average (private)	24,500

Percentage receiving financial aid: 84%

Above data applies to 1995–96 academic year.

Introduction

The state of New York chartered New York Medical College in 1860. It was originally located in New York City, but later moved to Westchester County. A relationship with the Archdiocese of New York was established in 1978, thus expanding the college's medical association with Catholic hospitals throughout the area. The institution was founded as the New York Homeopathic Medical College. In 1918 New York Medical College accepted students from the all-female New York Medical College for Women, which had closed, thereby becoming the first medical school to admit women.

In 1889 Flower Free Surgical Hospital was constructed as a place for hospital training. In 1938 the college and Flower Hospital merged with the Fifth Avenue Hospital and assumed the name New York Medical College. The Graduate School of Medical Sciences was founded in 1963.

Admissions (AMCAS)

Requirements include the basic premedical science courses and 1 year of English. Residence is not a factor in the admissions decision. *Transfer and advanced standing:* Transfer is possible in special instances from U.S. or Canadian schools to the second- or third-year class. Foreign transfers may apply to the third-year class.

Curriculum

4-year semitraditional. Classes will be held for 9 months of the year, with the last 3 months allotted for vacation. *Preclinical:* Basic medical sciences for first 2 years. Subjects are presented by lectures and conferences supplemented by laboratory exercises and demonstrations. In addition, lectures in the areas of immunology, clinical genetics, and behavioral sciences are presented. The lab-centered programs move in a gradual transition toward patient-centered program of clinical science. *Clinical:* Case method of instruction is used. Students are rotated as clerks in major clinical specialties. They also gain experience in management of geriatric and chronic diseases. Elective clinical or laboratory courses give seniors opportunities for advanced instruction in subspecialties and other areas. Opportunities for research also exist.

Grading and Promotion Policies

An Honors/Pass/Fail system is used. Students who pass all courses in a given year are recommended for promotion. Students who have failed courses may have to do remedial work, repeat a year, or be subject to dismissal. Students must take both steps of the USMLE and record scores.

Facilities

Teaching: The preclinical program is taught in the Basic Sciences Building at Valhalla in Westchester County. The clinical program utilizes facilities of 35 hospitals in New York, in the counties of Westchester, Rockland, and Ulster, and in Fairfield County in Connecticut. *Other:* The Mental Retardation Institute and the Institute of Environmental Sciences are affiliated. *Library:* The library occupies space in the Medical College Building at Westchester Medical Center and houses about 100,000 volumes and subscribes to 1500 periodicals. *Housing:* Arrangements for renting 1- and 2-bedroom garden apartments are possible for all students.

Special Features

Minority admissions: Highly motivated students from educationally deprived backgrounds are encouraged to apply. A pre-entrance summer program providing an intensive review of the basic sciences is available to such students. *Other degree programs:* The Graduate School offers combined MD-PhD programs in the basic medical sciences.

New York University School of Medicine

550 First Avenue
New York, New York   10016

Phone: 212-263-5290   *Fax:* 212-725-2140
WWW: http://www.med.nyu.edu/homepage.html

Application Filing		Accreditation
Earliest:	August 15	LCME
Latest:	December 1	
Fee:	$75	**Degrees Granted**
AMCAS:	no	MD, MD-PhD

Enrollment: 1996–97 First-Year Class

Men:	105	65%	Applied:	4840
Women:	57	35%	Interviewed:	871
Minorities:	58	36%	Enrolled:	162
Out of State:	87	54%		

1996–97 Class Profile

Mean MCAT Scores		*Mean GPA*
Physical Sciences:	11	3.5
Biological Sciences:	11	
Verbal Reasoning:	11	

Tuition and Fees

Resident	24,620
Average (public)	9500
Average (private)	22,500
Nonresident	24,620
Average (public)	20,500
Average (private)	24,500

(in thousands of dollars)

Percentage receiving financial aid: n/av%

Introduction

New York University, a nondenominational private institution was established in 1831; the School of Medicine was founded in 1841. The Bellevue Hospital Medical College, established in 1861, merged in 1898 with New York University to form the University and Bellevue Hospital Medical College, which became New York University College of Medicine in 1935. The present name was adopted in 1960. The School of Medicine boasts a host of distinguished alumni including Walter Reed, William Gorgas, Jonas Salk, and Albert Sabin.

Admissions

Requirements include the minimum premedical science courses and 1 year of English. Recommended are biochemistry, genetics, and embryology. *Transfer and advanced standing:* Not available.

Curriculum

4-year traditional. Basic sciences are introduced with interdepartmental correlations. *First year:* Concerned with the normal pattern of cellular and organ dynamics. An introduction to the physiologic and pathologic basis of human disease is provided that sets the stage for principles of clinical science and psychiatry. *Second year:* Devoted to general and organ pathology and neurological sciences. Continuation of the introduction to clinical science is correlated closely with studies in special pathology. Advanced basic sciences and principles of physical diagnosis provide the basis for clinical clerkships. *Third year:* Clinical clerkships in the major areas of medicine. *Fourth year:* A subinternship in a clinical area of interest for 6 weeks. An elective program of approved research or clinical studies at the school, at another U.S. school, or at a school abroad makes up the balance of the year.

Grading and Promotion Policies

A Pass/Fail system is used in the basic sciences and a letter or number in required clinical sciences. Advancement from 1 year to the next is made by a Faculty Committee that can approve advancement or require the student to repeat. Taking Steps 1 and 2 of the USMLE is optional.

Facilities

Teaching: The School of Medicine is located adjacent to the East River, between 30th and 34th Streets in Manhattan. The preclinical program is carried out in the Medical Science Building. Clinical teaching facilities are provided by the University Hospital (622 beds), Bellevue Hospital (3000 beds), and New York Veterans Hospital (1218 beds). *Other:* The off-campus Goldwater Memorial Hospital (1250 beds) is also affiliated. *Library:* The library houses more than 100,000 volumes and 1600 periodicals. In addition, the Institute of Environmental Medicine at Sterling Forest offers another reference library. *Housing:* Residence halls on campus provide single rooms or shared apartments for all students.

Special Features

Minority admissions: The school has an active recruitment program. *Other degree programs:* The school offers the Medical Scientist Training Program for an MD-PhD in all basic science disciplines.

SUNY Health Science Center at Brooklyn College of Medicine

450 Clarkson Avenue
Brooklyn, New York   11203

Phone: 718-270-2446
E-mail: imontano@netmail.hscbklyn.edu
WWW: http://www.hscbklyn.edu/

Application Filing		Accreditation	
Earliest:	June 1	LCME	
Latest:	December 15		
Fee:	$65	**Degrees Granted**	
AMCAS:	yes	MD, MD-PhD	

Enrollment: 1996–97 First-Year Class

Men:	108	58%	Applied:	5000
Women:	77	42%	Interviewed:	800
Minorities:	26	14%	Enrolled:	185
Out of State:	1	1%		

1996–97 Class Profile

Mean MCAT Scores		*Mean GPA*
Physical Sciences:	10	n/av
Biological Sciences:	10	
Verbal Reasoning:	9	

Tuition and Fees

Resident	11,060
Average (public)	9500
Average (private)	22,500
Nonresident	22,160
Average (public)	20,500
Average (private)	24,500

(in thousands of dollars)

Percentage receiving financial aid: n/av

Introduction

In 1860 the Long Island College Hospital became the Health Science Center at Brooklyn. It subsequently was called the Downstate Medical Center because of its role as a major provider of health care in the downstate New York region. It is located on a 13-acre urban campus in Brooklyn. The medical school is now part of SUNY Health Science Center of Brooklyn, which also includes colleges of Nursing, Health-Related Professions, School of Graduate Studies, and University Hospital.

Admissions (AMCAS)

In addition to the basic premedical sciences, requirements include 1 year of English. One mathematics course and courses in biochemistry and anatomy are recommended. Admissions preference is given to New York State residents. *Transfer and advanced standing:*

Students are considered for admission to the third-year class. Those wishing to transfer must take Step 1 of the USMLE.

Curriculum

4-year semitraditional. *First and second years:* Cover the basic medical sciences and include free half-days throughout the first 2 years for electives, correlation clinics in the second year to show relationships of basic sciences to clinical work, and introduction to patients during second-year Problem-Based Learning (PBL) Track. Second-year curriculum organized into organ system approach. *Third year:* Clerkship rotation in the major clinical specialties. *Fourth year:* Individualized selective programs making available a variety of courses and clinical experiences.

Grading and Promotion Policies

A High Pass/Conditional/Honors/Pass/Fail system is used; the USMLE Step 1 is required for promotion to third year.

Facilities

Teaching: The Health Science Education Building houses state-of-the-art classrooms, laboratories, an auditorium, and 2 floors of study carrels. Clinical teaching takes place at University Hospital (350 beds), Kings County Hospital (1234 beds), and several other affiliated institutions. *Other:* Facilities for research are located in the Basic Sciences Building. *Library:* The Medical Research Library, one of the largest medical school libraries in the country, occupies 3 floors of the Health Science Education Building. The Bibliographic Retrieval Service has 150 data bases. *Housing:* Two 11-story residence halls provide housing for both single and married students.

Special Features

Minority admissions: The school has an active recruitment program aimed at the Northeast. It offers a summer enrichment program for college sophomores and one for prematriculating students. *Other degree programs:* Combined MD-PhD programs are available in some of the basic sciences.

SUNY at Buffalo School of Medicine and Biomedical Sciences

Biomedical Education Building
Bailey Avenue
Buffalo, New York   14214

Phone: 716-829-3466   *Fax:* 716-829-2798
E-mail: jresso@ubmedc.buffalo.edu
WWW: http://www.wings.buffalo.edu

Application Filing		Accreditation
Earliest:	June 1	LCME
Latest:	November 1	
Fee:	$65	**Degrees Granted**
AMCAS:	yes	MD, MD-PhD

Enrollment: 1996–97 First-Year Class

Men:	71	53%	Applied:	3400
Women:	64	47%	Interviewed:	408
Minorities:	8	6%	Enrolled:	135
Out of State:	1	1%		

1996–97 Class Profile

Mean MCAT Scores		*Mean GPA*
Physical Sciences:	10	3.62
Biological Sciences:	10.2	
Verbal Reasoning:	9.3	

Tuition and Fees

Resident	11,190
Average (public)	9500
Average (private)	22,500
Nonresident	22,290
Average (public)	20,500
Average (private)	24,500

(in thousands of dollars)

Percentage receiving financial aid: n/av

Introduction

The School of Medicine and Biomedical Sciences of the State University of Buffalo was a private institution when it was established in 1846; it merged with the SUNY system in 1962. Instrumental in organizing the medical school was Millard Fillmore, the first chancellor, who later became the thirteenth president of the United States. The University of Buffalo has the most comprehensive campus in the SUNY system.

Admissions (AMCAS)

Requirements include the basic premedical science courses and 1 year of English. Only 1 semester of organic chemistry is required, although 1 year is recommended. Mathematics through calculus and quantitative and physical chemistry are also recommended.

High priority is given to residents of western New York as well as the entire state. Applications are accepted from children of alumni regardless of state of residence, but no preferential priority is accorded.

Curriculum

A comprehensive 4-year curriculum designed to prepare each graduate in the fundamentals of medicine. Patient experience is offered throughout the 4 years. A strong basic science course is combined with experience in preventive medicine and contemporary issues in medicine and health care. Research and preceptorship experiences are offered during the summer months between the first and second and the second and third years. Students may take as many as 4 elective experiences away from Buffalo.

Grading and Promotion Policies

An Honors/Pass/Fail system is used. A Promotion Committee reviews the progress of students at the end of each year and is responsible for recommendations based on all aspects of the student's work and departmental appraisals. Successful completion of Steps 1 and 2 of the USMLE is optional, but strongly encouraged.

Facilities

Teaching: The preclinical years are taught in totally modern facilities completed in 1986, which provide an environment conductive to informal experiences, small group teaching, and student enrichment. A modern computer-assisted learning laboratory, together with study carrels, is located in the school and the Health Science Library. The library is "world class" with a fine collection of textbooks and journals, an excellent reading room, and a history of medicine collection. Clinical teaching is coordinated in 9 hospitals located in Buffalo and the suburbs of Amherst, and at rural sites in the Buffalo area.

Special Features

Minority admissions: The school is committed to the educational preparation of students from minority or underrepresented population groups. *Other degree programs:* The medical school offers early-assurance guarantees to exceptional students at the end of the third semester of college. The school also offers an integrated 7-year MD-PhD program limited to a maximum of 4 students per year.

SUNY at Stony Brook School of Medicine

Health Sciences Center
Stony Brook, New York   11794

Phone: 516-444-2113   *Fax:* 516-444-2202
E–mail: admissions@dean.som.sunysb.edu
WWW: http://www.sunysb.edu/

Application Filing		Accreditation	
Earliest:	June 1	LCME	
Latest:	November 15		
Fee:	$65	**Degrees Granted**	
AMCAS:	yes	MD, MD-PhD	

Enrollment: 1996–97 First-Year Class

Men:	57	57%	Applied:	3982
Women:	43	43%	Interviewed:	836
Minorities:	13	13%	Enrolled:	100
Out of State:	8	8%		

1996–97 Class Profile

Mean MCAT Scores		*Mean GPA*
Physical Sciences:	n/av	n/av
Biological Sciences:	n/av	
Verbal Reasoning:	n/av	

Tuition and Fees

Resident	10,970
Average (public)	9500
Average (private)	22,500
Nonresident	22,070
Average (public)	20,500
Average (private)	24,500

(in thousands of dollars)

Percentage receiving financial aid: n/av

Above data applies to 1995–96 academic year.

Introduction

The School of Medicine opened in 1971 and is one of 5 professional schools, in addition to the hospital, that make up the Health Sciences Center at Stony Brook. Originating in 1957 as a small college in Oyster Bay, Long Island, with a mission to develop math and science teachers, the goal was dramatically altered by the State Board of Regents 3 years later. They mandated the establishment of a comprehensive research university, a goal that has been fulfilled. The school is located 60 miles east of Manhattan on Long Island's wooded north shore.

Admissions (AMCAS)

The basic premedical science courses are required. Few out-of-state residents are accepted. *Transfer and advanced standing:* Transfers to the third-year class are considered for students from other LCME-accredited schools.

Curriculum

4-year semimodern. The courses in the first 2 years are integrated by subject matter. *First year:* Courses include preventive medicine, the body, molecules, genes and cells, organ systems, introduction to clinical medicine I, basic cardiac life support, neuroscience, medicine in contemporary society, human behavior, and pathology. *Second year:* Interdepartmental courses in organ systems are taught in a multidisciplinary manner. In addition, introduction to clinical medicine, medicine in contemporary society, and courses in microbiology and pharmacology are also taught. *Third year:* Consists of clinical clerkships in medicine, surgery, pediatrics, psychiatry, obstetrics/gynecology, and primary care. *Fourth year:* Consists of 8½ months, of which 4 months are electives from a short list, and 4½ months are elective.

Grading and Promotion Policies

Honors/Pass/Fail system is used. The USLME Steps 1 and 2 are recommended but not required for promotion.

Facilities

Teaching: Clinical teaching takes place at the University Hospital (540 beds), Nassau County Medical Center (800 beds), Northport VA Hospital (480 beds), Winthrop University Hospital (533 beds), and other institutions. *Library:* The Health Science Library is located in the Health Science Center. Presently the collection totals about 130,000 volumes; periodicals received number about 2400. *Housing:* Residence halls are arranged in quadrangles, each having single and double rooms and 4- or 6-person suites.

Special Features

Minority admissions: SUNY Stony Brook encourages applications from members of groups that have historically been underrepresented in medicine. *Other degree programs:* The Medical Scientist Training Program (MSTP) is a fully funded MD-PhD program.

SUNY Health Science Center at Syracuse
College of Medicine

155 Elizabeth Blackwell Street
Syracuse, New York 13210

Phone: 315-464-4570   *Fax:* 315-464-8867
E-mail: compserve@vax.cs.hscsyr.edu
WWW: http://www.hscsyr.edu/

Application Filing		Accreditation	
Earliest:	June 15	LCME	
Latest:	December 1		
Fee:	$60	**Degrees Granted**	
AMCAS:	yes	MD, MD-PhD	

Enrollment: 1996–97 First-Year Class

Men:	90	60%	Applied:	3800
Women:	60	40%	Interviewed:	608
Minorities:	30	20%	Enrolled:	150
Out of State:	9	6%		

1996–97 Class Profile

Mean MCAT Scores		*Mean GPA*
Physical Sciences:	9	3.5
Biological Sciences:	9	
Verbal Reasoning:	9	

Tuition and Fees

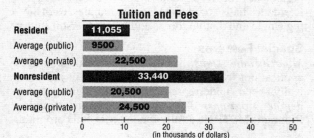

Resident	11,055
Average (public)	9500
Average (private)	22,500
Nonresident	33,440
Average (public)	20,500
Average (private)	24,500

(in thousands of dollars)

Percentage receiving financial aid: n/av

Introduction

The State University of New York College of Medicine at Syracuse can trace its origin to the establishment in 1834 of the General Medical School at the site of a small liberal arts college in Geneva, in upstate New York. This school, from which Elizabeth Blackwell, the first female physician, graduated, joined the newly formed Syracuse University in 1871. Expansion of the facilities took place in the 1930s and in 1950 the College of Medicine was transferred to the then newly organized State University of New York.

Admissions (AMCAS)

Required courses include 1 year of English. Preference will be given to New York State residents. Applications are accepted from U.S. citizens and from permanent residents who have completed at least 3 years of college study (90 semester hours) in the United States or Canada; applicants from foreign schools must complete at least 1 year of study at an accredited American or Canadian institution prior to application, and must demonstrate competency in English composition and expression. Preference also is given to applicants who have completed the required premedical science courses. Achieving excellence in the sciences is essential; however, academic work in the humanities and social sciences is equally important, as is experience in interacting with people.

Curriculum

4-year modern. The peculiarly human aspects of human biology are emphasized by encouraging students to think constructively about the comprehensive care of individuals and communities of people of all ages and socioeconomic backgrounds. *First year:* The first term is devoted to the study of gross anatomy, embryology, microscopic anatomy, and cell biology. The clinical applicability of anatomical information is demonstrated by presenting correlation conferences at regular intervals. Psychological effects of aging are studied at the cellular level. Neuroscience and biochemistry are presented in the second term. In the third term, students take genetics and physiology. *Second year:* Preventive medicine and behavioral sciences are offered concurrent with microbiology, pathology, and pharmacology. A large portion of the second year is devoted to an extended course in pathology, with which topics in microbiology and pharmacology are coordinated. Physical diagnosis or an introduction to clinical medicine is offered throughout the second year. This program is intended to prepare the student for clinical medicine and to integrate the basic sciences as they relate to problems in this area. Courses are also offered in nutrition and in endocrinology. *Third and fourth years:* The third and fourth years are considered a single unit. Every student is required to complete 50 weeks of clerkships and 26 weeks of electives. Forty-two weeks of required clerkship and 6 weeks of electives are included in the third year; 8 weeks of required time and 20 weeks of electives are included in the fourth year. Required courses are: medicine—12 weeks; general surgery—6 weeks; opthalmology, otorhinolaryngology, radiology, anesthesiology, and orthopedic surgery—6 weeks; psychiatry—6 weeks; obstetrics and gynecology—6 weeks; neuroscience—4 weeks; and preventive medicine and neurology—4 weeks.

Grading and Promotion Policies

The grading system used is Honors/Pass/Fail. Taking Steps 1 and 2 of the USMLE is required.

Facilities

Teaching: Facilities for instruction and research are in Weiskotten Hall, 766 Irving Avenue. Most of the hospital affiliates are adjacent to the basic science building at Weiskotten Hall. St. Joseph's Hospital Health

Center, Community General, and Van Duyn Home and Hospital are in other parts of Syracuse. *Other:* Affiliates are the State University Hospital (350 beds), U.S. Veteran's Administration Medical Center (379 beds), Crouse-Irving Memorial Hospital (490 beds), Community-General Hospital (350 beds), Richard H. Hutchings Psychiatric Center, and St. Joseph's Hospital and Health Center (472 beds). The Clinical Campus at Binghamton, a branch campus, offers clinical educational programs for the third and fourth years. Community health resources include the United Health Services, Our Lady of Lourdes Hospital, and the Robert Packer Hospital. The Clinical Campus program is designed to provide a quality education for medical students in their clinical years by developing a curriculum that defines attitudes and skills essential to every medical student regardless of subsequent career choice. The community orientation of the program fosters close working relationships with practicing physicians and other community professionals. Through emphasis on the "patient caring" function, the curriculum provides experiences in primary care and the ambulatory setting. *Library:* The library's collection numbers more than 130,000 volumes. About 2200 rare books, such as the library of the Geneva Medical College, early American medical imprints, and an archival collection containing numerous artifacts pertaining to the history of the Medical Center and of medicine in Syracuse, are included. The library also has access to 2 large online bibliographic services—Bibliographic Retrieval Services, Inc. (BRS) and the Online Services of the National Library of Medicine (NLM). *Housing:* Two modern 10-story residence halls on campus provide dormitory rooms, studios, and one-bedroom apartments for single and married students.

Special Features

Minority admissions: The college established Project 90, which includes a matriculation summer program and an extended curriculum, to increase opportunities for disadvantaged applicants. *Other degree programs:* Research is an important aspect of medical education at SUNY Health Science Center at Syracuse. Four common options are Academic Research Track, MD-PhD Program, Research Electives, and Summer Research.

University of Rochester School of Medicine

601 Elmwood Avenue
Rochester, New York   14642

Phone: 617-273-4539   *Fax:* 617-273-1016
E-mail: dadmish@urmc.rochester.edu
WWW: http://www.miner.lib.rochester.edu/

Application Filing		Accreditation	
Earliest:	June 15	LCME	
Latest:	October 15		
Fee:	$65	**Degrees Granted**	
AMCAS:	no	MD, MD-PhD, MD-MS	

Enrollment: 1996–97 First-Year Class

Men:	59	59%	Applied:	4088
Women:	41	41%	Interviewed:	654
Minorities:	11	11%	Enrolled:	100
Out of State:	65	65%		

1996–97 Class Profile

Mean MCAT Scores		*Mean GPA*
Physical Sciences:	10.4	3.54
Biological Sciences:	10.3	
Verbal Reasoning:	9.3	

Tuition and Fees

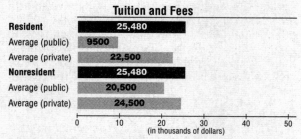

Resident	25,480
Average (public)	9500
Average (private)	22,500
Nonresident	25,480
Average (public)	20,500
Average (private)	24,500

(in thousands of dollars)

Percentage receiving financial aid: 87%

Introduction

The University of Rochester, founded in 1850, originated as a small liberal arts college for men and is now an independently supported, nonsectarian institution. The University of Rochester Medical Center consists of the School of Medicine and Dentistry, School of Nursing, and Strong Memorial Hospital. The School of Medicine and Dentistry was established in 1920.

Admissions

Required courses include the basic premedical sciences, 1 year of English, and courses in the humanities and/or social sciences. The MCAT is required. *Transfer and advanced standing:* Vacancies in the third-year class are open only to students enrolled in good standing in a U.S. or Canadian medical school, who have compelling personal reasons to be in Rochester.

Curriculum

4-year modern. *First year:* Courses deal with normal structure, function, and adaptation, arranged in 3 major blocks: Block I covers Gross Structure and Function. Block II covers Cell Structure and Function, and Block III covers Adaptive and Regulatory Mechanisms. Biopsychosocial medicine, medical humanities, ethics, and community medicine are covered. Students are introduced to the whole spectrum of human health and illness. *Second year:* Divided into a general and systems section. The general section covers genetics, pathology, pharmacology, and microbiology and immunology. The systems section is a multidisciplinary approach to 9 organ systems. Case studies and clinical correlations emphasize pathophysiology and an introduction to clinical medicine. Physical diagnosis is woven into these systems programs. Biopsychosocial medicine and the introduction to human health and illness course continue to run throughout the year. Electives are available. *Third year:* Encompasses a general clerkship followed by 6 clerkships rotating through the major clinical specialties. Electives are available. *Fourth year:* Required clerkships in emergency medicine, neurology, and surgical subspecialties. Ambulatory care and a 4-week block of case studies prepares students for residency experience in the evaluation and care of patients, and gives students additional experience in the application of laboratory medicine to clinical diagnosis and case management. Emphasis on evidence-based medicine characterizes the third and fourth year curriculum. Broad range of elective programs also is offered.

Grading and Promotion Policies

Pass/Fail at beginning of first year; Honors/Pass/Fail for remainder of preclinical years, 5-point grading system for the clinical years. The USMLE is not used in promotion decisions.

Facilities

Teaching: The school is situated on 60 acres adjacent to the undergraduate campus. The basic sciences are taught in the Medical Education Wing; clinical teaching takes place in Strong Memorial Hospital (720 beds), at 5 affiliated community hospitals, in a new Ambulatory Care Center, and in the offices of many practicing physician-teachers. *Other:* Research laboratory space for basic science departments is in the Medical Education Wing. *Library:* The Edward G. Miner Library houses more than 200,000 volumes and subscribes to 3000 periodicals. The historical collection contains about 10,000 rare books. *Housing:* 1 to 2 bedroom apartments are available near the Medical Center.

Special Features

Minority admissions: The Office of Ethnic and Multicultural Affairs coordinates an active recruitment program involving a Summer Research Fellowship Program for upper-level students. *Other degree programs:* A BA-MD program is offered. Combined degree programs are available for MD-MS and MD-PhD candidates. A MD-MPH combined degree program is available through Community and Preventive Medicine. MPH-MS programs are offered, and an MBA program is available in the Simon School of Business Administration. Community outreach programs, year-out research fellowships, and an active international medicine program are available. The school participates in the Medical Scientist Training Program.

NORTH CAROLINA

Bowman Gray School of Medicine
Wake Forest University
Winston-Salem, North Carolina   27157

Phone: 910-716-4264   *Fax:* 910-716-5807
E-mail: medadmit@bgsm.edu
WWW: http://www.is.bgms.edu

Application Filing		Accreditation	
Earliest:	June 1	LCME	
Latest:	November 1		
Fee:	$55	**Degrees Granted**	
AMCAS:	yes	MD, MD-PhD, MD-MBA	

Enrollment: 1996–97 First-Year Class

Men:	71	66%	Applied:	7884	
Women:	37	34%	Interviewed:	552	
Minorities:	11	10%	Enrolled:	108	
Out of State:	49	45%			

1996–97 Class Profile

Mean MCAT Scores		*Mean GPA*
Physical Sciences:	9.8	n/av
Biological Sciences:	9.9	
Verbal Reasoning:	10	

Tuition and Fees

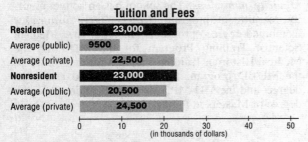

Resident	23,000
Average (public)	9500
Average (private)	22,500
Nonresident	23,000
Average (public)	20,500
Average (private)	24,500

0   10   20   30   40   50
(in thousands of dollars)

Percentage receiving financial aid: 85%

Introduction
In 1834 the Wake Forest Institute opened, and became a university in 1967. The Bowman Gray School of Medicine originally opened in 1902 as the Wake Forest Medical School. It was renamed the School of Medical Sciences in 1937 and operated as a 2-year medical school until 1941, when it was moved from Wake County to Winstom-Salem as a 4-year medical school in association with the North Carolina Baptist Hospitals, Inc. At this time, it was renamed the Bowman Gray School of Medicine of Wake Forest College in recognition of the benefactor who made the expansion possible.

Admissions (AMCAS)
The basic premedical courses are required. English and history are strongly recommended. Completion of 90 semester hours is necessary, but 120 are advised. A total of 108 students enter annually, with approximately half the class coming from North Carolina. Admission is without regard to race, creed, sex, religion, age, physical handicap, marital status, or national origin. *Transfer and*

advanced standing: Transfer to the second- or third-year classes is dependent upon vacancies.

Curriculum
4-year traditional and modern. *First year:* Morphology, including gross anatomy and histology, and biochemistry are taught in unit courses and correlated with clinical problems. Factors contributing to the doctor-patient relationship are stressed in behavioral sciences, ethics, and a course on patient interviewing. Physiology, aspects of community medicine, and neuroscience are also presented during the first year. *Second and third years:* Introduction to medicine, microbiology, an integrated course in physiology, pharmacology, and pathology; and clinical clerkships. *Fourth year:* Consists of eleven 4-week rotations: 2 in community medicine; 4 in basic clinical fields—medicine, surgery, pediatrics, or obstetrics-gynecology; and emergency medicine. The remainder are elective. Since 1987 part of the class is admitted to the Parallel Curriculum, which uses an integrated problem-based approach rather than the discipline-oriented approach of the traditional curriculum. Using the case-study method, small group tutorials led by faculty members address both basic and clinical sciences. Participation is voluntary, and the emphasis is upon independent, self-directed learning to develop sound clinical reasoning and problem-solving skills.

Grading and Promotion Policies
Grading is on a 0 to 4 scale. Students are provided with progress evaluations at the end of each course or rotation. The Promotion Committee meets regularly to evaluate student performance and make evaluations. Students must record total passing scores on Step 1 of the USMLE for promotion and on Step 2 for graduation.

Facilities
Teaching: Much of the basic science instruction takes place in the renovated James A. Gray Building and Hanes Research Building. The main teaching hospital is the North Carolina Baptist Hospital (806 beds). *Other:* Affiliated institutions include Forsyth Memorial Hospital (896 beds), the Kate Bitting Reynolds Health Center, and the Northwest Area Health Education Center. *Library:* The Coy C. Carpenter Library contains more than 126,000 volumes including approximately 2200 medical and scientific journals. It has on-line access to various computerized bibliographic services. *Housing:* The school maintains no housing facilities, but apartments and rooms are available in the surrounding residential area.

Special Features
Minority admissions: An active recruitment program is sponsored by the school through its Office of Minority Affairs. It provides a summer enrichment program for accepted students prior to matriculation. Also, there is a tuition-free post-baccalaureate program through Wake Forest University for students who have not achieved admission to medical school. *Other degree programs:* MD-MS in epidemiology, MD-MBA, and MD-PhD are offered.

Duke University School of Medicine

Box 3710, Medical Center
Durham, North Carolina   27710

Phone: 919-684-2985   *Fax:* 919-684-8893
E-mail: medadm@ mc.duke.edu
WWW: http://www.mc.duke.edu/depts/som

Application Filing		Accreditation	
Earliest:	June 15	LCME	
Latest:	October 15		
Fee:	$55	**Degrees Granted**	
AMCAS:	yes	MD, MD-PhD, MD-MPH	

Enrollment: 1996–97 First-Year Class

Men:	61	62%	Applied:	7181
Women:	38	38%	Interviewed:	670
Minorities:	14	14%	Enrolled:	99
Out of State:	61	62%		

1996–97 Class Profile

Mean MCAT Scores		*Mean GPA*
Physical Sciences:	12	n/av
Biological Sciences:	11	
Verbal Reasoning:	11	

Tuition and Fees

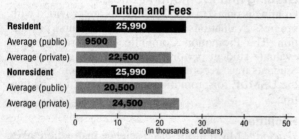

Resident	25,990
Average (public)	9500
Average (private)	22,500
Nonresident	25,990
Average (public)	20,500
Average (private)	24,500

0   10   20   30   40   50
(in thousands of dollars)

Percentage receiving financial aid: 76%

Introduction

The School of Medicine at Duke University was founded in 1930. The Medical Center, which includes the School of Medicine, the School of Nursing, and a hospital, is located on Duke's west campus. These health care facilities are all part of Duke University, an institution established in 1924 by James Buchanan Duke, industrialist and philanthropist. His original endowment served to transform Trinity College in Durham, North Carolina into Duke University.

Admissions (AMCAS)

Required courses include the basic premedical science courses, 1 year of calculus, and 1 year of English (consisting primarily of expository English composition). An introductory course in biochemistry is also helpful. Residence does not influence admissions decision. *Transfer and advanced standing:* None, except in unusual circumstances.

Curriculum

4-year modern. *First year:* Consists of 2 terms that are devoted to the introductory and advanced basic sciences. *Second year:* Consists of a 6-week introduction to clinical diagnosis course, followed by 6 blocks of 8 weeks in the major clinical disciplines. *Third and fourth years:* Made up of electives selected by student. Time is divided equally between basic sciences in the third year and clinical sciences in the fourth. There is a research requirement in the third year.

Grading and Promotion Policies

The Honors/Pass/Fail system is used. The USMLE is not required for promotion or graduation. Records of students are reviewed periodically by promotion committees consisting of course directors.

Facilities

Teaching: Preclinical teaching takes place in the Thomas D. Kinney Central Teaching Laboratory. Clinical instruction takes place at Duke Hospital (1008 beds), and at the Durham VA Hospital (489 beds). *Library:* The Medical Center Library houses more than 200,000 volumes and subscribes to 5000 periodicals. The Trent Collection includes books on the history of medicine, and is considered noteworthy for the Southeast. *Housing:* Off-campus housing is easily available and affordable.

Special Features

Minority admissions: The school has an active minority recruitment program. *Other degree programs:* Combined-degree programs include the Medical Scientist Training Program for the MD-PhD, the Medical Historian Training Program for the MD-PhD, the MD-JD program for a joint medical and legal degree, and the MD-MPH for a medical degree and a degree of Masters in Public Health.

East Carolina University School of Medicine

Greenville, North Carolina   27858

Phone: 919-816-2202   *Fax:* 919-816-3192
E-mail: webmstr@ecuvm.cis.ew.edu
WWW: http://www.med.ccu.edu/deptmenu.ktur

Application Filing		Accreditation
Earliest:	June 1	LCME
Latest:	November 15	
Fee:	$35	**Degrees Granted**
AMCAS:	yes	MD, MD-PhD

Enrollment: 1996–97 First-Year Class

Men:	36	50%	Applied:	1881
Women:	36	50%	Interviewed:	621
Minorities:	19	26%	Enrolled:	72
Out of State:	0	0%		

1996–97 Class Profile

Mean MCAT Scores		*Mean GPA*
Physical Sciences:	8.1	n/av
Biological Sciences:	8.4	
Verbal Reasoning:	8.6	

Tuition and Fees

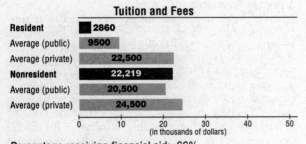

Resident	2860
Average (public)	9500
Average (private)	22,500
Nonresident	22,219
Average (public)	20,500
Average (private)	24,500

(in thousands of dollars)

Percentage receiving financial aid: 66%

Introduction

The School of Medicine at East Carolina University, located in the Health Sciences Center in Greenville, was founded in 1977. Educational facilities are located on a 100-acre Health Science Center Campus. The school has a 3-fold mission: training physicians for primary care, recruiting and educating minority students, and community service.

Admissions (AMCAS)

Only the basic premedical science courses and English are required. Strong preference for admission is given to qualified residents of North Carolina. *Transfer and advanced standing:* Applications for advanced standing are considered only if vacant positions exist, and such openings are infrequent.

Curriculum

4-year semitraditional. *First year:* In addition to the introductory basic sciences of anatomy, biochemistry, and physiology, courses in microbiology, genetics, psychosocial basis of medical practice, medical ethics, and a primary care preceptorship are offered. The 2-year clinical skills course begins early in the first semester. *Second year:* In addition to the advanced basic sciences of immunology, pathology, and pharmacology, courses are offered in substance abuse, human sexuality, clinical pathophysiology, pediatrics, and social issues in medicine. Primary care preceptorships and the clinical skills course continue throughout the second year. *Third year:* There are 6 major clinical rotations that last 8 weeks each, and together include at least 10 weeks of ambulatory experience. *Fourth year:* There are 36 weeks of clinical and basic science selectives. Of these, 2 months must be spent in primary care, and 1 month each in a surgical selective and an internal medicine selective.

Grading and Promotion Policies

Letter grades are used in evaluating students. Both steps of the USMLE must be taken and students must pass Part I prior to the start of the fourth year.

Facilities

Teaching: The Brody Medical Science Building contains lecture halls, classrooms, conference rooms, and well-equipped laboratories as well as an auditorium and library. The primary affiliated clinical teaching institution is the 725-bed Pitt County Memorial Hospital. *Other:* The Regional Cancer Center, Heart Center, Radiation Therapy Center, Eastern Carolina Family Practice Center, Biotechnology Building, Life Sciences Building, and various other clinical and technological facilities are all located on the medical school campus. *Library:* The Health Sciences Library has 300,000 volumes and receives more than 1800 periodicals. *Housing:* Ample private housing is available in the area.

Special Features

Minority admissions: An active recruitment program is coordinated by the Academic Support and Counseling Center (ASCC). *Other degree programs:* MD-PhD programs can be arranged on an individual basis.

University of North Carolina School of Medicine

Chapel Hill, North Carolina   27599

Phone: 919-962-8331
WWW: http://www.med.unc.edu/

Application Filing		Accreditation
Earliest:	June 1	LCME
Latest:	November 15	
Fee:	$55	**Degrees Granted**
AMCAS:	yes	MD, MD-PhD, MD-MS

Enrollment: 1996–97 First-Year Class

Men:	91	57%	Applied:	3420
Women:	69	43%	Interviewed:	855
Minorities:	38	24%	Enrolled:	160
Out of State:	17	11%		

1996–97 Class Profile

Mean MCAT Scores		*Mean GPA*
Physical Sciences:	9.1	n/av
Biological Sciences:	9.3	
Verbal Reasoning:	9.8	

Tuition and Fees

Resident	2680
Average (public)	9500
Average (private)	22,500
Nonresident	21,199
Average (public)	20,500
Average (private)	24,500

(in thousands of dollars) 0 10 20 30 40 50

Percentage receiving financial aid: 60%

Above data applies to 1995–96 academic year.

Introduction

Located on the Chapel Hill campus of the University of North Carolina, the School of Medicine was founded in 1879. It did not become a 4-year school until 1952. Adjacent to the School of Medicine on the university campus are: schools of Dentistry, Pharmacy, and Public Health. Clinical training is provided by several major, on-campus facilities, as well as health education centers located in community settings throughout the state.

Admissions (AMCAS)

The basic premedical courses plus 1 year of English are required. Recommended are advanced courses in chemistry, biology, and mathematics. A limited number of places may be available to nonresidents. *Transfer and advanced standing:* A very limited number of places are available for transfer to the third year. Students in good standing at accredited U.S. medical schools are considered.

Curriculum

4-year modern. The goals of the curriculum are to build problem-solving and communicative skills and to develop habits of self-assessment and continual learning that will remain with the physician throughout his/her professional life. *First year:* Consists of the introductory basic sciences and microbiology-virology, immunology, neurobiology, introduction to medicine, and social and cultural issues in medical practice, as well as a selective seminars program. *Second year:* Consists of several major courses: mechanisms of disease (includes 11 organ systems courses), pathology, pharmacology, epidemiology, psychiatry, and physical diagnosis, as well as selective seminars. *Third year:* Rotation through clerkship of major clinical specialties extending over 48-week period. *Fourth year:* A 4-week acting internship and a 4-week ambulatory care selective are 2 required selectives of the senior year. In addition, there are 24 weeks divided into 6 periods of electives. Opportunities for specialized clinical activities are offered as well as opportunities for in-depth study and investigation in special areas of interest to the student.

Grading and Promotion Policies

The system used is Honors/Pass/Fail. The Student Promotions Committee recommends promotion or dismissal to the dean.

Facilities

Teaching: The school is part of the medical center located on campus. Berryhill Basic Medical Sciences Building and preclinical Education Facilities Building provide facilities for the basic sciences. Clinical teaching takes place at the North Carolina Memorial Hospital (607 beds) and AHEC facilities throughout the state. The newest building is the 11-story Faculty Laboratory and Office Building. Affiliation for teaching purposes has been established with a number of community hospitals. *Other:* The Medical Sciences Research Building provides facilities for research. *Library:* The Health Sciences Library houses more than 202,000 volumes and 4000 periodicals. *Housing:* Residence halls are available on campus for single as well as some married students.

Special Features

Minority admissions: The school has an active recruitment program and sponsors an 8-week Medical Education Development program for minority college students. *Other degree programs:* Combined MD-PhD programs are available in a variety of disciplines including biomedical engineering, genetics, mathematics, neurobiology, and toxicology. MD-MS and MD-MPH programs are also offered.

NORTH DAKOTA

University of North Dakota School of Medicine

501 Columbia Road
Box 9037
Grand Forks, North Dakota   58203

Phone: 701-777-4221   *Fax:* 701-777-4942
E-mail: mmartin@mail.med.und.nodak.edu
WWW: http://www.med.und.nodak.edu/

Application Filing		Accreditation	
Earliest:	July 1	LCME	
Latest:	November 1		
Fee:	$35	**Degrees Granted**	
AMCAS:	no	MD, MD-PhD	

Enrollment: 1996–97 First-Year Class

Men:	32	56%	Applied:	370
Women:	25	44%	Interviewed:	155
Minorities:	11	19%	Enrolled:	57
Out of State:	12	21%		

1996–97 Class Profile

Mean MCAT Scores		*Mean GPA*
Physical Sciences:	8.8	3.56
Biological Sciences:	9	
Verbal Reasoning:	9.1	

Tuition and Fees

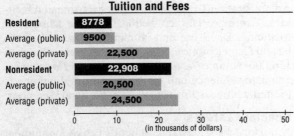

Resident	8778
Average (public)	9500
Average (private)	22,500
Nonresident	22,908
Average (public)	20,500
Average (private)	24,500

(in thousands of dollars) 0 10 20 30 40 50

Percentage receiving financial aid: 84%

Introduction

Established in 1884, the University of North Dakota includes 8 colleges. The School of Medicine at the University of North Dakota was opened in 1905. Until 1981, it offered only the first 2 years of medical education with arrangements made with other schools for the last 2 years of clinical training. The school emphasizes the training for providing primary care in a rural setting.

Admissions

The equivalent of 3 academic years or a minimum of 90 semester hours from an approved college is required for admission. Preference is given to applicants who have earned a bachelor's degree. Required coursework includes the basic premedical science courses and courses in college algebra, psychology or sociology, and English composition and literature. Students should be computer literate. The only out-of-state stu-

dents admitted in recent years are through the minority program INMED (Indians-into-Medicine), through the Professional Exchange Program of WICHE, or through the reciprocity agreement with the state of Minnesota.

Curriculum

4-year. The University of North Dakota School of Medicine is a university-based, community-integrated medical education program. A 5-phase curriculum is utilized and includes 3 transitional phases. *Phase I:* Occurs in Grand Forks and is a 2-week transition period from undergraduate study into medical school. *Phase II:* Also occurs on the Grand Forks campus over the next 2 academic years and includes basic and behavioral science courses as well as introductory clinical science courses. *Phase III:* A 3-week transition from the basic sciences to the clinical sciences. Occurs in rural communities throughout North Dakota. *Phase IV:* Encompasses the majority of the next 2 years and includes the third-year core clerkships of medicine, surgery, pediatrics, obstetrics and gynecology, and psychiatry and the fourth-year family medicine core clerkships, as well as 6 electives of 4 weeks' duration. *Phase V:* During this phase students return to their original Phase III site for a final 4-week transitional period geared to final preparation for beginning residency training.

Grading and Promotion Policies

The curriculum is criterion-referenced and evaluations are based on stated learning objectives. The minimum pass level is established at 75%. The grading system used is Honors/Satisfactory/Unsatisfactory. Honors are limited to 20% or fewer of the students enrolled in any specific course. Promotion from phase to phase and within a particular phase (such as, Phase II, Year 01 to Year 02) requires satisfactory completion of all courses, clerkships, and/or phase objectives.

Facilities

Teaching: The school is part of the North Dakota Medical Center. Courses in the first 2 years are taught in the Medical Sciences North buildings that contain classrooms, laboratories, administrative offices, and the library. Clinical teaching is coordinated through the 4 regional campuses in Bismarck, Fargo, Grand Forks, and Minot. *Other:* Community hospitals throughout the state are affiliated with the school as well as the VA Hospital in Fargo, the USAF Hospitals in Grand Forks and Minot, and the PHS Hospitals and Clinics that are part of the Indian Health Service. *Library:* The Health Sciences Library houses more than 50,000 volumes and about 1000 periodicals. Specialized biomedical research is conducted in the Edwin C. James Research Facility and the USDA Human Nutrition Research Center. *Housing:* A variety of on-campus housing is available.

Special Features

Minority admissions: The INMED (Indians-into-Medicine) program admits up to 7 fully qualified American Indian students to medical school each year. The Center for Rural Health serves both the school and rural communities throughout the state. *Other degree programs:* A combined MD-PhD program is offered.

OHIO

Case Western Reserve University School of Medicine

10900 Euclid Avenue
Cleveland, Ohio   44106

Phone: 216-368-3450   *Fax:* 216-368-4621
WWW: http://www.cwrv.edu/I/class/med

Application Filing		Accreditation	
Earliest:	June 1	LCME	
Latest:	October 15		
Fee:	$60	**Degrees Granted**	
AMCAS:	yes	MD, MD-PhD	

Enrollment: 1996–97 First-Year Class

Men:	77	56%	Applied:	7900
Women:	61	44%	Interviewed:	1185
Minorities:	25	18%	Enrolled:	138
Out of State:	55	40%		

1996–97 Class Profile

Mean MCAT Scores		*Mean GPA*
Physical Sciences:	10	3.5
Biological Sciences:	10	
Verbal Reasoning:	10	

Tuition and Fees

Resident	25,290
Average (public)	9500
Average (private)	22,500
Nonresident	25,290
Average (public)	20,500
Average (private)	24,500

0   10   20   30   40   50
(in thousands of dollars)

Percentage receiving financial aid: 77%

Introduction

Case Western Reserve University originated in 1967, when Western Reserve College and Case Institute of Technology combined to form the largest biomedical research institution in Ohio. The School of Medicine was established in 1943, when a medical department was added to Western Reserve College. In 1952 the school pioneered the introduction of a new innovative medical curriculum that was adopted by other institutions.

Admissions (AMCAS)

The basic premedical science courses and 1 year of English are required. More than half the places are filled by residents. Applicants from minority groups are encouraged. *Transfer and advanced standing:* Transfer students are not accepted routinely; each candidate is considered individually.

Curriculum

4-year modern. *First year:* Consists of instruction in subject areas of cell biology, differentiated cell, metabolism, biostatistics, cardiovascular-respiratory and renal systems, tissue injury, and mechanisms of infection. *Second year:* Consists of instruction in the organ systems as well as biometry and legal medicine. *Third year:* Consists of clerkship rotation through the major clinical specialties. *Fourth year:* Consists of neurosciences, surgical subspecialties, primary care, and 5 months of electives selected by the student.

Grading and Promotion Policies

Evaluation of a student is based on interim examinations, comprehensive examinations at the end of the year, and instructor's observations of performance in laboratory and clinical work. Grading is Pass/Fail in the basic sciences and Honors/Pass/Fail in the required clinical sciences. The Committee on Students determines whether or not it is desirable to refuse further registration to any student. Taking Step 1 of the USMLE is required. A passing total score must be obtained on Step 2 to graduate.

Facilities

Teaching: The school is located on the university campus about 5 miles east of the center of Cleveland. The Health Science Center is the site of teaching of the basic sciences. Clinical teaching is done at University Hospitals of Cleveland, Metro Health Medical Center, the Cleveland Veterans Administration Hospital, St. Luke's Hospital, and Mt. Sinai Hospital. *Other:* The Mather Memorial Building, the East Wing and Sears Administration Tower provide space for research facilities. *Library:* The collections of the schools of Medicine, Dentistry, and Nursing are located in the Health Center Library. The collection totals more than 150,000 volumes and 3000 periodicals. *Housing:* A graduate residence hall for single men and women is located within a 10-minute walk of the central campus.

Special Features

Minority admissions: The school's active recruitment program is conducted by its Office of Minority Student Affairs. A 6-week summer enrichment program is offered to incoming students. *Other degree programs:* Combined MD-PhD degree programs are offered in a variety of disciplines including biomedical engineering, developmental genetics and anatomy, molecular biology, pathology, pharmacology, physiology, and biophysics.

Medical College of Ohio

C.S. No. 10008
Toledo, Ohio   43699

Phone: 419-381-4229   *Fax:* 419-381-4005
WWW: http://www.mco.edu/

Application Filing		**Accreditation**
Earliest:	June 1	LCME
Latest:	November 1	
Fee:	$30	**Degrees Granted**
AMCAS:	yes	MD, MD-PhD

Enrollment: 1996–97 First-Year Class

Men:	84	62%	Applied:	4818
Women:	51	38%	Interviewed:	723
Minorities:	19	14%	Enrolled:	135
Out of State:	19	14%		

1996–97 Class Profile

Mean MCAT Scores		*Mean GPA*
Physical Sciences:	8.4	3.48
Biological Sciences:	8.7	
Verbal Reasoning:	9	

Tuition and Fees

Resident	9813
Average (public)	9500
Average (private)	22,500
Nonresident	13,242
Average (public)	20,500
Average (private)	24,500

(in thousands of dollars)

Percentage receiving financial aid: n/av

Above data applies to 1995–96 academic year.

Introduction

The Medical College of Ohio, which graduated its first class in 1972, is part of a health science center that includes a Graduate School, a School of Allied Health, and a School of Nursing. The Medical Center is located on a 475-acre campus in a residential/commercial area of south Toledo. The school serves as a center for medical education, community service, and research.

Admissions (AMCAS)

The basic premedical science courses and 1 year of English are required and additional courses in biology are recommended. Nonresidents with a superior background are considered for acceptance. *Transfer and advanced standing:* Ohio residents from LCME-accredited schools are considered.

Curriculum

4-year semitraditional. *First year:* In addition to the introductory basic sciences and behavioral sciences, 1 course titled introduction to clinical medicine is pre-

sented. *Second year:* Advanced basic sciences and continuation of freshman introductory clinical courses. *Third year:* Major clinical clerkships. *Fourth year:* Electives at university and non-university settings.

Grading and Promotion Policies

The system used is Honors/High Pass/Pass/Fail. Step 1 of the USMLE must be passed to be promoted and to graduate.

Facilities

Teaching: The basic sciences are taught in the Health Sciences Teaching and Laboratory Building and the Health Education Building. The primary teaching hospital is the Medical College of Ohio Hospital. *Other:* Associated hospitals in the city of Toledo participate in the undergraduate and residency training programs. The Eleanor Dana Center for Continuing Medical Education and the Child and Adolescent Psychiatric Hospital provide additional training facilities. *Library:* The Mulford Library contains a large collection of bound books and journals. *Housing:* None available.

Special Features

A special admissions program was established with Bowling Green State University and the University of Toledo. Ten students from each institution are accepted after the completion of their third undergraduate year. *Minority admissions:* The school has an active recruitment program directed by its Associate Dean of Minority Affairs. A 5-year curriculum is available for some minority and disadvantaged students. A 5-week summer prematriculation program is offered on an optional basis for all students. *Other degree programs:* Combined MD-PhD programs.

Northeastern Ohio Universities College of Medicine

4209 State Route 44
P.O. Box 95
Rootstown, Ohio   44272

Phone: 216-325-2511   *Fax:* 216-325-8372
E-mail: admission@nevocom.edu
WWW: http://www.neoucom.edu/

Application Filing	Accreditation
Earliest: June 1	LCME
Latest: November 1	
Fee: $30	**Degrees Granted**
AMCAS: yes	MD, MD-PhD

Enrollment: 1996–97 First-Year Class

Men:	14	56%	Applied:	1378
Women:	11	44%	Interviewed:	124
Minorities:	2	6%	Enrolled:	25
Out of State:	1	4%		

1996–97 Class Profile

Mean MCAT Scores		*Mean GPA*
Physical Sciences:	8.8	3.4
Biological Sciences:	9.1	
Verbal Reasoning:	9.4	

Tuition and Fees

Resident	10,416
Average (public)	9500
Average (private)	22,500
Nonresident	20,133
Average (public)	20,500
Average (private)	24,500

0   10   20   30   40   50
(in thousands of dollars)

Percentage receiving financial aid: 75%

Above data applies to 1995–96 academic year.

Introduction

The Northeastern Ohio University College of Medicine was established in 1973, and received full accreditation in 1981. The goal of the school is to train physicians to have knowledge of principles and practices of primary care in a community setting as well as the potential for specialization. Graduates receive a BS degree from the consortium university and an MD degree from the College of Medicine. The principal teaching site is in Rootstown on a 55-acre site in northeastern Ohio, located 35 miles southeast of Cleveland.

Admissions (AMCAS)

A BS-MD program is available to students entering directly from high school. The MD program is available to students who already have a premedical back-ground. For the MD program, the required courses are 1 year of organic chemistry and 1 year of physics at the college level. Recommended courses are biochemistry, calculus, embryology, physiology, microbiology, psychology, sociology, and statistics. Very strong preference is given to Ohio residents. *Transfer and advanced standing:* A small number of places are available for applicants entering the sophomore year of the MD (4-year) portion of the program based on attrition from the freshman year.

Curriculum

The first year of the medical curriculum covers the basic medical sciences; the second year is devoted to clinical correlation; the third year is the core clinical year; and the fourth year consists of electives and a primary care preceptorship.

Grading and Promotion Policies

The system used is Honors/Satisfactory/Conditional-Unsatisfactory/Unsatisfactory. Steps 1 and 2 of the USMLE must be taken and a total passing score recorded to be promoted into the clerkship years and to graduate.

Facilities

Teaching: The academic base consists of the University of Akron, Kent State University, and Youngstown State University, with the Basic Medical Sciences campus in Rootstown. Clinical facilities are utilized at 18 associated community hospitals in Akron, Canton, and Youngstown. *Library:* Located at the Basic Medical Sciences Center. *Housing:* Available for first- and second-year medical students on all 3 campuses.

Special Features

Minority admissions: Qualified minority and disadvantaged rural students are encouraged to apply. *Other degree programs:* Combined MD-PhD programs are offered in the basic sciences and in biomedical engineering.

Ohio State University College of Medicine

370 West Ninth Avenue
Columbus, Ohio   43210

Phone: 614-292-7137   *Fax:* 614-292-1544
E-mail: admiss-med@osu.edu
WWW: http://www.med.ohio-state.edu

Application Filing		Accreditation	
Earliest:	June 15	LCME	
Latest:	November 1		
Fee:	$30	**Degrees Granted**	
AMCAS:	yes	MD, MD-PhD, MD-MS	

Enrollment: 1996–97 First-Year Class

Men:	132	63%	Applied:	4607	
Women:	78	37%	Interviewed:	645	
Minorities:	17	8%	Enrolled:	210	
Out of State:	42	20%			

1996–97 Class Profile

Mean MCAT Scores		*Mean GPA*
Physical Sciences:	10.3	3.5
Biological Sciences:	10.3	
Verbal Reasoning:	10	

Tuition and Fees

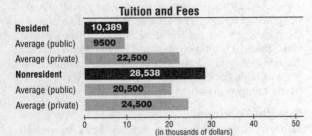

Resident	10,389
Average (public)	9500
Average (private)	22,500
Nonresident	28,538
Average (public)	20,500
Average (private)	24,500

(in thousands of dollars)

Percentage receiving financial aid: n/av

Introduction

Ohio State University consists of 5 campuses in Columbus, Lima, Mansfield, Marion, and Newark. The College of Medicine was founded in 1913 and has 19 different medical departments. It can trace its origin back to the Starling-Ohio Medical College of Columbus, which was absorbed into the present College of Medicine. The school is located on the south edge of the main university campus.

Admissions (AMCAS)

A baccalaureate degree is expected, but 3-year candidates are considered. Only the basic premedical science courses are required. Recommended courses include physical or analytical chemistry, cellular or molecular biology, genetics, comparative anatomy, modern physics, and advanced mathematics. *Transfer and advanced standing:* Transfer applicants are considered for entrance into the third year, from LCME-accredited, MD-granting institutions in the United States.

Curriculum

4-year. Body systems basic science presentation, independent study, problem-based learning, and lecture discussion, tracts for preclinical study. *First year:* Introduction to professional problems in service to the patient and community, along with the introductory basic sciences. *Second year:* Advanced basic sciences and patient-oriented interdisciplinary study of life processes by means of history taking, physical examinations, and diagnostic techniques, including a study of patients' diseases and treatment thereof. Disease mechanisms, correlation of abnormalities of structure and function with cardinal systems, and manifestations of disease. *Third and fourth years:* This segment begins with a 4-week introduction to clinical medicine and 6 required clerkships, including an 8-week clerkship in the major disciplines of medicine, surgery, pediatrics, psychiatry, and obstetrics-gynecology, and a primary care block of 4 weeks of family and general internal medicine. This is followed by 32 weeks of electives and selectives, allowing a 4-week vacation during these final months of medical school.

Grading and Promotion Policies

The nongrading system used is Pass/Fail. Faculty Appraisal Committee recommends promotions. Students must record a passing score on Step 1 of the USMLE in order to move on to required clerkships and a passing score on Step 2 to graduate.

Facilities

Teaching: The Nisonger Center for Mental Retardation is in McCampbell Hall. The Graves Hall and Hamilton Hall Medical Science buildings house the departments of anatomy, medical microbiology, pathology, pharmacology, physiological chemistry, and physiology. Starling Loving Hall houses the School of Public Health. University hospitals include Means Hall, Rhodes Hall, Wiseman Hall, Upham Hall, Dodd Hall, the Arthur James Cancer Research Hospital, and the Ambulatory Clinical Facility. *Other:* Nine hospitals in Columbus are affiliated for teaching, research, and patient care. A clinical Medical Sciences Educational Facility provides additional hospital support. Wiseman Hall provides laboratories for research. *Library:* The Health Sciences Library contains more than 200,000 books and bound journals and subscribes to more than 2200 periodicals. *Housing:* Campus and off-campus housing is available.

Special Features

Minority admissions: The college conducts an active minority recruitment program. It also offers a pre-entry summer enrichment program and a postbaccalaureate for underepresented minority students. *Other degree programs:* Combined MD-PhD programs. A Master of Science in Medical Science program is available. Applicants must have their MD degree and be concurrently pursuing training in an approved Ohio State clinical residency.

University of Cincinnati College of Medicine

P.O. Box 670552
Cincinnati, Ohio   45267

Phone: 513-558-7314   *Fax:* 513-558-1165
E-mail: clarice fooks@uc.edu
WWW: http://www.med.uc.eduu

Application Filing		Accreditation	
Earliest:	June 1	LCME	
Latest:	November 15		
Fee:	$25	**Degrees Granted**	
AMCAS:	yes	MD, MD-PhD	

Enrollment: 1996–97 First-Year Class

Men:	88	63%	Applied:	4787
Women:	63	42%	Interviewed:	622
Minorities:	23	15%	Enrolled:	151
Out of State:	25	17%		

1996–97 Class Profile

Mean MCAT Scores		*Mean GPA*
Physical Sciences:	9.7	3.45
Biological Sciences:	9.9	
Verbal Reasoning:	9.4	

Tuition and Fees

Resident	11,982
Average (public)	9500
Average (private)	22,500
Nonresident	26,043
Average (public)	20,500
Average (private)	24,500

(in thousands of dollars) 0 10 20 30 40 50

Percentage receiving financial aid: 78%

Introduction

The University of Cincinnati College of Medicine was established in 1819. It is part of the university's Medical Center, which also includes colleges of Pharmacy, Nursing, and Health. The school has introduced the innovative concept of early clinical exposure to medical students and was the first to establish a family medical residency program.

Admissions (AMCAS)

A minimum of 3 years at an accredited college is required. Baccalaureate degree is preferred, but not required. About 20% of each class are non-Ohio residents. The admission prerequisites are the basic premedical science courses and English. Applicants are expected to have a basic understanding of the social, cultural, and behavioral factors that influence individual's families and communities. *Transfer and advanced*

standing: Applicants are considered for second and third year positions. Students applying for the third year must take and pass the USMLE Step 1 in June to receive consideration. Acceptance is based on positions available in the class.

Curriculum

4-year. *First and second years:* Basic sciences, introduction to clinical practice I and II, and noncredit electives. *Third year:* Four 8-week clerkships (internal medicine, obstetrics/gynecology, pediatrics, and surgery); one 6-week clerkship (psychiatry); 4 weeks of family practice; 2 weeks of radiology; and 4 weeks of clinical specialty clerkships selected from a limited menu. *Fourth year:* 8-week acting internship in internal medicine, 4-week neuroscience selective, and 24 weeks of electives.

Grading and Promotion Policies

Grades of Honors, High Pass, Pass, Remediate, or Fail are used. Students must pass USMLE Step 1 before advancement to the third year. Students must pass the USMLE Step 2 before graduating.

Facilities

Teaching: The College of Medicine, housed in the Medical Sciences Building, is located in the center of the University of Cincinnati Medical Center (UCMC). The UCMC includes the Pharmacy and Nursing colleges, 2 research institutes, and a university hospital. *Other:* In close proximity are 6 associated teaching hospitals. *Library:* The Health Sciences Library is in the Medical Sciences Building, where 3 floors contain more than 125,000 volumes and 2800 current journals. *Housing:* A limited number of on-campus apartments are available for single and married students. A variety of off-campus housing is available.

Special Features

Minority admissions: The school actively recruits minority applicants on a state and national level. A 6-week summer prematriculation program is available for accepted applicants who are educationally disadvantaged. *Other degree programs:* A combined MD-PhD program is available in conjunction with any of the basic science departments.

Wright State University School of Medicine

P.O. Box 1751
Dayton, Ohio   45401

Phone: 513-873-2934   *Fax:* 513-873-3322
E-mail: speterson@desire.wright.edu
WWW: http://www.med.wright.edu/

Application Filing		Accreditation	
Earliest:	June 1	LCME	
Latest:	November 15		
Fee:	$30	**Degrees Granted**	
AMCAS:	yes	MD, MD-PhD	

Enrollment: 1996–97 First-Year Class

Men:	41	46%	Applied:	3582
Women:	49	54%	Interviewed:	430
Minorities:	19	21%	Enrolled:	90
Out of State:	15	17%		

1996–97 Class Profile

Mean MCAT Scores		*Mean GPA*
Physical Sciences:	n/av	n/av
Biological Sciences:	n/av	
Verbal Reasoning:	n/av	

Tuition and Fees

Resident	10,314
Average (public)	9500
Average (private)	22,500
Nonresident	14,862
Average (public)	20,500
Average (private)	24,500

0   10   20   30   40   50
(in thousands of dollars)

Percentage receiving financial aid: 85%

Introduction

Wright State University, located in Dayton, was founded in 1964; the School of Medicine was founded 10 years later. It is located on the main university campus in the city of Fairborn, a community within the metropolitan area of Dayton. The school's goal is to provide physicians with a strong foundation in primary care and comprehensive training in critical, acute, and chronic care as well as preventive medicine. A very substantial percentage of the school's graduates enter family medicine.

Admissions (AMCAS)

The basic premedical science courses are required. The school seeks students with diverse social, ethnic, and educational backgrounds. Secondary applications and letters of recommendation are requested upon receipt of the AMCAS application. Dedication to human concerns, communication skills, maturity, motivation, letters of recommendation, and academic qualifications are considered when reviewing applications. One-on-one interviews are by invitation only with Ohio residents receiving very strong preference. Women, minorities, and applicants from rural Ohio are particularly encouraged to apply. *Transfer and advance standing:* Students may transfer from LSMC — or AOA— accredited schools at the third year level. The number accepted depends upon space availability.

Curriculum

4-year modern. Major courses are designed to prepare students for lifelong learning and service in primary care fields. *Biennium I:* Students are taught in an interdisciplinary fashion using didactic teaching, large group lectures, small group discussions, computer-based instruction, and case-based/problem-based learning. Throughout the first 2 years, normal structure and functioning, behavioral sciences, health promotion, and disease prevention are integrated into the curriculum. Students are introduced to basic principles and mechanisms of disease in the spring of the first year. Instruction progresses through various organizational levels from molecular to organ systems. From the beginning of the freshman year, students acquire clinical skills through direct patient contact and interaction with clinical faculty preceptors. To provide additional opportunities for clinical exposure and enrichment, clinically based electives are offered as immersion experiences between academic periods in the first 2 years. Students rotate through 6 core clerkships during the third year. Individualized electives, mandatory clerkships, junior internships, and time for board study complete the fourth year.

Grading and Promotion Policies:

Information not available.

Facilities

Teaching: Educational programs are conducted in the Medical Sciences, Biological Sciences, and Health Sciences buildings on the main campus. Clinical instruction takes place in the 8 local affiliated teaching hospitals and institutions, in free-standing ambulatory health centers, and in physicians' offices. *Library:* The Fordham Health Sciences Library contains a large collection of books and journals, audiovisual and computer programs, access to on-line data base searching, quiet study areas, and after-hour study space.

Special Features

Minority Admissions: The school has a stated policy of providing educational opportunities to students from underrepresented minority groups. An Office of Minority Affairs is coordinated by an Assistant Dean for Minority Affairs. A 6-week prematriculation program, minority physician mentoring, big brother/big sister peer tutoring, board preparation courses, and assistance in development of critical thinking and learning are available. Resident and nonresident minority students are strongly encouraged to apply. *Other degree programs:* After matriculation students may apply for admission to the biomedical sciences PhD program.

OKLAHOMA

University of Oklahoma College of Medicine

P.O. Box 26901
Oklahoma City, Oklahoma   73190

Phone: 405-271-2331   *Fax:* 405-271-3032
E-mail: dotty-shaw@uokhsc.edu
WWW: http://www.online.vokhsc.edu/colleges/
medicine/

Application Filing		Accreditation	
Earliest:	June 1	LCME	
Latest:	October 15		
Fee:	$50	**Degrees Granted**	
AMCAS:	yes	MD	

Enrollment: 1996–97 First-Year Class

Men:	86	58%	Applied:	1701
Women:	63	42%	Interviewed:	374
Minorities:	25	17%	Enrolled:	149
Out of State:	17	11%		

1996–97 Class Profile

Mean MCAT Scores		*Mean GPA*
Physical Sciences:	8.8	3.57
Biological Sciences:	9	
Verbal Reasoning:	9.6	

Tuition and Fees

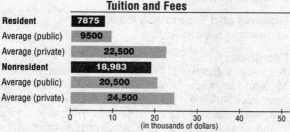

Resident	7875
Average (public)	9500
Average (private)	22,500
Nonresident	18,983
Average (public)	20,500
Average (private)	24,500

(in thousands of dollars)

Percentage receiving financial aid: 90%

Above data applies to 1995–96 academic year.

Introduction

Established in 1900 the University of Oklahoma College of Medicine combined with Epworth Medical College in 1910. The College of Medicine is one of 7 colleges belonging to the Health Sciences Center. The other schools are the colleges of Dentistry, Nursing, Pharmacy, Public Health, Allied Health, and the Graduate College. The College of Medicine offers programs in Oklahoma City and Tulsa. In Oklahoma City it is situated on the 200-acre Oklahoma Health Center.

Admissions (AMCAS)

Requirements include 3 semesters of English; 1 semester of general zoology; 1 semester (any one) of cell biol-

ogy, histology, embryology, genetics, or comparative anatomy; 3 semesters (any combination) of anthropology, psychology, sociology, philosophy, humanities, or foreign language; 2 semesters of physics; 2 semesters of general chemistry; and 2 semesters of organic chemistry. Strong preference is given to residents. Nonresidents can make up no more than 15% of each class. *Transfer and advanced standing:* Applicants from other medical schools may be admitted with advanced standing. Priority is given to those completing 2 years of study at an accredited medical college.

Curriculum

4-year. *First and second years:* Each of these years is 36 weeks. The program provides an integrated overview of the basic sciences and is accented by clinical correlation demonstrations. Patient contact begins in the first year in a wide variety of settings, including physicians' private offices. Interdepartmental courses in clinical medicine are offered. *Third and fourth years:* These make up a 23-month continuum, which is subdivided into 1-month blocks. Eight months in the third year are devoted to required clerkships in major clinical specialties; 5 months in the fourth year are devoted to required internships in major clinical specialties. Five months must be utilized for elective coursework.

Grading and Promotion Policies

The letter grading system is used. All courses must be completed with a grade of C or better (D or better in courses of fewer than 30 clock hours). The promotions committee is responsible for reviewing the academic performance of all students and for making recommendations to the dean regarding promotions, probation, or remedial work. Steps 1 and 2 of the USMLE must be taken to record a score.

Facilities

Teaching: The college is located on the university's Oklahoma City and Tulsa campuses. Basic sciences are taught in Oklahoma City. Clinical teaching takes place at 5 hospitals and numerous clinics located on campus and at 14 affiliated hospitals. In the beginning of the third year, 25% of the class may transfer to the Tulsa campus. *Library:* The Health Sciences Library in Oklahoma City contains more than 156,000 books, journals, and audiovisual material. *Housing:* There are no university-operated housing facilities on either campus.

Special Features

Minority admissions: The university seeks to identify and recruit underrepresented minorities, and applicants from this group or candidates with a disadvantaged background are encouraged to apply. *Other degree programs:* There is an opportunity for Honors Research.

OREGON

Oregon Health Sciences University School of Medicine

3181 S. W. Sam Jackson Park Road
Portland, Oregon   97201

Phone: 503-494-2998   *Fax:* 503-494-3400
WWW: http://www.ohsu.edu/

Application Filing		Accreditation	
Earliest:	June 1	LCME	
Latest:	October 15		
Fee:	$60	**Degrees Granted**	
AMCAS:	yes	MD, MD-PhD, MD-MPH	

Enrollment: 1996–97 First-Year Class

Men:	48	50%	Applied:		2100
Women:	48	50%	Interviewed:		168
Minorities:	8	8%	Enrolled:		96
Out of State:	30	31%			

1996–97 Class Profile

Mean MCAT Scores		*Mean GPA*
Physical Sciences:	10	3.6
Biological Sciences:	10	
Verbal Reasoning:	10	

Tuition and Fees

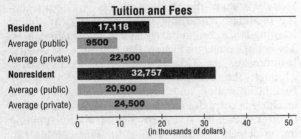

Resident	17,118
Average (public)	9500
Average (private)	22,500
Nonresident	32,757
Average (public)	20,500
Average (private)	24,500

(in thousands of dollars)

Percentage receiving financial aid: 92%

Introduction

As part of the Oregon State System of Higher Education, Oregon Health Sciences University is an independent collegiate health center. It was established in 1887 as the University of Oregon Medical School. Reorganization took place in 1974 when the schools of Medicine, Dentistry, and Nursing joined together to form the University of Oregon Health Science Center, which was renamed the Oregon Health Sciences University in 1981. The university is located on a 101-acre campus in Sam Jackson Park, a short distance from downtown Portland.

Admissions (AMCAS)

A bachelor's degree is required prior to matriculation. The basic premedical science courses, 1 college level course in mathematics, and 1 year each of humanities, social sciences, and English (including 1 semester of composition) are required. Courses in biochemistry and genetics are recommended. For those considering the MD-PhD program, advanced chemistry and molecular biology courses are recommended. *Transfer and advanced standing:* Availability decided yearly. Preference is given to Oregon residents.

Curriculum

4-year semitraditional. *First and second years:* Primarily devoted to the sciences basic to medicine, focusing initially on the normal structure and function of the human body and continuing with the study of the pathological basis of disease and its treatment. The course principles of clinical medicine is presented concurrently to develop fundamental knowledge and skills in patient interviewing and physical diagnosis. Socioeconomic, behavioral population health issues are also introduced during this period. *Third and fourth year:* Consists of clinical clerkships. A 6-week rural primary care experience is required and there are opportunities to pursue elective courses in clinical and basic sciences.

Grading and Promotion Policies

Grades are Honors, Near Honors, Marginal, or Fail. The Preclinical and Clinical Promotion Boards consist of faculty members and determine promotion. Students must take Step 1 and Step 2 of the USMLE to graduate.

Facilities

Teaching: The Oregon Health Sciences University includes more than a dozen buildings used for medical education, research, and patient care. The preclinical curriculum is provided in the Basic Sciences and Education buildings, which are designed for teaching in small group settings, as well as containing adequate space for lectures and laboratories. Clinical teaching is provided at the University Hospital and Clinics, Doernbecher Children's Hospital, and Portland Veteran's Administration Medical Center, as well as several affiliated hospitals and clinical teaching sites. In addition to research facilities, teaching space, and patient care facilities, the campus includes a computer center, library, and a fitness and sports center. *Library:* The library and auditorium afford facilities for lectures and scientific meetings. The library contains about 150,000 volumes of books and periodicals and subscribes to 2500 current periodicals. *Housing:* The Women's Residence Hall houses 170 women students from the Medical, Nursing, and Dental Schools.

Special Features

Minority admissions: Active recruitment of ethnic or educationally disadvantaged minorities is carried out through the Office of Minority Student Affairs. *Other degree programs:* Combined MD-PhD degree programs are offered in a variety of disciplines including medical genetics, medical psychology, and pathology. An MPH-MD program is also available.

PENNSYLVANIA

MCP/Hahnemann School of Medicine of Allegheny University

2900 Queen Lane
Philadelphia, Pennsylvania   19129

Phone: 215-991-8202   *Fax:* 215-843-1766
WWW: http://www.voicenet.com/voicenet/homepage/
avkaji/index.html

Application Filing		Accreditation	
Earliest:	June 1	LCME	
Latest:	December 1		
Fee:	$55	**Degrees Granted**	
AMCAS:	yes	MD, MD-PhD, BA-MD	

Enrollment: 1996–97 First-Year Class

Men:	132	55%	Applied:	13,602
Women:	108	45%	Interviewed:	1224
Minorities:	n/av	n/av	Enrolled:	240
Out of State:	105	44%		

1996–97 Class Profile

Mean MCAT Scores		*Mean GPA*
Physical Sciences:	n/av	3.5
Biological Sciences:	n/av	
Verbal Reasoning:	n/av	

Tuition and Fees

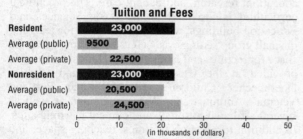

Resident	23,000
Average (public)	9500
Average (private)	22,500
Nonresident	23,000
Average (public)	20,500
Average (private)	24,500

(in thousands of dollars)

Percentage receiving financial aid: 85%

Above data applies to 1995–96 academic year.

Introduction

The Medical College of Pennsylvania (MCP), the first medical school for women, was established in 1850 and became coeducational in 1969. Established in 1948, Hahnemann University includes the School of Medicine, the Graduate School, the School of Health Sciences and Humanities, and the Hahnemann University Hospital. In 1988 MCP joined Allegheny Education, Health, and Research Foundation. In 1993 Hahnemann joined this organization, resulting in the MCP/Hahnemann School of Medicine. The merger has provided students with an opportunity for gaining their basic science education at a custom-designed facility on a 15-acre site in Philadelphia. Clinical training opportunities are provided through an extensive statewide network of hospitals linked with the Allegheny Foundation.

Admissions (AMCAS)

In addition to the basic premedical science courses, 1 year of English is required. *Transfer and advanced standing:* Applications are considered for the second and third years if openings are available.

Curriculum

4-year traditional. *First year:* Basic sciences and medical decision making. *Second year:* Pathology, pharmacology, molecular and human genetics, psychopathology, and introduction to clinical medicine. *Third year:* Clinical clerkships in each of the major divisions of medical practice. *Fourth year:* Clinical experience in ambulatory care, neurology, as well as subinternships and electives. In addition to the traditional curriculum, the school offers a group of selected students a Program for Integrated Learning, a problem-based curriculum track involving interactive medical education. Clinical problem solving and communication skills are learned in a similar manner.

Grading and Promotion Policies

A pass/fail system is used.

Facilities

Teaching: In 1992 the college opened a new Educational and Research facility. The building includes state-of-the-art research labs, modern teaching facilities, a learning resource center, a clinical learning lab, a computer center, and student amenities. The college manages Eastern Pennsylvania Psychiatric Institute for the Commonwealth of Pennsylvania. Through the college's membership in Allegheny Health, Education, and Research Foundation, clinical teaching is carried out in a number of diverse clinical settings within the Allegheny organization, including the principal teaching hospital in Philadelphia, St. Christopher's Hospital for Children, and Allegheny General Hospital. *Other:* The teaching program provides opportunities for additional clinical experience at many affiliated hospitals. An additional 2500 beds are provided by other hospitals that were affiliated with Hahnemann. *Library:* The Florence A. Moore Library of Medicine contains more than 37,000 volumes, and more than 1050 serial publications are received regularly. These holdings are supplemented by the Mental Health and Neurosciences Library on the EPPI campus. *Housing:* The Office of School/College Relations assists students in finding local housing.

Special Features

Minority admissions: The school has an active recruitment program. *Other degree programs:* The college offers a combined MD-PhD degree in which students spend 4 years in the medical curriculum and 2 to 3 years in advanced study in basic research. There is a BA-MD in conjunction with Lehigh University and a BS-MD program with Villanova University.

Jefferson Medical College
Thomas Jefferson University

1025 Walnut Street
Philadelphia, Pennsylvania   19107

Phone: 215-955-6983   *Fax:* 215-923-6939
WWW: http://www.tju.edu

Application Filing	Accreditation
Earliest: June 1	LCME
Latest: November 15	
Fee: $65	**Degrees Granted**
AMCAS: yes	MD, MD-PhD, MD-MBA

Enrollment: 1996–97 First-Year Class

Men:	152	68%	Applied:	11,600
Women:	71	32%	Interviewed:	696
Minorities:	18	8%	Enrolled:	223
Out of State:	124	56%		

1996–97 Class Profile

Mean MCAT Scores		*Mean GPA*
Physical Sciences:	10	3.4
Biological Sciences:	9.8	
Verbal Reasoning:	9.8	

Tuition and Fees

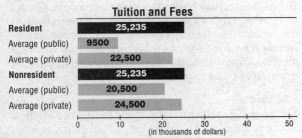

Resident	25,235
Average (public)	9500
Average (private)	22,500
Nonresident	25,235
Average (public)	20,500
Average (private)	24,500

(in thousands of dollars)

Percentage receiving financial aid: 70%

Introduction

Jefferson Medical College was established in 1824, almost 150 years before Thomas Jefferson University was founded. Located in Philadelphia, Jefferson Medical College is the largest private medical school in the United States. A Postgraduate College of Graduate Studies is affiliated with the university. The Medical College is located on a 13-acre urban campus in Philadelphia. In recent years there has been a significant expansion in research programs at the school.

Admissions (AMCAS)

The basic premedical science courses are recommended. *Transfer and advanced standing:* A very limited number of applications for transfer into the third year may be considered if compelling reasons exist.

Curriculum

4-year semimodern. *First year:* Basic sciences and courses in life cycle, ethics, genetics, health policy, and physiological approach to patient care. *Second year:* Medicine and society, introduction to clinical medicine, microbiology, pathology and cell physiology, and pharmacology. *Third and fourth years:* The clinical years are divided into 2 phases. Phase I consists of 6 weeks each of family medicine, general surgery, pediatrics, psychiatry and human behavior, and obstetrics/gynecology, and 12 weeks of internal medicine. Phase II consists of 6-week combination of anesthesiology, orthopedic surgery and urology; 6-week combination of neurology/neurosurgery, ophthalmology, and otolaryngology; 4-week combination of oncology/radiation and rehabilitation medicine; 4 weeks of advanced basic science; 4 weeks of inpatient subinternship in either internal medicine, general surgery, or pediatrics; 6 weeks of an outpatient subinternship in either family medicine, internal medicine, pediatrics, or psychiatry and human behavior; and 12 weeks of electives.

Grading and Promotion Policies

First and second years: Courses in the basic medical sciences are given numerical grades; 70 is passing. *Third and fourth years:* Clinical courses for all Phase I and Phase II required courses and all electives will be recorded as High Honors, Above Expected Competence, Expected Competence, Marginal Competence, Incomplete—I, Failure—F. An examination grade will also be recorded for all required Phase I courses. A written evaluation report is made a part of a student's permanent academic record. Students must record passing total scores on Step 1 and 2 of the USMLE.

Facilities

Teaching: The Jefferson Alumni Hall houses all basic science departments (and recreational facilities). College Building houses administrative and clinical department offices, laboratories, and lecture rooms and connects with the Curtis Building, in which are located additional clinical faculty offices, research laboratories, and classrooms. Bridges connect the College and Curtis buildings with the 4 Jefferson Hospital structures: the Gibbon Building, the Foerderer Pavilion, the Thompson Building, and the main building. The Gibbon Building is a facility with four 100-bed minihospitals, each with its own diagnostic and therapeutic facilities, teaching rooms, and physicians' offices, and the Bodine Center for Radiation Therapy. The outpatient Surgical Center contains physicians' offices, operating rooms, and surgical facilities for same-day surgery. *Other:* The college is affiliated with 19 hospitals. *Library:* The Scott Library Building contains 170,000 volumes and receives 2300 periodicals. *Housing:* Orlowitz, Barringer, Belmont, and Martin buildings provide apartment rentals.

Special Features

Minority admissions: The college encourages applications from minority and other disadvantaged students. *Other degree programs:* Selected students can earn BS and MD degrees in 6 calendar years from Jefferson Medical College in cooperation with Pennsylvania State University. There is a combined MD-PhD program with the College of Graduate Studies, Thomas Jefferson University and a joint 5-year MD-MBA (and MHA) program with Widener University.

Pennsylvania State University College of Medicine

P.O. Box 850
Hershey, Pennsylvania   17033

Phone: 717-531-8755   *Fax:* 717-531-6225
E-mail: jbwb@oas.psu.edu
WWW: http://www.psu.edu/psu/hershey/hershey.html

Application Filing		Accreditation
Earliest:	June 1	LCME
Latest:	November 15	
Fee:	$40	**Degrees Granted**
AMCAS:	yes	MD, MD-PhD

Enrollment: 1996–97 First-Year Class

Men:	62	57%	Applied:	7443
Women:	47	43%	Interviewed:	744
Minorities:	21	19%	Enrolled:	109
Out of State:	60	55%		

1996–97 Class Profile

Mean MCAT Scores		*Mean GPA*
Physical Sciences:	9.9	3.61
Biological Sciences:	9.9	
Verbal Reasoning:	9.4	

Tuition and Fees

Resident	17,010
Average (public)	9500
Average (private)	22,500
Nonresident	24,031
Average (public)	20,500
Average (private)	24,500

(in thousands of dollars)

Percentage receiving financial aid: 84%

Introduction

The Pennsylvania State University College of Medicine is part of the Milton S. Hershey Medical Center that was founded in 1935. Work on the College of Medicine was begun in the 1960s. The first class was enrolled in 1967. The Medical Center is located 12 miles east of Harrisburg, the state capital, and about 100 miles from the University Park Campus. The college occupies 550 acres on the western edge of Hershey.

Admissions (AMCAS)

Three years of college and the basic premedical science courses are required. Recommended courses include behavioral science, genetics, and physical chemistry. Courses in the humanities and social sciences are also encouraged. *Transfer and advanced standing:* Transfer students are considered from LCME-accredited institutions.

Curriculum

4-year semimodern. *First year:* An integrated approach to the teaching of organ systems and correlations between scientific principles and patient material. First-year courses include microscopic anatomy, embryology, biological chemistry, gross anatomy, family and community medicine, molecular and human genetics, physiology, neurobiology, physical diagnosis, behavioral science, and radiobiology. *Second year:* Interdisciplinary organ system approach to clinical science and pathology integrated with microbiology, pharmacology, and physical diagnosis. Longitudinal courses in behavioral science and psychiatry with particular emphasis on preventive medicine. An organized system of health care delivery is scheduled. A track in problem-based learning for first- and second-year volunteer students exists. Problem-based learning is offered as an alternative educational method for students who wish to work in smaller groups with faculty tutors. The learning objectives for students on the PBL track will be similar to those for students in the traditional track. *Third year:* Consists of required clinical clerkship experiences distributed between medicine, obstetrics and gynecology, surgery, pediatrics, psychiatry, and family and community medicine. *Fourth year:* 42 weeks devoted to selectives and electives.

Grading and Promotion Policies

Examinations may be written, oral, or practical. Grades of Honors, High Pass, Pass or Fail are determined by the faculty. The faculty is also responsible for recommendations for promotion and graduation. Students must take Steps 1 and 2 of the USMLE and have a score reported in order to graduate.

Facilities

Teaching: The principal structure is the 9-story Medical Sciences Building and Hospital, which contains basic teaching facilities, clinical sciences facilities, the teaching hospital, and research laboratories. *Other:* The Animal Research Farm is used for both teaching and research. The Central Animal Quarters, located in the Medical Sciences Building, is designed for teaching and experimentation. A Biomedical Research Building provides space for faculty and students. *Library:* The Harrell Library serves the Medical Sciences Building and the teaching hospital. Holdings total more than 100,000 volumes. This includes more than 3200 medical history, humanities, and rare books. About 2000 journal titles are currently received. *Housing:* There are 1-, 2-, and 3-bedroom apartments.

Special Features

Minority admissions: The school is strongly committed to and actively involved in the recruitment of minority applicants. *Other degree programs:* Combined MD-PhD programs are available in a number of disciplines. An overseas study program is available to selected students in their fourth year. Educational innovations include teaching by the Department of Humanities and the Department of Behavioral Science within the medical curriculum.

Temple University School of Medicine

3400 North Broad Street
Philadelphia, Pennsylvania   19140

Phone: 215-707-3656   *Fax:* 215-707-6932
E-mail: webmaster@www.temple.edu
WWW: http://www.temple.edu/

Application Filing		Accreditation	
Earliest:	June 1	LCME	
Latest:	December 1		
Fee:	$55	**Degrees Granted**	
AMCAS:	yes	MD, MD-PhD	

Enrollment: 1996–97 First-Year Class

Men:	109	58%	Applied:	8784
Women:	78	42%	Interviewed:	791
Minorities:	22	12%	Enrolled:	187
Out of State:	80	43%		

1996–97 Class Profile

Mean MCAT Scores		*Mean GPA*
Physical Sciences:	9.4	n/av
Biological Sciences:	9.7	
Verbal Reasoning:	9	

Tuition and Fees

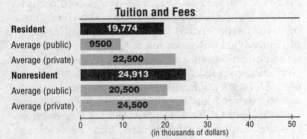

Resident	19,774
Average (public)	9500
Average (private)	22,500
Nonresident	24,913
Average (public)	20,500
Average (private)	24,500

(in thousands of dollars)

Percentage receiving financial aid: 81%

Above data applies to 1995-96 academic year.

Introduction

Temple University School of Medicine originated as the College of Temple University in 1901. The campus contains in addition to the School of Medicine other health-related schools of the university as well as Temple University Hospital. The school is located in the heart of Philadelphia, providing its students access to a large number of affiliated hospitals.

Admissions (AMCAS)

Only the basic premedical courses are required. Preference is given to Pennsylvania residents, but about 45% of the class are nonresidents. Strong preference is given also to students with 4 years of college. *Transfer and advanced standing:* Transfer students are accepted for the second and third years; on a space-available basis to qualified candidates from other LCME-approved schools.

Curriculum

4-year semitraditional. *First and second years:* Fundamentals of basic medical sciences. In addition, courses are offered in human genetics, behavioral science, molecular biology, endocrinology, and nutrition. Early patient contact is provided in fundamentals of clinical care. *Third year:* Rotation through clerkships in the major clinical specialties. *Fourth year:* Electives for 20 weeks in 4-week blocks in addition to required rotations in emergency medicine, neuroscience, a surgical subspecialty, and a subinternship in medicine, pediatrics, or surgery.

Grading and Promotion Policies

Honors/High Pass/Pass/Conditional Fail. A written evaluation of each student is required for each clinical clerkship and is encouraged for each basic science course. Steps 1 and 2 of the USMLE must be taken and passed.

Facilities

Teaching: Medical school activities during the first 2 years are housed in the School of Medicine and Kresge Science Hall. The latter is a teaching structure with student laboratories, demonstration classrooms, and a library. Clinical teaching takes place at Temple University Hospital, Albert Einstein Medical Center, Reading Hospital, St. Luke's Hospital, St. Christopher's Hospital for Children, and Abington Hospital. *Other:* There are formal agreements of affiliation with other general and specialty hospitals and letters of agreement with a number of institutions in Philadelphia, other parts of Pennsylvania, and New Jersey. The Fels Research Institute and Thrombosis Research Center are integral parts of the school. *Library:* A modern library is available to students and faculty. It houses a large number of books and periodicals and a computer center. *Housing:* No university-related dormitories are available.

Special Features

Minority admissions: The school has an active recruitment program and offers an 8-week summer enrichment program for incoming students. *Other degree programs:* Combined MD-PhD programs are available in the basic sciences.

University of Pennsylvania School of Medicine

Suite 100, Stemmler Hall
Philadelphia, Pennsylvania   19104

Phone: 215-898-8001   *Fax:* 215-573-6645
WWW: http://www.med.upenn.edu

Application Filing		Accreditation	
Earliest:	June 1	LCME	
Latest:	November 1		
Fee:	$55	**Degrees Granted**	
AMCAS:	yes	MD, MD-PhD, MD-MBA	

Enrollment: 1996–97 First-Year Class

Men:	72	48%	Applied:	8552
Women:	78	52%	Interviewed:	941
Minorities:	29	19%	Enrolled:	150
Out of State:	43	29%		

1996–97 Class Profile

Mean MCAT Scores		*Mean GPA*
Physical Sciences:	11	3.62
Biological Sciences:	11	
Verbal Reasoning:	11	

Tuition and Fees

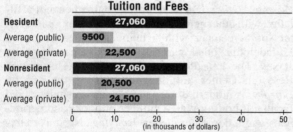

Resident	27,060
Average (public)	9500
Average (private)	22,500
Nonresident	27,060
Average (public)	20,500
Average (private)	24,500

(in thousands of dollars)

Percentage receiving financial aid: 76%

Introduction

The University of Pennsylvania School of Medicine was originally known as the College of Philadelphia. Founded in 1765, it was the first medical school established in the United States. It is a private, nondenominational school, located on the Irwin campus of the University of Pennsylvania in Philadelphia. The clinical training facilities such as the Hospital of the University of Pennsylvania and Children's Hospital of Philadelphia are located adjacent to the school.

Admissions (AMCAS)

Required courses are the basic premedical science courses. Recommended courses include mathematics (students should have a basic knowledge of logarithms, college-level algebra, analytical geometry, and differential calculus), and English (2 years of college-level work are suggested). Students are encouraged to prepare themselves broadly in the arts, the humanities, and in the social and behavioral sciences. Some preference is given to Pennsylvania students. *Transfer and advanced standing:* Information is not available.

Curriculum

4-year. *First year:* Consists of 40 weeks of basic sciences emphasizing normal form and function and an integrated clinical program. *Second year:* Begins with 6 months of coordinated teaching of pharmacology, pathophysiology, infectious disease, and continuation of the clinical program. This is followed by clinical clerkships. *Third and fourth years:* Programs consist of a mixture of required and elective courses chosen from over 100 offered which cover all basic and clinical sciences. New programs using seminars and minicourses help the student learn psychosocial and behavioral aspects of medicine, reinforce the student's knowledge of basic science, and reinforce an attitude favorable to later continuing self-education.

Grading and Promotion Policies

Each department submits a grade of Honors, Pass, or Fail for a student along with a description of the student's characteristics. The additional grade of High Pass is used by clinical departments. At the end of 3 academic years, the student's performance is evaluated and recommendations for postgraduate training are made. Students must obtain total passing scores on Steps 1 and 2 of the USMLE in order to graduate.

Facilities

Teaching: Students receive clinical instruction and experience in the hospitals of the University of Pennsylvania Medical Center as well as in other hospitals in Philadelphia and its vicinity. The chief source of clinical experience is the Hospital of the University of Pennsylvania. Besides teaching facilities, it houses research institutions and laboratories. Students serve clerkships and preceptorships at the Graduate Hospital of the University of Pennsylvania. A program for teaching and training has been established at Philadelphia General Hospital. Teaching privileges at Pennsylvania Hospital are reserved for clerkships in medicine, obstetrics, and surgery and for certain electives. Services at the Children's Hospital of Philadelphia are used for pediatric and surgical teaching. Students are assigned to the services of medicine and surgery at Presbyterian-University of Pennsylvania Medical Center. In addition, certain elective courses are offered there. *Other:* Courses, clerkships, and research facilities are offered at several other closely affiliated hospitals in the vicinity and at the Alfred Newton Richards Medical Research Building. *Library:* The library, which is housed in the Johnson Pavilion, contains more than 100,000 volumes and receives more than 2000 periodicals and other publications. *Housing:* On campus, Graduate Towers and High Rise North offers apartments and suites on a 12-month basis.

Special Features

Minority admissions: The school has short- and long-term recruitment programs to recruit underrepresented minority groups, which are directed by its Office of Minority Affairs. *Other degree programs:* Combined MD-PhD programs are available in the basic medical sciences; MD-JD and MD-MBA programs are also offered.

University of Pittsburgh School of Medicine

Pittsburgh, Pennsylvania 15261

Phone: 412-648-8975 *Fax:* 412-648-1236
E-mail: admissions@fsl.dean-med.pitt.edu
WWW: http://www.omed.pitt.edu/-omed/
homepage2.html

Application Filing		Accreditation	
Earliest:	June 1	LCME	
Latest:	December 9		
Fee:	$60	**Degrees Granted**	
AMCAS:	yes	MD, MD-PhD	

Enrollment: 1996–97 First-Year Class

Men:	85	58%	Applied:	5904
Women:	61	42%	Interviewed:	768
Minorities:	9	6%	Enrolled:	146
Out of State:	55	38%		

1996–97 Class Profile

Mean MCAT Scores		*Mean GPA*
Physical Sciences:	10.3	3.59
Biological Sciences:	10.5	
Verbal Reasoning:	10.2	

Tuition and Fees

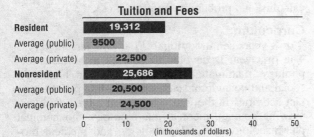

Resident	19,312
Average (public)	9500
Average (private)	22,500
Nonresident	25,686
Average (public)	20,500
Average (private)	24,500

(in thousands of dollars)

Percentage receiving financial aid: n/av

Introduction

In 1886 a charter was granted for the establishment of the Western Pennsylvania Medical College. In 1892 this school became affiliated with the Western University of Pennsylvania, which later became the University of Pittsburgh. The School of Medicine is located in the Oakland district of Pittsburgh and has extensive research facilities.

Admissions (AMCAS)

Applicants must have completed the basic premedical science courses including 1 year of English composition. Courses in the behavioral sciences, biostatistics, calculus, and computer sciences are recommended. Preference is given to residents. *Transfer and advanced standing:* Transfer students are considered when vacancies occur.

Curriculum

4-year semimodern. The curriculum emphasizes general principles and self-learning based on actual cases. *First and second years:* A multidisciplinary approach organized by organ will be used. Its aim is to develop communication and problem-solving skills; learning will be in small groups, rather than in large lectures. The curriculum will mainstream social, cultural, and ethical issues, and introduce the student to clinical medicine. *Third year:* Covers the major clinical specialties in the form of clerkships. *Fourth year:* Consists of 4 to 8 electives and a required subinternship.

Grading and Promotion Policies

Students are graded on the basis of their practical work and oral and written examinations. The system used is Honors/Pass/Fail. Students must record total passing scores on Step 1 and Step 2 of the USMLE for graduation.

Facilities

Teaching: All of the teaching in the basic science areas is conducted in the 12-story Alan Magee Scaife Hall of the Health Professions. The office and research space of the basic science departments and some of the clinical departments are also located there. Clinical teaching is conducted in the Health Center Hospitals as well as in hospitals in other parts of the city. The Western Psychiatric Institute and Clinic is a part of the university. The University Health Center at Pittsburgh is composed of 5 hospitals and the university. *Other:* The Terrace Village Health Center is an extension of the University Health Center into the community. Five hospitals and the Tuberculosis League are affiliated. *Library:* The Maurice and Laura Falk Library of the Health Professions is the main library. It has approximately 175,000 volumes and receives more than 2000 periodicals; there are 8 other libraries in which students have full privileges. *Housing:* No on-campus housing is available.

Special Features

Minority admissions: The school has an active recruitment program and offers an 8-week Summer Research Program for undergraduate college minority students. *Other degree programs:* Students selected for academic promise will be admitted to joint MD-PhD study programs in a variety of disciplines including biomedical engineering, epidemiology, and pathology. Also offered is a joint MD-MA Ethics degree.

RHODE ISLAND

Brown University School of Medicine

97 Waterman Street, Box 6A 212
Providence, Rhode Island   02912

Phone: 401-863-2149   *Fax:* 401-863-2666
E-mail: medschool_admissions@brown.edu
WWW: http://www.biomedcs.biomed.brown.edu/
medicine

Application Filing		Accreditation	
Earliest:	August 15	LCME	
Latest:	March 1		
Fee:	$60	**Degrees Granted**	
AMCAS:	no	MD, MD-PhD	

Enrollment: 1996–97 First-Year Class

Men:	32	51%	Applied:	2202
Women:	31	49%	Interviewed:	2202
Minorities:	8	12%	Enrolled:	63
Out of State:	58	92%		

1996–97 Class Profile

Mean MCAT Scores		*Mean GPA*
Physical Sciences:	n/av	n/av
Biological Sciences:	n/av	
Verbal Reasoning:	n/av	

Tuition and Fees

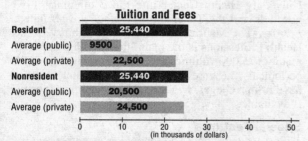

Resident	25,440
Average (public)	9500
Average (private)	22,500
Nonresident	25,440
Average (public)	20,500
Average (private)	24,500

(in thousands of dollars)

Percentage receiving financial aid: 65%

Above data applies to 1995–96 academic year.

Introduction

Brown University was established in 1764 in Providence, Rhode Island. It has offered a medical program since the 1880s, but its medical education program did not actually begin until 1963, when a 6-year course leading to a Masters of Medical Science degree was established. In 1975 a program leading to the MD degree was accredited. The Brown University program is an 8-year continuum of college and medical school. The enrollment is largely from high school seniors. Limited places are set aside for admission for the first year of medical school.

Admissions

Openings for the first-year class are reserved primarily for students enrolled in the 8-year program leading to both the bachelor's degree and the MD degree. The remaining openings are limited to individuals admitted to the MD-PhD program; to those admitted from a premedical postbaccalaureate program at Brown University, Bryn Mawr College, or Columbia University; to those admitted through the Early Identification Program at Providence College, Rhode Island College, the University of Rhode Island, or Tougaloo College; and to undergraduate or graduate students at Brown University. In addition, 20 students are admitted each year to the Brown-Dartmouth program. These students spend the first 2 years at Dartmouth Medical School and the last 2 years at Brown University, with the MD degree being awarded by Brown. Students who are interested in this program should contact Dartmouth Medical School at (603) 650-1505 for more information. Applications are considered from students who have or expect to receive a baccalaureate degree. Students admitted to the School of Medicine are expected to attain competence in the sciences basic to medicine. Although the majority of students demonstrate competence through coursework, such preparation may also be demonstrated through individualized study, research, or work experience. The following areas of study are recommended as guidelines to be used in selecting courses: 2 semesters of biology; 2 semesters of physics; 2 semesters in the social and behavioral sciences; and 1 semester each in general chemistry, organic chemistry, biochemistry, calculus, and probability and statistics.

Curriculum

4 or 8 years semitraditional. *First and second years:* The first year is devoted to courses in human morphology, mammalian physiology, human histology, social and behavioral sciences (including patient contact activities in the first semester in a medical interviewing course), medical microbiology, biochemical pharmacology, general pathology, and medical biochemistry. The second year curriculum consists of pathophysiology, neurosciences, systematic pathology, organ system pharmacology, and introductory courses in psychiatry and physical diagnosis. *Third and fourth years:* Students must satisfactorily complete 48 weeks of clinical clerkships and 32 weeks of electives. The clinical clerkships include internal medicine (12 weeks), surgery (12 weeks), obstetrics and gynecology (6 weeks), pediatrics (6 weeks), psychiatry (6 weeks), and community health (6 weeks). An advanced clinical clerkship (subinternship) is strongly recommended and a longitudinal ambulatory clerkship (6 months) is required.

Grading and Promotion Policies

Students are graded on an Honors/Pass/Fail basis. There is no numerical class ranking. Step 2 of the USMLE must be passed for graduation.

Facilities

Teaching: The medical school is located on the main university campus and all university facilities are available to medical students. The first 2 years of instruction take place in the biomedical building, which includes research laboratories, animal care facilities, student laboratories, and computer and audiovisual resources for students in addition to classrooms. Clinical training occurs in 9 affiliated hospitals in the Providence area. These hospitals include 4 general acute care hospitals, a specialty hospital for women and infants, a children's hospital, a Veterans Administration medical center, a general psychiatric hospital, and a child psychiatric hospital. More than half of the hospital beds in the state are part of the Brown medical community. *Other:* Two separate facilities house research laboratories in the medical sciences and neural sciences. *Library:* An 11-story sciences library on campus complements the libraries located in each affiliated hospital. The 2-million-volume Brown library system is available to medical students as is computerized literature searching. *Housing:* Most students live off campus, but residence halls for single students are available. A medical student co-op is also available on a limited space basis.

Special Features

Minority admissions: Applications from members of medically underrepresented minority groups are strongly encouraged. *Summer research:* Summer research assistantships are available on a competitive basis in both biomedical sciences and medically related social sciences. In addition, a summer research program is offered for members of underrepresented minority groups who wish to consider careers in the biological and medical sciences. *International studies:* Foreign studies fellowships offer an opportunity to study in any of more than a dozen different countries. Fellowships, which are awarded on a competitive basis, cover transportation costs and, if needed, living expenses for medical students. *Other degree programs:* Combined MD-PhD programs are offered in a variety of disciplines including ecology and evolutionary biology, molecular and cell biology, biochemistry, neuroscience, and pathobiology. The master of medical science degree is also available in conjunction with the MD degree.

SOUTH CAROLINA

Medical University of South Carolina College of Medicine

171 Ashley Avenue
Charleston, South Carolina   29425

Phone: 803-792-2055   *Fax:* 803-792-2967
E-mail: martinst@musc.edu
WWW: http://www.2.musc.edu/

Application Filing		Accreditation	
Earliest:	June 1	LCME	
Latest:	December 1		
Fee:	$45	**Degrees Granted**	
AMCAS:	yes	MD, MD-PhD	

Enrollment: 1996–97 First-Year Class

Men:	94	62%	Applied:	3181	
Women:	58	38%	Interviewed:	414	
Minorities:	46	30%	Enrolled:	152	
Out of State:	12	8%			

1996–97 Class Profile

Mean MCAT Scores		Mean GPA
Physical Sciences:	9	3.46
Biological Sciences:	9	
Verbal Reasoning:	9	

Tuition and Fees

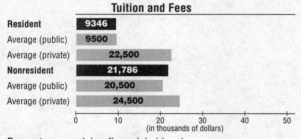

Resident	9346
Average (public)	9500
Average (private)	22,500
Nonresident	21,786
Average (public)	20,500
Average (private)	24,500

0   10   20   30   40   50
(in thousands of dollars)

Percentage receiving financial aid: n/av

Introduction

The Medical University of South Carolina is the oldest medical school in the South. There are 5 other medical education institutions besides the College of Medicine, namely colleges of Dental Medicine, Graduate Studies, Health Professions, Nursing, and Pharmacy. The institution was founded in 1824 by the Medical Society of South Carolina, a Charleston medical organization, as the Medical College of South Carolina. In 1913 ownership of the school was transferred to the state of South Carolina, committing it to provide financial support as a public institution for health education.

Admissions (AMCAS)

While there are no specific course requirements, adequate performance on the MCAT presupposes exposure to college-level basic premedical science courses. Students are advised to pursue any college studies that they find intellectually challenging and satisfying. *Transfer and advanced standing:* Students in good standing at other U.S. medical schools will be considered for transfer as space permits. Students enrolled in foreign medical schools must be South Carolina residents and must score in the top 50% of those taking Step 1 of the USMLE to be considered for advanced standing.

Curriculum

4-year. *First and second years:* There are 2 areas of emphasis in the first 2 academic periods, the traditional basic medical sciences and an umbrella course for all preclinical courses—introduction to clinical medicine (ICM) I-IV. This course includes ethics, human behavior, introduction to clinical reasoning, analytic and community medicine, laboratory medicine, and physical diagnosis. The use of small-group teaching is increasing. Emphasis is placed on clinical reasoning and issues of humanistic concern. The Parallel Curriculum is an alternative track that emphasizes acquiring basic science knowledge through problem-based learning and small-group interaction. *Third and fourth years:* The third academic period consists of rotating clerkships through the major clinical specialties. The fourth academic period consists of 36 weeks of selectives/electives.

Grading and Promotion Policies

A merit grading system is used. Passing Step 1 of the USMLE is required for advancement to the third year.

Facilities

Teaching: The college is in the center of a 45-acre medical complex. Clinical teaching is at the Medical University Hospital (510 beds), VA Hospital (431 beds), Charleston Memorial Hospital (175 beds), Children's Hospital (150 beds), and Psychiatric Institute (47 beds). *Library:* The Health Affairs Library is located in the Administration Building and contains 170,000 volumes and receives more than 2700 periodicals. *Housing:* Student housing on campus is not available.

Special Features

Minority admissions: The college has an active recruitment program directed by the College of Medicine Office of Diversity. It also conducts an 8-week Summer Health Careers Program for upper-level minority undergraduates matriculating in South Carolina colleges. *Other degree programs:* The MSTP offers a combined MD-PhD degree. Students conduct basic research leading to the PhD degree and, if appropriate, a companion clinical research project. The MSTP seeks to integrate the best qualities of medical and graduate school programs into a cohesive training experience.

University of South Carolina School of Medicine

Columbia, South Carolina   29208

Phone: 803-733-3325   *Fax:* 803-733-3328
E-mail: witch@dcsmserver.med.sc.edu
WWW: http://www.med.sc.edu/

Application Filing		Accreditation	
Earliest:	June 1	LCME	
Latest:	December 1		
Fee:	$45	**Degrees Granted**	
AMCAS:	yes	MD, MD-PhD	

Enrollment: 1996–97 First-Year Class

Men:	41	57%	Applied:	1878	
Women:	31	43%	Interviewed:	338	
Minorities:	13	18%	Enrolled:	72	
Out of State:	8	11%			

1996–97 Class Profile

Mean MCAT Scores		*Mean GPA*
Physical Sciences:	n/av	3.39
Biological Sciences:	n/av	
Verbal Reasoning:	n/av	

Tuition and Fees

Resident	10,090
Average (public)	9500
Average (private)	22,500
Nonresident	21,420
Average (public)	20,500
Average (private)	24,500

0   10   20   30   40   50
(in thousands of dollars)

Percentage receiving financial aid: 85%

Above data applies to 1995–96 academic year.

Introduction

As the most recent school at the University of South Carolina, the School of Medicine was not established until 1977. Located in the state capital, the school offers a wide range of educational and professional opportunities to its students. This includes small class size and an emphasis on the correlation between basic science and clinical science training. The school works closely with its 7 affiliated hospitals to provide students valuable clinical experience.

Admissions (AMCAS)

The basic premedical science courses plus 1 year of English (composition and literature) and 1 year of mathematics are required. Courses in integral and differential calculus and advanced natural science courses are recommended. *Transfer and advanced standing:*

Transfer from other accredited U.S. medical schools into the second or third year is possible if space is available.

Curriculum

4-year traditional. *First and second years:* These 2 years are devoted to the introductory and advanced basic sciences that are integrated with clinical correlations. An Introduction to Clinical Practice Continuum includes family medicine, clinical medicine, preventive medicine, psychiatry, and behavioral science components in a small-group format. *Third year:* This consists of 8-week clerkships in the major clinical sciences. *Fourth year:* Consists of rotations in medicine and surgery subspecialties and neurology with the remainder of the year devoted to a selective/elective program.

Grading and Promotion Policies

A letter grading system is used. Students are required to pass Step 1 of the USMLE before being promoted to the third year, and Step 2 before graduation.

Facilities

Teaching: The courses during the first 2 years are taught in the Medical Sciences Building, which also houses various departmental offices. Clinical training takes place at the VA Medical Center, Richland Memorial Hospital, Hall Psychiatric Institute, Greenville Memorial Hospital, and other affiliated hospitals. *Library:* The Medical School library is located on the grounds of the VA Center and has a collection of more than 67,000 volumes and subscribes to more than 1200 periodicals. *Housing:* On-campus housing is available to married students only.

Special Features

Minority admissions: The school has an active minority recruitment program. *Other degree programs:* A combined MD-PhD program is offered.

SOUTH DAKOTA

University of South Dakota School of Medicine

414 East Clark Street
Vermillion, South Dakota   57069

Phone: 605-677-5233   *Fax:* 605-677-5109
E-mail: gyutrzen@sunbird.usd.edu
WWW: http://www.usd.edu/med/index.html

Application Filing		Accreditation	
Earliest:	June 1	LCME	
Latest:	November 15		
Fee:	$15	**Degrees Granted**	
AMCAS:	yes	MD	

Enrollment: 1996–97 First-Year Class

Men:	24	46%	Applied:	965
Women:	28	54%	Interviewed:	174
Minorities:	3	6%	Enrolled:	52
Out of State:	2	4%		

1996–97 Class Profile

Mean MCAT Scores		*Mean GPA*
Physical Sciences:	8.5	3.58
Biological Sciences:	8.9	
Verbal Reasoning:	8.3	

Tuition and Fees

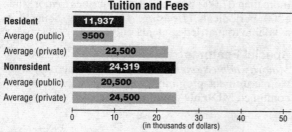

Resident	11,937
Average (public)	9500
Average (private)	22,500
Nonresident	24,319
Average (public)	20,500
Average (private)	24,500

(in thousands of dollars)

Percentage receiving financial aid: 87%

Introduction

The University of South Dakota was established in 1882. The School of Medicine began as a 2-year school for the basic medical sciences. An MD degree-granting program was initiated in 1975. The objective of the medical school is to train family practice physicians in South Dakota.

Admissions (AMCAS)

The basic premedical science courses plus 1 year of mathematics are required. Courses in genetics, developmental biology, cell physiology and behavioral sciences are recommended. *Transfer and advanced standing:* Candidates for transfer are accepted only under exceptional circumstances.

Curriculum

4-year semitraditional. The aim of this program is to provide a firm foundation in the basic medical sciences and to correlate these disciplines with clinical teaching and practical medical experience. *First year:* Introductory basic sciences as well as introduction to clinical medicine. *Second year:* Advanced basic sciences as well as laboratory medicine and continuation of introduction to clinical medicine. At the end of year two each student is assigned to a one-month practical preceptorship with a physician in private practice. *Third year:* 52 weeks of required clerkships. *Fourth year:* 4 weeks of family practice clerkship, 7 weeks of surgical subspecialties, 4 weeks of emergency medicine, and electives for 25 weeks in blocks of 4, 8, or 12 weeks.

Grading and Promotion Policies

The grading system of A to F is used. Promotion to the sophomore class is determined by the judgment of the faculty and not solely by the student's academic record. Students with one grade of D or F will be considered scholastically deficient. Students must take both steps of the USMLE as candidates and record passing total scores to graduate.

Facilities

Teaching: Preclinical instruction takes place in the Lee Memorial Medical Sciences Building on the USD campus in Vermillion. Clinical teaching takes place at the 3 VA hospitals in the state and at community general hospitals in Sioux Falls, Yankton, and Rapid City. *Library:* The Christian P. Lommen Health Science Library contains approximately 79,000 volumes and subscribes to about 1000 national and international medical and scientific periodicals. *Housing:* Both university residence halls and off-campus housing are available.

Special Features

Minority admissions: The school has a program designed to identify and assist Native Americans interested in medicine. *Other degree programs:* PhD programs are offered in the basic medical sciences.

TENNESSEE

East Tennessee State University James H. Quillen College of Medicine

P.O. Box 70580
Johnson City, Tennessee   37614

Phone: 423-439-6221   *Fax:* 423-929-6616
E-mail: kirkland@etsuserv.etsu-tn.edu
WWW: http://www.etsu.east-tenn-st.edu:80/-med com/

Application Filing		Accreditation
Earliest:	June 15	LCME
Latest:	December 1	
Fee:	$25	**Degrees Granted**
AMCAS:	yes	MD, MD-PhD, MD-MS

Enrollment: 1996–97 First-Year Class

Men:	39	65%	Applied:	1826
Women:	21	35%	Interviewed:	274
Minorities:	15	25%	Enrolled:	60
Out of State:	6	10%		

1996–97 Class Profile

Mean MCAT Scores		*Mean GPA*
Physical Sciences:	9	3.4
Biological Sciences:	9	
Verbal Reasoning:	9.7	

Tuition and Fees

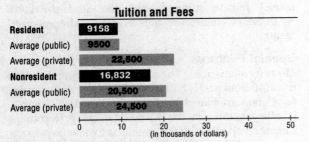

Resident	9158
Average (public)	9500
Average (private)	22,500
Nonresident	16,832
Average (public)	20,500
Average (private)	24,500

(in thousands of dollars)

Percentage receiving financial aid: n/av

Introduction

James H. Quillen College of Medicine is situated on the main campus of East Tennessee State University and it is one of the most recent fully accredited medical schools in the country. It graduated its first class in 1982. The school provides a community-based program with an emphasis on the education of primary care physicians. Small class size is another characteristic of this school. The College of Medicine is located in a naturally beautiful environment adjacent to 3 small rural communities in East Tennessee: Johnson City, Kingsport, and Bristol.

Admissions (AMCAS)

The basic premedical sciences plus 3 communications skills courses are required. Preference is given to residents of Tennessee. *Transfer and advanced standing:* Transfer to the second or third year is possible but extremely rare (LBA).

Curriculum

4-year semitraditional. Primary care-oriented. Rural primary care track available. *First and second years:* Devoted to the study of introductory and advanced basic science courses. In addition, courses are offered in biostatistics, personality development, medical genetics, psychopathology, and practicing medicine. *Third year:* Provides for rotations through the major clinical specialties including family practice. *Fourth year:* Involves required clerkships in internal medicine and surgery and 24 weeks of electives.

Grading and Promotion Policies

Letter grades are used for all work except for clinical electives, where a Pass/Fail system is used.

Facilities

Teaching: Teaching facilities are located on the ETSU campus and on the grounds of the adjacent VA Medical Center. Affiliation with the VA Medical Center, Johnson City Medical Center, Bristol Regional Medical Center, Holston Valley Hospital and Medical Center, and the Woodridge Psychiatric Hospital provides access to more than 2300 beds for clinical teaching. *Library:* The medical library has more than 50,000 volumes in its collection. *Housing:* Available on and near the campus.

Special Features

Minority admissions: The Office of Student Affairs coordinates recruitment. The school participates in a summer Premedical Enrichment Program and the Tennessee Preprofessional Program for minorities. *Other degree programs:* An integrated BS-MD program is available to ETSU students. Combined MD-PhD and MD-MS programs are offered in the basic sciences.

Meharry Medical College School of Medicine

1005 D. B. Todd Jr. Boulevard
Nashville, Tennessee 37208

Phone: 615-327-6223   *Fax:* 615-327-6228
WWW: http://www.ccmc.mmc.edu

Application Filing		Accreditation
Earliest:	June 1	LCME
Latest:	December 15	
Fee:	$25	**Degrees Granted**
AMCAS:	yes	MD, MD-PhD

Enrollment: 1996–97 First-Year Class

Men:	42	53%	Applied:	5548
Women:	38	48%	Interviewed:	444
Minorities:	64	80%	Enrolled:	80
Out of State:	71	89%		

1996–97 Class Profile

Mean MCAT Scores		*Mean GPA*
Physical Sciences:	7.2	3
Biological Sciences:	7.8	
Verbal Reasoning:	7.7	

Tuition and Fees

Resident	18,400
Average (public)	9500
Average (private)	22,500
Nonresident	18,400
Average (public)	20,500
Average (private)	24,500

(in thousands of dollars)

Percentage receiving financial aid: n/av

Above data applies to 1995–96 academic year.

Introduction

Established in 1876, Meharry Medical College educates about half of all African-American doctors and dentists in the United States. It was founded as the medical department of Central Tennessee College of Nashville, which later became Walden University. In 1915 a new charter was granted to the school from the state, establishing Meharry as an independent institution. Presently it includes schools of Medicine, Dentistry, Graduate Study and Research, and Allied Health. Its mission is the education of primary care physicians, for service in medically underserved areas.

Admissions (AMCAS)

Requirements include 1 year of English composition in addition to the basic premedical science courses. Preference given to those students who have more than 3 years of premedical training. *Transfer and advanced standing:* None.

Curriculum

4-year semitraditional. *First year:* An introduction to cell biology is followed by a progression from the cell through organ systems in the teaching of biochemistry, anatomy, and physiology. *Second year:* Includes courses in family and community health, genetics, and physical diagnosis. *Third and fourth years:* The clinical clerkships, beginning in the junior year and extending into the senior year, consist of six 8-week blocks in each of the following: internal medicine, pediatrics, surgery, obstetrics-gynecology, family and preventive medicine, and psychiatry. The fourth-year students take three 4-week blocks of surgery, Area Health Education Center, and radiology; two 4-week blocks in internal medicine; and three 4-week blocks of guided electives.

Grading and Promotion Policies

Grades of A, B, C, and F and a summary of the student's work are issued. Receiving total passing scores on Steps 1 and 2 of the USMLE is required for promotion to the third year and graduation, respectively.

Facilities

Teaching: The School of Medicine is housed primarily in a building that contains basic science departments and teaching laboratories, a teaching hospital with clinical departments, and research facilities. Hubbard Hospital houses the basic and clinical sciences departments including laboratories, classrooms, an amphitheater, teaching laboratories, and other facilities. *Library:* The library contains more than 50,000 volumes and 1000 journal titles and is located in the Learning Resources Center. *Housing:* Dorothy Brown Hall houses female students, and the Student-Faculty Apartment Complex contains 1- and 2-bedroom apartments.

Special Features

Minority admissions: The college, which over the years has turned out nearly half of the 7000 African American physicians graduated from American medical schools, is offering through the Kresge Learning Resources Center an opportunity for alumni and other physicians to continue their education. Several 8-week summer programs are available for undergraduates. *Other degree programs:* Combined MD-PhD programs in a variety of disciplines.

University of Tennessee, Memphis College of Medicine

800 Madison Avenue
Memphis, Tennessee   38163

Phone: 901-448-5559   *Fax:* 901-448-7255
WWW: http://www.utmgopher.utmem.edu/utm.htm/

Application Filing		Accreditation	
Earliest:	June 1	LCME	
Latest:	November 15		
Fee:	$25	**Degrees Granted**	
AMCAS:	yes	MD, MD-PhD, MD-MS	

Enrollment: 1996–97 First-Year Class

Men:	95	58%	Applied:	1959
Women:	70	42%	Interviewed:	392
Minorities:	21	13%	Enrolled:	165
Out of State:	13	8%		

1996–97 Class Profile

Mean MCAT Scores		*Mean GPA*
Physical Sciences:	9	3.5
Biological Sciences:	10	
Verbal Reasoning:	9	

Tuition and Fees

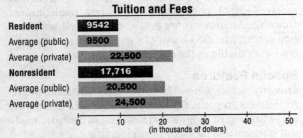

Resident	9542
Average (public)	9500
Average (private)	22,500
Nonresident	17,716
Average (public)	20,500
Average (private)	24,500

(in thousands of dollars)

Percentage receiving financial aid: n/av

Introduction

Established in 1851, the University of Tennessee at Memphis has a complete health science center that includes the colleges of Medicine, Graduate School of Health Sciences, Dentistry, Nursing, Pharmacy, and Allied Health Sciences. The school originated from the Medical Department of the University of Nashville, which in 1909 consolidated with the Medical Department of the University of Tennessee to form the University of Tennessee Department of Medicine. Further mergers took place with other institutions resulting in the formation of the present College of Medicine.

Admissions (AMCAS)

The basic premedical science courses as well as courses in English composition and literature are required. Preference is given to state residents; very few nonresidents are accepted. *Transfer and advanced standing:* Students are accepted only into the third year of the curriculum. They must be residents of Tennessee at the time they enter medical school or be children of alumni, must pass the USMLE Step 1, and must have completed the biomedical science portion of the curriculum.

Curriculum

The program is approximately 36 months of instruction over a 45-month period. It is divided into 3 major areas: biomedical sciences, clerkships, and electives. The biomedical science portion is 18 months in duration, consisting of 9 months in each of the first and second years. Clinical clerkships during the third year require that all students rotate through medicine, surgery, pediatrics, obstetrics-gynecology, family medicine, and psychiatry. Programs are available at facilities in Memphis, Knoxville, Chattanooga, and Nashville. The senior year consists of 1-month required clerkships in neurology, ambulatory medicine, surgical subspecialties, junior internship (medicine), junior internship (in any third-year clerkship discipline), and 3 months of electives.

Grading and Promotion Policies

An A to F grading policy is used. Students must achieve a 2.0 GPA for promotion, and must record total passing scores on Step 1 of the USMLE for promotion to the third year, and on Step 2 for graduation.

Facilities

Teaching: The college is part of the University of Tennessee Memphis Health Science Center. Students may spend 10 of the 20 clinical months at the units in Knoxville and Chattanooga. No more than 2 months may be spent at other institutions. *Library:* The C.P.J. Mooney Memorial Library holds more than 172,000 bound volumes. *Housing:* Two on-campus dormitories are available.

Special Features

Minority admissions: The school maintains a long-term program for recruiting disadvantaged students. It also sponsors 3 summer enrichment programs for undergraduate college as well as high school students. Scholarships for African-American students are available. *Other degree programs:* Combined MD-PhD programs are offered in the basic medical sciences.

Vanderbilt University School of Medicine

21st Avenue South at Garland Avenue
Nashville, Tennessee   37232

Phone: 615-322-2145   *Fax:* 615-343-8397
E-mail: medsch.admis.@msado
WWW: http://www.mc.vanderbilt.edu/medschool/

Application Filing		Accreditation
Earliest:	June 1	LCME
Latest:	October 15	
Fee:	$50	**Degrees Granted**
AMCAS:	yes	MD, MD-PhD

Enrollment: 1996–97 First-Year Class

Men:	67	64%	Applied:	6436
Women:	37	36%	Interviewed:	644
Minorities:	5	5%	Enrolled:	104
Out of State:	90	87%		

1996–97 Class Profile

Mean MCAT Scores		*Mean GPA*
Physical Sciences:	11.5	3.6
Biological Sciences:	11.4	
Verbal Reasoning:	10.7	

Tuition and Fees

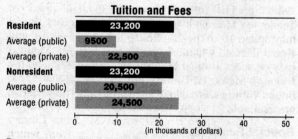

Resident	23,200
Average (public)	9500
Average (private)	22,500
Nonresident	23,200
Average (public)	20,500
Average (private)	24,500

0   10   20   30   40   50
(in thousands of dollars)

Percentage receiving financial aid: n/av

Introduction

Vanderbilt University was established in the late 1800s. The School of Medicine has been part of Vanderbilt University since it opened. This private university is located 1½ miles from the business center of Nashville; it consists of 10 schools. The School of Medicine is part of the Vanderbilt University Medical Center whose affiliated hospitals provide students with an opportunity for comprehensive, diversified clinical training.

Admissions (AMCAS)

The basic premedical science courses and 6 semester hours of English are required. Advanced Placement and pass/fail credits are not considered for required courses. A bachelor's degree is required. The present student body comes from a wide variety of states. *Transfer and advanced standing:* None.

Curriculum

4-year semitraditional. *First year:* Anatomy, biochemistry, physiology, cell biology, neurobiology, and electives. *Second year:* Advanced basic sciences with additional courses in laboratory diagnosis, preventive medicine, epidemiology, and psychiatry. Exposure to patients takes place during an interdepartmental course, introduction to clinical science, wherein history taking, physical examination, and laboratory study of patients are taught. One day per week is open for electives. *Third year:* Clerkships in the major clinical areas, including neurology. *Fourth year:* Selectives in medical and surgical areas and ambulatory medicine plus electives.

Grading and Promotion Policies

Letter grades A, B, C, and F and Pass/Fail grading systems are used (the latter for electives in the first 2 years). Promotion is considered by a committee composed of the faculty at the end of each academic year.

Facilities

Teaching: The basic sciences are taught at the Medical Center, and clinical teaching takes place primarily at the 514-bed Vanderbilt University Hospital and affiliated hospitals, including the Nashville VA Medical Center, Nashville Metropolitan General Hospital, and St. Thomas Hospital. *Library:* The Medical Center Library contains more than 155,000 volumes and receives 2000 periodicals and serial publications. *Housing:* Apartments are available for single and married students in the 11-story Lewis House, and are otherwise available in the community.

Special Features

Minority admissions: The school conducts an active recruitment program. *Other degree programs:* Combined MD-PhD degree programs are offered in the basic medical sciences and biomedical engineering.

TEXAS

Baylor College of Medicine

One Baylor Plaza
Houston, Texas   77030

Phone: 713-798-4841   *Fax:* 713-798-5563
E-mail: melodym@bcm.tmc.edu
WWW: http://www.bcm.tmc.edu

Application Filing		Accreditation	
Earliest:	June 1	LCME	
Latest:	November 1		
Fee:	$35	**Degrees Granted**	
AMCAS:	no	MD, MD-PhD	

Enrollment: 1996–97 First-Year Class

Men:	101	60%	Applied:	3671
Women:	67	40%	Interviewed:	624
Minorities:	39	23%	Enrolled:	168
Out of State:	41	24%		

1996–97 Class Profile

Mean MCAT Scores		*Mean GPA*
Physical Sciences:	11	3.7
Biological Sciences:	11	
Verbal Reasoning:	11	

Tuition and Fees

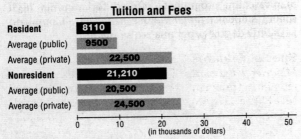

Resident	8110
Average (public)	9500
Average (private)	22,500
Nonresident	21,210
Average (public)	20,500
Average (private)	24,500

(in thousands of dollars)

Percentage receiving financial aid: n/av

Introduction

Baylor College of Medicine was chartered by the state of Texas and organized in 1900 as an independent, nonsectarian institution in Dallas. In 1903 it became affiliated with Baylor University and in 1943 the school relocated to Houston and became the medical school for the newly formed Texas Medical Center. The college separated from Baylor University in 1969.

Admissions

To be considered for admission, an applicant must have satisfactorily completed, by the time of enrollment in medical school, not less than 90 semester hours (or an equivalent number of quarter hours) at a fully accredited college in the United States. The following courses must have been completed satisfactorily: the basic premedical science courses and 1 year of English. *Transfer and advanced standing:* Admission into the first clinical year from fully accredited medical colleges in the U.S. is on a competitive basis, and the number admitted depends upon the availability of adequate faculty and facilities. No specific number of spaces is set aside.

Curriculum

4-year semimodern. *First year:* Basic medical sciences, and patient, physicians, and society and integrated problem solving. *Second year:* Finish basic sciences in December; begin clinical rotations in January. *Third year:* Required rotations through clinical science disciplines; patient care in both hospital and ambulatory settings; electives; clerkships in the major and some minor specialities, as well as primary care. *Fourth year:* Required rotations through clinical science disciplines; patient care in both hospital and ambulatory settings; electives; clerkships in the major and some minor specialties, as well as primary care.

Grading and Promotion Policies

Grades for the basic science courses and basic science electives are recorded as Honors, Pass, Marginal Pass, and Fail; required clinical clerkships and clinical electives are recorded as Honors, High Pass, Pass, Marginal Pass, and Fail. Students may not begin clinical clerkships until they have completed all the basic science courses. Steps 1 and 2 of the USMLE is optional.

Facilities

Teaching: The basic sciences are taught at the DeBakey Biomedical Research Building, which also contains auditoriums with a seating capacity of about 735. Five more buildings, the Jesse H. Jones Building for Clinical Research, the M. D. Anderson Basic Science and Research Building, the Jewish Institute for Medical Research, the Roy and Lillie Cullen Building, and the Ben Taub Research Center, provide additional space for the basic science departments. Clinical teaching and research take place in 8 general and specialized hospitals in the area. *Library:* The Jesse H. Jones Library includes an audiovisual resource center from which medical educational broadcasts are received. The library contains more than 180,000 volumes and receives a wide variety of periodicals. *Housing:* A student dormitory, belonging to the Texas Medical Center, offers accommodations for single and married students without children and is located across the street from the college. Women students can seek housing in the Nurses' Dormitory of Texas Women's University.

Special Features

Minority admissions: The school has an active recruitment program for minority students. *Other degree programs:* Combined MD-PhD degree HSTP is offered in a variety of disciplines: audiology and bioacoustics, biochemistry, biotechnology, cell biology, cell and molecular biology, developmental biology, microbiology and immunology, molecular genetics, neurosciences, physiology, cardiovascular sciences, and molecular biophysics, pharmacology, virology and epidemiology. A combined MD-PhD degree in biomedical engineering is also offered with Rice University.

Texas A&M University College of Medicine

College Station, Texas 77843

Phone: 409-845-7744 *Fax:* 409-847-8663
E-mail: med-stu-aff@tamu.edu
WWW: http://www.thunder.tamu.edu/

Application Filing		Accreditation
Earliest:	May 1	LCME
Latest:	November 1	
Fee:	$45	**Degrees Granted**
AMCAS:	yes	MD, MD-PhD

Enrollment: 1996–97 First-Year Class

Men:	40	63%	Applied:	1519
Women:	24	38%	Interviewed:	471
Minorities:	9	14%	Enrolled:	64
Out of State:	1	2%		

1996–97 Class Profile

Mean MCAT Scores		*Mean GPA*
Physical Sciences:	n/av	3.65
Biological Sciences:	n/av	
Verbal Reasoning:	n/av	

Tuition and Fees

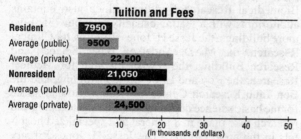

Resident	7950
Average (public)	9500
Average (private)	22,500
Nonresident	21,050
Average (public)	20,500
Average (private)	24,500

0   10   20   30   40   50
(in thousands of dollars)

Percentage receiving financial aid: 89%

Above data applies to 1995–96 academic year.

Introduction

Texas A&M University College of Medicine enrolled its first class of students in 1977. The College of Medicine is part of the Texas A&M University Health Sciences Center and is located on the university campus. The clinical campus is located in Temple, Texas with the basic sciences center located in College Station.

Admissions

In addition to the basic premedical science courses, calculus, English, and 1 advanced biology course are required. Strong preference is given to Texas residents. A number of those accepted have only 3 years of college, but have outstanding academic records. *Transfer and advanced standing:* Transfer is rare.

Curriculum

4-year semitraditional. *First year:* Consists of the introductory basic sciences, medical humanities, epidemiology/biomeasurements, environmental medicine, and working with patients. *Second year:* Consists of the advanced basic sciences and an introduction to the clinical disciplines and clinical psychiatry as well as a preceptorship. *Third year:* Involves rotating clerkships through the major clinical specialties. *Fourth year:* Made up of selective clerkships, a clerkship in neurology, medical jurisprudence, and electives.

Grading and Promotion Policies

Letter grades are used for the first 3 years and Satisfactory/Unsatisfactory for the fourth.

Facilities

Teaching: The basic sciences are taught in College Station, while clinical training is obtained at the Olin E. Teague Veterans Center (630 beds), Scott and White Memorial Hospital and Clinic (125 beds), and other affiliated institutions. *Library:* The Medical Library has 63,000 books and subscribes to 1900 journals. *Housing:* On-campus housing is limited. Some apartments are available at the Veterans Center for students completing the last 2 years.

Special Features

Minority admissions: Recruitment is coordinated by the School Relations Office (Admissions), and a summer research program is offered for minority high school students. *Other degree programs:* Combined MD-PhD degree programs are available.

Texas Tech University School of Medicine

Lubbock, Texas 79430

Phone: 806-743-2297
E-mail: webmaster@ttuhsc.edu
WWW: http://www.ttuhsc.edu/

Application Filing		Accreditation	
Earliest:	June 1	LCME	
Latest:	November 1		
Fee:	$40	**Degrees Granted**	
AMCAS:	no	MD, MD-PhD	

Enrollment: 1996–97 First-Year Class

Men:	90	75%	Applied:	1697
Women:	30	25%	Interviewed:	458
Minorities:	26	22%	Enrolled:	120
Out of State:	3	3%		

1996–97 Class Profile

Mean MCAT Scores		*Mean GPA*
Physical Sciences:	9.1	3.52
Biological Sciences:	9.4	
Verbal Reasoning:	9.4	

Tuition and Fees

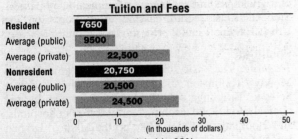

Resident	7650
Average (public)	9500
Average (private)	22,500
Nonresident	20,750
Average (public)	20,500
Average (private)	24,500

(in thousands of dollars)

Percentage receiving financial aid: 66%

Introduction

The Texas Tech University Health Sciences Center School of Medicine was opened in 1972 as a multi-campus regional institution with Lubbock as the administrative center and Armadillo, El Paso, and Odessa as regional centers. The School of Medicine is one of 4 schools in the Health Sciences Center, the other 3 being schools of Nursing, Pharmacy, and Allied Health. The major objective of the School of Medicine is to provide quality medical education and develop programs to meet health care needs for about 100 counties of West Texas.

Admissions

The basic premedical science courses are required, as is the MCAT. Only residents of Texas, eastern New Mexico, and southwestern Oklahoma are considered. *Transfer and advanced standing:* Applicants who have passed the USMLE Step 1 or the Basic Science part of the ECFMG will be considered for third-year placement when vacancies occur.

Curriculum

4 years. *First year:* Consists of 2 terms. In addition to basic science courses, medical ethics and electives are offered. *Second year:* Consists of 2 terms that cover the advanced basic science courses as well as an introduction to clinical medicine, psychiatry, and preventive medicine. *Third year:* 48 weeks, rotating through clinical clerkships. *Fourth year:* 8 required months including neurology (1 month), primary care (2 months), and 5 months of electives.

Grading and Promotion Policies

A numerical grading system is used for years 1–3. The fourth year is Honors/ Pass/Fail. Taking Step 1 of the USMLE is required.

Facilities

Teaching: Basic sciences are taught at the Health Sciences Center in Lubbock. The clinical sciences are taught in Lubbock and at the Regional Academic Health Centers in Amarillo and El Paso. There are well over 1000 teaching beds. *Other:* Senior electives can also be completed at the Regional Academic Health Center in Odessa. *Library:* The Library of the Health Sciences contains more than 100,000 volumes and receives more than 1600 periodicals regularly. Library facilities are available on all teaching campuses. *Housing:* None available on campus.

Special Features

Minority admissions: The school encourages minority students to apply and recruits through Texas colleges and universities. *Other degree programs:* A combined MD-PhD program is offered.

University of Texas Medical School at Galveston

Galveston, Texas   77555

Phone: 409-772-3517   *Fax:* 409-772-5753
E-mail: inet:jad@paa.utmb.edu
WWW: http://www.utmb.edu/

Application Filing		Accreditation	
Earliest:	May 1	LCME	
Latest:	October 15		
Fee:	$60	**Degrees Granted**	
AMCAS:	no	MD, MD-PhD	

Enrollment: 1996–97 First-Year Class

Men:	128	64%	Applied:	3335
Women:	72	36%	Interviewed:	1234
Minorities:	108	54%	Enrolled:	200
Out of State:	45	23%		

1996–97 Class Profile

Mean MCAT Scores		*Mean GPA*
Physical Sciences:	9	3.5
Biological Sciences:	9	
Verbal Reasoning:	9	

Tuition and Fees

Resident	6977
Average (public)	9500
Average (private)	22,500
Nonresident	20,077
Average (public)	20,500
Average (private)	24,500

0   10   20   30   40   50
(in thousands of dollars)

Percentage receiving financial aid: n/av

Introduction

A public university established in 1892, the University of Texas Medical Branch includes the School of Medicine, the School of Nursing, the Graduate School of Biomedical-Sciences, and the School of Allied Health Sciences. Galveston, a barrier reef island of approximately 47 square miles, has about 70,000 residents.

Admissions

Undergraduate degree waived only in exceptional cases. Besides the basic premedical science courses, an additional year of biological sciences and English, and 1 half-year of calculus are required. A very limited number of nonresidents accepted. *Transfer and advanced standing:* Transfer students accepted into third year.

Curriculum

4-year modern. *First academic period:* (32 weeks) Includes gross and developmental anatomy, microscopic anatomy, biochemistry, cells and genes, physi-

ology and biophysics, neuroscience, plus medical ethics, integrated functional laboratories, and introduction to patient evaluation. *Second academic period:* (42 weeks) Includes pathology, microbiology, endocrinology, immunology, pharmacology and toxicology, preventive medicine and community health, and introduction to clinical medicine, continuation of introduction to patient evaluation and integrated functional laboratories from the first year. *Third academic period:* (52 weeks) Covers clerkships in internal medicine, surgery, obstetrics-gynecology, family medicine, pediatrics, and psychiatry. Lectures and clinical exposure in anesthesiology, dermatology, medical jurisprudence, ophthalmology, and otolaryngology are given during the clerkships. Each student is assigned a faculty advisor to assist in developing individualized experience in clinical medicine. *Fourth academic period:* This period consists of 40 weeks; 36 weeks are elective courses. Electives may be taken either on campus or at other institutions with approval of the faculty advisor. The elective experience is flexible and can be designed to meet individual career goals. Two weeks clerkship in neurology and a 2-day certification in advanced cardiac life support are required.

Grading and Promotion Policies

Letter/number grades in required courses and Pass/Fail in electives. No student will be promoted until all work of a given grading sequence is completed and passed. Students must record passing total scores on the USMLE Steps 1 and 2 prior to graduation.

Facilities

Teaching: The basic sciences are taught at the Libby Moody Thompson Basic Sciences and Clinical Sciences Buildings. John Sealy Hospital (the principal clinical service and teaching facility), 6 other hospitals, and 2 outpatient clinics make up the Medical Branch Hospitals Complex. Other separately owned and operated hospitals offer educational and research opportunities. *Other:* The Clinical Study Center is an independent 12-bed unit located in the John Sealy Hospital. The Shriners Hospital for Crippled Children, Galveston Burn Unit is located on the campus and staffed largely by faculty members. The Birth Defects Center is involved in research and provides programs to help afflicted children under 15. *Library:* The Moody Medical Library houses about 240,000 bound books and subscribes to about 3000 biomedical periodicals. *Housing:* Limited dormitory rooms and housing are available through fraternities on campus.

Special Features

Minority admissions: An active recruitment program is conducted by the school's Office of Special Programs. A summer Medical School Familiarization Program, a postbaccalaureate program, and a Hispanic Center for Excellence in Medical Education program are available to assist minority disadvantaged college students interested in a career in medicine. *Other degree programs:* Combined MD-PhD programs are available in the basic sciences and medical humanities.

University of Texas—Houston Medical School

P.O. Box 20708
Houston, Texas 77225

Phone: 713-500-5116 *Fax:* 713-500-0604
E-mail: ves@dean.med.uth.tmc.edu
WWW: http://www.med.uth.tmc.edu/

Application Filing		Accreditation
Earliest:	June 15	LCME
Latest:	October 15	
Fee:	$45	**Degrees Granted**
AMCAS:	no	MD, MD-PhD, MD-MPH

Enrollment: 1996–97 First-Year Class

Men:	106	53%	Applied:	3471
Women:	94	47%	Interviewed:	1041
Minorities:	42	21%	Enrolled:	200
Out of State:	55	28%		

1996–97 Class Profile

Mean MCAT Scores		*Mean GPA*
Physical Sciences:	8.8	3.44
Biological Sciences:	9.3	
Verbal Reasoning:	9	

Tuition and Fees

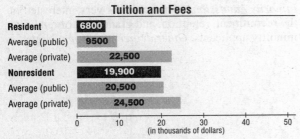

Resident	6800
Average (public)	9500
Average (private)	22,500
Nonresident	19,900
Average (public)	20,500
Average (private)	24,500

0   10   20   30   40   50
(in thousands of dollars)

Percentage receiving financial aid: 62%

Introduction

The University of Texas, which opened in 1883, consists of numerous schools, colleges, divisions, and branches distributed among 15 campuses in Texas. The University of Texas Health Science Center at Houston was established in 1972 and consists of the Medical School, Texas Dental College, schools of Nursing and Allied Health Sciences, and other institutions.

Admissions

In addition to the basic premedical science courses, 1 year of advanced biology, 1 year of English, and one-half year of college calculus are required. *Transfer and advanced standing:* None.

Curriculum

4-year traditional. Technical skills course through all 4 years. *First year:* Basic sciences plus courses in genetics and immunology. *Second year:* Integrated problem-based learning curriculum in behavioral science, pathology, pharmacology, fundamentals of clinical medicine, physical diagnosis, and reproductive biology. *Third year:* Required clerkships in the major specialties. *Fourth year:* Required clerkships in neurology, family practice, internal medicine, and surgery, and a 4-week period in epidemiology, clinical medicine, medical ethics, and medical jurisprudence. Also, electives consisting of four 1-month blocks.

Grading and Promotion Policies

System used is 5-cohort: Honors/High Pass/Pass/Marginal Performance/Fail.

Facilities

Teaching: The basic sciences are taught in the Medical School Building. Clinical teaching takes place at Hermann Hospital, Lyndon Baines Johnson County Hospital, University of Texas M. D. Anderson Cancer Center, Shriner's Hospital, St. Joseph Hospital, and Southwest Memorial Hospital. *Library:* The Houston Academy of Medicine-Texas Medical Center Library has more than 100,000 volumes; the 25,000-volume M.D. Anderson Cancer Center Library is another valuable asset. *Housing:* The UT student housing complex is located at Cambridge and El Paso, approximately 1 mile from the Texas Medical Center. Two student resident halls are located within the medical center.

Special Features

Minority admissions: There is an active recruitment program. *Other degree programs:* Combined MD-PhD programs are available through the UT-Houston Graduate School of Biomedical Sciences, in a variety of disciplines. A combined MD-MPH program is also available.

University of Texas Medical School at San Antonio

7703 Floyd Curl Drive
San Antonio, Texas 78284

Phone: 210-567-2665   *Fax:* 210-567-2685
E-mail: eliker@uthscsa.edu
WWW: http://www.uthscsa.edu/

Application Filing		Accreditation	
Earliest:	April 15	LCME	
Latest:	October 15		
Fee:	$35	**Degrees Granted**	
AMCAS:	no	MD	

Enrollment: 1996–97 First-Year Class

Men:	111	56%	Applied:	3400
Women:	89	45%	Interviewed:	1020
Minorities:	30	15%	Enrolled:	200
Out of State:	15	8%		

1996–97 Class Profile

Mean MCAT Scores		*Mean GPA*
Physical Sciences:	10	3.38
Biological Sciences:	10	
Verbal Reasoning:	10	

Tuition and Fees

Resident	6825
Average (public)	9500
Average (private)	22,500
Nonresident	19,925
Average (public)	20,500
Average (private)	24,500

(in thousands of dollars)

Percentage receiving financial aid: 85%

Introduction

The University of Texas Medical School is part of the University of Texas Health Science Center at San Antonio, which is located within the South Texas Medical Center. The Health Science Center consists of the Medical School, Dental School, and Graduate School of Biomedical Sciences. The school is located in the northwest section of the city in an area preserved to provide a rural-type setting.

Admissions

Aside from the basic premedical science courses, 1 additional year of biology, 1 year of English, and 1 semester of calculus are required. A few nonresidents are admitted. *Transfer and advanced standing:* Not possible at the present time.

Curriculum

4-year semimodern. *First year:* Spans the disciplines of biochemistry, anatomy, and systems physiology, to human ecology and the rudiments of human and clinical relationships. *Second year:* Pathology and pharmacology are covered, and 5 introductory courses are given for the major clinical disciplines (medicine, surgery, obstetrics-gynecology, pediatrics, and psychiatry). *Third year:* Clerkship rotation through the major clinical specialties and surgical subspecialties. *Fourth year:* Consists of 2 months of didactic courses, 28 weeks of electives, and 8 weeks of optional vacation time.

Grading and Promotion Policies

All final grades are reported as letter grades. Any student encountering academic difficulty shall be provided an opportunity to make up deficiencies and improve performance.

Facilities

The basic sciences are taught in the Medical School Building. Clinical teaching takes place at the University Hospital, the Brady/Green Community Health Center, the VA Hospital, and 3 other affiliated institutions. Research laboratories are located in the Medical School Building. *Library:* The library is also located in the Medical School Building. *Housing:* Information not available.

Special Features

Minority admissions: The school is very interested in the recruitment, retention, and graduation of qualified minority applicants. *Other degree programs:* None.

University of Texas Southwestern Medical School at Dallas

5323 Harry Hines Boulevard
Dallas, Texas 75235

Phone: 214-648-2670 *Fax:* 214-648-3289
E-mail: admissions@mednet.swmed.edu
WWW: http://www.swmed.edu/

Application Filing		Accreditation	
Earliest:	April 15	LCME	
Latest:	October 15		
Fee:	$45	**Degrees Granted**	
AMCAS:	no	MD, MD-PhD	

Enrollment: 1996–97 First-Year Class

Men:	120	60%	Applied:	3418
Women:	81	40%	Interviewed:	1367
Minorities:	22	11%	Enrolled:	201
Out of State:	32	16%		

1996–97 Class Profile

Mean MCAT Scores		*Mean GPA*
Physical Sciences:	10	3.6
Biological Sciences:	10	
Verbal Reasoning:	10	

Tuition and Fees

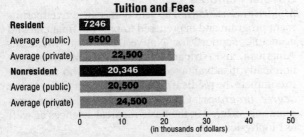

Resident	7246
Average (public)	9500
Average (private)	22,500
Nonresident	20,346
Average (public)	20,500
Average (private)	24,500

(in thousands of dollars)

Percentage receiving financial aid: n/av

Introduction

The University of Texas Southwestern Medical School was established in 1943. In 1949 the medical college became the Southwestern Medical School of the University of Texas, and in 1954 it was changed to the University of Texas Southwestern Medical School at Dallas. In 1972 the name and scope of the medical school were changed with its reorganization into the University of Texas Health Sciences Center at Dallas consisting of the Southwestern Medical School, Graduate School of Biomedical Sciences, and the School of Allied Health Sciences.

Admissions

In addition to the basic premedical science courses, an extra year of biology (or zoology), 1 semester of calculus, and 1 year of English are required. *Transfer and advanced standing:* Usually none.

Curriculum

4-year semitraditional. *First year:* Medical biochemistry, biology of cell and tissues, human anatomy and embryology, human behavior, medical physiology, neurobiology, introduction to clinical medicine I, endocrinology and human reproduction. *Second year:* Introduction to clinical medicine II, immunology and medical microbiology, anatomic and clinical pathology, medical pharmacology, and psycopathology. *Third and fourth years:* Divided into blocks and allocated to internal medicine, surgery, obstetrics/gynecology, pediatrics, neurology, family practice, and psychiatry. All instruction pertaining to these departments is given within its own block of time. About half of the fourth year is open to electives.

Grading and Promotion Policies

Traditional letter grading system within which D and F are failing grades. Each student's performance is computed on the basis of a system of quantitative and qualitative weighting. A student incurring a failing grade may be asked by the Promotions Committee to withdraw from school, to repeat the year's work, or to remove the deficiency by some other means. Satisfactory performance on Step 1 of the USMLE is required prior to promotion to the fourth year.

Facilities

Teaching: The 60-acre main campus serves as the focus of a large medical complex that includes Parkland Memorial Hospital, Children's Medical Center, St. Paul Hospital, Zale Lipshy University Hospital, City of Dallas Health Department, and Southwestern Institute of Forensic Sciences. *Other:* James W. Aston Ambulatory Care Center, Animal Resources Center, and Fred F. Florence Bioinformation Center. A 20-year master plan for 30 acres north of the main campus calls for 6 research towers, a support services building, an energy plant and underground parking, in addition to the Mary Nell and Ralph B. Rogers Magnetic Resonance Center. Affiliated teaching facilities include Baylor University Medical Center, John Peter Smith Hospital (Fort Worth), Charlton Methodist Hospital, Presbyterian Hospital of Dallas, Timberlawn Psychiatric Hospital, University of Texas Health Science Center at Tyler, and Veterans' Administration Medical Center. *Library:* The library has a collection of 175,000 volumes and receives 2400 serials annually. *Housing:* No on-campus housing is available.

Special Features

Minority admissions: The school has an active minority student recruitment program. *Other degree programs:* Combined MD-PhD programs are offered in a variety of disciplines including molecular biophysics, cell regulation, genetics and development, molecular microbiology, neuroscience, biochemistry and molecular biology and immunology. A combined MD-Oral Maxillofacial Surgery residency program is offered to candidates who have graduated from dental school.

UTAH

University of Utah School of Medicine

50 North Medical Drive
Salt Lake City, Utah   84132

Phone: 801-581-7498   *Fax:* 801-585-3300
E-mail: mylonakis@deans.med.utah.edu
WWW: http://www.med.utah.edu/

Application Filing		Accreditation	
Earliest:	June 1	LCME	
Latest:	October 15		
Fee:	$50	**Degrees Granted**	
AMCAS:	yes	MD, MD-PhD	

Enrollment: 1996–97 First-Year Class

Men:	61	61%	Applied:	1409
Women:	39	39%	Interviewed:	437
Minorities:	2	2%	Enrolled:	100
Out of State:	25	25%		

1996–97 Class Profile

Mean MCAT Scores		*Mean GPA*
Physical Sciences:	10.5	3.6
Biological Sciences:	10.6	
Verbal Reasoning:	10	

Tuition and Fees

Resident	7362
Average (public)	9500
Average (private)	22,500
Nonresident	15,111
Average (public)	20,500
Average (private)	24,500

(in thousands of dollars) 0 10 20 30 40 50

Percentage receiving financial aid: n/av

Above data applies to 1995–96 academic year.

Introduction

The University of Utah School of Medicine is part of the University of Utah Health Sciences Center along with the University of Utah Hospital, the College of Pharmacy, the College of Nursing and Health, and the Spencer S. Eccles Health Sciences Library. The School of Medicine was originally founded as a 2-year school in 1905, and expanded to a 4-year program in 1943.

Admissions (AMCAS)

Requirements include the basic premedical science courses and 1 year of English. Also, inorganic chemistry should include work in qualitative and quantitative analysis. About 75% of entering students are Utah residents; approximately 50% of out-of-state students are from WICHE states.

Curriculum

4-year semitraditional. *First year:* Major courses in anatomy, biochemistry, and physiology and their relationships to clinical application. *Second year:* Major courses include pharmacology, pathology, microbiology, nutrition, and introductory courses in physical diagnosis. Electives are available. *Third year:* Rotation in the major clinical specialties. Student is assigned patients for study and is responsible for the patient's history, physical examination, and the laboratory work necessary to make the diagnosis. *Fourth year:* Entirely composed of elective time during which independent programs are arranged for each student.

Grading and Promotion Policies

An evaluation on an Honors Pass/Pass/Fail basis and a description of student performance are submitted by the faculty. Students must take Steps 1 and 2 of the USMLE and record scores.

Facilities

Teaching: All preclinical instruction can be received within the Medical Center. Most of the clinical training is obtained in the University Hospital and the VA Hospital. *Other:* Five hospitals in Salt Lake City and 2 in Ogden are affiliated. *Library:* The library contains more than 100,000 volumes and 1750 current medical journal subscriptions. *Housing:* Board and room are available in residence halls for single students; there are also apartments for married students.

Special Features

Minority admissions: The school has an active recruitment program and is prepared to provide financial and academic support for Native American, Mexican-American, and African-American students from economically disadvantaged communities who are likely to complete the medical curriculum successfully. *Other degree programs:* Combined MD-PhD degree programs are offered in the basic medical sciences as well as biophysics.

VERMONT

University of Vermont College of Medicine

Burlington, Vermont 05405

Phone: 802-656-2154
WWW: http://www.salus.uvm.edu/

Application Filing		Accreditation
Earliest:	June 1	LCME
Latest:	November 1	
Fee:	$75	**Degrees Granted**
AMCAS:	yes	MD, MD-PhD

Enrollment: 1996–97 First-Year Class

Men:	38	41%	Applied:	8362
Women:	55	59%	Interviewed:	585
Minorities:	12	13%	Enrolled:	93
Out of State:	54	58%		

1996–97 Class Profile

Mean MCAT Scores		*Mean GPA*
Physical Sciences:	9	3.34
Biological Sciences:	9	
Verbal Reasoning:	9.2	

Tuition and Fees

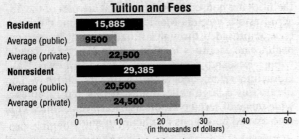

Resident	15,885
Average (public)	9500
Average (private)	22,500
Nonresident	29,385
Average (public)	20,500
Average (private)	24,500

(in thousands of dollars)

Percentage receiving financial aid: n/av

Introduction

The University of Vermont College of Medicine was founded in 1822 and is the seventh oldest college in the United States. The school acknowledges the need for primary care physicians, clinical specialists, and research scientists; thus, the curriculum provides for a fundamental background in the basic and clinical sciences and structured training to meet individual goal should students wish to specialize.

Admissions (AMCAS)

In addition to the required premedical science courses, applicants are urged to pursue a broad and balanced educational program during their undergraduate years. Priority for admission is given to residents of Vermont, but there are usually a significant number of places available for applicants from other states. *Transfer and advanced standing:* The makeup of the curriculum, the limited clinical facilities, and the minimal student attrition generally precludes accepting transfer students.

Curriculum

4-year. *Basic Science Core:* (57 weeks) Both introductory and advanced basic sciences are covered during this period. *Clinical Science Core:* (48 weeks) Instruction in clinical sciences and work within the hospitals and clinics. Instruction is based on the care of patients by means of clerkships in the major specialties. *Selective period:* (72 weeks) This final academic period is devoted to a combination of electives and requirements. Individually designed experiences fulfill chosen-pathway requirements and student needs.

Grading and Promotion Policies

System used is Honors/Pass/Fail. Taking Steps 1 and 2 of the USMLE is optional.

Facilities

Teaching: There is a 3-building medical college complex: a 492-bed teaching hospital (the Fletcher Allen Health Care) and 2 affiliated teaching hospitals in Plattsburgh, New York and in Portland, Maine. *Other:* Research facilities are located within the medical school complex and off campus. *Library:* The medical library has approximately 100,000 bound volumes and receives 1400 periodicals. *Housing:* Limited dormitory accommodations are available on campus for medical students. The majority of students find furnished rooms or furnished/unfurnished apartments and houses within easy walking or bicycling distance of the campus.

Special Features

Minority admissions: The College of Medicine is committed to increasing cultural diversity in the academic community. All people, regardless of ethnic background, are encouraged to apply for admission. *Other degree programs:* Combined MD-PhD programs are offered in a variety of basic science disciplines.

VIRGINIA

Eastern Virginia Medical School of the Medical College of Hampton Roads

721 Fairfax Avenue
Norfolk, Virginia   23507

Phone: 804-446-5812   *Fax:* 804-446-7468
E-mail: sic@worf.evms.edu
WWW: http://www.evms.edu

Application Filing		Accreditation
Earliest:	June 1	LCME
Latest:	November 15	
Fee:	$80	**Degrees Granted**
AMCAS:	yes	MD

Enrollment: 1996–97 First-Year Class

Men:	50	50%	Applied:	7278
Women:	50	50%	Interviewed:	560
Minorities:	4	4%	Enrolled:	100
Out of State:	19	19%		

1996–97 Class Profile

Mean MCAT Scores		*Mean GPA*
Physical Sciences:	10	3.32
Biological Sciences:	10	
Verbal Reasoning:	10	

Tuition and Fees

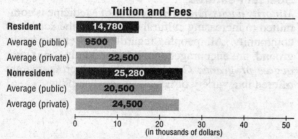

Resident	14,780
Average (public)	9500
Average (private)	22,500
Nonresident	25,280
Average (public)	20,500
Average (private)	24,500

0   10   20   30   40   50
(in thousands of dollars)

Percentage receiving financial aid: 91%

Introduction

The Eastern Virginia Medical School's purpose was to provide the Hampton Roads community with health care and offer students a quality medical education; consequently, major focus has been on the training of potential primary care physicians. This goal is achieved by the school's affiliations with more than 35 community-based health care facilities in the area.

Admissions (AMCAS)

Applicants must have a minimum of 100 semester hours from an accredited American or Canadian college or university, which must include the basic premedical science courses. Applicants are expected to have grades of C or better in all required courses. Credits earned in advanced placement programs or CLEP are acceptable. No application will be considered complete without scores of the MCAT taken within 2 years prior to application. *Transfer and advanced standing:* Transfer students for second and third years are considered. Applicant must be currently enrolled in an LCME-approved medical school. Applicants are considered to fill places vacated by attrition.

Curriculum

4-year. *Years 1 and 2:* The basic sciences are presented as a basis for the practice of medicine. Small-group, problem-based sessions with basic and clinical scientists as facilitators are utilized. Students receive introductory education in clinical and interpersonal skills and attend preceptorships with a physician in private practice. *Years 3 and 4:* Students rotate through clinical clerkships in family medicine, internal medicine, obstetrics and gynecology, pediatrics, psychiatry, and surgery, and through selectives designed to meet special interests and career goals.

Grading and Promotion Policies

Students are promoted on the basis of their ability to complete required objectives satisfactorily, with achievement being designated as Honors, High Pass, Pass, Fail, or Incomplete.

Facilities

Teaching: The school's primary teaching and research facilities are housed in buildings that are part of the 33-acre Eastern Virginia Medical Center. Clinical experience is provided through affiliation with 29 medical health care facilities located within Hampton Roads. *Other:* Research facilities are located in Lewis Hall, Hofheimer Hall, and South Campus. *Library:* The library has a large collection of books and receives a wide range of serial periodicals. *Housing:* Limited college-owned housing is available for students.

Special Features

Minority admissions: Educationally disadvantaged students are encouraged to apply and scholarships are available. *Special programs:* No combined programs are currently available.

Medical College of Virginia Virginia Commonwealth University

MCV Box 565
Richmond, Virginia   23298

Phone: 804-828-9629   *Fax:* 804-828-7628
E-mail: mack@som1.vcu.edu
WWW: http://www.vcu.edu

Application Filing		Accreditation	
Earliest:	June 1	LCME	
Latest:	November 15		
Fee:	$75	**Degrees Granted**	
AMCAS:	yes	MD, MD-PhD	

Enrollment: 1996–97 First-Year Class

Men:	101	59%	Applied:	5302	
Women:	71	41%	Interviewed:	318	
Minorities:	15	9%	Enrolled:	172	
Out of State:	50	29%			

1996–97 Class Profile

Mean MCAT Scores		*Mean GPA*
Physical Sciences:	9.5	3.45
Biological Sciences:	9.7	
Verbal Reasoning:	9.6	

Tuition and Fees

Resident	10,677
Average (public)	9500
Average (private)	22,500
Nonresident	25,288
Average (public)	20,500
Average (private)	24,500

0   10   20   30   40   50
(in thousands of dollars)

Percentage receiving financial aid: n/av

Introduction

This school originated when Hampden-Sidney College created a medical department in Richmond in 1837, which in 1854 became the Medical College of Virginia, an independent institution. In 1893 the College of Physicians and Surgeons was established, which consolidated with Medical College of Virginia in 1913. Currently this institution consists of schools of Medicine, Dentistry, Nursing, Pharmacy, and Allied Health Professions.

Admissions (AMCAS)

Requirements include the basic premedical science courses, 1 year of mathematics, and 1 year of English. Preference is given to those with baccalaureate degrees; residents preferred. *Transfer and advanced standing:* Transfer students are considered only into the third year when vacancies occur. Residents are given preference.

Curriculum

4-year semimodern. *First and second years:* The basic sciences are covered in the first 2 years. The body is divided into organ systems to permit integration of the basic science disciplines with one another and with the clinical aspects. Behavioral science, preventive medicine, public health, pathogenesis, emergency care, and physical diagnosis are also taught during this interval. *Third year:* This year is devoted to rotation through the major clinical specialties. Also included are courses in community practice and in neurology. *Fourth year:* Consists of 4 weeks devoted to clinical rotation in emergency room, and 4 weeks in an acting internship. A 3-week update course in clinical science is offered at the end of the year. The balance of the year consists of 4-week rotations in various electives.

Grading and Promotion Policies

Grades of Honors/High Pass/Pass/Fail are determined by the faculty. Steps 1 and 2 of the USMLE must be taken to record a score.

Facilities

Teaching: Classrooms and laboratories for the basic medical sciences are in Sanger Hall, McGuire Hall Annex, and the Egyptian Building. Clinical teaching is done at the Medical Center, which consists of the West, Main, and North Hospitals, at the A. D. Williams Memorial Clinic and at the VA Hospital. *Other:* Students in their third year spend a month in 1 of 5 community hospitals located in Richmond or in nearby cities or towns. *Library:* The comprehensive collections of the Tompkins-McCaw Library support study and research needs. *Housing:* Cabaniss Hall, a 432-bed dormitory, and 4 residence halls provide for student housing needs.

Special Features

Minority admissions: The director of the college's Health Careers Opportunity Program (HCOP) is actively involved in recruitment of minority students. The college also offers a Pre-Admissions Study Skills Workshop and a Summer Institute. *Other degree programs:* Combined MD-PhD programs are available in a variety of disciplines including biometry, biophysics, and genetics.

University of Virginia School of Medicine

Charlottesville, Virginia 22908

Phone: 804-924-5571 *Fax:* 804-982-2586
WWW: http://www.med.virginia.edu/home.html

Application Filing		Accreditation
Earliest:	June 1	LCME
Latest:	November 1	
Fee:	$50	**Degrees Granted**
AMCAS:	yes	MD, MD-PhD

Enrollment: 1996–97 First-Year Class

Men:	73	53%	Applied:	4879
Women:	66	47%	Interviewed:	1122
Minorities:	21	15%	Enrolled:	139
Out of State:	48	35%		

1996–97 Class Profile

Mean MCAT Scores		*Mean GPA*
Physical Sciences:	10.5	3.54
Biological Sciences:	10.2	
Verbal Reasoning:	10	

Tuition and Fees

Resident	10,598
Average (public)	9500
Average (private)	22,500
Nonresident	22,982
Average (public)	20,500
Average (private)	24,500

(in thousands of dollars) — scale 0 to 50

Percentage receiving financial aid: 81%

Introduction

Thomas Jefferson established the University of Virginia in 1819. As one of the 8 original schools, the School of Medicine was established in 1900 with a full 4-year instructional plan. The School of Medicine and the University of Virginia Hospital are both located on the same campus in Charlottesville. Its location is within driving distance of Richmond and Washington, D.C. The university ranks high in published surveys.

Admissions (AMCAS)

The basic premedical science courses are required. Preference is given to residents. *Transfer and advanced standing:* State residents receive preference for transfer into the third year.

Curriculum

4-year modern. The curriculum is divided into 4 major components. *Basic sciences:* (18 months) Provides a basic knowledge, both psychological and physical, of the structure of the normal and diseased human.

Clinical clerkships: (11 months) Provides a learning experience by direct contact with patients. *Electives:* (8 months) Offers clinical rotations, graduate courses, or research activities.

Grading and Promotion Policies

A letter grading system is used except in the fourth year, where Pass/Fail is used in grading electives. Students who have satisfactorily completed all the work of the session are eligible for promotion. Those who have incurred deficiencies that can be reasonably removed by the opening of the next session may be provisionally promoted. Students with serious deficiencies may be required to repeat the session's work. Students who are not considered competent to continue training in medicine may be required to withdraw. Students must record a score only on Step 1 of the USMLE, but must record a passing total score on Step 2 to graduate.

Facilities

Teaching: Students join faculty members in conducting basic and clinical research to help solve some of today's medical problems. They are aided by special facilities, including the central electron microscope facility, lymphocyte culture center, and protein and nucleic acid sequencing center. Many of these facilities are located in Harvey E. Jordan Hall, which also houses classrooms and laboratories for the 5 basic sciences. *Other:* Other facilities include several vivarium sites and research buildings in the Medical Center complex, adjacent to historic Central Grounds, and the University of Virginia Hospitals, licensed for 900 beds, including the main hospital, Blue Ridge Hospital, and Children's Rehabilitation Center. Students also receive clinical training at other hospitals in Virginia. *Library:* The Claude Moore Health Sciences Library contains 140,000 volumes and receives approximately 3000 publications. *Housing:* Limited housing is available for married students who may or may not have children.

Special Features

Minority admissions: The school has an active recruitment program. It also offers a Summer Enrichment Program for senior college students and graduates and applicants who have been accepted for admission. *Other degree programs:* Combined MD-PhD degree programs are offered in the basic sciences and jointly with other departments of the Graduate School or School of Engineering.

WASHINGTON

University of Washington School of Medicine

Seattle, Washington 98195

Phone: 206-543-7212
E-mail: patf@u.washington.edu
WWW: http://www.hslib.washington.edu/hsc/
som.html

Application Filing		Accreditation	
Earliest:	June 15	LCME	
Latest:	January 15		
Fee:	$35	**Degrees Granted**	
AMCAS:	yes	MD, MD-PhD	

Enrollment: 1996–97 First-Year Class

Men:	82	49%	Applied:	3603
Women:	84	51%	Interviewed:	829
Minorities:	18	11%	Enrolled:	166
Out of State:	75	45%		

1996–97 Class Profile

Mean MCAT Scores		*Mean GPA*
Physical Sciences:	10	3.58
Biological Sciences:	10.4	
Verbal Reasoning:	10	

Tuition and Fees

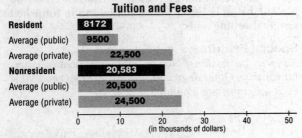

Resident	8172
Average (public)	9500
Average (private)	22,500
Nonresident	20,583
Average (public)	20,500
Average (private)	24,500

0   10   20   30   40   50
(in thousands of dollars)

Percentage receiving financial aid: 80%

Introduction

As the only medical school that directly provides educational service to Washington, Alaska, Montana, and Idaho (WAMI), the University of Washington School of Medicine was established in 1945. In 1971 the School of Medicine instituted a program to provide a decentralized medical education and a variety of educational opportunities. Through the WAMI program, basic science education and clinical training is offered in sites throughout the 4 states.

Admissions (AMCAS)

The basic premedical science courses and proficiency in mathematics and English are required. Preference is given to legal residents of the states of Washington, Alaska, Montana, and Idaho (WAMI Program). In addi-

tion, out-of-region minority group applicants will be considered. *Transfer and advanced standing:* None.

Curriculum

4-year modern. *First year:* The introductory basic sciences are taught in relation to their clinical relevance. Courses in epidemiology, psychology, and molecular and cellular biology are offered as well as an introduction to clinical medicine course. *Second year:* The advanced basic sciences are taught within a systems context. In addition, courses are offered in genetics, hematology, and health care systems. *Third and fourth years:* Students select from a variety of elective clerkships after completing the prescribed clerkships.

Grading and Promotion Policies

A system of Honors/Satisfactory/Not satisfactory is used. A passing total score must be recorded on Steps 1 and 2 of the USMLE to graduate.

Facilities

Teaching: Clinical teaching programs are conducted in the Health Sciences Building and in the University Hospital. *Other:* Other affiliated hospitals in the city and throughout the Pacific Northwest provide opportunities for clinical training. *Library:* A comprehensive medical library is available for students and staff. *Housing:* Information not available.

Special Features

Minority admissions: No students are admitted to the medical school on a preferential basis, but the school is interested in considering as many qualified applicants as it can from minority groups regardless of residence. *Other degree programs:* Combined MD-PhD programs are available in the basic sciences.

WEST VIRGINIA

Marshall University School of Medicine

1542 Spring Valley Drive
Huntington, West Virginia 25704

Phone: 304-696-7312 *Fax:* 304-696-7272
WWW: http://www.medicus.marshall.edu/

Application Filing		Accreditation
Earliest:	June 1	LCME
Latest:	November 15	
Fee:	$30	**Degrees Granted**
AMCAS:	yes	MD, MD-PhD, MD-MS

Enrollment: 1996–97 First-Year Class

Men:	31	65%	Applied:	1156
Women:	17	35%	Interviewed:	289
Minorities:	9	19%	Enrolled:	48
Out of State:	3	6%		

1996–97 Class Profile

Mean MCAT Scores		*Mean GPA*
Physical Sciences:	8.7	3.4
Biological Sciences:	8.8	
Verbal Reasoning:	9.6	

Tuition and Fees

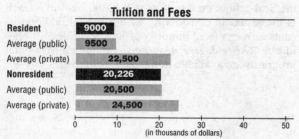

Resident	9000
Average (public)	9500
Average (private)	22,500
Nonresident	20,226
Average (public)	20,500
Average (private)	24,500

(in thousands of dollars)

Percentage receiving financial aid: 80%

Introduction

Marshall University was founded in 1837, but the School of Medicine was not established until 1978. The Marshall University School of Medicine was established under the Veteran's Administration Medical School Assistance and Health Training Act. The school offers a community-based program with emphasis on the education of primary care physicians.

Admissions (AMCAS)

The basic premedical science courses, English composition and rhetoric, and social or behavioral science are required. Preference is given to state residents. Some positions may be available to well-qualified nonresidents from states contiguous to West Virginia or to nonresidents who have strong ties to West Virginia. *Transfer and advanced standing:* Not available.

Curriculum

4-year semitraditional. *First year:* The basic medical sciences courses of anatomy, physiology, medical cell and molecular biology, neurosciences, and biochemistry are supplemented by a clinical interdepartmental course entitled introduction to patient care, which covers physical diagnosis and behavioral medicine. *Second year:* Includes pharmacology, pathology, microbiology, genetics, psychopathology, biostatistics, epidemiology, community medicine, physical diagnosis, immunology, and introduction to clinical medicine. *Third year:* 8-week rotations in 6 clinical specialties. Several rural health care programs are available for students who demonstrate special interest in primary care medicine. *Fourth year:* Consists of 4-week blocks in medicine, surgery, rural ambulatory care, and emergency medicine, and 19 weeks of electives.

Grading and Promotion Policies

A letter grading system is used. The Academic Standards Committee administers promotions. Students must record passing total scores on Steps 1 and 2 of the USMLE for promotion to the third year and graduation, respectively.

Facilities

Teaching: The school is affiliated with the Cabell Huntington Hospital (363 beds), St. Mary's Hospital (440 beds), VA Medical Center, and hospitals and clinics in other communities. *Library:* The medical library collection is available to students as well as faculty and is constantly expanding its holdings. *Housing:* Housing is available in university dormitories and in furnished family dwelling units.

Special Features

Minority admissions: No special recruitment program is available. *Other degree programs:* MS-MD and MD-PhD programs are available.

West Virginia University School of Medicine

Morgantown, West Virginia   26506

Phone: 304-293-3521   *Fax:* 304-293-7968
E-mail: dhall@wvu.edu
WWW: http://www.wvu.edu/som/

Application Filing		Accreditation	
Earliest:	June 1	LCME	
Latest:	November 15		
Fee:	$30	**Degrees Granted**	
AMCAS:	yes	MD, MD-PhD	

Enrollment: 1996–97 First-Year Class

Men:	44	50%	Applied:	1448
Women:	44	50%	Interviewed:	290
Minorities:	7	8%	Enrolled:	88
Out of State:	3	3%		

1996–97 Class Profile

Mean MCAT Scores		*Mean GPA*
Physical Sciences:	8.9	3.4
Biological Sciences:	9.3	
Verbal Reasoning:	9.1	

Tuition and Fees

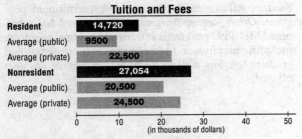

Resident	14,720
Average (public)	9500
Average (private)	22,500
Nonresident	27,054
Average (public)	20,500
Average (private)	24,500

(in thousands of dollars)

Percentage receiving financial aid: 80%

Introduction

The West Virginia School of Medicine first opened in 1902, but did not begin to provide a 4-year program until 1960 when the University Hospital opened. The school became known as the West Virginia University Health Sciences Center, Charleston Division, in 1972 when the Charleston Area Medical Center joined the university. In 1974 the Wheeling Division of the Health Sciences Center was established. It is currently known as the Robert C. Byrd Sciences Center of West Virginia University. Beside the School of Medicine, the Center contains schools of Dentistry, Nursing, and Pharmacy.

Admissions

Requirements include the basic premedical science courses and 1 year each of English and of behavioral or social sciences. Minimum of 3 years of college work. *Transfer and advanced standing:* Transfer applications for admission to the third-year class are accepted from medical students who are in good academic and professional standing at LCME-accredited schools.

Curriculum

4-year semitraditional. *First and second years:* Introductory and advanced basic sciences. Student is introduced to community medicine and clinical medicine, including the foundations for histories and physicals. The first-year basic science courses are integrated through common test methods and through problem-based learning clinical applications. *Third year:* The traditional clerkships, including neurology and family practice. *Fourth year:* 50% required rotations, 50% electives. Third- and fourth-year experiences are primarily based in Ruby Memorial Hospital or Charleston Area Medical Center, with some approved rotations at other institutions. During the third and fourth years, students spend a minimum total of 3 months in rural clinic locations.

Grading and Promotion Policies

All courses are graded on an Honors/Satisfactory/Unsatisfactory grading system. These designations are accompanied by a narrative report of the student's progress. Taking and passing Steps 1 and 2 of the USMLE is required.

Facilities

Teaching: The Basic Sciences Building opened for instructional purposes in 1957. Ruby Memorial Hospital opened in 1988; adjoining is the new Physician Office Center. Also on the Health Sciences Campus are the Chestnut Ridge Psychiatric Hospital, Mountainview Regional Rehabilitation Hospital, and a cancer center. *Library:* The Health Sciences Center Library has more than 265,000 bound volumes and 60,000 monograph titles, and receives 2227 journals. The Library and Health Sciences Center provide free internet access to National Library of Medicine data bases for affiliated students, faculty, and staff. Special services are offered to support medical students on rural rotations. *Housing:* The university maintains 7 residence halls, 2 for men and 5 for women, as well as efficiency and 1-bedroom apartments.

Special Features

Minority admissions: The school has a minority recruitment program and offers a 1-month summer enrichment program. *Other degree programs:* Combined MD-PhD programs are offered in the basic medical sciences and 3 other disciplines.

WISCONSIN

Medical College of Wisconsin

8701 Watertown Plank Road
Milwaukee, Wisconsin   53226

Phone: 414-456-8246

Application Filing		Accreditation	
Earliest:	June 1	LCME	
Latest:	November 1		
Fee:	$60	**Degrees Granted**	
AMCAS:	yes	MD, MD-PhD	

Enrollment: 1996–97 First-Year Class

Men:	133	65%	Applied:	7772
Women:	71	35%	Interviewed:	622
Minorities:	8	4%	Enrolled:	204
Out of State:	110	54%		

1996–97 Class Profile

Mean MCAT Scores		*Mean GPA*
Physical Sciences:	9.6	n/av
Biological Sciences:	9.6	
Verbal Reasoning:	9.5	

Tuition and Fees

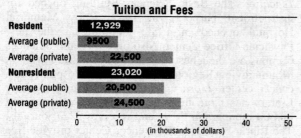

Resident	12,929
Average (public)	9500
Average (private)	22,500
Nonresident	23,020
Average (public)	20,500
Average (private)	24,500

(in thousands of dollars)

Percentage receiving financial aid: n/av

Above data applies to 1995–96 academic year.

Introduction

The Medical College of Wisconsin, originally part of Marquette University, was founded in the 1890s. It is the educational division of the Milwaukee Regional Medical Center, which also contains 6 other health care institutions. The college relocated its educational facilities in 1978, from downtown Milwaukee to the Medical Center campus in the west suburban section of the city.

Admissions (AMCAS)

Required courses include minimum premedical science courses plus 1 year each of college English and algebra (if not taken in high school). A significant number of nonresidents are accepted. *Transfer and advanced standing:* Data not available.

Curriculum

4-year semitraditional. *First and second years:* Basic medical sciences, in addition to a new course that pro-vides first- and second-year students with integrated early generalist experiences, the foundation skills and attitudes of professional development, and knowledge in the following disciplines: human behavior, bioethics and care of the terminally ill, information management, physical diagnosis, and health care systems. *Third and fourth years:* This time is devoted to rotating clerkships in major and some minor specialties. Two months of electives, including study at another school, are offered during senior year.

Grading and Promotion Policies

A 5.0 grading system (Honors/High Pass/Pass/Low Pass/Fail) is used. Students must take Step 1 of the USMLE and record a passing total score for promotion to the fourth year. Step 2 must be taken and a score reported.

Facilities

Teaching: Clinical instruction takes place at 5 major hospitals: John L. Doyne Hospital, Froedtert Memorial Lutheran Hospital, VA Hospital, Children's Hospital of Wisconsin, and Milwaukee Psychiatric Hospital. *Library:* A comprehensive medical library is available for student and staff use. *Housing:* Information not available.

Special Features

Minority admissions: The school's Office of Minority Student Affairs conducts an active recruitment program. *Other degree programs:* The school has combined MD-PhD programs in the basic medical sciences, including biophysics. MS programs in biostatistics and epidemology, as well as an MA in bioethics are also offered.

University of Wisconsin Medical School

1300 University Avenue
Madison, Wisconsin 53706

Phone: 608-263-4925 *Fax:* 608-262-2327
E-mail: janice,waisman@mail.admin.wisc.edu
WWW: http://www.biostat.wisc.edu/homepage.html/

Application Filing			Accreditation	
Earliest:	June 1		LCME	
Latest:	November 1			
Fee:	$38		**Degrees Granted**	
AMCAS:	yes		MD, MD-PhD, MD-MS	

Enrollment: 1996–97 First-Year Class

Men:	71	50%	Applied:	3034
Women:	72	50%	Interviewed:	212
Minorities:	21	15%	Enrolled:	143
Out of State:	25	17%		

1996–97 Class Profile

Mean MCAT Scores		*Mean GPA*
Physical Sciences:	9.5	3.51
Biological Sciences:	9.7	
Verbal Reasoning:	9.4	

Tuition and Fees

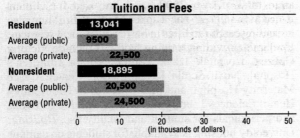

Resident	13,041
Average (public)	9500
Average (private)	22,500
Nonresident	18,895
Average (public)	20,500
Average (private)	24,500

(in thousands of dollars)

Percentage receiving financial aid: n/av

Above data applies to 1995–96 academic year.

Introduction

In 1907 the University of Wisconsin Medical School was established as a 2-year program and did not become a 4-year program until 1924. At present, the University of Wisconsin Center for Health Sciences incorporates the Medical School, University Hospital, Clinics, Psychiatric Research Institute, schools of Pharmacy, Nursing, and Allied Health Sciences, and the State Hygiene Laboratory.

Admissions (AMCAS)

The basic premedical sciences are required as well as 1 year of mathematics. An advanced biology course is required. English, biochemistry, and calculus are recommended. Few nonresidents are accepted. *Transfer and advanced standing:* Very few transfers accepted into third-year class.

Curriculum

4-year semimodern. The curriculum emphasizes active learning; interdisciplinary teaching by the basic science and clinical faculty throughout the first year and second year; a 4-year generalist curriculum with a focus on health risk assessment, prevention, common illnesses and outcomes; clinical clerkships around the state, including inner city and rural sites with an 8-week community-based outpatient primary care clerkship in the third year and an 8-week preceptorship with an experienced clinician in the fourth year. The senior year provides extensive elective opportunities for study at other institutions and abroad.

Grading and Promotion Policies

Examinations are given at the end of each semester during the first and second years and at the end of the third and fourth years. Grades, recorded by letter or number, are given by a committee of faculty members. Students must record a passing total score on Step 1 of the USMLE for promotion to the third year and on Step 2 for graduation.

Facilities

Teaching: The school's major teaching facility is the University of Wisconsin Hospitals, consisting of 6 hospitals under one administration. There are also Bardeen Laboratories for teaching and research and the McArdle Laboratory for cancer research. *Other:* The Medical Science Building provides research laboratories, and the Service Memorial Institute houses research laboratories, teaching laboratories, and lecture rooms. The State Hygiene Laboratory is concerned with the diagnosis, control, and eradication of communicable diseases, and the Genetics Building accommodates classrooms and laboratories. *Library:* The William S. Middleton Medical Library holds about 150,000 volumes and receives about 2000 serial publications. *Housing:* Students live in either rooms or apartments with other students. Married students are eligible for housing in the University Eagle Heights Apartments.

Special Features

Minority admissions: Recruitment is coordinated by the Office of Student Services. Accepted students can enter a summer program. *Other degree programs:* Combined MD-PhD and MD-MS degrees are offered in the basic sciences.

CANADA

Dalhousie University Faculty of Medicine

Halifax, Nova Scotia, Canada   B3H 4M4

Phone: 902-494-1874   *Fax:* 902-494-8884
E-mail: brenda-deticane@ dal.ca.

Application Filing		Accreditation	
Earliest:	October 1	LCME, CACMS	
Latest:	November 15		
Fee:	$55	**Degrees Granted**	
AMCAS:	no	MD	

Enrollment: 1996–97 First-Year Class

Men:	49	53%	Applied:		800
Women:	43	47%	Interviewed:		800
Minorities:	1	1%	Enrolled:		92
Out of State:	15	16%			

1996–97 Class Profile

Mean MCAT Scores		*Mean GPA*
Physical Sciences:	10	n/av
Biological Sciences:	10	
Verbal Reasoning:	10	

Tuition and Fees

Resident	5745
Average (public)	9500
Average (private)	22,500
Nonresident	8145
Average (public)	20,500
Average (private)	24,500

0   10   20   30   40   50
(in thousands of dollars)

Percentage receiving financial aid: n/av
Average tuition shown is for U.S. schools.

Introduction

Dalhousie University is a nondenominational, privately endowed, coeducational university that was founded in 1818. It is located in a residential area of Halifax on the Atlantic coast of Canada. The Faculty of Medicine was established in 1868 and is responsible for providing physicians for the 3 maritime provinces of Nova Scotia, New Brunswick, and Prince Edward Island.

Admissions

In addition to the basic premedical science courses, requirements include a minimum GPA of 3.30, 1 year of English and taking the MCAT. Individuals are regularly accepted who have had other careers and choose to enter medicine later in life. Preference is given to residents of the Maritime Provinces of Nova Scotia, New Brunswick, and Prince Edward Island. *Transfer and advanced standing:* Transfer students are accepted only under special circumstances.

Curriculum

4-year semimodern. *First year:* (37 weeks) Core courses in the introductory basic sciences, some advanced basic sciences, some clinical and system courses, and electives. *Second year:* (37 weeks) Several systems courses, psychiatry, preventive medicine, pharmacology, patient contact, and electives. *Third year:* Mostly systems courses with a pathophysiological perspective. Also courses in genetics, ophthalmology, otolaryngology, human sexuality, and electives. *Fourth year:* (52 weeks) 8-week clerkships in major specialties and 4-week clerkships in subspecialties. Also, a 4-week elective.

Grading and Promotion Policies

A letter or number is given in basic and clinical sciences, but a Pass/Fail system is used for electives. Students are assessed each year on aptitude and fitness for the medical profession. In addition, all required exams must be passed in order that a student may progress from one year to the next. Taking Step 1 of the USMLE is optional, but Step 2 is required.

Facilities

Teaching: The Tupper Medical Building provides facilities for basic science instruction, while hospitals in the area (total of over 2500 beds) are used for clinical instruction. *Other:* The Tupper Medical Building also houses research facilities in basic and clinical sciences. Hospitals providing training facilities include Victoria General Hospital, Izaak Walton Killam Children's Hospital, Nova Scotia Rehabilitation Center, Grace Maternity Hospital, and others. *Library:* The Kellogg Health Sciences Library has a large volume of books and periodicals for student and faculty use. *Housing:* University housing is available for students on campus as single rooms or shared apartments.

Special Features

There are no combined degree programs at this time.

Laval University Faculty of Medicine

Sainte-Foy, Quebec, Canada   G1K 7P4

Phone: 418-656-2492   *Fax:* 418-656-2733
E-mail: admission@facmed@ulaval.ca
WWW: http://www.fmed.ulaval.ca

Application Filing		Accreditation	
Earliest:	January 1	LCME, CACMS	
Latest:	February 1		
Fee:	$55	**Degrees Granted**	
AMCAS:	no	MD, MD-PhD, MD-MSc	

Enrollment: 1996–97 First-Year Class

Men:	41	38%	Applied:	1850
Women:	71	65%	Interviewed:	370
Minorities:	n/av	n/av	Enrolled:	109
Out of State:	4	4%		

1996–97 Class Profile

Mean MCAT Scores		*Mean GPA*
Physical Sciences:	n/av	n/av
Biological Sciences:	n/av	
Verbal Reasoning:	n/av	

Tuition and Fees

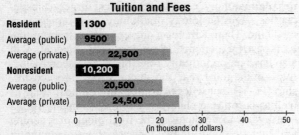

Resident	1300
Average (public)	9500
Average (private)	22,500
Nonresident	10,200
Average (public)	20,500
Average (private)	24,500

(in thousands of dollars)

Percentage receiving financial aid: n/av

Average tuition shown is for U.S. schools.

Introduction

Named after the first Bishop of Quebec, this private institution was established in 1852, after being granted a royal charter by Queen Victoria. Teaching instruction is in French.

Admissions

The basic premedical science courses plus mathematics through calculus are required. Applicants should have a good command of the French language as it is the language of instruction. Priority is given to residents of Quebec, but outstanding French-speaking students from other provinces and countries are considered. *Transfer and advanced standing:* Applications for transfer are not accepted.

Curriculum

4-year nontraditional. *First and second years:* One trimester of basic sciences, followed by 3 trimesters with an organ system-integrated approach plus courses in ethics, epidemiology, and the psychosocial aspects of medicine. Most teaching is done through small group discussion. *Third and fourth years:* Eleven weeks of primary clerkship followed by 18 months of clerkship rotation through the major clinical specialties including family medicine and social and preventive medicine. During this period, 3 months are devoted to electives.

Grading and Promotion Policies

Letter grades in basic sciences, required clinical sciences, and electives. Taking the USMLE is optional.

Facilities

Teaching: Clinical instruction takes place at 1 academic health center, 1 affiliated hospital, and 1 institute. Research facilities in most fields are available. *Library:* A comprehensive medical library is at the disposal of students and faculty. *Housing:* Accommodations are available for many students.

Special Features

Six combined MD-MSc and MD-PhD programs are available.

McGill University Faculty of Medicine

3655 Drummond Street
Montreal, Quebec, Canada   H3G 1Y6

Phone: 514-398-3517
E-mail: marlene@medusa.medcor.mcgill.ca

Application Filing		Accreditation	
Earliest:	September 1	LCME, CACMS	
Latest:	November 15		
Fee:	$60	**Degrees Granted**	
AMCAS:	no	MD, MD-PhD	

Enrollment: 1996–97 First-Year Class

Men:	56	51%	Applied:	1040
Women:	53	49%	Interviewed:	354
Minorities:	n/av	n/av	Enrolled:	109
Out of State:	29	27%		

1996–97 Class Profile

Mean MCAT Scores		*Mean GPA*
Physical Sciences:	10.8	3.55
Biological Sciences:	10.8	
Verbal Reasoning:	10	

Tuition and Fees

Resident	2660
Average (public)	9500
Average (private)	22,500
Nonresident	8454
Average (public)	20,500
Average (private)	24,500

(in thousands of dollars) 0 10 20 30 40 50

Percentage receiving financial aid: n/av

Average tuition shown is for U.S. schools.

Introduction

In 1823, 4 staff members of the recently opened Montreal General Hospital founded the Montreal Medical Institution where they gave lectures for medical students. The Faculty of Medicine was established in 1829. World-renowned physician William Osler taught from 1874 to 1884. McGill is located in the heart of Montreal.

Admissions

The faculty offers 4-year and 5-year programs of undergraduate medical education. Entrance to the 5-year program is restricted to Quebec residents enrolled in one of the Quebec Colleges of General and Professional Education. Entrants to the 4-year program are not restricted geographically and include approximately 19 U.S. students and 6 foreign students each year. Applicants must have a bachelor's degree or be in the final year of study leading to the degree, and must take the MCAT. *Transfer and advanced standing:* No transfer opportunities are foreseen in the future.

Curriculum

4-year. McGill University introduced a new curriculum for undergraduate medical education in August 1994. The new curriculum is composed of 4 components entitled Basis of Medicine (BOM), Introduction to Clinical Medicine (ICM), Practice of Medicine (POM), and Back to Basics (BTB). The BOM component occupies the first 18 months of medical school, ICM occurs in the second half of the second year, and POM is given in the third year and half of the fourth year. The BTB component occupies the remainder of the fourth year. Each component is composed of individual units of interdisciplinary basic science and clinical teaching. The BOM component consists of 10 system-based units and focuses on normal structure and function with a progression to abnormal structure and function, disease prevention, and therapy. There will be a significant interdisciplinary coordinated clinically based aspect to all of this teaching. In addition, 2 units, Introduction to the Patient and Introduction to the Practice of Medicine, will permit early introduction of students into the hospital. In January of the second year, the students will begin their full-time activity in the hospitals (ICM). This will commence with a course devoted to clinical skills, physical diagnosis, medical ethics and jurisprudence, and doctor-patient communication skills. The students will subsequently participate in clinical rotations in medicine, medical subspecialties, dermatology, neurology, surgery, surgery subspecialties, anesthesiology, radiology, and emergency medicine. There will be an ongoing ambulatory outpatient-based experience in primary care. Students will also have an opportunity for clinical or research electives. In the third year, the students will enter a clerkship (POM) that will cover all major clinical areas as well as permitting elective time. From January of the fourth year to graduation, the final block of teaching will include opportunities to learn about medicine in society, molecular medicine, and selected topics in basic science as applied to clinical medicine.

Grading and Promotion Policies

Grading is on a Pass/Fail basis. A student is evaluated by each unit and students with academic difficulties are reviewed by a Faculty Promotions Committee.

Facilities

Teaching: There are 5 university teaching hospitals, 3 specialty teaching hospitals, and 14 special research centers and units. Classroom instruction is carried out mainly in the McIntyre Medical Sciences Building. Research opportunities are provided in all of the basic medical sciences and in many fields of clinical medicine. *Library:* The Medical Library contains approximately 200,000 volumes and an excellent journal collection. The Osler Library has a large collection in medical history and biography. *Housing:* Housing for approximately 1000 students is available.

Special Features

An MD-PhD program is available in a variety of disciplines for students planning careers involving research.

McMaster University School of Medicine

1200 Main Street West
Hamilton, Ontario, Canada   L8N 3Z5

Phone: 905-525-9140   *Fax:* 905-527-2707
E-mail: otrosinacfhs.csu.mcmaster.ca
WWW: http://www.fhs.mcmaster.ca/nd prog

Application Filing		Accreditation	
Earliest:	July 1	LCME, CACMS	
Latest:	November 1		
Fee:	$25	**Degrees Granted**	
AMCAS:	yes	MD	

Enrollment: 1996–97 First-Year Class

Men:	27	27%	Applied:	2900
Women:	73	73%	Interviewed:	203
Minorities:	n/av	n/av	Enrolled:	100
Out of State:	n/av	n/av		

1996–97 Class Profile

Mean MCAT Scores		*Mean GPA*
Physical Sciences:	n/app	n/av
Biological Sciences:	n/app	
Verbal Reasoning:	n/app	

Tuition and Fees

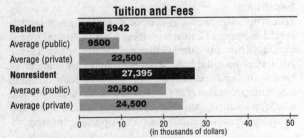

Resident	5942
Average (public)	9500
Average (private)	22,500
Nonresident	27,395
Average (public)	20,500
Average (private)	24,500

(in thousands of dollars)

Percentage receiving financial aid: n/av

Average tuition shown is for U.S. schools.

Introduction

The School of Medicine at McMaster University admitted its first student in 1969. It offers both undergraduate and postgraduate medical education programs. The McMaster University Health Sciences Center provides extensive hospital and ambulatory facilities for the clinical training of its students.

Admissions

Completion of at least 3 years of university degree credit work and an overall B average are required. Priority is given to Ontario, out-of-province, and then out-of-country applicants for purposes of determining the pool of those to be interviewed. Applicants need not take the MCAT. Nonbiology majors are given the same consideration as students with a more scientific orientation. *Transfer or advanced standing:* Not available.

Curriculum

3-year (130 weeks) semimodern. Small-group tutorials, self-directed problem-based learning. The curriculum is divided into 6 units as follows: *Unit 1* (16 weeks): Introduction. *Units 2, 3, 4* (39 weeks): Comprehensive analysis of human structure, function, and behavior organized around the organ systems of the body. *Unit 5* (12 weeks): Life cycle dealing with health care problems along the conception to death continuum. *Unit 6* (48 weeks): The clerkships. There is also a 6-week period of revision at the end of the programs. *Electives:* The program includes 26 weeks of electives designed to encourage in-depth study in portions of the medical program. The program also includes horizontal electives that run concurrently with the 3-year program. The entire program works on a full-year schedule.

Grading and Promotion Policies

A Pass/Fail system is used. Taking the USMLE is optional.

Facilities

Teaching: The Health Sciences Centre provides classroom area for basic sciences instruction and contains a 371-bed teaching hospital. The major hospitals in Hamilton also provide clinical teaching for the McMaster program. *Other:* The Health Sciences Centre also houses research facilities. *Library:* The Health Science Library provides a large number of periodicals, clinical science references, and audiovisual materials for student use. *Housing:* Information not available.

Special Features

No combined programs are currently available.

Memorial University of Newfoundland Faculty of Medicine

Prince Phillip Drive
St. John's, Newfoundland, Canada   A1B 3V6

Phone: 709-737-6615   *Fax:* 709-737-5186
E-mail: munmed@morgan.ucs.mun.ca
WWW: http://www.aorta.library.mun.ca./med/
admission/

Application Filing		Accreditation
Earliest:	July 1	LCME, CACMS
Latest:	January 15	
Fee:	$50	**Degrees Granted**
AMCAS:	no	MD, MD-PhD

Enrollment: 1996–97 First-Year Class

Men:	35	57%	Applied:	654
Women:	26	43%	Interviewed:	183
Minorities:	n/av	n/av	Enrolled:	61
Out of State:	18	30%		

1996–97 Class Profile

Mean MCAT Scores		*Mean GPA*
Physical Sciences:	9	n/av
Biological Sciences:	9	
Verbal Reasoning:	9	

Tuition and Fees

Resident	6450
Average (public)	9500
Average (private)	22,500
Nonresident	33,440
Average (public)	20,500
Average (private)	24,500

0   10   20   30   40   50
(in thousands of dollars)

Percentage receiving financial aid: n/av

Average tuition shown is for U.S. schools.

Introduction

Memorial University of Newfoundland was established in St. John's, Newfoundland in 1925; it was granted full university status in 1949. The campus extends over 220 acres and the university offers a broad range of programs.

The Faculty of Medicine awarded its first degrees in 1973. It is located in the Health Sciences Centre, on the northwest corner of the main university campus along with the schools of Nursing and Pharmacy, and St. John's General Hospital.

Admissions

A bachelor's degree is required. In exceptional circumstances, an application may be considered from someone who does not hold a bachelor's degree; such an applicant will have completed at least twenty 1-semester courses at a recognized university or university college, and be a student who has work-related or other experience acceptable to the admissions committee. The course of study must include 2 courses in English. All applicants must take the MCAT. Preference is given to residents of Newfoundland, Labrador; however, a number of places are available for residents of other parts of Canada as well as non-Canadians. *Transfer and advanced standing:* Only in exceptional circumstances.

Curriculum

4-year. *First year:* Courses are offered in cell and whole body structure and function, behavioral science, and community medicine. Patient contact is established in work in varied medical settings in the community. *Second and third years:* Instruction is based on a systems approach with an integration of anatomy, physiology, pathology, and introductory clinical studies. *Fourth year:* Rotating clerkships through the major specialties. Four months of elective study are included in the 4-year course. Elective study may be either research or clinical in nature.

Grading and Promotion Policies

A Pass/Fail system is used. Taking the USMLE is optional.

Facilities

Teaching: The medical school complex includes the Health Sciences Centre with its medical sciences teaching facilities and the General Hospital (531 beds). Affiliated hospitals in St. John's and other areas of Newfoundland participate in the school's clinical teaching programs. *Library:* A biomedical library and research facilities are also part of the medical complex. *Housing:* Accommodations on campus are limited.

Special Features

Combined MD-PhD programs are available on request.

Queen's University Faculty of Medicine

Kingston, Ontario, Canada   K7L 3N6

Phone: 613-545-2542   *Fax:* 613-545-6884
E-mail: cumpsona@post.queensu.ca

Application Filing		Accreditation	
Earliest:	July 1	LCME, CACMS	
Latest:	November 1		
Fee:	$75	**Degrees Granted**	
AMCAS:	yes	MD	

Enrollment: 1996–97 First-Year Class

Men:	46	61%	Applied:	1548
Women:	29	39%	Interviewed:	433
Minorities:	n/av	n/av	Enrolled:	75
Out of State:	n/av	n/av		

1996–97 Class Profile

Mean MCAT Scores		*Mean GPA*
Physical Sciences:	11	n/av
Biological Sciences:	11	
Verbal Reasoning:	10.4	

Tuition and Fees

Resident	4273
Average (public)	9500
Average (private)	22,500
Nonresident	n/app

0   10   20   30   40   50
(in thousands of dollars)

Percentage receiving financial aid: n/av

Average tuition shown is for U.S. schools.

Introduction

One of the integral components of this university is the Faculty of Medicine, established in 1954. The city of Kingston, in which the campus is located, is on Lake Ontario at the origin of the St. Lawrence River. The goal of the school is to provide a broad medical education and to train medical students for specialized postgraduate education.

Admissions

Candidates must be Canadian citizens, Canadian landed immigrants prior to the closing date for receipt of applications, or the children of Queen's University alumni who reside outside Canada.

Curriculum

4-year semimodern. The curriculum emphasizes a great degree of independent student learning and the promotion of the art and the science of medicine, in order to prepare students for a changing health care system. A systems-based approach integrating biomedical and clinical sciences is used in order to emphasize rel-evance and avoid undue repetition. There is a decreased emphasis on lectures and an increase in independent study time and electives. *Phase I:* Emphasizes selected principles and concepts in the sciences basic to medicine both for an understanding of these sciences and for their relevance and importance to clinical medicine. *Phase II:* Uses clinical-based learning, such as selected clinical topics that will provide a framework for integrating basic and clinical sciences. Instruction in clinical skills is integrated with each systems-based component of Phase II. *Phase III:* The clinical clerkship is an integral part of the MD program, with structured elements that build upon Phase I and II and an additional phase, as well as specific elements and clinical experiences unique to Phase III. *Additional Phase:* Introduces broad themes and specific topics and integrates these where appropriate into Phases I, II, and III.

Grading and Promotion Policies

An Honors/Pass/Fail system is used. Taking the USMLE is optional.

Facilities

Teaching: Botterell Hall is the major facility, housing the library, some student facilities, and major classrooms; the departments of anatomy, biochemistry, microbiology and immunology, pharmacology and toxicology, and physiology; a national cancer institute research group of the department of pathology; and animal facilities. The department of pathology has its major facility in the Richardson Laboratory, which is connected to Kingston General Hospital. Etherington Hall, devoted to clinical teaching and research, is also connected to KGH and contains a major auditorium. *Other:* Other major facilities include Abramsky Hall, major research space in the Hotel Dieu Hospital, and in the LaSalle Building. *Library:* The Health Sciences Library contains about 100,000 volumes and more than 1400 serials, and offers interlibrary loan service. *Housing:* Information not available.

Special Features

There are no combined degree programs at this time.

Université de Sherbrooke Faculté de Médecine

Sherbrooke, Quebec, Canada   J1H 5N4

Phone: 819-564-5208   *Fax:* 819-564-5378
E-mail: mmoreau@courrier.usherb.ca

Application Filing		Accreditation	
Earliest:	November 1	LCME, CACMS	
Latest:	March 1		
Fee:	$30	**Degrees Granted**	
AMCAS:	no	MD, MD-MS, MD-PhD	

Enrollment: 1996–97 First-Year Class

Men:	37	38%	Applied:	1562
Women:	51	52%	Interviewed:	1562
Minorities:	n/av	n/av	Enrolled:	98
Out of State:	16	16%		

1996–97 Class Profile

Mean MCAT Scores		*Mean GPA*
Physical Sciences:	n/app	n/av
Biological Sciences:	n/app	
Verbal Reasoning:	n/app	

Tuition and Fees

Resident	3014
Average (public)	9500
Average (private)	22,500
Nonresident	11,697
Average (public)	20,500
Average (private)	24,500

(in thousands of dollars)

Percentage receiving financial aid: n/av

Average tuition shown is for U.S. schools.

Introduction

Admitting its first class in 1966, this French-speaking institution is part of the developing Health Sciences Centre, which includes a modern teaching hospital and a department of nursing.

Admissions

Admission is based primarily on ability and premedical achievement as demonstrated by scholastic records. A learning skills test will also be included in selection for admission in 1997. Seventy-four places are reserved for applicants from the province of Quebec. Fifteen additional places are reserved for applicants from New Brunswick for admission in 1997 and 20 places will be reserved for admission in 1998. There is also 1 place available for an applicant from Prince Edward Island. Two places are available for qualified foreign applicants with a student visa. Applicants must be fluent in both written and spoken French. The school is a French-teaching institution. *Transfer and advanced standing:* Information not available.

Curriculum

The form of teaching is a problem-based learning program. Formal lecturing has been reduced to a minimum. Audiovisual facilities, seminars, small group discussions, panels, field work, and case studies are used extensively. Most learning sessions integrate many disciplines representing various departments. Students work in the hospital from the beginning of their first year.

Grading and Promotion Policies

Grading is on a 4-point basis, A = 4. Evaluations are made by examination results and reports of professors on student progress. A grade of C, based on these exams and evaluation reports, must be obtained for promotion at fourth year's end. Taking the USMLE is optional.

Facilities

As required by modern medical teaching, the Faculté de Médecine is integrated into a developing Health Sciences Centre to serve all members of the health team. This centre includes a modern 700-bed teaching hospital. Twelve hospitals, many health centres, and CLSC are affiliated with the Faculté de Médecine. *Library:* An on-campus biomedical library containing a large number of bound volumes and periodicals is available for use by students and faculty. *Housing:* On campus housing is available.

Special Features

Combined degree programs are available at the MS-MD and MD-PhD levels to students with outstanding academic records.

University of Alberta Faculty of Medicine

2-45 Medical Sciences Building
Edmonton, Alberta, Canada   T6G 2H7

Phone: 403-492-6350
E-mail: silvia.franklin@ualberta.ca

Application Filing		Accreditation	
Earliest:	July 1	LCME, CACMS	
Latest:	March 1		
Fee:	$60	**Degrees Granted**	
AMCAS:	no	MD, MD-MS, MD-PhD	

Enrollment: 1996–97 First-Year Class

Men:	54	51%	Applied:	900
Women:	51	49%	Interviewed:	342
Minorities:	n/av	n/av	Enrolled:	105
Out of State:	10	10%		

1996–97 Class Profile

Mean MCAT Scores		*Mean GPA*
Physical Sciences:	n/av	n/av
Biological Sciences:	n/av	
Verbal Reasoning:	n/av	

Tuition and Fees

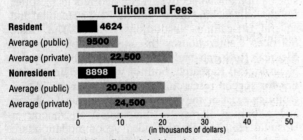

Resident	4624
Average (public)	9500
Average (private)	22,500
Nonresident	8898
Average (public)	20,500
Average (private)	24,500

(in thousands of dollars)

Percentage receiving financial aid: n/av

Average tuition shown is for U.S. schools.

Introduction

The university, established in 1908, is located in Edmonton, the capital of the province of Alberta. The Faculty of Medicine was founded in 1913 with a 3-year program. It subsequently became a 4-year MD degree program whose first class was graduated in 1925. In addition to the Medical School, the university has professional programs in dentistry, law, and library science.

Admissions

Requirements include the basic premedical sciences and courses in statistics and English. Preference is given to Alberta residents. Five percent of places are allocated to visa students. *Transfer and advanced standing:* School accepts transfer students only under exceptional circumstances and only from LCME-accredited institutions.

Curriculum

4-year semimodern. The first 2 years consist of instruction from September to May, while the last 2 years are a combined 86-week program with a 4-week vacation break. *Phase I:* One academic year of instruction covering most of the basic sciences and an introduction to clinical skills. *Phase II:* A 1-year program of interdepartmental teaching in a clinical setting relating clinical and basic medical sciences to human diseases. *Phase III:* Consists of rotating clerkships in affiliated hospitals with 10 weeks devoted to electives in a wide range of fields, also a selective in either geriatrics or rural family medicine. Students are encouraged to organize individual programs with career and special interests in mind.

Grading and Promotion Policies

Evaluations of student work are made at the conclusion of each phase of the program on the basis of performance on final, course, and interdisciplinary examinations. A number grading system is used. Each student must attain a GPA of at least 5.0 to progress to the next level of study. Taking both or any steps of the USMLE is optional.

Facilities

Teaching: The Faculty of Medicine is located on the campus of the University of Alberta. The Basic Sciences Building houses facilities for the teaching of basic science, and the 843-bed W. C. MacKenzie Health Sciences Centre provides for most of the clinical instruction. There are also several other hospitals affiliated with the school. *Other:* Facilities for research in experimental medicine are available at the Surgical-Medical Research Institute. The Cancer Research Institute is housed at the McEachern Cancer Research Laboratory. *Library:* A comprehensive medical library contains a large number of bound volumes and periodicals. *Housing:* There are residence halls available for single students and a 299-unit apartment building for married students.

Special Features

Combined MD-PhD programs are available in a variety of disciplines including immunology and pathology. An MD-MS program is also offered.

University of British Columbia Faculty of Medicine

2194 Health Sciences Mall
Vancouver, British Columbia, Canada   V6T 1Z3

Phone: 604-822-4482   *Fax:* 604-822-6061
E-mail: mark@medd.med.ubc.ca
WWW: http://www.med.ubc.ca

Application Filing		Accreditation	
Earliest:	August 15	LCME, CACMS	
Latest:	December 15		
Fee:	$105	**Degrees Granted**	
AMCAS:	no	MD, MD-PhD	

Enrollment: 1996–97 First-Year Class

Men:	61	51%	Applied:	597
Women:	59	49%	Interviewed:	597
Minorities:	n/av	n/av	Enrolled:	120
Out of State:	4	3%		

1996–97 Class Profile

Mean MCAT Scores		*Mean GPA*
Physical Sciences:	10.6	3.25
Biological Sciences:	10.4	
Verbal Reasoning:	9.8	

Tuition and Fees

Resident	4177
Average (public)	9500
Average (private)	22,500
Nonresident	n/app

0   10   20   30   40   50
(in thousands of dollars)

Percentage receiving financial aid: n/av
Average tuition shown is for U.S. schools.

Introduction

This school was initiated in 1950 and it is one component of the university, which has a variety of faculties and schools. The Health Sciences Center is located on the university campus, which contains an instructional resources center, and acute care and psychiatric hospitals.

Admissions

Required courses include the basic premedical sciences, 1 year of English, and 1 year of general biochemistry or cell biology. Residents of British Columbia are given priority. Applicants must have 3 years of college work and take the MCAT. A personal interview is advisable. Recommended courses include those in the humanities and behavioral sciences. *Transfer and advanced standing:* None.

Curriculum

4-year semitraditional. *First and second years:* For the first 2 years the program concentrates on the basic medical sciences. Instruction is given mainly on the university campus with some hospital teaching taking place during the second year. *Third and fourth years:* Instruction shifts entirely to the hospitals. The third year provides the essentials of modern diagnosis and treatment that students use in their work with hospital patients. By the fourth year, students have received enough experience through clerkships in major clinical specialties to enable them to practice medicine under supervision with increasing responsibility for patient care. A 6-week elective program is offered.

Grading and Promotion Policies

Grades are letter or percentage. Promotion is determined by the Faculty Committee at the end of each session. The committee also decides whether unsatisfactory work can be corrected by a special examination or by repeating the course, or if the failing student must withdraw from studies completely. Taking the USMLE is optional.

Facilities

Teaching: The Health Sciences Center on campus provides for teaching basic sciences. Included in the complex are research facilities, classrooms, and audiovisual equipment. Vancouver Hospital offers its facilities for clinical teaching along with St. Paul's Hospital and several off-campus institutions. *Other:* The Basic Sciences Center houses the Strong Laboratory for Medical Research and the Kinsman Laboratory for Neurological Research, both of which provide facilities for special research. *Library:* On-campus library facilities exist at the Woodward Biomedical Library and a branch library is maintained at Vancouver Hospital. *Housing:* Single student accommodations are available on a room or room-and-board basis. Married students can find a limited number of unfurnished suites.

Special Features

MD-PhD program offered.

University of Calgary Faculty of Medicine

3330 Hospital Drive, N.W.
Calgary, Alberta, Canada   T2N 4N1

Phone: 403-220-4262   *Fax:* 403-283-4740
E-mail: meyers@med.ucalgary.ca
WWW: http://www.med.ucalgary.ca/ume/infoda.html

Application Filing		Accreditation	
Earliest:	July 15	LCME, CACMS	
Latest:	November 30		
Fee:	$60	**Degrees Granted**	
AMCAS:	no	MD	

Enrollment: 1996–97 First-Year Class

Men:	27	39%	Applied:	1035
Women:	42	61%	Interviewed:	279
Minorities:	n/av	n/av	Enrolled:	69
Out of State:	1	1%		

1996–97 Class Profile

Mean MCAT Scores		*Mean GPA*
Physical Sciences:	10.2	3.62
Biological Sciences:	10.4	
Verbal Reasoning:	9.5	

Tuition and Fees

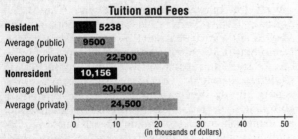

Resident	5238
Average (public)	9500
Average (private)	22,500
Nonresident	10,156
Average (public)	20,500
Average (private)	24,500

(in thousands of dollars)

Percentage receiving financial aid: n/av

Average tuition shown is for U.S. schools.

Introduction

The University of Calgary began in 1945 when the Calgary Normal School became a branch of the University of Alberta's Education Faculty. It moved to its current campus in northwest Calgary in 1960 and gained full autonomy as a degree-granting institution in 1966. The Faculty of Medicine was initiated in 1970 and established its facilities in the Calgary Health Science Centre in 1972.

Admissions

Priority is given to residents of Alberta, and non-Canadian citizens are not encouraged to apply. Applicants need not have a strict premedical background if their academic record is superior. The basic premedical science courses and biochemistry, cell biology, and physiology are recommended. The MCAT must be taken by the fall of the year before the one for which admission is sought. Final applicants will be required to attend an interview at Calgary. *Transfer and advanced standing:* Applications are considered from students attending LCME-accredited medical schools, but only for the final or clerkship year.

Curriculum

3-year (11 months). After graduation, the student usually takes at least 2 years of postgraduate work. The initial program provides a basic education, while the graduate work furnishes opportunity for specialization. The main emphasis is on problem solving, with patient contact and responsibility throughout the entire program. *First and second years:* A short introductory course prepares the student for the 9 body systems courses. In January of the second year, the Human Development block commences, covering topics from infancy to aging. An independent study program of 16 hours per week is time set aside secure from encroachment by scheduled curricular activities. Four hours a week are allotted for electives. *Third year:* Consists of clinical clerkships where the concepts taught in the first 2 years are applied. Elective programs are available.

Grading and Promotion Policies

Evaluation is made on a multidisciplinary basis and will test the student's factual knowledge and his/her ability to solve problems. Grading is on a Pass/Fail basis.

Facilities

Teaching: The Calgary Health Sciences Centre, which includes the University of Calgary Medical Clinic, provides a model of health care services, teaching and research areas, an audiovisual center, and space for labs, lecture halls, and study areas. Clinical teaching takes place at Foothills Hospital, Calgary General Hospital, and Alberta Children's Hospital. *Library:* The Health Sciences Library contains about 50,000 volumes and subscribes to about 2000 periodicals. An interlibrary loan service also exists. *Housing:* Both single and married student housing is available.

Special Features

A combined degree program is contemplated for the future.

University of Manitoba Faculty of Medicine

753 McDermot Avenue
Winnipeg, Manitoba, Canada   R3E 0W3

Phone: 204-789-3569   *Fax:* 204-774-8941
E-mail: porogge cc.umarituhc.ca

Application Filing		Accreditation	
Earliest:	September 1	LCME	
Latest:	November 30		
Fee:	$50	**Degrees Granted**	
AMCAS:	no	MD, MD-PhD	

Enrollment: 1996–97 First-Year Class

Men:	48	67%	Applied:	360	
Women:	24	33%	Interviewed:	244	
Minorities:	n/av	n/av	Enrolled:	72	
Out of State:	7	10%			

1996–97 Class Profile

Mean MCAT Scores		*Mean GPA*
Physical Sciences:	10.1	3.6
Biological Sciences:	10.1	
Verbal Reasoning:	9.7	

Tuition and Fees

Resident	4913
Average (public)	9500
Average (private)	22,500
Resident	4913
Average (public)	20,500
Average (private)	24,500

(in thousands of dollars)

Percentage receiving financial aid: n/av

Average tuition shown is for U.S. schools.

Introduction

The Manitoba Medical College was founded in 1883 and from its outset was affiliated with the University of Manitoba. Its name was changed to the Faculty of Medicine of the University of Manitoba. Its teaching facilities lie adjacent to the Health Sciences Centre in Winnipeg, and is some distance from the main university campus.

Admissions

Applicants must have completed a bachelor's degree. Coursework should include the basic premedical sciences plus a full course in English. Undergraduates and graduates of the universities in Manitoba are given preference. The MCAT is required. Only Canadian citizens or landed immigrants are eligible.

Curriculum

4-year semimodern. *First year:* Devoted to a study of normal human biology, both by individual disciplines and in an integrated manner, and the general mechanisms of disease. *Second year:* During the second year, the clinical sciences are studied. *Third and fourth years:* Consists of clinical clerkships in the major specialties, electives, and basic sciences review.

Grading and Promotion Policies

The Pass/Fail system is used. Taking the USMLE is optional.

Facilities

Teaching: The medical buildings are adjacent to the Health Sciences Centre, which contains the teaching hospitals General Centre (750 beds) and Children's Hospital (220 beds). Other hospitals are also utilized in the clinical training program and include the Deer Lodge Veterans Hospital (500 beds), St. Boniface General Hospital (570 beds), Seven Oaks Hospital (336 beds), Misericordia Hospital (409 beds), Grace Hospital (300 beds), and Victoria Hospital (254 beds). *Library:* A comprehensive medical library serves student and faculty needs. *Housing:* Not available.

Special Features

Combined MD-PhD programs are offered in immunology, pharmacology, and physiology.

University of Montreal Faculty of Medicine

P.O. Box 6128, Station A
Montreal, Quebec, Canada   H3C 3J7

Phone: 514-343-6265

Application Filing		Accreditation	
Earliest:	May 15	LCME, CACMS	
Latest:	March 1		
Fee:	$55	**Degrees Granted**	
AMCAS:	yes	MD	

Enrollment: 1996–97 First-Year Class

Men:	65	40%	Applied:	2202
Women:	96	60%	Interviewed:	n/av
Minorities:	n/av	n/av	Enrolled:	161
Out of State:	10	6%		

1996–97 Class Profile

Mean MCAT Scores		*Mean GPA*
Physical Sciences:	n/av	n/av
Biological Sciences:	n/av	
Verbal Reasoning:	n/av	

Tuition and Fees

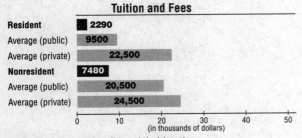

Resident	2290
Average (public)	9500
Average (private)	22,500
Nonresident	7480
Average (public)	20,500
Average (private)	24,500

(in thousands of dollars)

Percentage receiving financial aid: n/av

Above data applies to 1995–96 academic year.

Average tuition shown is for U.S. schools.

Introduction

The Faculty of Medicine was established in 1843. In 1891 the school merged with the Faculty of Medicine of the Montreal branch of Laval University. In 1920 the latter institution was granted independent status and the school became known by its present name. Instruction in the medical school is in French.

Admissions

A thorough knowledge of the French language is a prerequisite. All candidates accepted must be either Canadian citizens or landed immigrants. Under the present Quebec educational system, the minimum requirement is 2 years of college (Sciences Program). The college curriculum should provide a wide cultural background. Coursework must include philosophy, behavioral and social sciences, French, English, mathematics (analytical geometry, calculus, college algebra, and trigonometry), and the basic premedical sciences courses.

Curriculum

4-year. The first year of a 4-year program is devoted to basic biological and behavioral sciences. Clinical experience begins with this year. During the second year, morphology and function, both normal and abnormal, will be presented. Students must take 90 hours of elective learning. The third and fourth years consist of a clerkship of 80-week duration. Formal lecturing will be reduced to a minimum and replaced by active methods, especially problem-based learning and small-group discussion.

Grading and Promotion Policies

A letter grade system is used in basic sciences and in clinical sciences; Pass/Fail in electives.

Facilities

Teaching: Clinical instruction is carried out at 14 affiliated teaching hospitals and research centers. *Library:* A comprehensive medical library containing numerous bound volumes and periodicals is at the disposal of students and faculty. *Housing:* Information not available.

Special Features

Residency training in the teaching hospitals is under the direction of the Faculty of Medicine. Various courses and symposia are organized by the continuing medical education division.

University of Ottawa Faculty of Medicine

451 Smyth Road
Ottawa, Ontario, Canada   K1H 8M5

Phone: 613-787-6463
E-mail: admissions dlessqrd@ottawa.ca

Application Filing		Accreditation
Earliest:	July 1	LCME, CACMS
Latest:	November 1	
Fee:	$50	**Degrees Granted**
AMCAS:	yes	MD, BSc-MD

Enrollment: 1996–97 First-Year Class

Men:	39	46%	Applied:	1903
Women:	45	54%	Interviewed:	585
Minorities:	n/av	n/av	Enrolled:	84
Out of State:	9	11%		

1996–97 Class Profile

Mean MCAT Scores		*Mean GPA*
Physical Sciences:	10	3.4
Biological Sciences:	10	
Verbal Reasoning:	9	

Tuition and Fees

Resident	4040
Average (public)	9500
Average (private)	22,500
Nonresident	n/app

0   10   20   30   40   50
(in thousands of dollars)

Percentage receiving financial aid: n/av

Average tuition shown is for U.S. schools.

Introduction

This school began as a 2-year medical science program in 1926; a 4-year curriculum was introduced in 1953. In 1988 a 6-year curriculum was initiated, which includes a 2-year premedical program. The school prepares its students for careers in family medicine, specialty practice, and research.

Admissions

Successful completion of the first 2 years of a university program and of the basic premedical science courses is required. Only Canadian citizens or landed immigrants are considered for admission except in the case of children of alumni. *Transfer and advanced standing:* Not possible.

Curriculum

4-year semitraditional. *First and second years:* Stage 1 includes 70 weeks of study of essential biomedical principles and consists of 13 multidisciplinary blocks. The students learn clinical skills in an integrated fashion with the study of body systems. Stage 2, also 2 years, is devoted to clinical clerkships, and 16 weeks are available for elective study.

Grading and Promotion Policies

An Honors/Pass/Fail system is used. Taking the USMLE is optional.

Facilities

Teaching: The university's Health Science Building houses the facilities for basic science instruction. Clinical instruction takes place at Ottawa General Hospital (450 beds) and Ottawa Civic Hospital (900 beds). *Other:* Other facilities include Children's Hospital of Eastern Ontario (300 beds), Royal Ottawa Hospital (150 beds), and several smaller institutions. *Library:* The Health Sciences Library has 40,000 volumes and subscribes to about 2000 journals. *Housing:* Information is not available.

Special Features

A combined BSc-MD program is available.

University of Saskatchewan College of Medicine

Saskatoon, Saskatchewan, Canada   S7N 0W0

Phone: 306–966-8554   *Fax:* 306-966-6164
E-mail: pitzel@skyfox.usask.ca

Application Filing		Accreditation	
Earliest:	September 1	LCME, CACMS	
Latest:	December 1		
Fee:	$40	**Degrees Granted**	
AMCAS:	no	MD, BSc-MD	

Enrollment: 1996–97 First-Year Class

Men:	34	62%	Applied:	463
Women:	21	38%	Interviewed:	207
Minorities:	n/av	n/av	Enrolled:	55
Out of State:	5	9%		

1996–97 Class Profile

Mean MCAT Scores		*Mean GPA*
Physical Sciences:	n/av	n/av
Biological Sciences:	n/av	
Verbal Reasoning:	n/av	

Tuition and Fees

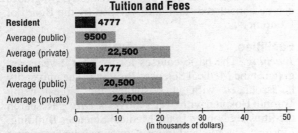

Resident	4777
Average (public)	9500
Average (private)	22,500
Resident	4777
Average (public)	20,500
Average (private)	24,500

0   10   20   30   40   50
(in thousands of dollars)

Percentage receiving financial aid: n/av

Average tuition shown is for U.S. schools.

Introduction

The University of Ottawa received its charter in 1866. Originally operated by a missionary order, it is presently managed by a board of governors representing the community. The Faculty of Medicine was established in 1945 and is now a component of the Faculty of Health Sciences, which also includes schools of Nursing and Human Kinetics. In 1989 the Faculty of Medicine resumed its independent status as an academic unit.

Admissions

Requirements include 2 full premedical years and the basic premedical science courses, English, and an elective in the social sciences or humanities. Priority is given to residents of Saskatchewan; however, 5 positions may be offered to out-of-province students. All applicants must be Canadian citizens or landed immigrants. Applicants are not required to take the MCAT.

Transfer and advanced standing: Not applicable at this college. For detailed information, contact the Admissions Secretary at the above address.

Curriculum

4-year. The curriculum is aimed at educating doctors for entrance into any phase of the medical profession. *First year:* Largely devoted to basic sciences and introductory clinical sciences. *Second year:* Includes bridging sciences—pathology, microbiology, immunology, pharmacology, and nutrition—and systems, clinical sciences, and concurrent courses. *Third year:* Continuation of systems, clinical sciences, and concurrent courses. *Fourth year:* Rotation clerkship through internal medicine, surgery, obstetrics/gynecology, pediatrics, psychiatry, family medicine, anesthesia, neurology, geriatric medicine, and electives.

Grading and Promotion Policies

Percentage grades are assigned for most courses; Pass/Fail for the others.

Facilities

Teaching: Basic sciences are taught in the Medical Building. Clinical instruction takes place at the University Hospital, connected with the Medical Building. *Other:* Other affiliated hospitals are St. Paul's, Saskatoon City Hospital, Regina General Hospital, and Plains Health Centre in Regina. *Library:* The Medical Building also houses the school library. *Housing:* Information not available.

Special Features

A BSc(medicine)-MD combined program is available.

University of Toronto Faculty of Medicine

Toronto, Ontario, Canada   M5S 1A8

Phone: 416-979-4901   *Fax:* 416-979-4936
E-mail: judy-irvine@utoronto.ca.
WWW: http://www.medicine.uti2.library.utoronto.ca.

Application Filing		Accreditation	
Earliest:	August 1	LCME, CACMS	
Latest:	November 1		
Fee:	$150	**Degrees Granted**	
AMCAS:	no	MD, MD-PhD	

Enrollment: 1996–97 First-Year Class

Men:	105	59%	Applied:	1759
Women:	72	41%	Interviewed:	352
Minorities:	n/av	n/av	Enrolled:	177
Out of State:	27	15%		

1996–97 Class Profile

Mean MCAT Scores		*Mean GPA*
Physical Sciences:	10.3	3.6
Biological Sciences:	10.3	
Verbal Reasoning:	10	

Tuition and Fees

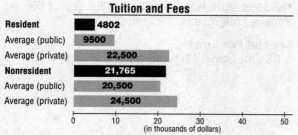

Percentage receiving financial aid: n/av

Average tuition shown is for U.S. schools.

Introduction

The Faculty of Medicine is the largest in all of Canada. It belongs to a university that can trace its origin back to Kings College, which was founded in 1843. The school is affiliated with 10 teaching hospitals. It was a site of several major medical breakthroughs that have had a profound impact on society. This includes the discovery of insulin, which facilitated the management of diabetes, and the development of the cardiac pacemaker, which permits an artificial regulation of the heart rate.

Admissions

Requirements include completion of 3 years at a Canadian university or, for applicants registered in a non-Canadian university, a recognized bachelor's degree. All applicants must have the following prerequisites: 2 full courses in the life sciences and 1 full course in humanities, social science, or language. Preference is given to residents of Ontario. Applicants must take the MCAT and have a personal interview. No preference for admission is given to science majors. *Transfer and advanced standing:* Transfer students from other medical schools are not considered because of enrollment limitations.

Curriculum

4-year semimodern. The curriculum is focused on student-centered learning. The pre-clerkship phase consists of 6 multidisciplinary courses, each of which is built upon a series of patient-based cases. Selected lectures, seminars, and laboratory exercises will complement small-group, problem-based learning sessions. The remainder of the 4 years is dedicated to the clinical clerkship, which will include a basic or junior component and specialty or senior component. During the clerkship phase, education occurs on the wards, in the laboratories, and in ambulatory care units of affiliated teaching hospitals.

Grading and Promotion Policies

Grades are given in both letter and percentage form, with in-course evaluations and examination scores being the principal means of determination. Each system and topic is graded. All evaluations must be passed for promotion to the next program of study. No grades can be considered final until verified by the Board of Examiners.

Facilities

Teaching: The basic courses for the first 2 years are given at the Medical Sciences Building. The university is associated with 11 hospitals, the largest being Toronto Hospital with over 1400 beds. *Other:* Research facilities are housed in the Medical Sciences Building. *Library:* The medical library contains a large volume of books and subscribes to many periodicals. *Housing:* Some university housing is available. For students unable to find accommodations on campus, the school maintains a list of local housing.

Special Features

A combined MD-PhD program is offered by the Faculty of Medicine and the School of Graduate Studies.

University of Western Ontario Faculty of Medicine

London, Ontario, Canada   N6A 5C1

Phone: 519-661-3744   *Fax:* 519-661-3797
E-mail: admissions@do.med.uwo.ca
WWW: http://www.med.uwa.ca

Application Filing		Accreditation	
Earliest:	November 1	LCME, CACMS	
Latest:	November 1		
Fee:	$50	**Degrees Granted**	
AMCAS:	yes	MD, MD-PhD, MSc-MD	

Enrollment: 1996–97 First-Year Class

Men:	63	64%	Applied:	1845	
Women:	36	36%	Interviewed:	387	
Minorities:	n/av	n/av	Enrolled:	99	
Out of State:	n/av	n/av			

1996–97 Class Profile

Mean MCAT Scores		*Mean GPA*
Physical Sciences:	8	n/av
Biological Sciences:	8	
Verbal Reasoning:	9	

Tuition and Fees

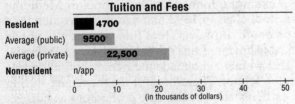

Resident	4700
Average (public)	9500
Average (private)	22,500
Nonresident	n/app

0   10   20   30   40   50
(in thousands of dollars)

Percentage receiving financial aid: n/av
Average tuition shown is for U.S. schools.

Introduction

The university originated in 1878 as the Western University of London, Ontario. The Faculty of Medicine was initiated in 1882 and became affiliated with the university in 1912, by which time the name had changed to the University of Western Ontario. The Medical School underwent various stages of growth and became closely associated with the Dental School, which was established in 1965. The university is a private school, but receives some government grants.

Admissions

Applications are considered only from Canadian citizens or permanent residents. Requirements include MCAT scores. Special detailed information should be secured from the Admission Office of the Faculty of Medicine.

Curriculum

4-year semitraditional. *Phase I:* Includes three 12-week trimesters, and work with patients begins early. Courses include the basic medical sciences and studies of the relationship between medicine and society. *Phase II:* Includes three 12-week trimesters with a continuation of basic science courses with a consideration of their connection with body systems. *Phase III:* A single 7-week semester focused on clinical work, with an introduction to clerkship. *Phase IV:* Consists of an integrated clinical clerkship (51 weeks), basic science options (6 weeks), and clinical science option blocks (16 weeks).

Grading and Promotion Policies

An Honors/Pass/Fail grading system is used, and taking the USMLE is optional.

Facilities

Teaching: Clinical teaching facilities exist at Victoria Hospital, University Hospital, and several other affiliated institutions. *Library:* A comprehensive medical library is available for student and staff use. *Housing:* Information not available.

Special Features

Combined MD-PhD programs are available. The latter include programs in the basic medical sciences as well as in biophysics, epidemiology, and biostatistics.

Opportunities for Women

Historical overview
Women's health issues
Medicine: a career for women
Doors are open
Admission to medical school
The woman physician: a status report
Unique challenges for women in medicine
Financial aid and support sources

HISTORICAL OVERVIEW

A summary of the history of medical education in the United States reveals the surprising observation that, in terms of acceptance of women into medical school, there is no consistent pattern.

Acceptances of women fluctuated widely until 1970 when a sustained increase ensued. That the road to women gaining admission into medical school has been long and hard may not always be evident. For example, Johns Hopkins School of Medicine accepted women with its first medical school class in 1893 and had more women than men in their entering class. It should be noted, however, that this situation is not as straightforward as it seems. The initial establishment of this school involved a substantial endowment from a group of Baltimore-area women who made their contribution dependent upon the acceptance of women into the school. Therefore, for the most part, during the nineteenth century women primarily participated in health care professions as nurses.

The first American woman medical graduate was Elizabeth Blackwell, who received her degree from (the now defunct) Geneva Medical College in New York in 1849. Prior to that, Harriet Hunt began to practice medicine in 1835 after gaining professional training by serving as an apprentice to a Boston physician. She had been repeatedly denied admission into all of the male medical schools.

Blackwell's acceptance was followed by a handful of other women. Those women who succeeded in getting into medical school seldom received clinical experience, as hospitals did not want women treating their patients. On the other hand, homeopathic and other nontraditional schools were more liberal regarding admission.

The educational opportunities for women improved somewhat when Philadelphia's Quakers established a school in 1850 exclusively for women, Medical College of Pennsylvania, (which became coeducational in 1969). This event probably motivated some eminent and enlightened male physicians in New York, Boston, and Chicago to contribute money and use their influence to establish all-women institutions in those three cities.

Unable to gain admission to U.S. schools, starting in the 1880s, women in large numbers went to such European cities as Paris and Zurich to secure a first-rate medical education; however, the struggle was far from over after they completed their medical studies because hospitals would not hire them. Therefore, Elizabeth Blackwell and her sister opened a 24-bed infirmary. (She also opened a medical school, as she was dissatisfied with the caliber of some of the graduates of women's colleges who were working for her.) Some women doctors went west, where they were welcomed because of the rough lifestyle in which circumstances often required prompt treatment of many trauma cases.

After the turn of the century, financial problems as well as the 1910 Flexner report resulted in the closing of some of the all-women medical schools and the merger of others. By 1919 only the original Philadelphia Medical School for Women remained.

When Johns Hopkins introduced coeducational medical training in 1893, other medical schools were encouraged to do the same. However, the door to the admission of women opened only a crack and unofficial quotas existed that kept the numbers of women down to an insignificant amount.

The reduction of male manpower during World War I resulted in a small increase in the number of women accepted into American schools (from 5 to 6%, as compared with 4.4% in 1900).

The longstanding problem for women to secure hospital experience remained and by the 1920s more than 90% of U.S. hospitals did not accept women and women did not attend institutions run by men.

World War II lowered the barriers to women gaining admission, since the number of qualified male applicants was limited. After the war, the numbers were once again made smaller so that women were making up only 5 to 8% of entering classes.

Since 1970 there has been a dramatic increase in the enrollment of women due to court decisions and the intense impact of the feminist movement, which swept aside the unofficial quota system.

WOMEN'S HEALTH ISSUES

A slow but gradual increase in interest in women's health issues is currently taking place. This is due to three factors:

1. women are demanding more from their health care provider;
2. a record number of women are being admitted to medical school;
3. more women have risen to positions where they can influence policy.

The standard reference patient, used in medical school until recently, was the 70 kilogram male. The special health needs of women, (except for female reproductive organs) were not addressed. Now the NIH has an Office of Research on Women's Health (ORWH) and has funded a more than half-billion-dollar 15-year Women's Health Initiative. Increasing numbers of physicians are taking continuing education courses dealing with woman's health, and medical schools are slowly introducing women's health into their curricula.

At one time, it was common practice for research projects to omit women from research trials. This was encouraged by the Thalidomide and DES tragedies of the 1960s and 1970s, which resulted in pregnant women and those with childbearing potential being prohibited by the FDA from participating in most drug trials. Moreover, the belief that the monthly hormonal changes in women could destabilize research results further served to restrict research studies to males.

In the early 1980s it was noted that the death rate from heart disease and cancer was the same for both sexes. Nevertheless, the 1982 landmark study of coronary artery disease was restricted to 15,000 males. As a result of intervention by some women in Congress, a task force was established in 1983 to examine the status of American women's health. In 1985 the task force reported, among other things, that the lack of attention to women's health issues had indeed "compromised the quality" of women's health care. Subsequently it was learned that only 13.5% of NIH funds went for research on women's health issues. Although NIH issued new guidelines to include women in clinical research study pools, even by 1990 the situation had not significantly changed. The appointment of the first female NIH director in 1992 led to the establishment of the Office of Research on Women's Health, whose permanency was confirmed by being included in the 1993 NIH Revitalization Act. This act mandated the inclusion of subpopulations (women and minorities) in all NIH-funded studies.

In 1992 the Council on Graduate Medical Education (COGME) identified 42 training components considered essential to preparing physicians to provide comprehensive health care for women. Internists and ob/gyn specialists are currently the principal health care providers for women. Both groups are fully trained to provide all these components. This has prompted self-education on women's health issues by physicians through continuing education courses. The American Medical Women's Association (AMWA) has sponsored development of a two-part course based on the life phases of women, rather than on organs.

While universities in the 1960s and 1970s integrated women's studies into their curricula, medical schools are only now just beginning to focus on women's health issues. Several residency programs have also undertaken initiatives in this area.

One reason to feel there will be improvement in the area of women's health is the fact that it is easier to introduce these issues into problem-based curricula. Because this educational approach is becoming increasingly popular, the trend may impact favorably on helping resolve the question of women's health during the present decade.

Medical College of Pennsylvania (MCP), in cooperation with Hannemann Medical College, is doing the pioneering work in this area. Undoubtedly, as women become increasingly represented on medical school faculties, there will be an acceleration of interest in, and attempts to remedy the absence of, medical education on women's health issues at both the undergraduate and graduate levels. The fact that women now make up about half of each entering class will presumably also impact positively. These efforts will also be furthered by the National Academy on Women's Health Medical Education that was jointly formed by the MCP and AMWA.

There are some who advocate establishing a women's health specialty. Others argue that this would be a mistake, since it would suggest that only those specialists would then be knowledgeable about women's health needs and problems. This debate will ultimately be settled by the wishes of women medical students in terms of merely getting an education or wanting specialty training in the area of women's health, and by the choice of women patients.

In summary, there is a consensus that the time is right to introduce women's health education into the general curriculum but the process may take some time.

MEDICINE: A CAREER FOR WOMEN

The large number of women applying to medical school demonstrates how attractive this profession is for them. This career presents them with many opportunities. Women accepted to medical school are as likely to complete their studies as men and will also probably make a lifetime career in the profession.

The special attraction of medicine for women may stem from the following:

1. *Satisfaction.* Practicing medicine provides an opportunity to render a service.

2. *Opportunities.* A broad spectrum of possible roles are offered, such as patient care, teaching, laboratory research, community service, and administration.

3. *Independence.* Convenient hours and distribution of effort among multiple activities can be arranged.

4. *Flexibility.* There is an opportunity to change careers during different phases of life, such as additional educational opportunities, receiving a master's degree in public health, moving into the area of public policy by working for a state or federal agency, or serving health-care management.

5. *Stimulation.* The continuing challenge of practicing medicine provides for lifetime learning and is reinforced by the high prestige of the social role of a physician and the satisfaction of achievements attained through intellectual and physical efforts.

DOORS ARE OPEN

By 1975, enrollment of women in medical schools increased to 20%, and by 1980 to 29% of the total number of medical students. For the 1995–96 academic year, first-year women made up more than 38% of the entering class (see Table 7.1). About 50% of the women (and men) who applied in 1995–96 were admitted to medical school. Of the 126 U.S. medical schools, 121 currently have a total female enrollment greater than 30% and 88 have 40% or more.

The impact of increased enrollment of women is shown by the fact that in the 40-year span between 1930 and 1970 only 14,000 women graduated from medical school, while over the 10-year period between 1970 and 1980 more than 20,000 women graduated.

The increase in total enrollment that has taken place is not due to an improved aptitude on the part of women students applying or an increase in the number of women obtaining their baccalaureate degree. Rather the increase is probably due to the following reasons: (1) a perceptible change in society's attitude toward women in medicine, particularly in the educational climate; (2) the realization that women make up a vast and untapped source of medical talent; (3) the obvious difference between the proportion of female doctors in this country as against other countries; and (4) the increase in the trend for women to become wage earners, reflecting a changing cultural pattern.

ADMISSION TO MEDICAL SCHOOL

The dramatic change in the admission picture for women is reflected in two major ways. The first manifestation is evident in both the number of women being accepted (currently more than 40%) and the number of women in recent graduation classes (presently more than 30%). Second is the sustained character of the positive enrollment picture for women, which has extended for more than 15 years. Thus, while the year-to-year increases have been small over the last few years, they have maintained the forward momentum to the point where an average 40% enrollment level for women in U.S. medical schools becomes a realistic expectation. This is especially true since the white male segment of the applicant pool has decreased sharply over the past 15 years, from nearly 80% to less than 50%, while female applicants constitute nearly 40% of the pool, a threefold increase over the same period.

The prospects for women in medicine are more encouraging now than at any other time in the past century. This is clearly evident from a review of the percentages of women accepted in recent years, which establishes that an equal percentage of women to men were accepted from their respective applicant pools. Therefore, it can be anticipated that more women will continue to make up a large part of medical school classes in the coming years.

The obvious conclusion is that women now make up a major, permanent segment of the available freshman places.

THE WOMAN PHYSICIAN: A STATUS REPORT

The status of women will be discussed from three perspectives: (1) an overview, (2) residency choices, and (3) faculty appointments.

An Overview

A profile of the typical woman physician emerged from an early study that was conducted in 1957 covering graduates from a 15-year period. In terms of their personal life, it showed that 57% of all female doctors were married and that these women had, on the average, 1.8 children (as against the national average of 2.3 children in all medical families). Other findings were that half of the married physicians were part of a husband-wife doctor team and that women doctors were slightly more likely to be divorced than females in the general population. Recent studies updated this profile and showed that

Table 7.1 PERCENTAGE OF WOMEN IN THE 1996–97 FIRST-YEAR CLASS

School	%	School	%
Albany Medical College	54	Morehouse School of Medicine	77
Baylor College of Medicine	40	New Jersey Medical School, Univ of Medicine and Dentistry	34
Boston Univ School of Medicine	39	New York Medical College	40
Brown Univ School of Medicine	49	New York Univ School of Medicine	36
Case Western Reserve Univ School of Medicine	45	Northeastern Ohio Univ College of Medicine	42
Chicago Medical School, Univ of Health Sciences	42	Northwestern Univ Medical College	49
City Univ of New York, Mount Sinai School of Medicine	50	Ohio State Univ College of Medicine	37
Columbia Univ College of Physicians and Surgeons	46	Oregon Health Sciences Univ School of Medicine	50
Cornell Univ Medical College	50	Pennsylvania State Univ College of Medicine	42
Creighton Univ School of Medicine	32	Robert Wood Johnson Medical School, Univ of Medicine and Dentistry	37
Dartmouth Medical School	53	Rush Medical College	49
Duke Univ School of Medicine	38	St. Louis Univ School of Medicine	41
East Carolina Univ School of Medicine	50	Southern Illinois Univ School of Medicine	42
East Tennessee State Univ, James H. Quillen College of Medicine	35	Stanford Univ School of Medicine	43
Eastern Virginia Medical School	32	SUNY at Brooklyn College of Medicine	42
Emory Univ School of Medicine	38	SUNY at Buffalo School of Medicine and Biomedical Sciences	47
George Washington Univ School of Medicine	53	SUNY at Stony Brook School of Medicine	43
Georgetown Univ School of Medicine	42	SUNY at Syracuse College of Medicine	40
Harvard Medical School	51	Temple Univ School of Medicine	43
Howard Univ College of Medicine	58	Texas A&M Univ College of Medicine	38
Indiana Univ School of Medicine	41	Texas Tech Univ School of Medicine	25
Jefferson Medical College, Thomas Jefferson Univ	32	Tufts Univ School of Medicine	48
Johns Hopkins Univ School of Medicine	45	Tulane Univ School of Medicine	47
Loma Linda Univ School of Medicine	35	Uniformed Services Univ, F. Edward Hebert School of Medicine	28
Louisiana State Univ School of Medicine in New Orleans	38	Univ of Alabama School of Medicine	32
Louisiana State Univ School of Medicine in Shreveport	41	Univ of Arizona College of Medicine	51
Loyola Univ Chicago Stritch School of Medicine	43	Univ of Arkansas for Medical Sciences, College of Medicine	33
Marshall Univ School of Medicine	35	Univ of California — Davis, School of Medicine	37
Mayo Medical School	55	Univ of California — Irvine, College of Medicine	42
MCP/Hahnemann School of Medicine	45	Univ of California — Los Angeles, School of Medicine	47
Medical College of Georgia	36	Univ of California — San Diego, School of Medicine	40
Medical College of Ohio	38	Univ of California — San Francisco, School of Medicine	48
Medical College of Wisconsin	35	Univ of Chicago, Pritzker School of Medicine	41
Medical Univ of South Carolina College of Medicine	38		
Meharry Medical College School of Medicine	48		
Mercer Univ School of Medicine	36		
Michigan State Univ College of Human Medicine	51		

Table 7.1 PERCENTAGE OF WOMEN IN THE 1996–97 FIRST-YEAR CLASS (Continued)

School	%	School	%
Univ of Cincinnati College of Medicine	42	Univ of South Alabama College of Medicine	38
Univ of Colorado School of Medicine	48	Univ of South Carolina School of Medicine	43
Univ of Connecticut School of Medicine	47	Univ of South Dakota School of Medicine	54
Univ of Florida College of Medicine	43	Univ of South Florida College of Medicine	32
Univ of Hawaii Burns School of Medicine	48	Univ of Southern California School of Medicine	46
Univ of Illinois College of Medicine	29	Univ of Tennessee College of Medicine	42
Univ of Iowa College of Medicine	50	Univ of Texas Medical School at Galveston	36
Univ of Kansas School of Medicine	39	Univ of Texas Medical School at Houston	47
Univ of Kentucky College of Medicine	41	Univ of Texas Medical School at San Antonio	45
Univ of Louisville School of Medicine	46	Univ of Texas, Southwestern Medical School at Dallas	40
Univ of Maryland School of Medicine	49	Univ of Utah School of Medicine	39
Univ of Massachusetts Medical School	50	Univ of Vermont College of Medicine	59
Univ of Miami School of Medicine	48	Univ of Virginia School of Medicine	47
Univ of Michigan Medical School	42	Univ of Washington School of Medicine	51
Univ of Minnesota — Duluth, School of Medicine	52	Univ of Wisconsin Medical School	51
Univ of Minnesota — Minneapolis, Medical School	51	Vanderbilt Univ School of Medicine	36
Univ of Mississippi School of Medicine	30	Virginia Commonwealth Univ Medical School of Virginia	41
Univ of Missouri — Columbia, School of Medicine	41	Wake Forest Univ, Bowman Gray School of Medicine	34
Univ of Missouri — Kansas City, School of Medicine	61	Washington Univ School of Medicine	49
Univ of Nebraska College of Medicine	46	Wayne State Univ School of Medicine	35
Univ of Nevada School of Medicine	40	West Virginia Univ School of Medicine	50
Univ of New Mexico School of Medicine	56	Wright State Univ School of Medicine	56
Univ of North Carolina School of Medicine	43	Yale Univ School of Medicine	58
Univ of North Dakota School of Medicine	44	Yeshiva Univ, Albert Einstein College of Medicine	44
Univ of Oklahoma College of Medicine	44		
Univ of Pennsylvania School of Medicine	52		
Univ of Pittsburgh School of Medicine	42		
Univ of Rochester School of Medicine and Dentistry	41		

female doctors married in the same proportion as nonphysicians and that nearly 70% of them had children. Moreover, female physicians were much more likely to have had working mothers than male doctors, indicating the importance of role models in developing career decisions.

In terms of their professional lives, it was found that women tended to practice in larger cities and that a large number (over one-third) worked either on a fixed salary or in what could be characterized as "fixed-hours" positions. Also, women had a slightly higher tendency to specialize than men, with the most popular fields being pediatrics, psychiatry, anesthesiology, and pathology. Other fields having significant appeal to women were obstetrics-gynecology, internal medicine, family practice, and public health. About half were found to have been in full-time practice all of their professional lives and 87% in full- and part-time practice.

Since the early study was conducted, extensive change has occurred. Opinions about the importance of a career for a woman have changed, as well as attitudes concerning traditional family patterns.

Group practice and part- or full-salaried positions with hospitals, health departments, medical schools, or pharmaceutical companies are but some of the ways in which women can enjoy medical careers with regular and reasonable hours. With the increase in the number and size of Health Maintenance Organizations (HMOs) and the possibility of some form of national health insurance plan, the number of these positions most assuredly will increase.

A significant impact that will improve the status of women in medicine is the fact that many women physician leaders say that they feel a responsibility to mentor young women, because they have found that good mentors helped them excel in their own careers. Mentors can be a valuable asset during training. They advise and encourage and can provide inside information. Mentors can serve to nominate their proteges for committee assignments, awards, grants, and competitive positions, and facilitate research and publication. It is not unique to utilize mentoring as a tool for professional advancement, since it has been a primary career tool in medicine. Seeking guidance from a mentor should be a route to follow, even when there are obstacles to establishing such a relationship.

Residency Choices

With the doors being opened to women, they have moved out of the traditional fields of postgraduate training into all major specialty areas, to differing degrees. A recent survey of the distribution of women in the major residences shows that they can be grouped into six groups, which we categorize as a percentage of all residents:

1. above 50%: pediatrics, geriatric medicine, dermatology, obstetrics/gynecology;
2. above 40–50%: preventive medicine, psychiatry;
3. 30–40% family practice, internal medicine, pathology, pediatric subspecialties;
4. 20–30%: anesthesiology, emergency medicine, internal medicine subspecialties, diagnostic radiology;
5. 10–20%: surgery and its subspecialties; and
6. under 10%: orthopedic surgery, urology.

Faculty Appointments

With women assuming a larger role in medical practice, it is natural that some should elect to enter the field of medical education or academic medicine. They represent about 20% of the basic and clinical science faculties and make up more than 30% in such departments as family practice, obstetrician/gynecology, pediatrics, physical medicine, psychiatry, and public health. This matches the representation in residency training areas (see above).

UNIQUE CHALLENGES FOR WOMEN IN MEDICINE _____

There are three major issues facing women in medicine today, namely (1) professional acceptance, (2) gender bias, and (3) family.

Professional Acceptance

Many years ago, a two-day conference titled "Woman MD" was held at Johns Hopkins University School of Medicine. In attendance were 200 female doctors from across the country who met to study the impact of the increase in the number of women entering medicine. Among the major issues raised were that:

1. Women physicians were looked down upon for showing feelings of tenderness and sadness toward patients and their families, thereby violating what is considered implicit medical standards of behavior. It was pointed out, however, that demonstrating sensitivity and compassion is not incompatible with the need for the doctor to also demonstrate strength.

2. Women physicians often enter specialties they did not originally want because of various family obligations.

3. Women physicians, especially young ones, were concerned that they would not be able to have both a career and a family unless they found a mate who would help with the housework and child rearing—or unless they were untiring "superwomen."

In a summary of the symposium, the women doctors were warned of two separate "pitfalls": an intolerance of the emotional responses of the other sex in times of stress and possible discrimination if they tried to change the medical system too much.

In general, the attitude of young women physicians toward their professional futures is optimistic. The forces responsible for changes have been the trail-blazing efforts of older women, together with changes in societal values and laws. Having become firmly convinced that medicine is a suitable career choice, more and more women are applying to medical schools and discriminatory barriers are falling.

Gender Bias

In the early 1990s several medical journals published the results of surveys among female medical students and residents regarding harassment. The results indicate that between 50 and 75% experienced some form of gender discrimination. The offensive behavior took the form of denied professional opportunities, malicious gossip, sexist slurs, and even sexual advances. Surprisingly, harassment varied with different fields, being most prevalent in general surgery and least in pediatrics. Students were reportedly harassed by both faculty and residents. While harassment during medical training is quite common, women face this issue more intensely because of their gender. The hierarchical nature of the medical power structure, with men in the upper echelons, is thought to contribute to this problem.

Gender bias impacts on women negatively, both directly and indirectly. It may slow their advancement, thereby keeping them in a lower pay scale, and may also be psychologically damaging enough to lower self-confidence and sometimes work performance.

Efforts are being made to curtail harassment. This includes periodic publication by the medical school of its policy against discrimination, presenting "Gender Neutral Awards" to faculty who are especially sensitive to gender issues, establishing workshops where the relationship between genders are discussed, sponsoring lectures, publishing newsletters, and providing support groups.

Family

A recent survey indicated that about 10% of female medical graduates had one or more dependents. This represents about 3,000 medical school students. While the issue of childbearing during medical training years has long been known to educators, little progress has been made to satisfactorily resolve it. The problem is being addressed on an *ad hoc* basis, which may in some cases provide for flexibility, rather than by having written institutional policies addressing maternity leave. As the percentage of women medical students increases, this issue will probably be brought to the forefront.

There is conflicting advice being offered on preparing for parenting, with some advocating preparation, while others emphasizing the importance of the need to adapt as problems arise. Certainly, medical residents, who frequently are guaranteed about six weeks of parental leave, should advise their program directors well in advance so that adequate coverage during their absence can be provided. It should be noted that a substantial number of residency programs do not have written parental leave policies and that those that do vary.

Of special significance are the child-care arrangements that are made prior to delivery. In most cases where a day-care center or other facility has to be used, the availability of a backup care provider is still essential. A supportive spouse is a key element in the quest to attain successful parenting.

There appears to be no ideal time for a woman physician to have a child. Young children may make it difficult to pursue her studies and training, and she may be at a financial disadvantage during that part of her life. Conversely, delaying child bearing may result in infertility as a result of normal age-related changes. This is a highly personal choice, and individual circumstances will influence it. Young women, perhaps, should seek the advice of older women physicians as they make their plans.

For additional information see:

Journal of the American Medical Women's Association, May/June 1992.

Working and Parenting by B. Brazelton, Addison-Wesley, 1985.

Day-Care: Finding the Best Child Care for Your Family, American Academy of Pediatrics, Dept. C/H, 141 NW Point Blvd, Elk Grove, IL 60007.

Medicine and Parenting, 1991, and *Building a Stronger Women's Program*, 1993, AAMC Publication Sales, 2450 N Street NW, Washington, DC 20037.

FINANCIAL AID AND SUPPORT SOURCES

The following are financial aid sources specifically for women students. Additional details are available from the organizations listed below:

1. American Association of University Women Educational Foundation. Contact: Director, Fellowships Office, American Association of University Women, 1111 16th Street, NW, Washington, DC 20036.

2. American Medical Women's Association Loan Fund. Contact: American Medical Women's Association, Inc., 801 North Fairfax Street, Alexandria, VA 22314.

3. Educational Financial Aid Sources for Women. Contact: Clairol Loving Care Scholarship Program, 345 Park Avenue, New York, NY 10022.

In the past several years a number of support groups that aim to facilitate women's adaptation to the demands of residency have been established. They include:

Dual Doctor Families, 6900 Grove Road, Thorofare, NJ 08086.

Shared Residencies (Drs. Frazer and Somjen), 1125C Grant Boulevard, Woodlawn Gardens, Syracuse, NY 13203.

American Medical Student Association, Women in Medicine Task Force, 1902 Association Drive, Reston, VA 22091.

American Medical Women's Association, 2302 East Speedway #206A, Tucson, AZ 85719.

Association of American Medical Colleges, Special Assistant to the President on Women's Issues, 2450 N Street NW, Washington, DC 20037.

8 Opportunities for Minorities

Minorities in medicine: historical perspective
Doors are opening for minorities
Admission of minorities: a status report
Current challenges
Financial aid for minority students
Summer programs

MINORITIES IN MEDICINE: HISTORICAL PERSPECTIVE

Currently, a very substantial number of practicing African-American physicians are graduates of one medical school, Howard University College of Medicine, Washington, DC, one of the three predominantly black schools. At one time, virtually all African-American medical students attended these schools. By the end of World War II, one-third of medical schools were exclusively white and, as late as 1960, African-Americans were unable to gain admission to 12 schools. In 1968 the AAMC strongly urged medical schools to begin to admit increased numbers of minority students.

The three medical schools, Howard (Washington, DC), Meharry (Nashville, Tennessee), and Morehouse (Atlanta, Georgia), continue to play a major role in training the pool of minority medical students, admitting about 15% of all such students. From the other 123 allopathic schools, six account for another 15%. Thus, nine schools currently accept about one-third of all underrepresented students.

The three traditionally black medical schools remain attractive to minority students for a variety of reasons. Such schools tend to cost less than many predominantly white institutions. They also provide more role models, having many African-Americans on their faculties. Socialization problems, so common at nonminority schools, obviously do not exist. These schools seem to carefully monitor academic performance and provide assistance to their students, even those not at risk to fail. Thus, the three historically black schools have retained their pivotal position in the education of underrepresented minority physicians (even though they now contain a significant number of white students among their student bodies).

DOORS ARE OPENING FOR MINORITIES

The academic medical community has responded in a positive manner to provide greater opportunities for members of minority groups to secure admission. There are intensive efforts to enroll minority group members: African-Americans, Native Americans/Alaskan natives, Mexican Americans, mainland Puerto Ricans, Asians, or Pacific Islanders. This policy has been especially effective, as reflected by the fact that for 1995–96, minority group members made up 12% of both the first-year class (see Table 8.1) and the total medical student enrollment. This represents a significant increase over the less than 5% representation about two decades ago. Facilitating this process is the fact that many schools have a specific person to deal with minority affairs. Thus, if you are a member of a minority group, you should often address your inquiries to "Director of Minority Affairs."

A special service that has been initiated to assist such students is the Medical Minority Applicant Registry (Med-MAR). This service enables any minority student applying to medical school to have his or her basic biography (except GPA and MCAT scores) circulated to all U.S. medical schools without charge. A list of such students is published two times a year. To be put on this list, you should identify yourself on the questionnaire as a member of a minority group at the time you take the MCAT, or contact the Minority Student Information Clearing House, Association of American Medical Colleges, One Dupont Circle, NW, Suite 200, Washington, DC 20036.

You should also consider that some medical schools may waive their application fee for minority group students with economic need. The AMCAS fee can also be waived because of financial need, but the MCAT fee is never waived.

The increase in the number of African-Americans being admitted to medical school has had an impact on their total enrollment and on the number of African-Americans graduating. As expected, the number of African-Americans undertaking graduate education, that is, securing special training by means of residencies, has increased significantly over the past decade. The majority of African-Americans initiating residency training do so at hospitals located in California, Maryland, New Jersey, New York, and Pennsylvania. The majority of African-Americans in residency programs are being trained in five specialties: family practice, internal medicine, obstetrics-gynecology, pediatrics, and surgery.

To help disadvantaged or minority group students, some schools arrange special summer programs prior to the formal beginning of medical school for candidates already admitted. In addition, a variety of flexible curricular alternatives are available in some schools for such students as they progress through medical school. For specific information on these programs, contact the Office of Minority Students Affairs at the individual schools.

Summaries of special minority admissions programs are outlined for individual schools in the special features section of the medical school profiles, which begin on page 185.

ADMISSION OF MINORITIES: A STATUS REPORT

Minorities made up 12.4% of the 1995–96 entering class. This figure, representing a slight increase over the previous year, is the third successive annual increase in enrollment. This points up the fact that the movement to increase ethnic diversity in the nation's medical schools is accelerating.

Also on the positive side, the minority applicant pool has remained the same, and the chances of admission are 50%, as compared with 40% a decade ago. The mean MCAT scores for minority applicants have also improved. There remains, though, a discrepancy when compared with the acceptance rate for majority applicants, which currently stands at 55%. Also, the attrition rate among minority medical students has doubled over the past decade to 12%.

The cutback in educational funding has made acceptance into medical school a formidable challenge for underprivileged students; the dropout rate along the way is high from completion of elementary school through college. In addition, these students are being discouraged by the same factors that have generated a negative climate relative to choosing medicine as a career. These include talk of an oversupply of physicians, malpractice litigation publicity, rising tuition costs, and (for some) the need to treat AIDS patients.

CURRENT CHALLENGES

Over the past decade, the overall composition of the medical school class has changed from predominantly white male to a very substantial number of women and a modest, yet significant, number of minority members. This radical change is in response to the drastic alteration in the social climate of the United States. That further changes may be

Table 8.1 PERCENTAGE OF MINORITY STUDENTS IN THE 1996–97 FIRST-YEAR CLASS

School	%
Albany Medical College	1
Baylor College of Medicine	23
Boston Univ School of Medicine	11
Brown Univ School of Medicine	12
Case Western Reserve Univ School of Medicine	18
Chicago Medical School, Univ of Health Sciences	12
City Univ of New York, Mount Sinai School of Medicine	16
Columbia Univ College of Physicians and Surgeons	10
Cornell Univ Medical College	12
Creighton Univ School of Medicine	9
Dartmouth Medical School	12
Duke Univ School of Medicine	14
East Carolina Univ School of Medicine	26
East Tennessee State Univ, James H. Quillen College of Medicine	25
Eastern Virginia Medical School	4
Emory Univ School of Medicine	38
George Washington Univ School of Medicine	16
Georgetown Univ School of Medicine	6
Harvard Medical School	14
Howard Univ College of Medicine	79
Indiana Univ School of Medicine	6
Jefferson Medical College, Thomas Jefferson Univ	8
Johns Hopkins Univ School of Medicine	13
Loma Linda Univ School of Medicine	7
Louisiana State Univ School of Medicine in New Orleans	31
Louisiana State Univ School of Medicine in Shreveport	7
Loyola Univ Chicago Stritch School of Medicine	3
Marshall Univ School of Medicine	19
Mayo Medical School	19
MCP/Hahnemann School of Medicine	14
Medical College of Georgia	22
Medical College of Ohio	14
Medical College of Wisconsin	4
Medical Univ of South Carolina College of Medicine	30
Meharry Medical College School of Medicine	80
Mercer Univ School of Medicine	7
Michigan State Univ College of Human Medicine	19

School	%
Morehouse School of Medicine	91
New Jersey Medical School, Univ of Medicine and Dentistry	13
New York Medical College	11
New York Univ School of Medicine	7
Northeastern Ohio Univ College of Medicine	6
Northwestern Univ Medical College	4
Ohio State Univ College of Medicine	8
Oregon Health Sciences Univ School of Medicine	8
Pennsylvania State Univ College of Medicine	19
Robert Wood Johnson Medical School, Univ of Medicine and Dentistry	19
Rush Medical College	10
St. Louis Univ School of Medicine	2
Southern Illinois Univ School of Medicine	0
Stanford Univ School of Medicine	11
SUNY at Brooklyn College of Medicine	14
SUNY at Buffalo School of Medicine and Biomedical Sciences	6
SUNY at Stony Brook School of Medicine	13
SUNY at Syracuse College of Medicine	20
Temple Univ School of Medicine	12
Texas A&M Univ College of Medicine	14
Texas Tech Univ School of Medicine	22
Tufts Univ School of Medicine	8
Tulane Univ School of Medicine	7
Uniformed Services Univ, F. Edward Hebert School of Medicine	7
Univ of Alabama School of Medicine	10
Univ of Arizona College of Medicine	24
Univ of Arkansas for Medical Sciences, College of Medicine	10
Univ of California — Davis, School of Medicine	n/av
Univ of California — Irvine, College of Medicine	42
Univ of California — Los Angeles, School of Medicine	33
Univ of California — San Diego, School of Medicine	53
Univ of California — San Francisco, School of Medicine	22
Univ of Chicago, Pritzker School of Medicine	13

Table 8.1 PERCENTAGE OF MINORITY STUDENTS IN THE 1996–97 FIRST-YEAR CLASS (Continued)

School	%	School	%
Univ of Cincinnati College of Medicine	15	Univ of South Alabama College of Medicine	13
Univ of Colorado School of Medicine	14	Univ of South Carolina School of Medicine	18
Univ of Connecticut School of Medicine	11	Univ of South Dakota School of Medicine	6
Univ of Florida College of Medicine	7	Univ of South Florida College of Medicine	25
Univ of Hawaii Burns School of Medicine	2	Univ of Southern California School of Medicine	21
Univ of Illinois College of Medicine	27	Univ of Tennessee College of Medicine	13
Univ of Iowa College of Medicine	13	Univ of Texas Medical School at Galveston	54
Univ of Kansas School of Medicine	10	Univ of Texas Medical School at Houston	21
Univ of Kentucky College of Medicine	n/av	Univ of Texas Medical School at San Antonio	15
Univ of Louisville School of Medicine	n/av	Univ of Texas, Southwestern Medical School at Dallas	11
Univ of Maryland School of Medicine	16	Univ of Utah School of Medicine	2
Univ of Massachusetts Medical School	6	Univ of Vermont College of Medicine	13
Univ of Miami School of Medicine	12	Univ of Virginia School of Medicine	15
Univ of Michigan Medical School	18	Univ of Washington School of Medicine	11
Univ of Minnesota — Duluth, School of Medicine	7	Univ of Wisconsin Medical School	15
Univ of Minnesota — Minneapolis, Medical School	3	Vanderbilt Univ School of Medicine	5
Univ of Mississippi School of Medicine	14	Virginia Commonwealth Univ Medical School of Virginia	9
Univ of Missouri — Columbia, School of Medicine	5	Wake Forest Univ, Bowman Gray School of Medicine	10
Univ of Missouri — Kansas City, School of Medicine	11	Washington Univ School of Medicine	n/av
Univ of Nebraska College of Medicine	9	Wayne State Univ School of Medicine	15
Univ of Nevada School of Medicine	5	West Virginia Univ School of Medicine	8
Univ of New Mexico School of Medicine	40	Wright State Univ School of Medicine	21
Univ of North Carolina School of Medicine	24	Yale Univ School of Medicine	17
Univ of North Dakota School of Medicine	19	Yeshiva Univ, Albert Einstein College of Medicine	8
Univ of Oklahoma College of Medicine	17		
Univ of Pennsylvania School of Medicine	19		
Univ of Pittsburgh School of Medicine	6		
Univ of Rochester School of Medicine and Dentistry	11		

anticipated is implied in the fact that by the year 2000, one-third of all college students will be members of minorities.

Currently, although blacks make up 12% of the population, they account for only 3% of the physicians in the United States and 8% of the medical students in the country. Similarly, Hispanics comprise 9% of the population and 4% of the nation's physicians. Native Americans fare worse, making up 0.8% of the public and 0.1% of its doctors. These three groups are thus considered underrepresented minorities. The medical education establishment responds to these facts by maintaining an ambitious recruitment campaign. While this has had a positive impact on increasing minority class representation, it is now recognized that efforts need to be strengthened to encourage these students to endure the rigors of the training process and to complete their medical studies. This is indicated by the fact that the dropout rate for freshman minority students is close to 10%, as compared with 3% for all other students.

The cause of the increased dropout rate among minority students may not be exclusively academic, but, rather, due to cultural conflicts and lack of social adjustment. Many minority students are the first members of their family to have reached such an educational level and are under intense pressure to succeed. Many minority students have attained admission to medical school without encouragement, and may even have been advised against pursuing higher education or a professional career. Therefore, for most of them, medical school is a pioneering experience in a not too supportive environment. This makes the process an extremely challenging one. A major element influencing this situation is a lack of role models, since few minority members come from physician families. Moreover, only about 3% of all medical school faculty are minority physicians. (Included in this figure are those at predominantly black institutions.) There is the perception that minority faculty are more approachable and responsive to disadvantaged students. Such support can be critical to a student's progress. The number of minority residents is unfortunately not large enough to have them serve as role models. In all, the lack of role models is considered a critical issue in the retention of minority students.

Medical schools that have been successful in recruitment and retention of minorities have made use of mentoring programs. A mentor can provide a direct vision of what it means to be a physician. The mentor can not only offer support during difficult intervals, but also can help students make pivotal career choices relative to such issues as choosing electives, specialization, and where to do one's residency training. At some institutions, white faculty members have been used to serve as mentors, due to the shortage of minority faculty.

A lack of social interaction in medical school leads to a sense of isolation among minority students. This leads them to form their own networks, which helps to a degree. Having a chapter of a national minority student organization on campus also can be useful as a form of protection against social isolation.

Because of alienation early in their education, minority students frequently do not acquire desirable skills for group learning. Also, they often are not prepared for the demanding workload in medical school. For some minority students who lack adequate academic preparedness, improvement in study skills is essential.

Success in handling standardized tests—the SAT I or ACT exam, MCAT, or USMLE—is especially challenging for minority students. Hispanic students, who frequently speak English as a second language, are at a special disadvantage. Remaining in medical school is often closely tied to performance on Step 1 of the USMLE.

Many medical schools make special efforts to assist disadvantaged students. They provide summer enrichment programs for premeds to help prepare for MCATs, as well as an experience in basic premed science coursework and research. This is usually the first opportunity for premeds to meet an academic physician. Enrichment programs were found to improve subsequent academic performance. Many schools also offer postbaccalaureate and prematriculation programs to accepted minority students in order to prepare them academically before they must face the pressures of their first year in medical school. These programs are attractive because they have a small faculty-student ratio and provide early exposure to the basic medical sciences. In some schools, students are permitted to lighten the load of the first year by satisfactorily completing part of it in advance. Flexible curricula and five-year programs are becoming more common in medical schools. Many schools also make special efforts to prepare minority students for the USMLE. All of the aforementioned strategies enhance both recruitment and retention of disadvantaged students. In addition, such students have access to the wide variety of academic and social support services offered to all students.

The cost of medical education remains high and can reach $150,000 for four years of tuition and fees at some schools. This can be especially burdensome for minority students. The average debt of African-American students after college and medical school exceeds $55,000. Yet the dropout rate does not seem to have been heavily influenced by the financial demands of medical education. A potentially disturbing issue is the possibility that federally funded minority scholarships may be in danger of being curtailed.

Recognizing the demographic shift toward a multiethnic and multiracial society, the AAMC has established a special recruitment campaign—Project 3000 by 2000—to enhance science education in public schools, thus helping to nurture the potential pool of minority applicants.

Minority applicants can now explore the opportunities that are offered to them at the schools to which they are considering applying and can determine if they will feel comfortable there for four years.

FINANCIAL AID FOR MINORITY STUDENTS

The following listing gives a brief idea of the scholarships and loans available for minority group students. Additional information is available from each of the sources cited.

1. National Medical Fellowships, Inc. For minority group students. Contact: Executive Secretary, 254 West 31st Street, New York, NY 10001.

2. American Medical Association and Research Foundation. Contact: Foundation, 535 North Dearborn, Chicago, IL 60610.

3. National Scholarship Service and Fund for Negro Students. Contact: Executive Director, NSSFNS Application Department, 250 Auburn Avenue, Suite 500, Atlanta, GA 30303.

4. United Student Aid Funds, Inc. For low-income families. Contact: Executive Director, 11100 USA Parkway, Fishers, IN 46038.

5. Emergency Scholarships. For American Indian students. Contact: Association on American Indian Affairs, 432 Park Avenue South, New York, NY 10016.

6. Bureau of Indian Affairs. For American Indians and Eskimos. Contact: Director, Higher Education Program, 500 Gold, S.W., Albuquerque, NM 87103.

Additional information is available from the AAMC by writing to the Minority Student Opportunities in U.S. Medical Schools, AAMC, 2450 N Street NW, Washington, DC 20037.

Information on financial aid is also available from the following sources.

1. *Financial Aid for Minorities in Health Fields*, published by Garrett Park Press, PO Box 190, Garrett Park, MD 20896, 1993. It contains references to fellowships, loans, grants, and awards.

2. Office of Statewide Health Planning and Development, Health Profession Career Opportunity Program, 1600 Ninth Street, Sacramento, CA 95814. Upon request, you will receive a free copy of *Financial Advice for Minority Students Seeking an Education in the Health Professions*.

3. Office of the Associate Dean for Student Affairs, Boston University, School of Medicine, 80 East Concord Street, Boston, MA 02118. Ask for *Financing Medical Education*.

SUMMER PROGRAMS

Summer enrichment programs are designed to increase the minority applicant pool in medical schools. Participants obtain a variety of assistance, including concentrated science review courses. They also receive help in improving test taking, study and writing skills, and clinical research lab exposure.

California
Student Research Program
American Heart Association
1710 Gilbreth Road
Burlingame, CA 94010
(415) 259-6700

Minority Access to Health Careers Program
MAHC Program
California Polytechnic State University
San Luis Obispo, CA 93407
(805) 756-2840

HCOP Summer Enrichment Program
Program Coordinator
San Jose State University
College of Applied Arts and Sciences
One Washington Square
San Jose, CA 95192
(408) 924-2911

HCOP Summer Academic Program
College of Sciences LS204
San Diego State University
San Diego, CA 92187
(619) 594-4793

Summer Academic Study Program (*SASP*)
Office of Minority Affairs
School of Medicine
University of California, Davis
Davis, CA 95616
(916) 752-4808

Summer Premedical Program
Office of Educational and Community Programs
College of Medicine
University of California, Irvine
PO Box 4089
Irvine, CA 92717
(714) 824-4603

Enrichment Program
Office of Student Support Services, B-154 CHS
School of Medicine
University of California, Los Angeles
Los Angeles, CA 90024
(310) 825-3575

HePP Consortium for Health Care Preparation
Office of Minority Affairs
School of Medicine
University of Southern California
1333 San Pablo St., MCH 51-C
Los Angeles, CA 90033
(213) 342-1050

Summer Research Training Program for Undergraduate Minority Students
Graduate Division
513 Parnassus, S-140, Box 0404
University of California, San Francisco
San Francisco, CA 94143
(415) 476-8134

Summer MCAT Preparation Program
Center for Educational Achievement
Charles R. Drew University
School of Medicine and Science
1621 East 120th Street
Los Angeles, CA 90059
(213) 563-4926

Summer Interships
Hispanic Center of Excellence
University of California, San Francisco
145 Irving Street, Rm. 106
San Francisco, CA 94143
(415) 476-3667

Project Prepare
Medical Center
University of Southern California
1975 Zonal Avenue, KAM B-29
Los Angeles, CA 90033
(213) 342-1328

Connecticut
Pre-College/College Enrichment Program
Office of Minority Student Affairs
Health Center
University of Connecticut
Farmington, CT 06030
(203) 679-3483

District of Columbia
Summer Health Careers Advanced Enrichment Program
Director, Center for Preprofessional Education
Box 473, Administrative Building
Howard University
Washington, DC 20059
(202) 806-7231

Iowa
Summer Enrichment Program
Associate for Student Affairs
University of Iowa
College of Medicine
124 Medicine Administration Building
Iowa City, IA 52242
(319) 335-8056

Louisiana
Summer Reinforcement and Enrichment Program (SREP)
Office of MEDREP
Tulane Medical Center
1430 Tulane Avenue-SL 40
New Orleans, LA 70112
(504) 588-5327

Massachusetts
Summer Honors Undergraduate Research Program
Division of Medical Science
Harvard Medical School
260 Longwood Avenue
Boston, MA 02115
(617) 432-4980

Minority Summer Research Program
MIT Summer Research Program
Graduate School Office, Rm. 3-138
Cambridge, MA 02139
(617) 253-4869

Summer Enrichment Program
Office of Outreach Programs
University of Massachusetts
55 Lake Avenue N
Worchester, MA 01655
(508) 856-5541

Michigan
*Summer Enrichment Program in Health Administration for
Undergraduate Minority Students*
Department of Health Services, Management and Policy
M 3031 School of Public Health II
University of Michigan
Ann Arbor, MI 48109
(313) 763-9900

Minnesota
Summer Inorganic Chemistry and Precalculus Program
Summer Biology Program
Summer Organic Chemistry and Calculus Program
Summer Physics Program
515 Delaware Street SE
1-125 Moos Tower
Minneapolis, MN 55455
(612) 624-5904

Nebraska
Summer Research Enrichment Program
Director, Multicultural Affairs Office
600 South 42nd Street
Omaha, NE 68198
(402) 559-4437

New York
Summer Student Program
Science Education Center, Bldg. 438
Brookhaven National Laboratory
Upton (Long Island), NY 11973
(516) 282-4503

Travelers Summer Research Fellowship for Minority Premedical Students
Cornell University Medical College
1300 York Avenue, D-119
New York, NY 10021
(212) 746-1057

Summer Research Fellowship (SURF) Program
Director, Ethnic and Multicultural Affairs
School of Medicine and Dentistry
University of Rochester
Rochester, NY 14642
(716) 272-2175

North Carolina
College Phase Summer Program
Office of Minority Affairs
Bowman Gray School of Medicine
Medical Center Boulevard
Winston-Salem, NC 27157
(910) 716-4201

Ohio
Pre-Entry Program
MEDPATH
1178 Graves Hall
College of Medicine
Ohio State University
Columbus, OH 43210
(614) 292-3161
Fax (614) 688-4041

Summer Scholars Program
College of Osteopathic Medicine
Ohio University
Center for Excellence
930 Grosvenor Hall
Athens, OH 45701
(614) 593-0917

Summer Premedical Enrichment Program
Office of Student Affairs and Admissions
College of Medicine
University of Cincinnati
231 Bethesda Avenue
Cincinnati, OH 45267
(513) 538-7212

Oklahoma
Headlands Indian Health Careers Summer Program
Headlands Indian Health Careers
BSEB Rm 200
University of Oklahoma
Health Sciences Center
PO Box 26901
Oklahoma City, OK 73126
(405) 271-2250

Pennsylvania
Summer Premedical Academic Enrichment Program
Director of Minority Programs
School of Medicine
University of Pittsburgh
M-247 Scaife Hall
Pittsburgh, PA 15261
(412) 648-8987

Texas
Honors Premedical Academy
Project Coordinator
Division of School Based Programs
Baylor College of Medicine
1709 Dryden, Suite 545
Houston, TX 77030
(800) 798-8244

Bridge to Medicine Summer Program for Minority Disadvantaged College Students
Office of Student Affairs and Admissions
College of Medicine
Texas A&M University
106 Reynolds Medical Building
College Station, TX 77843
(409) 862-4065

Virginia
Medical Academic Advancement Program
Office of Student Academic Support
School of Medicine, Box 446
University of Virginia
Charlottesville, VA 22908
(804) 924-2189

Washington
Northwest Consortium Minority Medical Education Program (MMEP)
School of Medicine SM-22
University of Washington
Seattle, WA 98195
(206) 685-2489

Wisconsin
Summer Science Enrichment Program
School of Dentistry
Marquette University
PO Box 1881
Milwaukee, WI 53201
(414) 288-1533

9 Financing Your Medical Education

The current financial aid crisis
Successfully managing educational indebtedness
Scholarships and loans

Securing a medical education can be extremely expensive. The annual tuition at the costliest school has exceeded $28,000, and the national mean for private schools is more than $16,000 per academic year.

The reason for high tuition is many-faceted. Many schools are burdened with the major expense of sustaining commitments—from tenured faculty to capital improvements. Research, which requires a physical plant and equipment, is no longer as heavily subsidized by the government. Medical technology has created increasingly costly instrumentation that must be updated to maintain the state of the art.

Essentially, however, tuition constitutes only a very small part of the school's income. The bulk of the income comes from research grants, government funding, endowments, and medical practice fees. For most private schools the critical factor is the endowment. For public medical schools the allotment by the state legislature is the determining factor, with the state's economy and demographics being the key factors.

The only bright spot in the financial picture is that there is evidence that tuition levels may have peaked and recently, in a few cases, tuition reductions have taken place, perhaps in response to the decline in applicants during the late 1980s.

The high cost of medical education raises problems for many students. Various sources of financial assistance are presently available, so that, once accepted, a student can feel relatively assured that adequate financial support will be forthcoming, if not in scholarships, then in loans. Recent proposed cuts in the federal aid to medical schools have included mostly attempts to cut back on research and building grants. These cuts in funding would affect the research being done primarily by staff professors and would threaten the future of research and the training of research scientists. In addition, other proposals include the substitution of a loan program instead of scholarships for students. Needless to say, educators have been decrying these cuts and have been urging a reassessment of financial allocations.

How do medical students meet their expenses? Usually from multiple sources including gifts and loans from families, their own earnings, and, if married, their spouses' earnings. Scholarships and loans form another major source of financial assistance, with about 50% of all students currently being helped by either of these means. Employment during medical school is not advisable, but work during the summers is possible. In light of this situation, it is important that prospective medical students anticipating the need for financial assistance undertake long term planning early in their careers. Once the student has been accepted and has decided to attend a school, the financial aid office should be contacted for information and assistance. In most cases, financial aid is provided solely on the basis of need.

In determining how to finance your medical education, keep the following points in mind.

1. The most important sources of current financial information are the individual schools.

2. Students who are planning to apply to medical school should obtain current information as to tuition and fees (and any projected increases), room and board, and other expenses (see Table 5.1, Chapter 5).

3. Students who have been accepted and are considering enrolling at a school should request relevant information from the school's Financial Aid Office.

4. Students who have decided to enroll at a school should arrange to obtain specific information about a personal aid package by requesting an interview with the school's financial aid officer.

5. Some federally funded programs exist (see Scholarships and Loans section) that provide financial aid for medical school students in return for a specified number of years of service.

6. Students should realize that the financial aid picture is a changing one and that the general pattern of aid has been toward a declining level of support.

7. Financial aid awards are usually made on the basis of demonstrated need established by a financial analysis system. There are three national organizations that analyze the information provided by the students and their families. The results are sent to the individual medical schools. The schools then determine the award to be made.

8. Public medical schools are less expensive for residents and, generally, for nonresidents also than private schools. This applies to both tuition and fees as well as all other expenses.

9. In 1995–96, the *average* cost of tuition and fees for freshman medical students was about $9,500 for residents and $20,500 for nonresidents at a *public* school, and $24,000 at a *private* school.

10. The total *average* expenses (tuition, fees, living) for 1995–96 for a freshman thus can be estimated as $18,500 for a resident attending a state school and $30,000 for a nonresident. For a student attending a private school, the average total expenses were about $34,000.

Note that there is a range on both sides of all the above figures.

THE CURRENT FINANCIAL AID CRISIS

During the past several years, there has been a marked escalation in tuition and other costs related to medical education. This inflationary spiral may continue for the foreseeable future. It is taking place unfortunately at a time when financial aid programs are being cut. This situation has caused a rising deficit between what funds are needed by medical students and what financial aid is available to them. To aggravate the situation, in 1979, legislation reducing federal grants to medical and osteopathy schools by 20% was approved. These schools will receive approximately $1,100 per student. Congress is being asked to end the grants entirely, citing fears that there will be a surplus of health personnel soon. In addition, it has become increasingly difficult to receive bank loans through the Federally Insured Student Loan Program, and private sources of support to medical students are also on the decline. All this strongly suggests that very careful consideration be given to financing one's medical education well before one considers applying for admission. In 1976 a Health Manpower bill was passed that will require almost every recipient of a federally supported medical scholarship to serve at least two years with the National Health Service Corps in areas of need.

It is essential for prospective medical students to be fully aware of the high cost of a medical education and its possible consequences.

Medical school tuition and fees are the largest expense facing a medical student. The average cost of tuition in private schools is approximately $24,000 a year, while in-state residents at public schools pay about $9,500 per year. This represents an increase of more than 400% for private schools and 275% for public schools over the past 25 years. Thus, for a typical private school, the cost of four years of medical school (tuition, fees, and living expenses) can run $150,000 or more.

If the reasonable assumption is made that half of the total expenses are covered by borrowed money, loan repayment, which begins five years after graduation, will exceed $1,000 a month. In addition, interest, which begins at the time of borrowing and is due as "interest only" payments as early as two years after graduation, when added to the principal of the loan, would increase considerably the monthly repayment cost beyond $1,000 per month. Parenthetically, this interest is not tax deductible.

The next question then is, at what income level must one be in order to be able to comfortably repay a debt of approximately $75,000? Such a debt repayment level is estimated as 8% of one's *gross* income per year. This would require an income of $145,000, while an income of $97,000 would make repayment difficult, and an income of $70,000 would not allow for repayment. These income levels are to take place five years after graduation, namely at the time of completion of postgraduate (residency) training. To achieve the desirable upper income level at the initial stage of one's professional career is quite difficult.

These debt prospects suggest that, as time goes on, premedical students from less affluent backgrounds will find themselves unable to pursue medical careers or, if choosing to do so, will shun such lower remunerative specialties as family medicine, pediatrics, or general internal medicine. Particularly severe pressure would be felt under these conditions by qualified minority students who do not have access to special financial assistance.

In the light of this situation, prospective medical students should do as much research as possible about financing their education, debt service, and available resources. The apparent leveling off of tuition will also be helpful, even though the cost of living will continue to increase. If, as some anticipate, there are massive loan defaults, the impetus for aggressive governmental action to solve the financial aid crisis will be necessary.

An example of the direction that the issue of loan default is taking is the action by the Health Resources and Services Administration (HRSA) against the several thousand individuals who have not repaid federal Health Education Assistance Loans (HEAL). Hoping to pressure them into repayment, they have published their names and last known addresses in the *Federal Register*, the official government listing of federal actions and regulations. HRSA, in an effort to recover funds, can go further and alert credit bureaus, request that IRS withhold tax refunds, and bar defaulters from being eligible for Medicare or Medicaid reimbursement for their services. They can even arrange for the Department of Justice to litigate and withhold wages and property. They are also seeking to secure the cooperation of state agencies in getting them to withhold licenses to practice to such individuals until their loans are paid up.

SUCCESSFULLY MANAGING EDUCATIONAL INDEBTEDNESS ___

Most medical students take out loans to pay for the cost of their education. Borrowing means that they benefit by having access to someone else's money now because they agree to pay it back with interest later. This reimbursement is a legal obligation that they assume. Those defaulting on repayment can face serious financial and legal consequences, which can impact negatively on borrowers, both personally and professionally.

The majority of students are able to repay their loans. The two major ways to succeed in handling debt repayment is to participate in a loan repayment program (usually sponsored by the federal government), and or practice prudent debt management. The latter is outlined in the five advisory tips discussed below:

TIP 1   Avoid overspending

It is essential that you live within your budget so that your need to borrow will be under control and ultimately your debt load will be restricted to an absolute minimum.

TIP 2   Avoid using credit cards

You must recognize that this form of payment represents an expensive loan. Credit cards should certainly not be used to purchase items that you cannot afford; you should restrict yourself to one credit card and it should be held for identification purposes or emergency use.

TIP 3   Understand your loan

The terms of all loans are different. From the outset you should be aware of the interest rate, duration of your loan, deferment options, and consolidation conditions. You will then know how to handle your loan and avoid under- or overpayments and possible default.

TIP 4   Check your mail

Psychologically, some students try to avoid opening mail from lenders because they do not like to read "bad news." This attitude obviously can backfire and payments can be missed. Your loan is then passed on to another lender for collection. Also, you may be sending your payments to a wrong address and over a period of time this may result in loan default.

TIP 5   Keep accurate records

To be sure that your payment is properly credited to your account, it is obviously in your best interest to maintain a complete and up-to-date record of all your payments. You should also note the remaining balances and see if they correspond to that indicated on the lender's statement. If there is a discrepancy, contact the lender promptly and call their attention to the apparent possible error.

SCHOLARSHIPS AND LOANS

Scholarships largely come from two sources: medical schools and the federal government. All medical schools have some scholarships or tuition-remission grants available that are awarded on the basis of financial need and scholastic performance. The school catalogs usually give the necessary details. The federal government provides most of the funds that the medical schools, as well as banks and other lending institutions, make available to students.

Scholarships

Scholarships for First-year Students of Exceptional Financial Need

U.S. citizens or permanent residents who have been accepted and are planning to enroll as freshmen in medical school, and have exceptional financial need, can apply for such a scholarship. While funds under this program are very limited, they do provide for tuition as well as a stipend (currently about $6,000) for all other educational expenses. No service payback is required. School financial aid officers are the best sources of information concerning these scholarships.

Armed Forces Health Professions Scholarship Program

All three armed forces offer scholarships to U.S. citizens who have been accepted or are already enrolled at a medical school in the United States or Puerto Rico. These scholarships provide full tuition and payment of educational expenses, plus a substantial stipend (currently in excess of $6,000). Recipients must serve one year of active military duty for each year they receive support, with the usual minimum being three years. Premedical advisors generally have, or can secure, information concerning the individual programs sponsored by the Army, Navy, and Air Force. (See *Other loan sources,* #2, on page 355.)

National Health Service Corps Scholarship Programs (NHSC)

These scholarships are provided by the U.S. Public Health Service, on a competitive basis, to students enrolled at U.S. medical schools. They provide for tuition, educational expenses, and a substantial stipend (currently about $6,000). Support may be provided for up to four years, and the stipend is subject to annual cost-of-living adjustments. Recipients of such a scholarship, usually upon completion of postgraduate training, must provide one year of service in health manpower shortage areas for each year of financial support provided (two years minimum). The service may be fulfilled as salaried federal employees of the National Health Service Corps, or as self-employed private practitioners.

Loans

Health Education Assistance Loan Program (HEAL)

This program provides insured loans of up to $20,000 a year (with a maximum of $80,000 for four years). Interest is not to exceed 12% during the life of the loan, and the principal is repayable over a 10- to 25-year period starting nine months after completion of postgraduate training. It is also possible (if funds are available) to repay the loan in part or in whole by arranging a service contract through the Department of Health and Human Services.

Federal Stafford Loan

These loans are provided in two forms: subsidized and unsubsidized. For the former, the government pays the interest while the student is in school. The latter requires that the student pay interest throughout the life of the loan. These loans have a variable interest rate with 2.5% cap and provide a maximum of $8,500 (subsidized) and $10,000 (unsubsidized) annually. Repayment begins six to nine months after completing studies. Repayment can be extended up to ten years.

Health Professions Student Loan Program (HPSL)

This program is administered by the medical schools and gives a student who has exceptional need the opportunity to borrow the cost of tuition and up to $2,500 for other expenses per year. The interest rate is 5% and is applied after completion of residency training. The loan is repayable over a ten-year period.

Perkins Loans

Formerly known as the National Direct Student Loan Program (NDSL), it is administered by the U.S. Office of Education. This program enables a student to borrow up to $440,000 (including loans received as an undergraduate). The interest rate is 5% and repayment can extend over a ten-year period. Repayment begins six months after completing school.

Guaranteed Student Loan Program (GSL)

This program is also administered by the U.S. Office of Education. It permits a student to borrow up to $5,000 per year, the maximum not to exceed $25,000 (including undergraduate loans). The sources of these guaranteed funds are banks, savings and loan associations, or other participating lending institutions. Interest is at 9% and repayment begins 6 to 12 months after completing one's studies.

National Health Service Corps: Federal Loan Repayment Program

This program provides payment toward both government and commercial education loans. This can amount to $25,000 per year for the first two years and up to $35,000 for every year thereafter with a minimum two-year commitment.

Other loan sources

Medical schools have loan funds provided by philanthropic foundations, industry, or alumni. Interest rates and repayment policies are determined by the individual schools.

Funds in the form of scholarships and loans in varying amounts are available from many other sources. There are, however, restrictions as to eligibility based on residence, ethnic group, or other requirements. Sources of some of these programs are:

1. National Medical Fellowships, Inc., 250 West 57th Street, New York, NY 10019

2. Armed Forces Health Professions Scholarship Program. Commander, US Army Health Professions Support Agency SGPS-PD, 5109 Lessburg Pike, Falls Church, VA 22041; Commander, Navy Recruiting Command, 801 North Randolph, Arlington, VA 22203; United States Air Force, Recruiting Service, Medical Recruiting Division, Randolph Air Force Base, TX 78148

3. American Medical Association, Education and Research Foundation, 535 North Dearborn Street, Chicago, IL 60610

4. Educational and Scientific Trust of the Pennsylvania Medical Society, P.O. Box 8820, 777 East York Drive, Harrisburg, PA 17105

5. USA Funds Loan Information Services 8349, P.O. Box 6180, Indianapolis, IN 46209

6. National Health Service Corps Scholarship Program, U.S. Public Health Recruitment, 8201 Greensboro Drive, McLean, VA 22102

7. Robert Wood Johnson Student Loan Guarantee Program, 675 Hoes Lane, Piscataway, NJ 08854

There are many sources of information regarding specialized financial aid programs that are offered to state residents or to those entering particular specialty fields. For additional information on such programs, consult the following publications:

1. *Medical Scholarship and Loan Fund Program,* published by the AMA, 535 North Dearborn Street, Chicago, IL 60610.

2. *FIND: Financial Information National Directory—Health Careers,* published by the AMA, 535 North Dearborn Street, Chicago, IL 60610.

3. "The Health Education Assistance Loan Program: A New Way to Help Finance Your Health Professions Education." HEAL, 5600 Fishers Lane, Rockville, MD 20857.

4. "The Health Field Needs You! Sources of Financial Aid Information," published by the Bureau of Health Professions, Health Resources and Service Administration, DHHS, Parklawn Building, 5600 Fishers Lane, Rockville, MD 20857.

In addition, there are several programs for women and minority group students. Information on these programs is included in Chapters 7 and 8.

10 Medical Education

The traditional program
The curriculum in transition
Evolving new curricula
Attrition in medical school
Preparing for medical school
The making of a physician
United States Medical Licensing Examination

Until the early 1900s, medical education in the United States was unstructured and unregulated. A person wishing to become a doctor would usually seek some didactic training at a medical school and/or spend time as an apprentice with one or more physicians. Since a license to practice was not needed, many unqualified individuals were engaged in the healing arts. The caliber of many medical schools was also open to serious question.

In 1910, after an investigation into the state of affairs existing in medical education, Abraham Flexner proposed a program of reorganizing medical education in a way that would ensure that only qualified individuals would enter the profession. With the adoption of the Flexner report, many medical schools of borderline quality became defunct while others significantly improved their standards. Another result was that medical education became a structured four-year program consisting of two years of basic sciences or preclinical training followed by two years of clinical experience. This educational program was essentially the same in all medical schools.

To ensure the maintenance of high standards, today all medical schools must obtain and maintain legal accreditation. The status of their educational programs is periodically evaluated by the Liaison Committee on Medical Education (LCME) of the Association of American Medical Colleges. This has not restricted medical schools, however, from introducing modifications in their traditional programs. The traditional program, nonetheless, still forms the basis of the medical education process.

THE TRADITIONAL PROGRAM

The First Year

This introductory phase is devoted to the study of normal human biology, which includes anatomy, biochemistry, and physiology. The scope and emphasis within each of these areas are gradually being altered as new experimental approaches result in fresh data. Thus, for example, while the time allotted to gross anatomy is being diminished, the time spent on histology (microscopic anatomy) is being increased, and more emphasis is being placed on ultrastructural and histochemical findings. Most schools incorporate clinical demonstrations within basic science lectures so as to relate subject matter to actual medical problems. Many schools offer some introductory lectures in the behavioral sciences and genetics during the first year.

The first year is about 35 weeks long, with about 35 hours of required class work per week. Half or more of the class time is spent in lectures; the rest is spent in the laboratory.

The Second Year

The second year is the bridge between the preclinical sciences and the clinical subjects that occupy the bulk of the final two years of study. This year establishes the scientific basis for understanding abnormal states of human biology. The standard courses taken during the sophomore year are pathology, microbiology, pharmacology, physical diagnosis, clinical laboratory procedures, and introductions to certain specialty fields such as public health and psychiatry.

Pathology is probably the keystone course of the sophomore year. It provides an introduction to the essential nature of disease and, in particular, the structural and functional changes that cause or are caused by disease. During the second semester, the more common diseases of each organ system and each organ are studied. The teaching process in pathology involves formal lectures, clinical pathological conferences, and laboratory exercises in pathological histology.

Microbiology provides an introduction to disease processes. It involves a study of the microorganisms that invade the body. The basis of mechanisms of infection and immunity is analyzed. One of the most effective means of combating disease is through drugs. Pharmacology concerns itself with the chemistry of the natural and synthetic drugs and their action in the healthy and diseased human body. The full impact of this subject comes to the forefront during the lengthy laboratory exercises in which experimental animals are frequently used to measure the effects of drugs.

The groundwork provided by the aforementioned courses, together with those completed during the first year, provide a great deal of fundamental information about the human body in illness and in health. The next step is to become familiar with the practical techniques required to determine the nature of a patient's illness. An introduction to this procedure is provided by the course in physical diagnosis. This phase of preclinical study gives one a strong psychological lift. The student learns the art of taking a medical history and examining a sick patient. The sophomore year ends with a framework for the clinical years well established.

The Third Year

While the junior year is highlighted by considerable exposure to clinical experience, the formal educational process continues during this period with lectures, conferences, and seminars in medicine, surgery, pediatrics, obstetrics, and gynecology, as well as other specialties and subspecialties. The educational process is usually closely integrated with presentation of relevant patient cases. The emphasis in this early clinical training period is on the diagnosis of disease. The principles of treatment noted will be emphasized later.

Juniors are assigned various patients for a "workup," obtaining a history and physical examination. To carry out the former, the junior medical student learns to interrogate the patient so as to elicit and organize the chronological story of his or her present illness, obtain information as to the general state of his or her past and present health, secure vital data concerning the patient's family history, occupation, and social life. Supplementing this is a physical examination using manual manipulative and instrumental aids (stethoscope and ophthalmoscope). All the information is then integrated to provide preliminary diagnosis. The student then decides whether laboratory tests, X-rays, or special studies are needed. A faculty member reviews the entire "workup" and makes adjustments or confirms the order for diagnostic tests. This preliminary stage of clinical training, like all initial educational experiences, is of special importance. It helps develop a critical approach that tends to avoid the hazards that result from insufficient gathering of information, careless observation, or improper evaluation of the obtained data.

The initial diagnostic training is provided as part of service in the outpatient clinics and in the hospital wards. Later in the year, having attained proficiency in working up new patients, the student serves as a full-time clinical clerk in various clinical departments and in their outpatient clinics. As an apprenticing diagnostician, he or she is introduced to a variety of specialties. The aim of these experiences is not only to introduce the student to possible areas of specialization, but to teach the techniques of detecting all kinds of illness, regardless of specialization. Generally, the student will spend one quarter on medicine, another on surgery, a third on obstetrics-gynecology and pediatrics, and a fourth on electives.

As a clerk in medicine the student will rotate among various outpatient clinics and become familiar with groups of diseases that are classified as cardiovascular, allergic, infectious, rheumatic, neurological, gastrointestinal, and dermatological. Teaching clinics in these subspecialties are conducted by members of the medical school's faculty.

Short periods of time (several weeks each) are usually allotted to otolaryngology (diseases of the ear and throat) and ophthalmology. The student learns the basic diagnostic techniques in these specialties and has an opportunity to study the medical and surgical treatments used in these areas.

The clerkship in surgery enables the student to apply their newly acquired diagnostical training. The student gains insight into the process of determining when an operation is required as well as the need for pre- and post-surgical care. If assigned to the emergency room, he or she may have an opportunity to perform, under supervision, minor surgery such as treatment for infections of fingers, draining of abscesses, or suturing of lacerations. Many institutions offer as an elective a course in operative surgery where animals are treated as patients. Participation by the third-year student in such a program provides him or her with an opportunity for training as a surgeon, first assistant, scrub nurse, and anesthetist.

The student develops a foundation in the physiology of the human female in the first year and in pathology of diseases of the female urogenital system in the second year; he or she is now prepared for clinical work in gynecological diseases, and during the third year, the student participates in conferences, ward rounds, lectures, surgery, and outpatient clinics. It is quite common for the student to deliver about a half dozen babies. These deliveries are naturally performed under the close supervision of a resident in obstetrics. Aside from the training in childbirth, the student learns about the medical and emotional problems of prenatal care. In the outpatient obstetric clinic the student has the opportunity to examine and counsel women in pregnancy. This provides an especially favorable opportunity to develop the doctor-patient relationship.

The clerkship in pediatrics is devoted to the study of children and their diseases. The life span covered is from shortly after birth to adolescence. The student is taught to recognize the need not only for diagnosis of the pediatric diseases but to anticipate them and thus better help to ensure that the child will develop into a healthy adult. The preparation for the pediatric clerkship is frequently initiated in the latter part of the second year with lectures and some clinical experience in the fundamentals, such as heart sounds, X-rays, and EEGs of infants and children. Work in the clinics and wards becomes more intensive in the third year when the student is exposed to varied medical and surgical problems of children's diseases. The fourth year then provides additional opportunity for pediatric training along with greater responsibility.

During the third year, the student-instructor relationship becomes more personalized and an exchange of views begins to take place; the student assumes the status of a junior colleague. The junior medical student's responsibilities are carefully demarcated and essentially restricted to taking medical history and carrying out a physical examination. The acute illnesses the student sees in the wards and the explicit problems he or she handles in the clinics are often "classical," and therefore the student is free from the necessity of coping with diagnostic and therapeutic uncertainties that fall outside a limited area.

The Fourth Year

In the fourth year, the student's activities are frequently divided into four quarters. One is devoted to surgery (including general, orthopedic, and urological), another to medicine, a third to pediatrics, psychiatry, neurology, and radiology, and a fourth to elective study. There is usually considerable latitude in the arrangement of the order in which the program may be carried out.

In the surgical clerkship, seniors may frequently be assigned their own cases. They will, under careful supervision, be responsible for the patient workup, help arrange for laboratory tests, and contribute to discussions involving the diagnosis. Students will participate in preparing the patient for surgery, and, in the operating room, can expect to serve as third or fourth surgical assistant. They may be assigned to keep watch over the patient in the recovery room and be responsible for routine postoperative check-ups until the patient is discharged. The aim of the limited surgical experience for the senior student is not to secure specialized training, but to gain diagnostic experience so as to have a balanced insight into the usefulness of surgical intervention in the process of healing the sick. The exposure in surgery will be a very wide one, ranging from tonsillectomy to cardiac surgery.

In the block of surgical time devoted to orthopedics, the senior is exposed to the diagnosis and treatment of diseases of the joints and vertebral column, as well as fractures and deformities of the bones of the body. In urology some surgical and medical experience is gained by coming into contact with patients suffering from diseases of the kidney, bladder, prostate gland, and reproductive organs.

The quarter devoted to clinical clerkship in medicine is rather similar to that in surgery; naturally, the nature of the patient's illness and the method of treatment differ. Nevertheless, for the fourth-year student, there are workups to be made, tests to be ordered, and diagnoses to be reached. Several times a week students and their supervisors will go on rounds and students will participate in the discussions about the patients' conditions, treatments, and prognoses. During the clerkship period, seniors will be on call 24 hours a day and must be ready to assist in emergencies and to comfort patients through periods of stress. Naturally, throughout this period, the house staff—the residents—will bear the direct responsibilities for prescribing treatment and directing emergency care. But senior medical students nevertheless gain firsthand insight into the responsibilities that must be assumed in postgraduate training.

THE CURRICULUM IN TRANSITION

Since the mid-1960s, there has been increased pressure from medical students to introduce greater flexibility into the course of study. In response to such pressure, most schools have established committees (sometimes including students) to periodically reevaluate and update their curricula. In many schools, new curricula have been introduced that have modified the traditional program using one or more of several different approaches:

1. Determination of a core curriculum that places the emphasis on principles rather than only on facts.

2. Greater correlation between basic and clinical sciences. In the first year, the student is exposed to some clinical experience by seeing patients having illnesses related to the subject being studied.

3. Greater emphasis placed on function than structure. This approach is reflected by a decrease in the amount of time allotted to morphological studies (anatomy, for example) and by an integration of material presented by different departments.

4. Introduction of multiple-track systems. This offers students who have completed the core curriculum, which is the required common experience of all stu-

dents, to choose one of several pathways having different emphases, depending upon their ultimate career goals. Thus, there is a differentiation of exposure depending upon interest, need, and ability.

5. Use of interdisciplinary and interdepartmental courses. These frequently replace departmental offerings, especially in the basic sciences. The combined viewpoints of several basic medical sciences are presented in an integrated fashion as each organ system is discussed, rather than being taught in the classical manner at varied times through separate courses. The organ systems are muscular, skeletal, nervous, cardiovascular, respiratory, gastrointestinal, hematopoetic, genitourinary, integumentary, endocrine, and reproductive. This type of teaching is known as "back to back"; that is, the normal aspects of the anatomy, chemistry, physiology, and pharmacology are considered in relation to abnormal or pathological principles.

6. Use of visual aids. These and other modern methods of instruction are much more widely used, although their effectiveness cannot yet be evaluated.

7. Taking qualifying examinations. In many schools students are encouraged to take such examinations before beginning certain basic science courses. If successful, they may proceed to other areas or disciplines without further coursework in the subject they demonstrated competence in.

8. Introduction of more elective time. This permits the student to spend additional time in areas of special interest, thus facilitating the choice of and preparation for a specialty or becoming more proficient in a selected area.

9. A slow national trend toward sweeping curricular change with an emphasis on communication skills. Thus far these changes have taken place at Harvard University, University of Pittsburgh, Johns Hopkins University, University of Michigan, University of Toronto, and Northwestern University. Consistent with national trends, the new curriculum emphasizes active self-directed learning rather than rote memorization. The supporters of this change feel that medical "facts" become obsolete so quickly that it is pointless to force students to memorize them. Rather, they believe students should be trained to be "lifelong learners."

10. Accelerating the program of studies. A very small number of schools have offered their most promising students opportunities to complete their studies in less than four years. The schools listed below have standard four-year programs with an acceleration option for a three-year program.

Baylor College of Medicine
Johns Hopkins University
Northwestern University
Ohio State University
SUNY at Buffalo
University of Illinois at Chicago
University of North Carolina
University of Texas Medical School at Galveston
University of Washington

The number of schools shortening their curriculum increased during the early 1970s. However, the enthusiasm for the three-year program has diminished markedly, and all schools now offer a four-year program.

11. Lengthening the program of studies. If it proves necessary, some medical schools permit students to extend their educational program for a year. Among such schools are:

Boston University
Creighton University
Howard University
Medical College of Wisconsin
Stanford University
University of California, San Diego
University of California, San Francisco
University of Hawaii

Since there now exists a diversity of curricula because of the many possible variations, it is advisable for the prospective applicant to become familiar with the programs offered by the school in which the applicant is interested (see individual school profiles, Chapter 6).

Alternative Medicine

Over the past two decades many alternative practitioners of healing have gradually gained some acceptance. In a recent survey it was found that about one-third of all Americans use some form of unconventional therapy, spending close to $14 billion annually on treatments.

U.S. medical schools have responded very slowly to this change. Thus far, only about half a dozen include information about alternative medicine in their curriculum. These include Georgetown, Harvard, Tufts, University of California in San Francisco, and the Universities of Arizona, Louisville, and Virginia. Among the reasons offered for doing so is that unconventional medicine can benefit patients, especially those suffering from chronic pain, as well as physicians. The latter may sometimes find using a holistic approach more stimulating than merely treating diseases.

The momentum behind the drive for alternatives to conventional medicine may have its roots in the longstanding undercurrent of unorthodox practice existing in medicine. The assertive spirit of social movements in our society, where the call is to take hold of one's destiny, has probably also impacted on the practice of medicine.

Within the medical community, there is strong opposition by some to alternative medical approaches, with the argument that their claims are not subject to rigorous scientific testing. Thus, physicians who desire to include alternative therapies in their practice run the risk of ostracism. However, intense public interest in alternative medicine is gradually forcing a change. In mid-1992, the National Institutes of Health opened an office for the study of unconventional medical practices, which will provide research grants. Establishing good clinical trials to test unorthodox treatments is not easy. When definitive positive results emerge, the possibility of including some alternative medical practice into the mainstream of allopathic medicine will become more likely. (For definitions of alternative medical practices, see Appendix E.)

In view of the large number of individuals using alternative modalities, it is desirable that future physicians be aware of the nontraditional practitioners and be sympathetic to patients who have sought help outside of conventional medicine.

Elective Programs

Almost all schools now offer opportunities for students to pursue such activities as independent study, honors programs, and special research projects, either at home or elsewhere during the academic year or in the summer.

Overseas Study

In the pre-World War II decades, it was common for U.S. physicians to travel overseas, usually to Europe, for specialty training. With the dramatic advances in U.S. medical education, this is no longer necessary. During the 1980s, however, it was noted that there was an increase in the number of U.S. medical students taking clinical electives abroad, especially in developing countries. It is thought that currently more than 15% of medical students participate in international health projects.

Overseas study is essentially a student-motivated undertaking. Finding an appropriate place abroad that has adequate funding can be quite difficult. The initiative to secure a position rests with students, although they may find a sympathetic faculty member to assist them.

The desire to have a unique life adventure while also serving as a goodwill ambassador is one of the motivating factors for overseas work-study endeavors. A more pragmatic motive is the desire by some students to determine which area of international health they should pursue. However, most of those who feel compelled to undertake such a project do so in order to contribute to improving health care resources of underserved people.

Medical students considering an overseas stint should be prepared to be flexible so far as living conditions are concerned, both in terms of accommodations and diet. Also, they should not consider their project a sight-seeing trip and they need to take time to learn about the culture of the elective country. They must be aware that there are negative aspects to service abroad. Some residency program directors view such an activity as time off from medicine. Frustrated by the inability to improve conditions in underdeveloped areas, some individuals may fail in their efforts to study and help overseas health care providers.

Obtaining permission from a medical school to study abroad should, in most cases, not prove difficult, since more than 90% of the schools allow third- or fourth-year students to do so for up to two months. However, only about 25% of the schools provide training in international health. This is regrettable, since preparation is the key to a successful overseas stay and typical university-based clinical training is inadequate for preparing students for service in underdeveloped areas. The University of Arizona Health Sciences Center in Tucson, Arizona, offers a free summer international health course that is held in high regard.

Medical Assistance Program International, Brunswick, Georgia, funded by the Reader's Digest International Fellowships, provides funding for 50 senior medical students to serve in overseas missions. It is one of the few programs offering overseas study support.

The following additional advice can be useful in trying to secure an overseas elective:

1. Seek an established program to ensure that it will be well organized.

2. Start the search for an elective country early; overseas correspondence is time consuming.

3. Get to know people in your elective country, since this can provide for meaningful future relationships.

4. Be prepared to deal with communication problems, loneliness, and frustration.

5. Consider yourself a collaborator for health improvement, rather than a savior.

6. Travel lightly, but be sure to take pure chlorine for water purification and a non-leaking water bottle in which to store it.

7. Respect the ways of the people you are visiting; this enhances respect on their part.

8. Before departing, read *Cross-cultural Medicine: What to Know Before You Go* (AMSA International Health Task Force) and *Where There Is No Doctor: A Village Health Care Handbook* (Chesperian Foundation, Palo Alto, California).

For an in-depth discussion of foreign medical study, see Chapter 12.

Community Service Activities

In the 1950s medicine emphasized the patient as an individual, rather than as part of a larger group. In the 1960s patients were introduced to students early in the educational process and medical ethics became a part of the curriculum. Currently, new concerns have emerged, such as the impact of technology on the terminally ill and the spiraling cost of and accessibility to health care.

In recent years there has been a growing awareness among health care professionals of the needs of the disadvantaged, which include nearly 40 million uninsured Americans. This has resulted in students volunteering their services, and some of these activities are gaining medical school recognition.

Service programs that students have initiated and led involve a very wide range of activities such as work in soup kitchens for the homeless, helping to build low-income housing, serving as health educators in local grade schools, or assisting in medical clinics. Increasing numbers of medical school administrators are beginning to view such activities as an integral component of medical education, rather than merely an extracurricular activity. Medical schools are starting to support such programs both financially and by granting academic credit for community service. Some schools are engaged in formally integrating community service into their curricula. Schools such as Dartmouth, University of California (Davis), and the University of Miami have large numbers of their first-year students participating in community service projects. Thousands of fourth-year students are involved in service as community health educators or as volunteers in clinics for underserved populations.

Community service is also reflected in the activities of medical students (and physicians) at the hundreds of free clinics located in urban and rural areas across the country. Medical students can thus gain hands-on experience under supervision in primary care. Both this and nonmedical-oriented service projects offer students an opportunity for a brief respite from the rigors of formal lectures, labs, and exams. It also serves as a reminder about the humanitarian goals of medicine as a caring profession.

Legislation that is part of the National Community Service Trust Act supports the award of grants to schools to facilitate service learning. The extent of funding for this and similar programs remains uncertain in an era of budget tightening.

EVOLVING NEW CURRICULA

A major consequence of the introduction of new medical curricula is the individualization of medical schools. From the time of the Flexner report in 1910 until Case Western Reserve University introduced organ-based learning in 1952, all medical schools were essentially the same in following the traditional two-year basic science courses plus a two-year clinical science curriculum. They differed only in the size, facilities, and quality of their teaching staff. With the introduction by McMaster University of problem-based learning in 1975, the option for wide-ranging curricula variations became feasible and has, in fact, taken place.

The major nontraditional approach to medical education in the basic and clinical sciences involves incorporating fact-intensive courses into an integrated curriculum. In this approach the focus is on general principles that usually cut across traditional disciplines, resulting in blocks of time devoted to a particular organ system in the context of various relevant sciences. Frequently coupled with this educational format is a technique known as problem-based learning, in which small groups of medical students analyze clinical case histories with the participation of a faculty member. Each student selects an aspect of the case to research and at the next session each discusses what was uncovered, thereby generating a collaborative learning system. This system is currently in effect on a limited basis in about 60 medical schools, about half the medical programs in the United States. While fully assessing the effectiveness of this approach is premature, preliminary findings indicate that students educated under the nontraditional system had overall lower scores on Step 1 of the USMLE, but generally scored higher on Step 2. Students seem to like the new system, perhaps because it is less demanding. A full day of lectures along with tedious lab work has been eliminated in favor of only a few lecture hours daily with streamlined labs.

There are some stresses in small group learning situations, such as one-upmanship to impress teachers and classmates by students who enjoy demonstrating their substantial pool of knowledge. Another problem is that some students do not pull their weight in meeting their assignments, making it more difficult for others. In addition, this new approach requires readjustment away from the competitive isolated learning experience. Learning to approach a problem in a "holistic" manner, rather than memorizing a mass of facts as was done during the premed years, involves drastic change, but may prove very worthwhile in the end.

ATTRITION IN MEDICAL SCHOOL

If you have been accepted to a U.S. medical school, you are one of a select group of students who have survived the successive academic prunings of elementary school, high school, college, and medical school selection procedures. In addition, you rank in the upper 50% of all students entering graduate and professional schools. Medical schools seek to graduate as many of their entrants as possible; therefore you stand a better chance of successfully completing your medical education than students in other professional schools in the United States or medical students in practically every other country. While the attrition rate in American professional schools is relatively high, that for medicine has consistently been relatively low. Nevertheless, any loss of medical students is a loss to society and is especially painful when one considers the many qualified applicants who were rejected and thus denied an opportunity to study medicine.

It is therefore encouraging to report that the overall dropout rate has remained very low over the past few years. The withdrawals from the total student enrollment in a recent year were 751, or 1.85% of the enrollment. Moreover, even this figure may in reality be artificially high because one-fifth of the students (143, or 0.35%) withdrew to pursue advanced study and are expected to return to medical school. In addition, less than one-third of the withdrawals or dismissals (223) were for academic reasons, the remainder (385, or 1%), for other reasons, making, in actuality, the true attrition rate closer to 0.5%. This means that admissions committees have been able to select from the large pool of qualified applicants those most likely to succeed. If accepted, you should feel confident that with consistent hard work you will most likely complete your course of studies.

An analysis of student records over an extended period has provided significant information regarding the relationship of various student characteristics to attrition that can help you assess your own chances for success and indicate when extra care and effort may be called for. Successful students are more likely to have attended an undergraduate college with a sizable premedical program that they found to be both difficult and competitive. The premedical grades of academic dropouts are substantially lower than are the grades of both successful students and nonacademic dropouts. The average test scores for dropouts are much lower than those of successful students. Unsuccessful students report almost twice as many personal problems as do successful students. Older students have a much higher dropout rate than do younger students. Women have a somewhat higher attrition rate than do men. It should be noted, however, that studies have shown that the academic dropout rate was the same for both sexes but the dropout rate for nonacademic reasons (marriage or pregnancy) was almost three times higher in women. The dropout rate did not differ significantly for married students or for those reporting similar time allocations to study, part-time employment, or extracurricular activities. Successful students tend to be influenced by a desire for independence and for prestige, whereas unsuccessful students are most likely to be influenced by such additional factors as reading and by religious and service motivation.

The following are some specific suggestions that can reduce your changes of dropping out of medical school. Prior to entering medical school you should obtain a strong background of fundamental knowledge in the sciences and develop good study habits; seek opportunities to test your motivation for a career in medicine by exposure to health science-related work (lab assistant, hospital aide, volunteer work with handicapped, visiting hospitals and medical schools); and seek admission to medical schools where you can most likely gain admission and that are most suited to your abilities and interests.

If you fail at the end of a year and are offered a chance to repeat, accept the opportunity to do so if you still want to study medicine. The chances are high that you, like many previous repeaters, will finally successfully complete your studies. Should you decide to withdraw voluntarily, do so only after consultation with appropriate faculty and administrative members of your school.

PREPARING FOR MEDICAL SCHOOL

The Transition

There are significant differences between attending college, especially a small one, and being enrolled in a medical school. It is thus desirable to first enumerate some of the characteristics of the learning environment in medical school so as to provide a better perspective as to what is involved in making the transition.

Medical school is characterized by:

1. a fast-paced, fact-oriented, and highly impersonal environment, especially during the first two years;

2. the keen competition that usually exists because the students have similar backgrounds as high achievers and are all taking the same required courses. The competition usually involves staying above the median class level, although striving for superior grades obviously exists;

3. the staggering amount of material that is usually presented and must be assimilated in a short amount of time;

4. multi-instructor course teaching, which inherently does not favor the establishment of meaningful student-faculty relationships; and

5. early exposure to human cadaver dissection, and subsequently to dying and death, without adequate preparation.

Retaining Idealism

The special challenge of medical school is retaining the sense of idealism premedical students usually bring with them at the outset of their studies. Medical school is an especially stressful interlude in a young person's life. It is not uncommon to find third- or fourth-year students speaking of the negative impact of the pressures of the first years. Cynicism and apathy appear to be replacing much of the idealism that was present at the beginning of a student's education.

Medical students frequently begin their education with many idealistic interests, strong views on the need for political and economic change, constructive thoughts on increasing the number of general practitioners, and positive attitudes toward medical ethics and eliminating bias. When their studies begin, stress also builds. During the initial years, students are expected to learn vast amounts of information, besides the regular school exams. Students face taking Step 1 of the USMLE, long clinical rotations, and, finally, the challenge of finding a suitable residency. Heightening the existing burden is the anxiety of student loan debt. Consequently, students begin to feel overwhelmed and start to prioritize the distribution of their interest and energy, with little idealism remaining for work to bring about change and progress.

In order to be maintained, idealistic beliefs need encouragement or they die. In theory, sustaining altruism should be a shared responsibility of student, school, and profession. Unfortunately, important fiscal concern for their institution or their constituents distracts school administrators or profession leaders from focusing on this issue. In reality, the responsibility for retaining idealism falls essentially on the students. While some feel that it is impossible to do, many have successfully accomplished it.

The key to nurturing one's sense of idealism as a medical student is to reinforce it. This can perhaps best be done by establishing close relationships with like-minded classmates. In addition, participation in the activities of student organizations, such as the American Medical Student Association, Student National Medical Association, American Medical Women's Association, or the Student Section of the American Medical Association, can be stimulating. The ideals generated and contacts made can serve to sustain one's altruistic impulses.

Domestic or overseas volunteer work in typical social settings can provide another opportunity for enhancing idealistic motives. Taking electives at rural community or similar locations can prove to be an enriching experience that will nourish service attitudes.

Coping with Stress

The inherent characteristics of medical school listed earlier clearly lend themselves to stimulating a stressful life for the medical student. This potential is enhanced by the natural insecurity that a major new phase in life can engender. Thus, a significant element in achieving success by a medical student is knowing how to cope with stress.

The ability to cope with stress is dependent upon your personality as well as your prior life experiences. Some people can withstand very intense stress before they feel the pressure, while others have a lower stress tolerance threshold. Mastering the art of coping with stress is essential in order to succeed in medical school.

Coping with stress is also essential in helping you maintain your health. Under stress, your breathing becomes shallow and uneven, your pulse speeds up, and your senses sharpen. Consequently, a stressful day frequently results in a feeling of tiredness. Prolonged stress has been demonstrated to contribute to headaches, skin rashes, or even more serious illness such as ulcers and asthma.

If you have any problems coping with stress, you should seek information about deep breathing, stretching, or regular aerobic exercises that can help you control the feelings produced by stress. Consulting a physician can also prove useful, especially in severely stressful situations where medication may be indicated.

At the very outset, it should be recognized that, if you have been admitted to medical school, you have already proven that you can probably cope rather effectively with stress induced by educational demands. A successful premedical stage clearly included securing appropriate grades in college, especially in the science courses, as well as on the MCAT exam, completing an application that was impressive, and adequately facing the challenge of admission interviews. These achievements should serve to reinforce your sense of confidence in being able to cope with stress while attending medical school.

The goal in coping with stress should be twofold: (1) to control the extent of your exposure to stressful situations; and (2) to learn how to respond to stress.

The following seven suggestions may be useful in coping with stress:

1. Maintain your health as optimally as possible. This includes following an appropriate diet and a suitable exercise regimen.

2. Meet pending responsibilities one at a time, if possible. Tasks and problems should be prioritized and addressed accordingly. When possible, subdivide large problems into small manageable tasks, which in turn should also be solved in a prioritized manner.

3. Utilize your time efficiently. This means budgeting time in an appropriate manner. Don't overextend yourself with an excessive number of scheduled activi-

ties, or underestimate the time they may require. Be flexible in meeting needed changes in planned activities.

4. Realize that some stressful situations are unavoidable (such as scheduled examinations, traffic delays, etc.). Since you cannot exercise control over certain potential stress-inducing problems, try to accept them calmly and matter-of-factly.

5. Find a wholesome outlet for stress and frustrations. This can include participation in some sports activities, or the use of a close friend to whom you can verbalize your frustrations and fears.

6. Avoid situations that you know will be stressful: if last minute cramming for an exam generates stress, schedule your study time so that you are fully prepared in advance of the test deadline and therefore can avoid cramming. Similarly, if getting to school is an erratic experience time-wise, schedule an adequate amount of time in order to avoid the frustration and stress created by the fear of arriving late.

7. Allow for several short periods of relaxation during the day (such as during mealtimes) and more extended ones on weekends. Periodic holiday vacations can help you to recover from long spells of even semi-stressful living.

First-year Guidelines

Special emphasis deserves to be placed on the freshman year of medical school, where attrition, if it will occur at all, is most likely. Like the first year of high school or college, it marks a year of transition from the triumph of graduation to the lowest rung of the school's hierarchical ladder. It frequently involves relocating and having a new group of peers.

The average freshman begins medical school with unresolved feelings about the level of achievement attainable in a new and unproven milieu. The nature of the academic environment, with its large volume of work and the presence of bright and hardworking classmates, makes it difficult to prove oneself and attain one's inner expectations. Students with a high degree of self-worth and those who can gain gratification from intrinsic rewards, such as the satisfaction derived by keeping up with and passing through the curriculum, will best respond emotionally to the existing stressful situation. Providing self-praise rather than seeking external sources of encouragement is helpful.

The special features of the freshman year that deserve to be brought to the attention of prospective medical students are as follows:

1. Students frequently have a wide range of emotional experiences during the course of the year, ranging from exhilaration to anxiety, frustration, and depression.

2. The academic program offered is usually uneven, with some courses being exciting and others dull. Taken as a whole, the program is exhausting.

3. A key to success is to organize one's time most effectively to meet one's specific needs. Allowance should be made for a reasonably fulfilling personal and social life.

4. Upperclass students may provide useful insights into the pressures to be faced and methods of coping, as well as helpful study tips. The advice given should not always be taken at face value, but must be adjusted to one's specific needs.

5. While attaining high grades is commendable, developing a competent grasp of the material presented should be the prime goal. This involves developing a priority system of study of the wide-ranging subject matter and the various topics, focusing on understanding concepts, and fitting the details into the conceptual framework so as to facilitate their retention.

6. Development of an objective approach to clinical problems should begin in the first year. This involves beginning to establish a flexible emotional balance between excessive sympathy for patients and exaggerated detachment.

7. It is important to avoid a feeling of complete isolation in an endless sea of information, some of which is esoteric and apparently irrelevant to one's specific career activities. To avoid losing one's perspective, it is useful to set aside some free time for clinical observation, such as attending rounds or conferences.

8. Although difficulties and setbacks may occur, they need not necessarily lead to failure.

9. Emotional self-care, using such methods as having planned breaks and regular exercise, utilizing preventive stress management techniques, and maintaining personal relationships, as well as providing oneself with rewards, is worthwhile.

10. Help should be sought if signs of trouble, in the form of depression, relationship problems, and increased use of alcohol or drugs, become evident.

11. To offset the decrease in overall physical activity due to the considerable time spent in the classroom and laboratory, an exercise schedule, even if at a limited level, should be maintained.

12. To help ensure good physical, mental, and emotional health and stamina, proper attention should be paid to nutrition and diet.

Finally, it should be kept in mind that, while there frequently is an increase in stress as the freshman school year progresses, there is also a tendency for coping effectiveness to improve. Associated with this improvement is a betterment in health and mood. Along with these changes comes a heightened enjoyment of medical school, with feelings of greater competence and reduced uncertainty about entering a medical career.

Second-year Guidelines

The second year marks a turning point on the student's road to becoming a physician. The focus is drastically altered, from what heretofore has been almost exclusively the normal state of the human body, to a consideration of the disease process, its consequences, and modes of therapy. While conceptual thinking continues to be required, the volume and the content of the information presented place a heavy premium on memorization. This year represents an equalization in potential between premeds and non-science majors.

For obvious reasons, pathology represents the key transitional course from the normal to the diseased. It is usually taught by means of formal lectures, exercises in laboratory medicine, seminars in clinical problem solving, and autopsy exposure. The interplay of anatomy, biochemistry, and physiology with pathology provides the intellectual challenge inherent in this subject. The linkage of clinical observations with autopsy findings as revealed in clinicopathologic conferences (CPCs) provides dramatic insights into the effects of the disease process.

Pharmacology complements pathology, since the actions of individual drugs and drug families can be learned in the context of the diseases they treat. This course stimulates a review of relevant basic science topics and, while heavy on memorization, also demands conceptual understanding.

A significant course of the upper sophomore semester is physical diagnosis. This is usually taught by formal lectures, at hospital teaching rounds, and by individual hospital assignments. This course provides an invaluable base upon which to build for the coming clinical years.

The major challenge of the second year is to balance all its demands, namely multiple-coursework, patient responsibilities, and preparation for tests and Step 1 of USMLE in June. The second year thus has all the components to generate a great deal of physical and emotional stress, and it usually does. The advice given as to stress management in the preceding section is obviously applicable for preventing and/or meeting this year's crises. The survival skills developed during the first year should help ensure satisfactory completion of the second.

Third-year Guidelines

The beginning of the third year marks a major turning point in professional medical education. It represents the onset of a lifelong involvement with the realities of clinical medicine.

The initial impact is reflected by the need to learn how to develop a relationship with patients. In this regard, students should clarify to the patient and/or the patient's family their position as being on the first rung in the medical hierarchy. This may desirably be reinforced by referring to oneself as "student Doctor Smith." This will limit the student's responsibilities to their appropriate level and permit unanswerable patient questions to be referred to the appropriate authority without embarrassment.

Concomitant with the introduction to patient care is the impact it has on the attitude of the medical student toward patients. There generally (and unfortunately) is a change in attitude from being service oriented to being self-education oriented. The goal that should be sought is the ability to view the patient simultaneously as a human being and as a source of biomedical knowledge.

Another special feature of the junior year is the development of a relationship with the house staff. There will be substantial learning opportunities as well as exposure to menial "scut" work. Thus the results can be both exhilarating and rewarding, and frustrating and depressing. The key to a meaningful experience is to determine what the patient's diagnostic or therapeutic plan is so that you can interact as intelligently as possible with the other members of the medical team.

During this year the opportunity to view the bedside manners of different attending physicians will be available, perhaps for the first time. Each will be found to have a distinctive style that can be instructive to the doctor-in-training.

Learning to chart, that is, to prepare a current, clear, concise, and complete record of the patient's progress, is a significant part of the educational experience. Finally, a central element of medical school experience, mainly the "workup," will be introduced during the junior year. Developing a positive attitude toward hospital work routine and critical skills in achieving a differential diagnosis is the key to professional success. To master the art of diagnosis, one must work out the rationale for every question and organize questions into logical groups. Leads should be followed up by additional questions and a search for specific physical findings. Thoroughness in taking a history and carrying out a physical examination will prove most rewarding for both the practitioner and the patient.

In summary, the junior year represents a relearning of the basic sciences in a clinical setting. Learning the biochemical and physiological bases of disease mechanisms in the context of living patients will facilitate developing the skills to provide therapeutic relief.

The onset of the clinical years is the appropriate time to learn how to avoid making mistakes. The three basic rules in this regard are:

1. Recognize your own limitations. Be prepared to admit when you feel unqualified to undertake an assigned task. Do not try to bluff your way through a challenge or develop an air of bravado that you can do anything.

2. Don't be afraid of new challenges, so long as you feel assured you are being adequately supervised.

3. Do not ignore the advice of residents and nurses. Their experience and judgment can be very helpful in avoiding costly errors.

A number of schools offer formal training in technical skills such as venipuncture. Such introductory courses most frequently teach "universal precautions," such as handling needles and wearing protective gear. Existing programs, however, vary from a five-day intensive course to ad hoc training at the hospital.

Fourth-year Guidelines

The fourth year represents the final stages before assuming the responsibilities of post-graduate education. The knowledge and experience acquired during the first three years will be put to use during this year of intensive clinical training.

A number of admonitions are in order as the student now proceeds toward the practice of medicine.

1. The principal goal in practicing medicine should be the satisfaction gained through service to others.

2. The essence of good medicine is to reach a diagnosis on the basis of a carefully secured, complete history and physical examination, supplemented, where necessary, by laboratory findings. The lab results should not be used, however, to negate the results of a good "workup," nor should they serve per se as a diagnostic tool.

3. Patients tend to place physicians on a pedestal. By recognizing that the majority of illnesses are self-limiting, physicians should realize that often the services they render only provide reassurance and make the patient comfortable. This should promote an attitude of humility that can counteract the ego-stimulating factor inherent in the practice of medicine.

4. While medicine is an inexact science, its practice nevertheless requires one to be as exact as possible. Nothing should be taken for granted; otherwise, unforeseen complications can ensue.

5. It should always be recognized that it is the patient who is ill, and that it is the patient, not the disease, that should be treated.

6. There is a critical need to remain up to date by reading the current literature and attending meetings. This will ensure quality health care and maintenance of an intellectually stimulating quality in the practice of medicine.

7. Responsibility to the profession calls for the practitioner to set the best possible example in appearance, speech, and action.

8. The goal should not be solely to gain an education by isolating oneself from world affairs and one's community. By remaining alert to what is transpiring and being as active as possible, one meets the broader responsibilities associated with the title "Doctor."

Goals to Strive for in Medical School

The premedical college years can have a negative impact because of the competition for a place in the entering class. Those gaining admission are usually achievers of high grades that have been attained by intensive studying. This generates an attitude where learning becomes a chore rather than a pleasure.

The goals in medical school should be associated with the learning process. They should be to:

1. learn how to develop and maintain a love for learning;

2. learn to develop a balanced lifestyle incorporating work, relaxation, rewarding relationships, and varying interests;

3. learn to be receptive to new concepts while at the same time being reserved in making definitive judgments, since not all that appears logical is proved correct in the end;

4. learn to develop a genuine interest in finding out more about people and the best ways to care for them as individuals;

5. learn to use one's imagination and not be overwhelmed by the mountain of information ingested;

6. learn how to acquire a serviceable foundation in the biomedical sciences during the preclinical years and how to secure additional information in each area when needed;

7. learn how to attain a secure base during the clinical years upon which to build during postgraduate training;

8. learn to accept the fact that practicing medicine requires a certain amount of personal sacrifice in terms of private life, time off, and other areas;

9. learn that one's goals are not only to acquire knowledge and skill, but also to retain an interest in society and the world; and

10. learn to accept the fact that medicine is a continual challenge and that it brings with it both the joy of triumph and the sorrow of defeat.

THE MAKING OF A PHYSICIAN

The premedical and medical school preparation and training intervals usually extend over an eight-year period. During this time, the student is, for the most part, preoccupied with coursework and then clinical training. The concerns are essentially with the mechanics of climbing from one rung to the next on the ladder of professional status. Little time is thus available to reflect upon the nature of the nonacademic aspects of medical education and medical practice, although these may be subtly realized as one journeys along the educational route. By enunciating them at this point and bringing them to the attention of prospective physicians, the metamorphosis from layperson to healer may be better understood and appreciated.

Two fundamental interpersonal characteristics must be understood to develop a proper perspective about the practice of medicine.

Physician-Patient Relationship

The basic strength of medicine has been, and undoubtedly will remain, the highly personalized one-to-one relationship between the patient and the physician. It involves establishing and maintaining a bond of trust and faith between an individual in pain and the doctor selected to diagnose and cure, or at least alleviate, the suffering. The interaction between these two human beings seeking a common goal is the cornerstone of the practice of medicine. Maintaining this unique interpersonal bond between patient and doctor, even if other members of the health team are interposed in the diagnostic and therapeutic phases, is one of the most essential elements of medical practice.

Physician-Patient Responsibility

The second key element in the care of, as well as in caring about, the patient is providing appropriate care. The trust placed in the hands of a physician needs to be reciprocated by his or her genuine concern for the patient. This involves the proper application of both the science and the art of medicine so that one achieves the goal of the maintenance of health, or easing of pain.

To meet one's responsibilities as a physician involves absorbing and assimilating a sound basis in human biology and acquiring and maintaining a high level of clinical expertise. Only a sound scientific basis for critical evaluation will enable the physician to incorporate or reject various items in the large volume of data obtained during the course of a patient's "workup" and thereby arrive at an appropriate diagnosis.

A better relationship may be facilitated if one has a view of what the patient seeks in a physician. A survey has shown that priority is given to: (1) being knowledgeable, (2) being competent, (3) answering questions honestly and completely, (4) providing clear explanations to medical problems, (5) making sure that patients understand what they have been told, (6) spending adequate time with them, and (7) demonstrating a genuine interest in the patient's health and welfare.

UNITED STATES MEDICAL LICENSING EXAMINATION

There is no national medical licensing body in the United States. It is the function of the individual states to determine who shall practice within their borders and to maintain high standards of medical practice in accordance with their own rules and regulations. In recognition of the thoroughness and widely accepted standards of the USML examinations, its certificate is accepted by the medical licensing authorities of the District of Columbia, Puerto Rico, and all states except Louisiana and Texas.

The National Board of Medical Examiners (NBME) has established three qualifying examinations which are referred to as Steps 1, 2, and 3 of the United States Medical Licensing Examination (USMLE). Step 1 is given in June and September and is a two-day multiple-choice examination. It seeks to assess the ability to apply knowledge and understanding of key concepts of basic biomedical science, with an emphasis on principles and mechanisms of disease and modes of therapy. Step 2 is given in March and September and has a similar format to Step 1. It seeks to assess the ability to apply the medical knowledge and understanding of clinical science considered essential for the provision of patient care under supervision, including emphasis on health care and disease prevention. Step 3 seeks to assess the ability to apply the medical knowledge and understanding of biomedical and clinical science considered essential for the supervised practice of medicine with emphasis on patient management in ambulatory settings. To be eligible to take Step 3, the individual must (a) have obtained the MD degree (or its equivalent) or the DO degree, (b) have successfully completed both Steps 1 and 2, (c) if a foreign medical school graduate, have successfully completed a Fifth Pathway Program, and (d) have met the requirements for taking Step 3 imposed by the medical licensing authority that is administering the examination, such as the completion of any postgraduate requirements. The latter generally is the near completion or completion of one full postgraduate training year in an accredited graduate program.

There are indications that the standard method of testing a future doctor's clinical competence will be computerized, using interactive simulations of physician-patient encounters. The reason is that computer-based examinations (CBX) are thought to be a more reliable method of testing clinical competence than the present multiple-choice and true-false exams. From a preliminary pilot study, the NBME concluded that CBX measures important qualities not measured by current testing modes.

The computer-based test links a personal computer and a video player. The examinee serves as the attending physician. Information on the patient's basic condition is displayed on the screen. The examinee can request additional information, such as EKG readings or X-rays. The "patient's" progress is continually updated in response to the examinee's medical care. The score reflects (1) whether the "physician" took the appropriate steps, (2) whether they were ordered in the appropriate sequence, and (3) whether the orders were timely.

While CBX is designed *ultimately* to replace patient management problems in Step 3 of the USMLE, which is taken by residents, it may in time be included in Step 2, of which third-year medical students are the usual examinees.

11 Postgraduate Education and Training

Incorporating the residency and internship
Resident matching program
Residency training
Fellowship training
Improving postgraduate training
Challenges in training
New trends in medical specialties
Physician employment opportunities

INCORPORATING THE RESIDENCY AND INTERNSHIP

When the internship first became an established part of medical education in the early part of this century, its purpose was straightforward and uniform: a *rotating* internship, with nearly equal portions devoted to medicine, surgery, pediatrics, and obstetrics-gynecology, which provided the first extended clinical experience and the first supervised responsibility for the welfare of patients. These experiences were deemed necessary, and usually sufficient, to complete the preparation of a younger physician for independent practice.

With advances in medicine, the purpose of an internship was no longer obvious nor uniform. The internship did not provide the student's first practical experience with problems of diagnosis and treatment; that function is served by undergraduate clinical clerkships. Nor was it sufficient to provide the final educational experience preceding independent practice; the additional training of a residency is generally considered necessary to fulfill that purpose.

The nature of the internship also changed over the years. Aside from the original rotating format, in time two other types came into use: *mixed* internships—providing training in two or three fields with prolonged concentration in one of them; and *straight* internships—devoting time entirely to single areas, such as medicine, surgery, or pediatrics.

While medical school curricula are the corporate responsibilities of faculties, internship programs were not the corporate responsibilities of hospitals. The responsibility of ensuring a truly educational internship was usually that of an individual head of a service or heads of several independent services. An inevitable result of such highly individualized and fragmented responsibility was that internship programs varied widely in the extent to which they duplicated the experience already gained in the clinical clerkship, in the amount of routine and sometimes menial service required, and in their educational quality.

As a result of the questionable value of the internship in the educational process and the very high percentage of physicians taking residencies, its usefulness as a distinct program came into serious question. At its annual convention in December 1968, the AMA adopted a resolution that "an ultimate goal is unification of the internship and residency years into a coordinated whole." Further steps toward implementation of this resolution were subsequently adopted and the goal was set that by July 1, 1978 all internship programs would be integrated with residency training to form a unified program of graduate medical education. This means that the internship year becomes the first year of residency and that one person is assigned as program director in a specialty at a given institution and is responsible for the entire program. That person has the option of requiring or recommending a specific type of first year (rotating, mixed, or straight) acceptable as part of the residency program, or even assigning trainees to an outside hospital for their first residency year. A significant amount of flexibility has been introduced so as to permit the graduating physician to secure postgraduate training that is specifically designed for individual interests and career goals. It will also facilitate long-term plans and ensure a more stable personal life.

RESIDENT MATCHING PROGRAM

Almost all graduates of U.S. and Canadian medical schools secure internship appointments in U.S. hospitals through the National Resident Matching Program (NRMP). Foreign medical graduates are eligible to participate if they have passed the USMLE in September or earlier. The matching is carried out in March for residencies that usually start July 1.

Currently, about 54,000 residents are training at U.S. civilian hospitals. The number of residency slots has increased slightly in recent years, particularly in the fields of anesthesiology, internal medicine, and, to a lesser degree, psychiatry and emergency medicine. There were decreases in positions for residents in the fields of pathology and plastic surgery.

In the fall of the senior year, all medical students apply to the hospitals to which they would like an appointment. Sometime during the winter, after the students' marks have been submitted to the hospital's chief of staff, they will be asked to visit the hospital. They may be interviewed by one or several attending physicians as well as the director of the training program. After the interviews are completed in the early spring, future interns make up a list of hospitals to which they have applied, with the number one choice at the top, the last choice at the bottom. All the participating hospitals submit similar lists of the students they have interviewed. The lists are gathered in a central office and fed into a computer, and pairings are made. Senior medical students then get an appointment at the hospital highest on their list that wants a particular student. This program, which was instituted in 1952, avoids a great deal of chaos and anguish, since previously neither students nor hospitals knew where they were until the last moment. The match rate for U.S. medical graduates is usually over 90%.

All specialty boards have made significant modifications in their requirements to adjust to the plan for integrated postgraduate training; senior medical students may now apply for a first year of graduate medical education (PGYI), either in one of the existing types of "internships" or in a first year of residency in most specialties. For additional information contact: National Resident Matching Program, 2450 N Street NW, Suite 201, Washington, DC 20037.

The current average salaries for residents are in the $20,000 to $45,000 range. However, as a result of the deterioration of their financial status because their salaries have not kept up with inflation and their education indebtedness has increased, many residents hold second jobs. Married people, especially those with children, are the most likely to be forced to supplement their incomes.

The rate of annual increase in house staff (resident) salaries has been slowing over the past few years. Some hospitals have not increased their stipends at all, and a number have even decreased them. In general, pay increases are higher at hospitals located in the Northeast and lowest for those in the South. Also, the pay for house staff at university-owned hospitals, because of their higher status as teaching institutions, tends to be lower than the national average, while that for hospitals with limited university affiliation tends to be higher.

Most hospitals offer hospitalization for house staff and their dependents as part of the benefit package. Vacation time varies from one to four weeks annually with the amount increasing by year of training.

Currently, somewhat more than half the hospitals have maternity leave policies but the types of programs vary considerably. One-third of the hospitals treat maternity leave as sick leave, another third have specific guidelines, and the others consider it as short-term disability leave, without pay or vacation.

RESIDENCY TRAINING

After the first postgraduate year comes specialization. The function of this extended period of training has changed greatly since its start a century ago. At that time a residency was a special period of additional clinical education for a few promising and scholarly young physicians who wished to become the teachers or leaders in medicine. Residency training in the past few decades has become standard for the average physician and more than 1500 American hospitals offer such programs. Completing an approved residency and passing a written and/or oral examination given by a specialty board are the basic requirements for certification as a specialist.

In the early 1900s, nearly half of all medical school graduates entered general practice. By the 1960s, this figure had shrunk to about 20%. A recent study concerning medical specialization showed that the distribution of entrants into specialty training has been relatively constant over the last decade. Economic factors are comparatively minor in determining medical specialization, while up to 87% of the sampling indicated intellectual interests to be a major determining factor. Most recruits are entering internal medicine, surgery, psychiatry, obstetrics/gynecology, and pediatrics. Women physicians have generally favored fixed-schedule specialties (anesthesiology, radiology, psychiatry, pediatrics, public health) and work settings (state hospitals and industry).

The length of residency training varies among the different specialties and is indicated in Table 11.1.

It should be noted that many of the specialties listed have subspecialties that may require two to three years additional training beyond that listed in Table 11.1. Among the many subspecialties of internal medicine are cardiology, critical care, endocrinology, gastroenterology, infectious diseases, nephrology, and hematology; of pathology are forensic and neuropathology; and of surgery are hand, plastic, and thoracic surgery.

Securing a Residency

Appointments to residency positions are competitive and usually made through the Residency Matching Program (page 374). Your ranking by the Residency Program Director largely depends on three considerations:

1. medical school performance;

2. summary of recommendations from clinical clerkship supervisor; and,

3. residency interview performance.

As when applying to medical school (see Chapter 3), the personal contact that takes place during the course of the interview can impact very decisively on your future professional career. For this reason, we offer advice on preparing for your residency interview in this section.

Obtaining a residency appointment is not a hit-or-miss affair. Careful planning can avoid many pitfalls and improves your chances for success. Medical students frequently underestimate the importance of residency selection. The training program determines the specialty tract, and within the program, the curriculum and its monitoring staff can profoundly influence your career path. You may be directed into a career in academic or rural medicine, or into a specific subspecialty. In addition, each program has its own philosophy and work environment. In selecting a program, a determination is made as to the amount of time that you will have to devote to meet the program's requirements over a period of several years. The residency interview provides a possible means of enhancing your chances for securing a house staff appointment as well as finding out if

Table 11.1 RESIDENCY TRAINING FOR VARIOUS SPECIALTIES

Specialty	Nature of Work	Prerequisite Training Year(s)	Prerequisite Training Area	Training Period (years) Minimum	Training Period (years) Maximum
Aerospace Medicine	Care for individuals involved in space travel	One	Preventive Medicine	Two	Two
Allergy and Immunology	Treatment of illness due to hypersensitivity to a specific substance or condition	Three	Medicine	Two	Three
Anesthesiology	Producing a partial or total loss of pain by use of drugs, gases, or other means	One	Clinical Base	Three	Four
Child and Adolescent Psychiatry	Treatment of emotional disorders of children and adolescents	One	General Psychiatry	Four	Four
Colon and Rectal Surgery	Treatment of diseases of the lower bowel	Three	General Surgery	Two	Two
Dermatology	Treatment of skin diseases	One	Medicine	Three	Three
Diagnostic Radiology	Use of specialized X-ray techniques for diagnosis	One	Clinical Base	Four	Five
Emergency Medicine	Diagnosis and treatment of acute and life-threatening illnesses	One	Medicine	Two	Three
Family Practice (Primary Care)	Evaluating total health needs and providing routine treatment	—	—	Three	Three
Forensic Pathology	Use of pathological methods in criminal investigations	Three	Pathology	One	Two
Internal Medicine	Treatment of diseases and organs with medications	—	—	Three	Three
Neurosurgery	Surgery of the nervous system	One	General Surgery	Five	Five
Neurology	Treatment of nervous system with medications	One	Clinical Base	Three	Four
Neuropathology	Diagnosis of pathological conditions of the nervous system	Four	Pathology	One	Two
Nuclear Medicine	Use of radioactive substances in the diagnosis and treatment of diseases	Three	Medicine, Pathology, or Radiology	Two	Three
Obstetrics and Gynecology	Care during pregnancy and labor and treatment of diseases of genital and reproductive system	One	Clinical Base	Three	Four
Ophthalmology	Care and treatment of eye diseases	One	Optional	Three	Four
Orthopedic Surgery	Treatment of skeletal deformities and injuries of the bones and joints	One	General Surgery	Three	Four
Otolaryngology	Treatment of ear, nose, and throat diseases	One	General Surgery	Three	Four
Pathology	Diagnosis of structural and functional changes in the body tissues due to diseases	One	Optional	Four	Four

Table 11.1 RESIDENCY TRAINING FOR VARIOUS SPECIALTIES (Continued)

Specialty	Nature of Work	Prerequisite Training Year(s)	Prerequisite Training Area	Training Period (years) Minimum	Training Period (years) Maximum
Pediatrics	Care of infants and children and treatment of their diseases	—	—	Three	Four
Pediatric Cardiology	Treatment of heart diseases in children	Three	Pediatrics	Two	Two
Physical Medicine and Rehabilitation	Treatment by physical and mechanical means to permit maximum restoration of function	One	Medicine and Surgery	Three	Three
Plastic Surgery	Surgery to repair or restore injured, deformed or destroyed parts of the body, especially by transferring tissue	Four	General Surgery	Two	Three
Preventive Medicine	Prevention of disease for individuals and the public	One	Public Health	Two	Two
Psychiatry	Treatment of mental disease	One	Clinical Base	Four	Four
Radiology	Diagnosis of disease by radioactive means	One	Clinical Base	Four	Four
Surgery	Treatment of diseases by surgical intervention	One	—	Four	Seven
Therapeutic Radiology	Treatment of diseases by radiation therapy	One	Clinical Base	Four	Four
Thoracic Surgery	Surgical treatment of chest diseases	Four	General Surgery	Two	Two
Urology	Treatment of kidney and bladder diseases	Three	General Surgery	Two	Two

it is the right one for you. Following are important suggestions to help you secure a suitable position. Many of the pointers noted in the premed interview discussion are relevant here as well.

Do Your Homework

Familiarize yourself with the program for which you are being offered an interview. It is risky to go unprepared into such a situation, since you can make poor choices of places to visit and appear uninformed at the interview. Carefully study published residency program material that was sent to you or a classmate or is on file at your medical school. Such material could provide information concerning faculty-resident ratio and the philosophy, curriculum, work hours, and support staff at the teaching hospital.

Setting up a card file on all prospective interview sites is useful. It will help you refresh your memory just prior to a visit. Add new information and your impressions after each visit for possible future reference. Sequence your interview schedule so that the interviews are not so close that you do not have time to recover from one before you present yourself for another and you can arrive fresh and enthusiastic for each interview. A practice interview at a program low on your acceptance list is a good way to develop self-confidence. Your highest priority interview should be scheduled in the middle of your interview cycle. By that time you should have an adequate amount of experience and will not be physically drained by this demanding process. Remember that making a good initial impression can be enhanced by a firm handshake and proper grooming.

Know Yourself

It is important at the outset of the entire interview process to define your goals career-wise. Completion of a personality test and discussion with faculty members with whom you are close about your goals, interests, and strengths can be helpful. After this process you should be able to clearly articulate your career plans and defend your choices. This should include knowledge of your choice of a clinical or academic career and the type of the residency you are seeking.

Anticipate Obvious Questions

Although interviews vary widely, many questions asked are standard ones. Among the most favorite ones are:

1. What are your short- and long-range goals?
2. What are your strengths and weaknesses?
3. Why do you seek admission to this program?
4. What do you want out of life?
5. Why did you choose medicine as a career?
6. What have been your most important accomplishments so far?

Practicing answers to these questions is advisable so long as they do not sound rehearsed when you deliver them. Mock interviews with fellow students can prove useful in preparing for the real ones.

Ask Tactful Questions About the Program

You should seek to learn about the program in the context of the interview session by inquiring as to the program's commitments to education versus service obligation. Tactful questions are appropriate; therefore, rather than asking about a program's weakness, phrase your question as an inquiry. You may wish to ask the interviewer if the program has received an unrestricted grant, what areas it would be invested in. The most appropriate questions to ask are those relevant to education and the quality of patient care. In any case, the questions you ask should be determined by the position of the person to whom you are speaking. In other words, when being interviewed by a department head, an inquiry relevant to salary or housing would not be appropriate but should be directed to a resident. Questions about the philosophy and curriculum of a program should obviously be presented to the program director and would suggest a more meaningful interest. Try to leave a distinct positive and memorable impression on your interviewer.

Sample the Residency

The best way to evaluate a program is to spend a senior year rotation at the hospital in which you might consider doing your residency. When this is not feasible, you may be able to spend a day as an observer with residents, following them on rounds (if possible, dressed in whites). First-hand observation on the wards and in the clinics will provide a good window to assess the value of the program. Questioning residents, especially those who are particularly positive or negative about the program, is useful.

Present a Team Player Image

The residency is quite different from medical school; therefore, it is desirable to leave an impression that you can make the transition from working independently to being part of a team. Projecting the sense that you will fit well into the existing team will enhance your chance of securing the residency appointment.

Be Yourself

While making a strong effort to project a favorable image, you should also strive to be sure that it is a realistic one. You must balance your desire to get the appointment with a candid assessment of whether the position will fill your own needs. When you leave the interview, you should go away with a positive feeling that this is the place you would like to spend the next several years training, to attain the proficiency you will require in order to succeed in your profession.

FELLOWSHIP TRAINING

After completing four years of medical school and several years of residency, many physicians consider seeking a fellowship for training in a subspecialty. While still in medical school, additional training beyond the residency is considered remote but this attitude is reversed in the course of time. By gaining an awareness of the advantages of subspecialization, trends in various medical disciplines, and the challenge involved in securing a suitable fellowship, one can more easily decide if this is an appropriate course to follow.

Motivating factors influencing residents to pursue fellowship training vary. For some, the issue is to enhance the marketability of their own specialty. Others are concerned with the issue of variety of work experience, while some seek the special challenge that certain subspecialties present, such as critical care, neonatology, etc.

Financial remuneration is also significant when considering subspecialization. While primary care physicians are now in increasing demand, specialty practices are financially more rewarding, as specialists perform more billable procedures. In addition, their patients are more likely to have medical insurance.

Subspecialization is also attractive to some because of its implied higher status within the medical community. Being interested in a limited area makes it easier to keep abreast of new information and technological advances in a particular field. A subspecialist also usually has a more routine work schedule. Thus, all the aforementioned features have resulted in the increased attractiveness of subspecialization in recent years. While the number of medical school graduates choosing an internal medicine residency has declined, the number of those electing to subspecialize in this field has remained high. Some subspecialties are attracting more candidates than others. There has been some decline in interest in hematology, rheumatology, endocrinology, geriatrics, and infectious diseases. On the other hand, the fastest growing subspecialty within internal medicine is critical care, due to the fact that it is an action-oriented area. The demand for this type of subspecialty will continue to grow as more hospitals offer high tech procedures such as open heart surgery and organ transplants.

Another very popular field is pediatric emergency medicine, with a substantial increase in the number of fellowships available. Orthopedic surgery is still another area where subspecialization is very common. Areas of special interest include orthopedic oncology, knee reconstruction, and hand and spine surgery. Subspecialization is also increasingly common among radiology residents.

During medical school and residency, the individual has to focus on the clinical side of medicine. After the residency, research becomes important. This includes developing a suitable project, collecting data, and analyzing and reporting the results. Potential fellows should determine in advance where research funding will come from or if they must secure it on their own. Candidates should determine the extent of interest of the fellowship program in generating publications, especially if the program is academically oriented. This can be ascertained by inquiring about the program's publication record and if it supports fellows in presenting abstracts of their research at academic meetings. Fellowship candidates should try to determine the strength of the director's commitment to the program, so as to judge the extent of support they can anticipate.

It is useful to determine in advance the role of the fellow in the program to find out if the staff position, while an important one, does not place an excessive burden on the individual. Knowing the number of attendings and residents available to assist can help determine if the fellowship will merely serve to fill a resident gap, or if it will be a genuine advanced training position. Obtaining a current copy of the conference and call schedule can provide a good insight into the nature of the position. The number of fellows in a program is also important, because the environment is more stimulating when a group that is on a similar educational level is working together.

Accreditation of fellowship programs varies. It usually takes place after being established at a large hospital that has an adequate number of fellowships. When a program is not accredited, it is important that the program director have a strong enough reputation to compensate for this liability. This is especially relevant in less traditional subspecialties, such as fertility.

Currently, there is increasing pressure to standardize subspecialty educational programs and create a matching process in this area, as for residencies. This effort is geared to enhance the overall quality control of fellowship offerings. It already exists in some of the internal medicine subspecialties and is now impacting on other areas, such as radiology and pediatrics. Gradually, the number of free-standing programs will be reduced as accreditation of fellowship programs increases.

Obtaining a Fellowship

To obtain an attractive fellowship requires careful strategic planning. Standards for fellowship applicants vary. Program directors are quite selective and competition for an appointment is keen. Completing a residency at an institution where the fellowship is offered can usually give the applicant an edge. The disadvantage in continuing at the same institution is that the fellow receives rather narrow training, since the fellow is in contact with the same attending as in the residency, and the opportunity to expand contacts is limited. If one anticipates ultimately seeking a fellowship, the residency training should at least be at an institution that has a good track record of its residents securing fellowships. Thus, the site of one's residency training is one major critical factor in the process of finding suitable subspecialty training.

A second strategic consideration is selecting appropriate faculty to provide letters of recommendation. The goal is to receive these from the people you worked with and who are prepared to write as strongly as possible in your behalf. The impact of a favorable letter is significantly influenced by the stature of the author of the letter. Obviously, a department chair's letter has greater credibility than one from a junior faculty member. Similarly, a positive impact can be made by a letter from a prominent person in the specialty or a known acquaintance of the fellowship program director. Completing an elective in the prospective area of subspecialization can facilitate obtaining helpful letters of recommendation.

Of special importance is the interview and interpersonal and communication skills that the candidate demonstrates. Showing that you are open-minded, flexible, and enthusiastic, and that you are amenable to open discussion of issues will enhance your chances to secure a fellowship.

IMPROVING POSTGRADUATE TRAINING

The long-established system of clinical education is one in which senior physicians serve as instructors to their junior colleagues. This apprentice system may be flawed by the fact that mentor physicians often lack formal training as educators. This weakness impacts directly on the atmosphere and ultimate success of the learning process. As a result of the increased awareness that many physicians are deficient in teaching skills, a few medical schools, residency programs, and continuing education seminars are providing opportunities to remedy this situation. Physicians are learning the basics of good teaching, such as how to create a positive learning climate, how to enhance learner retention, and how to evaluate learner performance.

There are many skeptics, especially among older physicians, who question the need and value of teaching physicians how to teach. Some of the younger doctors believe that clinical teaching is a basic medical skill that is as valuable as physical diagnosis or history taking.

Providing teaching skills to physicians is hampered by the fact that it is not a grant-funded area and does not generate patient revenue. In addition, it is not formally encouraged by the medical establishment but is the driving force of some individual medical school faculty members. While not yet widespread, support for their efforts is gaining momentum.

One of the approaches used, in addition to a discussion of teaching skills, is videotaped role-play exercises. Each role-play is a sort of skit that is designed to demonstrate common, yet troublesome, scenarios in clinical teaching. After the role-play is completed, participants review the tape and analyze their performance.

Since the majority of physicians-in-training do not yet have access to teaching skills training, they are forced to learn how to teach on their own. While this is difficult to accomplish, they can seek help at the Office of Medical Education at their hospital or school. Also, information on clinical teaching may be available in a medical library. The best sources are the following short books: *The Physician as Teacher and Residents as Teachers* by T.L. Schweml and N. Whitman and *Teaching during Rounds: A Handbook for Attending Physicians and Residents*, by J. Edwards and D. Weonholtz.

Finally, improvement in teaching skills can even be obtained by so simple an approach as identifying and listing the attributes of the most skilled clinical teachers one has been exposed to and trying to emulate them. Similarly, the weaknesses of poor clinical teachers can be identified so that those deficiencies can be avoided.

CHALLENGES IN TRAINING

For many years the postgraduate training interlude was looked upon as an initiation rite into the exclusive world of medical practice. Stress and a heavy workload have long been accepted as part of this process. In recent times, a growing number of educators, as well as many trainees, have emphasized the negative aspects of this process.

Already, competition, rather than team effort, may be fostered in medical school. The emphasis is strong on the science of medicine, with the human aspects of medical care often being neglected. In the residency, the heavy workload and its associated responsibilities overshadow educational goals. A further impact of these conditions is the tendency toward physician desensitivation, but reforms over the past few years have improved both the education and training systems. Nevertheless, unhealthy demands are still being placed upon prospective practitioners. Recently, it took a fatal error in judgment by a sleep-starved resident to bring about the 80-hour work week for New York State residents, which has also been adopted in other areas. Those outside the system are still astounded by such conditions, while some within the system regret that changes have been made.

The dehumanization effect may be initiated in medical school when patients are presented merely as abstract cases. Standardization of patients to 150-pound white male stereotypes makes it harder to think in terms of patient differences.

The negative impact of stress and long work hours was ignored for a long time. When its effects in human terms were evident, such as substance abuse or increased divorce rate, more attention began to be given to the problem. A number of approaches have been developed to cope with this problem, including formation of support groups. The consensus is that, while progress has been made, it will take time to alter long entrenched attitudes.

NEW TRENDS IN MEDICAL SPECIALTIES

In response to discoveries in research and changes in society, alterations within established medical specialties, as well as the evolution of new specialties, have resulted. A brief overview of several specialties that have taken new directions follows.

Family Practice (Primary Care)

Public demand for a single, competent physician for the entire family has grown as the availability of such physicians continues to diminish. To meet this need, the specialty of family practice evolved. This specialty differs from the others in that it is defined in terms of functions performed rather than limited by treatment of certain diseases or parts of the body or on the basis of the patient's chronological age.

The specialist in family practice must acquire a basic core of knowledge in all areas of medicine. Being the physician of first contact, he or she is responsible for evaluating the patient's total health needs over an extended period of time. Family practice is thus a specialty in breadth rather than a specialty in depth.

The family practice specialty will become especially important as the U.S. health care system undergoes changes. A suitable balance between specialists and generalists will be one of the ultimate goals to ensure the success of a new system. An overabundance of specialists makes the health care system more expensive, less accessible, and less focused on prevention. The imbalance is a principal cause of the high cost of health care.

Suggestions are being made for ways to shift the trend away from specialization by limiting funding for training in subspecialization and by creating incentives for entering the field of primary care. Among the attractive features of a primary care practice is the opportunity to treat patients ranging in age from children to the elderly. A primary care physician also sees a great variety of cases, from cardiology to rheumatology, and is responsible for providing continual care, creating a special bond between the patient and the physician.

Many physicians are becoming convinced of the value of preventive primary care. Health care reforms, emphasis on primary care, and the demand by women for more comprehensive health care have motivated obstetricians/gynecologists to seek recognition as primary care providers. Some groups, such as the American Academy of Family Physicians, strongly oppose granting such recognition, believing that it should be used for specially trained practitioners. Women frequently use ob/gyn specialists who sometimes also provide a general medical check-up. The American College of Obstetricians and Gynecologists has redefined its mission to include health care of women throughout their lifetime. They have even encouraged their members to subscribe to a journal containing generalist information.

Considerable efforts are being made to encourage medical students to choose primary care as their specialty but there is some uncertainty about the most effective means of achieving this goal. Some feel that having generalists serve as student mentors is the best approach but a medical school survey found that faculty can do little to influence student specialty choice. A different study, however, demonstrated that, where required family practice clerkships exist, the number of students electing to become primary care physicians has significantly increased. This should be of interest to those considering primary care as their career choice.

Interest in family practice over the past few years has risen significantly, with the number of fourth year students matched with this specialty at high levels, second only to internal medicine. There has been a concerted and successful effort by the American Academy of Family Physicians to market this specialty. They have targeted medical schools to set up departments of family practice, and most now have them. Students are encouraged to take primary care clerkships within family practice settings. Such exposure, as noted above, can profoundly alter one's career goals. When the number of physicians entering family practice, internal medicine, and pediatrics for residency training—namely the primary care specialties—combined, it makes up about half of all physicians receiving postgraduate training. Of these three groups, the overwhelming majority of those entering family practice will remain in primary care, while, of the other two segments, a portion go into subspecialty training.

While the federal government is interested in reforming medical education as part of altering the health care system, these efforts are slowed down by political in-fighting. A somewhat more meaningful effort in being made by state legislatures. Their focus is to encourage the training of more primary care physicians so as to promote cost-effective medicine and to encourage physicians to practice in underserved areas. Thus, 13 (out of 21) states succeeded in enacting legislation that offers medical students financial aid or scholarships as incentives to practice in remote areas or inner city ghettos. These states include Maryland, Rhode Island, North Carolina, and Nebraska. Some states, such as Pennsylvania, have increased their funding directly for programs in family practice training. Mandating the training of primary care physicians can be successful in a state like Washington, which serves a largely rural population locally, and in adjacent states. Most other states turned down quota systems. Some schools are voluntarily setting goals of steering students to become primary care physicians in the hope of avoiding legislative coercion later on.

Pediatrics

Although some serious infectious diseases of childhood have been conquered, children will always need care for the usual viral illnesses. Now, however, more attention is being focused on the patient as a whole, especially his or her behavioral problems. Thus such issues as child abuse, drug addiction, and suicide prevention are emerging areas of concern for pediatricians.

A developing subspecialty is pediatric emergency care. Increasing recognition of the need for specialists in this area is reflected by the fact that one-third of all emergency room visits involve children. They frequently present different problems than adults. Those specializing in pediatric emergency care usually complete a pediatric residency and an emergency medicine fellowship. A special five-year program for certification is under consideration.

The next frontier to become open to pediatricians will undoubtedly involve the treatment of genetic diseases with drugs that will come into being because of advances in genetic engineering technology.

Psychiatry

The field of psychiatry is undergoing "remedicalization" in that the emphasis is now on using medical therapy in the context of hospital practice and closer affiliations with other specialties. In addition, a strong move toward subspecialization is developing, and such areas as geriatric psychiatry, clinical psychopharmacology, and forensic psychiatry are emerging.

Diagnostic Radiology

New patterns of health care delivery coupled with advances in imaging technology are altering the professional schedules of radiologists. They are now more frequently on call, and more of them are practicing in outpatient settings.

The expanded use of magnetic resonance imaging (MRI), ultrasound, angioplasty, and other technologies has brought radiologists more intimately into the core of medical practice. Nevertheless, radiological techniques are used by other specialists as well, and an intense jurisdictional debate is in progress.

Subspecialization by means of fellowship training in such areas as ultrasound or pediatric radiology is increasing.

Emergency Medicine

The relatively new specialty is emerging as a distinct entity, as indicated by the fact that board certification now requires specialized training in this area rather than merely passing the qualifying examinations.

Academic emergency medicine centers are now aiming at securing high-quality physicians with four years of training. As more medical students are exposed to this area, a very substantial upswing in the numbers seeking admission to residency programs is expected.

Physical Medicine and Rehabilitation

War injuries and polio epidemics led to the development of physicians especially trained in treating pain and in rehabilitation therapy. Although debilitating diseases such as polio have been eradicated, accident and stroke victims and paralytics live much longer today, and thus the need for the services of physiatrists has increased.

Physiatrists are largely hospital based in terms of their practice, but more are moving into part-time private practice. Moreover, the approach of customizing treatment plans within the context of the patient's quality of life and maximal potential is becoming the norm. This specialty continues to use the multidisciplinary approach in patient care, which is an especially attractive feature for those who choose training in this area.

Sports Medicine

This specialty is still in its infancy, and there are as yet no formal residency programs. Nevertheless an increasing number of physicians, including those trained in orthopedics and family practice, are entering full-time sports medicine. This field is developing because of the dramatic increase in popularity of physical fitness. In addition, the field is expanding beyond treatment to an understanding of the disease process and to prevention. In time, certification and a clearer definition of this specialty will evolve.

Cosmetic Surgery

This developing field is an offshoot of reconstructive surgery. It comes in response to a more affluent society and the desire to obtain a greater degree of self-worth. Technical advances have also promoted cosmetic surgery as a distinct area of specialization. Breast reconstruction, liposuction, and certain kinds of laser surgery are but a few of the more recent developments that are encompassed by this field. In 1979 the American Board of Cosmetic Surgery was established; it certifies physicians from varying specialties who are primarily involved in cosmetic surgery.

Geriatrics

This emerging specialty deals with medical care of the aged, usually defined as being over 65. It involves review of a patient's medical and social history, marital status, and functional ability. The geriatrician aims to address the patient as a whole.

The need for geriatricians is great and will increase as the percentage of the aged in the population gradually increases. The aged spend more than double the nation's health care dollars in proportion to their group size.

Geriatricians are usually initially trained in a specialty such as internal medicine or other relevant area and spend a two-year fellowship training period. Standards for fellowships are being developed.

Career Placement

National trends in career placement are not directly available, and specialty imbalances change from year to year as well. The activities of the AMA Physician's Placement Service for the past few years do provide an insight into what is happening. The AMA's statistics show that there is a general pattern of undersupply of physicians for general and family practice and an oversupply of anesthesiologists, dermatologists, pediatricians, psychiatrists, radiologists, surgeons, and urologists. The only area other than general practice in which there currently seems to be a shortage is otolaryngology, with fewer specialists in this field in proportion to the opportunities available. Note, however, that the oversupply of particular specialists reflects the desires for prime locations, rather than a national oversupply.

Perhaps a good indicator of the current specialty trends is the residency choices of medical school graduates. For a very recent year these choices were approximately as follows:

Internal medicine, 27%
Pediatrics, 11%
Family practice, 12%
Surgery, 10%
Obstetrics and gynecology, 8%
Psychiatry, 6%
Orthopedic surgery, 5%
Radiology, 4%
Anesthesiology, 3%
Emergency medicine, 3%
Others, 11%

PHYSICIAN EMPLOYMENT OPPORTUNITIES

Because of the shortage of physicians in rural and inner city areas, it was decided in the late 1960s to increase the number of practicing physicians. It was assumed that this would bring about a surplus of urban physicians and induce a better geographical distribution of health professionals. This has not come about and the underserved areas have had only modest improvement in spite of a higher ratio of specialists to generalists of 70:30. Projections of a surplus of over 100,000 specialists and a shortage of 30,000 generalists by the year 2000 have been reported.

In partial response to this situation, the number of allotted residency slots have diminished from 135% to 100%. Medical schools are beginning to focus on training primary care physicians by giving students an opportunity to complete ambulatory clerkships. Nevertheless, greater emphasis on the changing health care scene has to be brought to the attention of prospective physicians so that they can find their appropriate place in the professional world.

## 12

Foreign Medical Study

Admission
Transfer to U.S. schools
Internship and residency
Fifth pathway opportunities
Requirements for practice
Selecting a foreign medical school
Foreign medical schools

During the early decades of this century it was relatively common to find Americans going to Europe for postgraduate medical training. Since World War II, significant numbers of Americans have gone overseas for their undergraduate medical education. At the peak of this trend, it was roughly estimated that as many as 10,000 were enrolled in foreign medical schools. Approximately 300 new students are thought to matriculate each year and this figure may be an underestimate.

The fact that a significant number of Americans are studying medicine abroad should not be taken to mean that if you fail to gain acceptance in the United States, you should automatically seek admission to a foreign school. You should first determine if rejection by American schools means that you genuinely lack the ability to complete your medical studies. You should realize that *only* well qualified and highly motivated students stand a good chance of overcoming the obstacles of studying medicine in a foreign language. They then face the difficulties of securing suitable postgraduate training and a license to practice in the United States. The obstacles to be faced in overseas medical study are reflected by the findings of a study that indicates that, of all the American students entering foreign medical schools, one-third will complete their studies after many years but cannot qualify to practice in the United States, and one-third will finish their studies within the standard period (five to eight years) and eventually enter the U.S. physician manpower pool (although they may not end up practicing in the state of their choice).

Current estimates are that about 100 foreign-trained American physicians become practitioners each year; that is, less than half of those who have gone overseas. If you are contemplating overseas study you should ask yourself if you really want to become a physician so much that you are willing to do so by this long and very arduous means, if you have a chance of gaining acceptance to a U.S. school if you reapply, and if you could be happy in some health science career other than medicine.

ADMISSION

The process of securing admission to a foreign medical school is cumbersome because there are no standard application procedures or forms, no standard documents required for submission, and no central clearing service for foreign schools. In spite of these difficulties, it is still advisable to avoid private placement agencies that advertise that they can get you into a foreign school. They provide their services at a high fee and you can gain admission on your own if you are qualified. The following sources of information will be of help:

1. *Foreign embassies and consulates.* They usually have catalogs of the medical schools in their countries. They frequently have staff members who are familiar with the current admission policies and procedures and whose advice should be sought. This source may have applications and descriptive literature or may provide the names and addresses of admissions officers.

2. *Institute of International Education,* 809 United Nations Plaza, NY 10017, maintains a library of foreign university catalogs.

3. *World Directory of Medical Schools* published by the World Health Organization, Geneva. This publication, while providing some helpful data, is not written especially for the potential American applicant and lacks such useful information as how to initiate an application, who is responsible for admissions at a particular school, and how many Americans are enrolled at the school. Therefore, this volume may not be worth purchasing but should nevertheless be examined at a reference library.

Most German, Austrian, and Belgian schools have relatively high admission standards and strict scholastic requirements. As many as from 30 to 50% of the students fail the basic science examination that is taken prior to beginning clinical studies. However, graduates from schools in these three countries have some of the best records for passing the ECFMG examination. Italian, Mexican, and Spanish schools have relatively low admissions requirements and accept and graduate relatively large numbers of students. Graduates from schools in these countries have had the most difficulty passing the ECFMG examination. (This possibly may be due to the poor quality of the students and not necessarily the standards of education at the schools.)

The course of studies in foreign medical schools varies from four to six years. At some schools, examinations are usually taken voluntarily at the end of one- or two-year periods and can be retaken a number of times. This system of academic freedom adds to the existing problem of studying medicine in a foreign language.

TRANSFER TO U.S. SCHOOLS

In 1970 the Coordinated Transfer Application System (COTRANS) was established on an experimental basis to facilitate the transfer of students studying abroad to U.S. medical schools. In the past, this system involved taking Part 1 of the National Board Examinations at a U.S. or foreign test center, a program terminated in 1979. During the decade of COTRANS's existence, less than half of those who took Part 1 of the NBME passed and only about half of those who passed managed to transfer to U.S. medical schools. This points up the inherent difficulties associated with overseas medical study.

In June 1980, a special examination was developed and administered by the NBME for U.S. citizens enrolled in foreign medical schools who wish to apply for transfer with advanced standing to a U.S. medical school. It was known as the Medical Sciences Knowledge Profile (MSKP). This two-day examination was designed to provide medical schools with a method of evaluating such an applicant's knowledge in the basic medical sciences and in introductory clinical diagnoses. Each part of the examination was graded on a nine-point scale. No total score or pass or fail was reported, but the difficulty of transferring to a U.S. medical school is reflected in the fact that less than 40% of students have succeeded in doing so each year. Moreover, the numbers transferring have declined. The MSKP was replaced by the USMLE Step 1 in June 1992.

INTERNSHIP AND RESIDENCY

There are five pathways for foreign graduates to follow in securing AMA-approved internship and residency appointments: (1) transferring with advanced standing to a U.S. medical school and repeating one or more years (the policies of U.S. medical schools regarding transfer and advanced standing are given in the profiles for the individual schools in Chapter 6); (2) certification by ECFMG on the basis of satisfying the ECFMG educational requirements as well as passing the ECFMG examination; (3) obtaining a full and unrestricted license to practice medicine, issued by a state or other U.S. jurisdiction authorized to license physicians; (4) successfully passing the complete licensure examination in any state or licensing jurisdiction where a full and unrestricted license is issued upon satisfactory completion of internship or residency without further examination; and (5) an approach that is especially popular among one segment of foreign medical students, and is for obvious reasons known as the Fifth Pathway, which is discussed in the next section.

Among the drawbacks of attending a foreign medical school is the difficulty in securing a residency appointment at a U.S. hospital upon graduation. A substantial number of Americans, after investing much effort, time, and money, are unable to secure a residency in this country due to a variety of reasons. First, they may have received a poor medical education at the school they elected to attend, which seriously weakens their candidacy for postgraduate training. Second, they are competing against other foreign graduates for the very limited number of places not filled by graduates of U.S. schools. Finally, the total number of residency openings is diminishing in response to the perceived over-supply of physicians that is anticipated. Consequently, the awareness of this potential problem in the educational program of foreign medical students should stimulate careful consideration of this career pathway.

FIFTH PATHWAY OPPORTUNITIES

Students who have completed all of the formal requirements of the foreign medical school except internship and/or social service may substitute a year of supervised clinical training for the required foreign internship (that is, clinical clerkship or junior internship) under the direction of an AMA-approved medical school. Upon successful completion, students may enter the first year of an approved residency program without having to complete the social service requirement of the foreign country. Before beginning the supervised clinical training, students must have their academic records reviewed and approved by the school supervising the clinical training and must pass a screening examination acceptable to the Council on Medical Education. The ECFMG examination and/or Step 1 of the USMLE are used for this purpose.

Currently only mainland U.S. medical schools offer Fifth Pathway clerkships. This option applies primarily to students in Mexican medical schools and is open only to physicians who have completed their undergraduate premedical studies in an acceptable manner at an accredited American college or university. The Fifth Pathway program allows U.S. students who have completed the requirements for a medical degree in Mexico to be eligible for a continuous academic year of supervised clinical training under the direction of a medical school approved by the Liaison Committee on Medical Education. The students who complete this supervised clinical training are then able to enter an AMA-approved graduate training program without completing the Mexican-required internship or social science obligation. This program allows graduates of Mexican medical schools to pass easily into graduate medical programs in this country. The following schools are associated with this Fifth Pathway program. They give preference to state residents. Inquiries should be addressed to the directors of these programs.

University of Arizona
College of Medicine
Tucson, AZ 85724
(Arizona residents only)

University of California, Irvine
California College of Medicine
Irvine, CA 92717
(Preference for California Residents)

Loma Linda University
School of Medicine
Loma Linda, CA 92354
(Out of state residents discouraged)

University of Colorado
School of Medicine
Denver, CO 80262
(Colorado residents only)

University of Illinois
College of Medicine
1737 West Polk, Room 204
Chicago, IL 60612
(Preference for Illinois residents)

Albert Einstein College of Medicine
The Bronx Lebanon Hospital Center
Fulton Avenue at 169th Street
Bronx, NY 10456

New York University
School of Medicine
Booth Memorial Medical Center
56-45 Main Street
Flushing, NY 11355
(New York residents only)

State University of New York
Downstate Medical Center
College of Medicine
The Brooklyn Hospital
121 Dekalb Avenue
Brooklyn, NY 11201

Mount Sinai School of Medicine
Fifth Ave. & 100 St.
New York, NY 10029

New York Medical College
Valhalla, NY 10595

Brown University
Division of Biology and Medicine
Providence, RI 02912

It should be noted that additional hospitals in California, Illinois, New Jersey, and Texas may also offer Fifth Pathway opportunities, and additional information can be obtained from the Council on Medical Education of the American Medical Association. Securing a Fifth Pathway appointment presents a significant challenge, because the numbers are very limited.

REQUIREMENTS FOR PRACTICE _____

FLEX Examination

The Federation Licensing Examination (FLEX), which has been replaced by the USMLE, was prepared by the Federation of State Medical Boards for administration by the state medical boards of examiners, which participate in the program. Admission to the examination for medical graduates, including foreign medical graduates, will depend upon the statutory regulatory requirements of the individual states. All states and the District of Columbia participate in the program except for Florida and Texas. Requests for applications should be addressed to the specific state boards.

ECFMG Examination

Students from the United States who are graduates of foreign medical schools and wish to secure an internship or residency in or practice in the United States must pass an examination given by the Educational Council for Foreign Medical Graduates (3930 Chestnut St., Philadelphia, PA 19104). This examination, which is given twice a year in many centers throughout the world, consists of 360 multiple-choice questions selected from a pool of questions previously used in Steps 1 and 2 of the USMLE. To pass, a student must attain a score of 75.

State Board Requirements

While the AMA recognizes a graduate of any foreign medical school who has been certified by the ECFMG as eligible for internship and residency training, licensure to practice in the United States is under the jurisdiction of state governments, each of which establishes its own standards. Some states accept no foreign graduates while others accept graduates from certain foreign schools. Information on the requirements in each state can be secured from the secretary of each of the State Boards of Medical Examiners. (Graduates of Canadian medical schools are considered equivalent to U.S. graduates but must meet the requirements for citizenship and internship.)

SELECTING A FOREIGN MEDICAL SCHOOL _____

In deciding to attend a foreign medical school, which, as discussed, is an awesome challenge, you should be certain that (1) you cannot gain admission to a U.S. school (2) you are not interested in an alternative career in the health sciences, and (3) you have adequate financial support. Electing to study outside of this country is a major decision and selecting a school to attend represents another critical hurdle.

Careful planning and considerable investigation should be made before you make any commitments. As a component of your planning, you should determine how best to meet the foreign language requirements that will enable you to secure your medical education and training. Only a few schools that accept foreign students teach in English (such as those in the Philippines and the Caribbean). By examining catalogs, you should seek to determine how the course of studies at an overseas school compares with that at a typical U.S. school. There should be an attempt to secure information about the adequacy of the clinical facilities, which is critical to be able to succeed in your residency training. This information may come from students who have been or are currently in attendance at the school in question. They (or their families) can provide useful information concerning the nature of the housing and cost of living expenses at their particular foreign school. A key piece of information is how well U.S. students perform after attending the foreign medical schools in question. Also, insight can be secured by finding out how U.S. citizens perform on the ECFMG. It should be realized that this data cannot be taken without allowing for a number of variables, such as the quality of the students in each country, the number of times the exam was taken, the time lapse between taking the exam and completing one's education, and other factors, such as the total number of applicants taking the exam.

FOREIGN MEDICAL SCHOOLS _____

The majority of Americans studying at overseas schools are located in four countries: Mexico, Italy, Belgium, and Spain.

Australia

It is difficult, but still possible, for a U.S. student to be admitted to an Australian medical school. The general policy is to encourage foreign applicants.

Austria

It is not recommended that students attempt to apply to any Austrian medical schools as none of the schools are currently accepting foreign students. However, it is possible that this situation may change.

Belgium

Belgium is a dual-language country: at the Universities of Ghent and Antwerp, courses are given in Flemish, while at Brussels, Liège, and Louvain, French is the standard language. A Flemish section, however, is also presented at Brussels and Louvain. Students can join the section they prefer, and most Americans enroll in the French schools. Students must apply individually to each school, preferably in the spring. Usually, Americans have had to start from the beginning of the six-year didactic program (which includes the premedical courses) and must also serve a year of internship in order to receive the medical degree. There is an unofficial 5% quota for non-Belgian students.

University of Antwerp
This school previously only offered the first three years of the medical curriculum, the basic sciences. The fourth year is now available and is similar to a rotating internship. *Contact:* Faculteit der Geneeskunde, Rijksuniversitair Centrum Antwerpen, Goemaerelei, 52, 2000 Antwerpen, Belgium.

University of Brussels
A request for admission can be directed to either the French or Flemish section or both. Proof of proficiency in either language will be required. Students spend approximately half their study time for the full four years in clinical areas. *Contact:* Faculté de Médecine, Université Libre de Bruxelles, Rectorat-Affaires Etudiantes, Avenue A. Buyl, 131, 1050 Bruxelles, Belgium.

University of Ghent
This school offers courses in Flemish for foreign students. It requires certified copies of diplomas and letters of recommendation in order to be considered. *Contact:* Faculteit der Geneeskunde, Rijksuniversiteit te Gent, Voldersstraat, 13, 9000 Ghent, Belgium.

University of Liège
This school considers applicants who have their bachelor's for admission to the first and possibly also the second year. The work at this school is considered especially difficult because there is an oral final for the entire term's work. *Contact:* Faculté de Médecine, Université de Liège, Service des Etudiants, Place de XX Août, 4000 Liège, Belgium.

University of Louvain
The French section is now located at Brussels. A language proficiency examination is required in both sections. In the French section, examinations are given in each course. *Contact:* (French) Faculté de Médecine, Université Catholique de Louvain, Secrétariat des Etudiants Etrangers, Avenue E. Mounier, 1200 Bruxelles, Belgium. (Flemish) Faculteit der Geneeskunde, Universiteit Katholik te Leuven, Studentensecretariaat, Universiteithal, Naamsestraat, 22, 3000 Leuven, Belgium.

Admission Requirements

Bachelor's degree. The documents required include: letter of recommendation from the premedical committee (or individual letters where a committee does not exist), transcript covering all four years of college, and a copy of the diploma from college.

Caribbean

In recent years several medical schools were established in the Caribbean with the aim of being profit-making institutions. Since their goal is to enroll rejected American students, they teach in English and have high tuition and fees. The academic standards of some of these schools have been subject to adverse criticism, and potential applicants are strongly urged to evaluate such schools *thoroughly* before committing themselves.

The three Caribbean medical schools noted below may be especially attractive to some potential applicants because their language of instruction is exclusively English. This important feature eliminates a major obstacle facing Americans studying overseas. It also permits the use of English language textbooks as a required component of the courses being given. In addition, the proximity of the Caribbean schools to the U.S. mainland permits students at these institutions to return home more frequently (and at a lower cost) than from a European medical school.

For additional information, *contact:* Ross University School of Medicine, 460 West 34th Street, New York, NY 10001; American University of the Caribbean, School of Medicine, 100 N.W. 37th Avenue, Miami, FL 33125.

St. George's University, Grenada, West Indies

St. George's University, Grenada, West Indies, was established more than two decades ago and offers a six-term sciences and three-term clinical sciences program. Admission to this school is handled by the Foreign Medical School Services Corp., One East Main Street, Bay Shore, NY 11706.

Dominican Republic

For a while, medical study by Americans in the Dominican Republic was fairly popular. The principal school accepting Americans was the Universidad Central del Este. The school accepted a large number of U.S. students and in particular a large number of Puerto Ricans. Unfortunately, a major scandal involving granting of fraudulent degrees has resulted in the closing of one school and has created a cloud of suspicion over the others.

Universidad Central del Este

The standard medical program of this school extends over 10 semesters. Each semester is 18 weeks long and this time is lengthened by holidays that occur within the semester. Students can be expected to complete their studies in four and one-quarter years. *Contact:* Admissions Office for Foreign Students, Universidad Central del Este, Tampico, Dominican Republic.

Admission Requirements

Bachelor's degree and minimum science courses plus two semesters each of English, philosophy, and one of sociology. School requires the following documents: official SAT and MCAT scores, high school and college transcripts, photocopy of birth certificate, and a certificate of good conduct from the local police department.

Universidad Nacional Pedro Henriquez Urena

The course of study takes 9 semesters and each semester is 20 weeks long. The first 2 years deal with the basic sciences, and the last 2½ years are devoted to clinical work. *Contact:* Director, Escuela de Medicina, Universidad Nacional Pedro Henriquez Urena, Santo Domingo, Dominican Republic.

Admission Requirements

Bachelor's degree and premedical average above 2.8. School requires the following documents: official college transcript, premedical committee evaluation, three letters of recommendation, MCAT scores, and a certificate of good conduct from the local police department.

France

U.S. students may not encounter too much trouble in being admitted to the first year at a French medical school. At the end of the first year, however, all medical students in France take a qualifying test in order to obtain entry to the second year. Since there are many more first-year medical students than second-year places, the competition is very stiff and it is unlikely that a U.S. student will fare well. For additional information, *contact:* Théraplix, Secrétariat du Guide Théraplix des Études Médicales, 46-52 rue Albert, 75640 Paris Cedex 13.

Germany

The probability of being accepted to a German medical school is very slight, owing to the limited number of places available to foreign students and to the great difficulty of the entrance examinations, which are language tests. For more information on German schools, *contact:* Cultural Division, Consulate General of the Federal Republic of Germany, 460 Park Avenue, New York, NY 10022.

Hungary

The medical school of the University of Pécs has introduced a six-year English-language program. *Contact:* Hungarian Consulate, 8 East 75th Street, New York, NY 10021.

Ireland

Ireland has one private institution that accepts foreign applicants, the Royal College of Surgeons. There is an entrance examination; the school also requires MCAT scores, academic courses, and a letter of recommendation. *Contact:* Royal College of Surgeons, 123 St. Stephen's Green, Dublin 2, Ireland.

Israel

Most students need not consider applying to an Israeli medical school because, although such applicants may be considered, few will be accepted. A program for U.S. and Canadian citizens exists at the Sackler School of Medicine of the University of Tel Aviv Medical School and English is the language of instruction. *Contact:* Office of Admissions, Sackler School of Medicine, 17 East 62nd Street, New York, NY 10021.

The Barry Z. Levine School of Health Sciences of Touro College (844 Avenue of the Americas, New York, NY 1001-4003, phone 212-463-0400) has a one-year program on Long Island, New York, that grants a master's degree in interdisciplinary science, which is equivalent to the first year of medical school. Students who have maintained a B average are then eligible to enter the Technion Medical School in Haifa, Israel as a second-year medical student. The latter is a five-year program.

Italy

Previously, Italy had a fairly open admissions policy. Americans were screened at the consulate office in New York and, if accepted, were allowed to attend any of the medical schools in the country. Meetings between the Italian medical schools and American counterparts have resulted in a law that requires the assignment of foreign applicants to particular schools. Until this law, most American students went to the universities at Bologna, Rome, and Padua. Another law requires all students to have a B average and to speak Italian. These laws have markedly reduced the number of Americans in attendance at Italian medical schools.

Preclinical coursework is characterized by overcrowded classrooms. After finishing their didactic coursework, students must pass a series of final examinations before they receive the degree of doctor of medicine and surgery. They must then complete a one-year internship to be eligible for admission to the Italian State Examination. The year of internship can be fulfilled by a year of clinical clerkship at an undergraduate medical school approved by the AMA Liaison Committee on Medical Education.

University of Bologna

This school enrolls the largest group of Americans studying in Italy. Its appeal over other schools appears to be the lack of "obstacle" courses along the path to the degree. In addition, the American students have organized an association that seeks to assist the membership to adjust to their new environment. *Contact:* Università degli Studi, Bologna, Italy.

University of Padua

This school enrolls a small number of Americans. Anatomy is strongly emphasized in preclinical teaching. The school has a reputation for being very demanding and, as a result, a significant number of students transfer to Bologna after three years at Padua. *Contact:* Università degli Studi, Padua, Italy.

University of Rome

This school enrolls a small number of Americans. Most seem to have little academic difficulty until they reach the third and fourth year when the pharmacology and pathology courses are taken. The cost of living in Rome is relatively high. *Contact:* Università degli Studi, Rome, Italy.

University of Turin

Contact: Università degli Studi di Torino, Turin, Italy.

University of Pisa

Contact: Università degli Studi, Pisa, Italy.

University of Pavia

Contact: Università degli Studi, Pavia, Italy.

University of Palermo

Contact: Università degli Studi, Palermo, Italy.

University of Forence

Contact: Università degli Studi, Florence, Italy.

University of Genoa

Contact: Università degli Studi di Genova, Genoa, Italy.

University of Milan

Contact: Università degli Studi, Milan, Italy.

University of Naples

Contact: Università degli Studi, Naples, Italy.

Address for Information
Italian Consulate, 690 Park Avenue, New York, NY 10021 (or the nearest consulate).

Admission Requirements
Bachelor's degree, minimum science courses, and adequate knowledge of Italian. The following documents are required and should be sent to the consulate between April 1 and September 15: official college transcript, letter of recommendation from the premedical committee or individual letters from the heads of science departments. If requirements are met, students will be asked to submit photographs (two, passport size), original high school diploma, and affidavit of support.

Mexico

All of the Mexican medical schools but one are state schools. They follow the six-year, European-style curriculum and the applicant may apply in person. The only nonstate school is the Universidad Autónoma de Guadalajara, a four-year school where a large number of American medical students have studied.

Autonomous University of Guadalajara

This school is located in Guadalajara, which is the second largest city in Mexico. The weather there is ideal almost year-round; though it does get hot in May and June, it generally cools off at night. All coursework and conversation with instructors is in Spanish. Americans are required to take special language instruction and must pass a language examination at the end of the first year. Spanish translations of most of the well-known English textbooks are available. Classes at the medical school are scheduled through most of the day, except between the hours of one and four in the afternoon. Attendance is required in 80% of all classes in order to be eligible to take the final examinations. While the didactic work is currently four years, a year of internship and a year of social service in a rural community, presentation of a thesis, and a final examination are required before the student is awarded the *Titulo de Medico Cirujano* (the title of physician and surgeon). The ECFMG Board of Trustees has approved the substitution of a year of clinical clerkship, under the sponsorship of an American medical school, for a year of internship that is a postgraduate requirement in certain foreign medical schools. The acceptability of an American clerkship in lieu of the internship by the Universidad Autónoma de Guadalajara is uncertain at this time. *Contact:* Oficina de Información a Extranjeros, Universidad Autónoma de Guadalajara, Apartado Postal 1-440, Guadalajara, Jalisco, Mexico.

Admission Requirements

Bachelor's degree and minimum science courses. The school requires the following documents: birth certificate (three copies), letters of recommendation (two), certificate of health, photographs, high school transcript and diploma, college diploma, letter of financial solvency, certificate of completion of premedical requirements, and MCAT scores. Of these, the following must be legalized by the Mexican Consulate: transcripts, diplomas, birth certificate, letter of financial solvency, and certificate of premedical studies.

Three other schools in Mexico enroll Americans:

Autonomous University of Ciudad Juarez

Contact: Universidad Autonoma de Ciudad Juarez, Instituto de Ciencias Biomedicas, Apartado Postal 21574, Sucursal "D," Ciudad Juarez, Chihuahua, Mexico.

University of Monterrey

Contact: Dirección de Admisiones, Seccion de Extranjeros, Apartado Postal 4435, Sucursal "J" de Correos, Monterrey, Nuevo Leon, Mexico.

University Del Noreste (Tampico)

Contact: Universidad del Noreste, Admissions Office, 120 East 41st Street, Suite 1000, New York, NY 10017.

The Netherlands

The Netherlands no longer accepts American students.

Philippines

Some Americans are seeking admission to medical schools in the Philippines. This is probably owing to the increasing difficulty in securing admission to European schools and the fact that the teaching methods and procedures employed in the Philippines are similar to those used in the United States. The language of instruction is English. The course of study is four years and the academic year is divided into two semesters. The following are the names and addresses of the six medical schools in the Philippines. An * indicates those schools that accept from 10 to 25 Americans each year; the others accept fewer than 10.

University of the Philippines
Taft Avenue, Ermita, Manila, 1000.

Pamantasan NC Lungsod NG Maynila
Ermita, Manila, 1000.

AGO Medical and Educational Center
Rizal Street, Legaspi City, Ricol, 4500.

Cebu Doctors
College of Medicine, Osmana Boulevard, Cebu City 6000.

De La Salle University
Dasmarinas Cavite, 4114.

Fatima Medical Science Foundation
MacArthur Highway, Valenzuela, MM, 3024.

*Far Eastern University
Institute of Medicine, N. Reyes Street, Quiapo, Manila, 1001.

Galang Medical Center College, Inc.
2151 Ipil, Sta Cruz, Manila, 1003.

Gullas College of Medicine
Mandau City, 6014.

*Manila Central University
College of Medicine, MGU Compound, Caloocan City, 1400.

Manila Doctors College
6667 UN Avenue, Ermita, Manila, 1000.

Our Lady of Fatima
College of Medicine, 120 MacArthur Highway, Valenzuela, MM, 1405.

Southwestern University
College of Medicine, Cebu City, 6000.

University of the East
College of Medicine, Aurora Boulevard, Quezon City, 1106.

University of Santo Thomas
Espana Street, Sampaloc, Manila, 1008.

Velez College
F. Ramos, Cebu City, 6000.

Address for Information
Consulate General of the Philippines, 556 Fifth Avenue, New York, NY 10036

Admission Requirements
Bachelor's degree with a premedical major or appropriate courses completed. Applications for admission can be secured from the individual universities and must be returned with a transcript and other required credentials. A student visa will be issued only after an official letter of acceptance is received.

Poland

Students in the United States with Polish ancestry will have the most success in being accepted to Polish medical schools. The schools are state-supported and therefore a very limited number of foreign applicants will be accepted. *Contact:* Embassy of the Polish People's Republic, 2640 16th NW, Washington, DC 20009.

Spain

Medical schools in Spain appear to be receptive to Americans. The majority of those attending are at the University of Madrid. A reform plan has gone into effect that has resulted in a 75% attrition rate for first-year students, and, therefore, students may want to attend a different school (for example, at Bilbao or Barcelona). Acceptance confers eligibility to attend the school you select. Spanish schools require a two-year internship. Medical facilities are to be found at the following universities:

Barcelona	**Murcia**
Bilboa	**Navarra**
Cardoba	**Oviedo**
Granada	**Salamanca**
Santander	**Sevilla in Cadiz**
Santiago de Compostela	**Valencia**
Sevilla	**Valladolid**
La Laguna	**Zaragoza**
Malaga	

In addition, there are several Colegios Universitarios that offer the first year of medical study. Eventually these schools will offer a full program:

Burgos	**Soria**
Vitoria	**Toledo**

Address for Information
Cultural Relations Department, Spanish Embassy, Columbia Road NW, Washington, DC 20001.

Admission Requirements
Bachelor's degree. Documents required include: birth certificates with city or county seal (two), college transcript with school seal, copy of high school diploma, and a college catalog. An application for admission (obtainable from the embassy or consulate) plus the required documents should be taken to the embassy or consulate for legalization and then submitted to the former for transfer to Madrid.

Expenses
The cost of living is higher in Madrid than in other Spanish cities. However, the cost of living in general is lower in Spain than in other European countries. The overall cost of travel plus tuition and living expenses is significantly less than the mean cost in the United States.

Switzerland

Swiss schools are no longer accepting U.S. students.

United Kingdom

There are very few openings for U.S. students at British medical schools but some students are occasionally accepted. *Contact:* Universities Central Council on Admissions, P.O. Box 28, Cheltenham GL50 1HY, England.

## 13

Osteopathic Medicine

Basic philosophy
Educational data
Admission prospects
Internship, residency, and practice
Relationship between osteopathic and allopathic medicine
Financial assistance
The osteopathic scene in a nutshell
Osteopathic medical school profiles

Aside from the 124 standard, or allopathic, medical schools, there are 17 osteopathic schools in the United States, which, in a recent year, had an enrollment of more than 8,100 students. There were more than 35,000 osteopathic physicians listed in the directory published by the American Osteopathic Association. Thus, this branch of medicine contributes a significant number of professionals to the physicians' pool. Over the past several years, interest in osteopathy has intensified significantly. This is reflected by an overall increase in enrollment, including women and minority students, and a new school—the seventeenth. For this reason, the philosophy, educational data, admission prospects, and training program leading to the Doctor of Osteopathy, or DO degree, are outlined.

BASIC PHILOSOPHY

The osteopathic approach was developed by a physician, Dr. Andrew Taylor Sill, in 1874 and is based upon a holistic view of the function of the human body. Osteopathic medicine is structured on the principles that the human body is an integrated organism and therefore abnormal function in one part of the body exerts unfavorable influences on other parts and on the body as a whole; a complex system exists in the body that tends to provide for self-regulation and self-healing in the face of stress; adequate function of all body organs and systems depends on the integrating forces of the nervous and circulatory system; the body's musculoskeletal system (such as bones, joints, connective tissues, skeletal muscles, and tendons) plays an important role in the body's continuous effort to resist and overcome illness and disease. Based on these principles, osteopathic medicine postulates that any stress—physical, mechanical, or emotional—that causes muscles to become tense (referred pain) intensifies the constant stream of sensory nerve impulses being sent *to* the central nervous system (CNS) by receptors in the muscles and tendons. If this neural barrage is severe enough, it may spill over and initiate an excessive volley of autonomic nerve impulses that pass *away* from the CNS to segmentally related organs and tissues. As a result, muscular responses to referred pain may trigger a neural feedback that can become a secondary source of irritation and pain. This, in turn, may induce responses by the internal organs that are referred back to the musculoskeletal system and a vicious cycle of sensory-motor nerve excitation can be created. Unless this cycle is interrupted, it may perpetuate itself until the somatic response to referred pain becomes more severe than the original visceral disease. The somatic response in effect becomes a secondary disease.

The musculoskeletal system is easily accessible and it is believed that the treatment of it may be beneficial in altering the disease process by interrupting the vicious cycle of neural exchange. In practice, osteopathic medicine involves the application of manipulative procedures to help tense muscles, tendons, and connective tissues to relax. The increase in muscle-fiber length resulting from the relaxation eases the tension on the impulse receptors in the muscles and tendons, reducing sensory bombardment to the spinal cord. This reduction may allow the entire body to return to more normal homeostatic levels and permit segmentally related visceral structures to repair themselves under more normal conditions. It is important to note that *the osteopathic system of diagnosis and therapy is used in conjunction with the standard medical procedures of drug and surgical therapy.* As part of the educational program, osteopathic colleges train their students in the standard medical diagnostic and therapeutic methods as well as those associated with osteopathic medicine. For additional information write the American Osteopathic Association, 142 E. Ontario Street, Chicago, IL 60611.

EDUCATIONAL DATA

In the United States, there are presently 17 osteopathic colleges. The establishment of colleges of osteopathic medicine is being discussed in other areas of the country, and there are two in development, in San Francisco and in Pikeville, Kentucky. In a recent year, the present 17 colleges admitted about 2,200 freshmen out of an applicant pool of about 10,200. Students from six states—Pennsylvania, Michigan, Ohio, Missouri, Texas, and Iowa—made up the largest segment of the enrollment of the first-year classes. The grade point average of the class was about 3.3 (where 4.0 = A). This is a lower average than that for the entering class at conventional medical schools. Thus borderline premedical students who are intrinsically qualified should seek to secure places in osteopathic medical schools.

Admissions committees are putting increased emphasis on grade point average, recommendations, and interviews, and less emphasis on test scores. The committees seek the same general characteristics in prospective students as allopathic medical schools (such as dependability, maturity, integrity), but they also look for special interest in and motivation to study osteopathic medicine. Letters of recommendation from osteopathic physicians (and even students) adequately acquainted with applicants can be helpful.

The number of women in a recent freshman class was about 35% of the total enrollment. This is relatively similar to the proportion of women enrolled in allopathic medical school. The number of entering students having less than four years of undergraduate education was a small percentage of the total entering class. This clearly reflects the fact that both osteopathic and allopathic medical schools still feel that the fourth year in the undergraduate college is desirable.

The average age of entering osteopathic students has been 26 years (range: 20–42); this is higher than for those accepted in allopathic medical schools. It may be because many matriculants were motivated to enter this field after exposure to related community service careers. Among the older freshmen, many have backgrounds in teaching, allied health fields, and research. As with the allopathic schools, applicants over 28 need not expect to have special difficulties in gaining admission. The basic science course requirements for admission to osteopathic schools are the same as those for allopathic schools. The majority of freshmen, as would be expected, were biology or chemistry majors and almost all of them took the MCAT.

The curriculum at an osteopathic school is almost identical with that offered at the allopathic schools. Study is divided into basic science and clinical science training. There is a required course in the basic theory and practice of osteopathic medicine. The philosophy of osteopathic medicine, with its emphasis on total health care, is incorporated where appropriate into the standard courses. Curriculum revision in line with that taking place at allopathic schools is also occurring at osteopathic schools.

ADMISSION PROSPECTS _____

The number of applicants to osteopathic schools continues to grow. Existing schools have responded by enlarging the size of classes so that currently there are over 8,000 osteopathic students being trained. At the same time, the number of graduates is also increasing. Consequently, there will be an increase in the approximately 5% of the physician population made up by osteopaths. Replacing IMGS with osteopathic residents will accelerate this growth.

INTERNSHIP, RESIDENCY, AND PRACTICE _____

After obtaining the DO degree, those planning to practice osteopathic medicine are expected to spend at least a year in internship training. There are about 130 osteopathic hospitals distributed in 24 states that have been accredited by the American Osteopathic Association and 53 of these have been approved for internship training. Some of these hospitals offer residency training in some medical specialty. Training for specialization can extend over a three- to five-year period in an osteopathic hospital having an approved program, or can be service as a trainee under a certified osteopathic specialist, or can be a combination of both types of training. After the completion of the formal training period, no added specialized practice is required before the applicant is eligible to take the examination for certification in a specialty field.

It should be noted that the majority of osteopathic physicians are general practitioners and only about 36% are engaged in specialty training or practice (full- or part-time). While many osteopathic physicians practice in large cities, others are found in small communities where there is a special need for family physicians and general practitioners. The income for osteopathic physicians is roughly comparable to that of allopathic physicians and depends on the location of the practice.

Note also that DOs are eligible for appointment and are serving as medical officers in the U.S. Public Health Service, Veterans Administration, and armed forces. They also serve as examiners or may prepare certificates of health examinations required by various federal agencies, as coroners, and as members of state, county, and city boards of health. They provide medical and surgical care for those insured under Blue Cross and Blue Shield as well as private health insurance plans. In other words, the same general opportunities are on the whole open to DOs as to MDs. With the pressure to increase family practice doctors, DOs should be in high demand.

An osteopathic physician may obtain a license to practice in one of three ways:

1. Examination administered by the state board, which is usually the USMLE.

2. Acceptance of the certificate issued by the National Board of Osteopathic Medical Examiners, which is issued after meeting their requirements.

3. Reciprocity of a license previously received from another state.

RELATIONSHIP BETWEEN OSTEOPATHIC AND ALLOPATHIC MEDICINE _____

Students who are interested in attending an osteopathic medical school should be aware that osteopathic medical schools, like many allopathic schools, utilize a centralized application service for processing student applications. To obtain the application packet, which contains an application form for the AACOMAS and procedures for applying as well as materials describing each college and its fees, write to the American Association of Colleges of Osteopathic Medicine Application Service, 6110 Executive Boulevard, Suite 405, Rockville, MD 20852. The AMA recommends that AMA-approved internship and residency programs be opened to qualified graduates of schools of osteopathy; that American boards for medical specialties accept for examination for certification those osteopaths who have completed AMA-approved internships and residency programs and have met the other regular requirements applicable to all board candidates; that accredited hospitals accept qualified osteopaths for appointment to the medical staffs of hospitals; and that determination of qualification be made at the level of the medical staff of a hospital, or the review committees and boards having appropriate jurisdiction.

The aforementioned recommendations have potentially opened the way for wider acceptance of DOs into the mainstream of medical training and practice. Twenty-four specialty boards have agreed to examine for certification osteopathic graduates who have completed AMA-approved internships and residency programs. Among the 24 are the American Boards of Pathology, Pediatrics, Physical Medicine and Rehabilitation, Preventive Medicine, Radiology, Anesthesiology, Dermatology, Internal Medicine, Obstetrics and Gynecology, Orthopedic Surgery, Psychiatry, and Neurology.

The application of the AMA proposals is indicated by the fact that in a recent year about 300 hospitals had appointed some 2,000 osteopathic physicians to their attending staff as house officers. These appointments were spread over 25 states with the largest number in Pennsylvania, New Jersey, California, Michigan, and Washington. These figures will probably rise steadily during the next few years.

FINANCIAL ASSISTANCE

1. *National Osteopathic Scholarships.* Annually 25 scholarships of $1,500 are awarded to entering osteopathic students. These will be applied to tuition at the rate of $750 per year for the first two years. (Information is available from the Office of Education, American Osteopathic Association, 142 East Ontario Street, Chicago, IL 60611.)

2. *Canadian Osteopathic Scholarships.* A $3,000 scholarship is available to a first- or second-year Canadian student enrolled in an osteopathic school. (Information is obtainable from Canadian Osteopathic Education Trust Fund, Suite 126, 3545 Cote des Neiges Road, Montreal 25, Quebec.)

3. *New Jersey Association of Osteopathic Physicians and Surgeons Scholarships.* Scholarships are awarded to assist in paying tuition for first-year students who are New Jersey residents. (Information is obtainable from the Executive Director, New Jersey Association of Osteopathic Physicians and Surgeons, 1 Distribution Way, Monmouth Junction, NJ 08852-3001.)

4. *National Osteopathic Foundation Student Loan Fund.* An approved candidate may borrow a sum not exceeding $1,000 annually. (Information is obtainable from the National Osteopathic Foundation 5775G Peachtree-Dunwoody Road, Suite 500, Atlanta, GA 30342.)

THE OSTEOPATHIC SCENE IN A NUTSHELL

Table 13-1 reflects the admissions picture at the osteopathic medical schools presently in operation.

Note: Applications for most osteopathic schools are processed by a centralized application service, the American Association of Colleges of Osteopathic Medicine Application Service (AACOMAS). To secure an application, write to AACOMAS, 6110 Executive Boulevard, Suite 405, Rockville, MD 20852.

OSTEOPATHIC MEDICAL SCHOOL PROFILES

In these school descriptions, the admissions requirement of the basic premedical science courses refers to one year each of inorganic and organic chemistry, biology, and physics, plus laboratory work.

Table 13.1 BASIC DATA FOR OSTEOPATHIC SCHOOLS (1996–97)

School	Total Number Applicants	Number 1st Year Enrolled			Applications Deadline	Tuition Res/ Nonres
		Men	Women	Out-of-State		
Arizona College of Osteopathic Medicine of Midwestern University	5400	70	33	87	2/1	$20,800 $20,800
Western University of Health Sciences	3500	393	241	38	2/1	$20,060 $20,060
*Nova Southeastern University College of Osteopathic Medicine	3300	88	52	60	2/1	$18,500 $21,750
*Chicago College of Osteopathic Medicine of Midwestern University	5400	94	59	84	2/1	$18,411 $22,374
*University of Osteopathic Medicine and Health Sciences	4490	132	73	159	4/1	$20,700
*University of New England College of Osteopathic Medicine	3186	71	41	1	1/1	$21,150
*Michigan State University College of Osteopathic Medicine	3089	70	56	17	12/1	$ 986 $31,876
*Kirksville College of Osteopathic Medicine	4577	99	48	125	2/1	$21,900 $21,900
University of Health Sciences College of Osteopathic Medicine (Kansas City)	4809	165	55	156	2/1	$22,200 $22,200
*New Jersey School of Osteopathic Medicine	3211	148	142	30	2/1	$14,492 $22,679
*New York College of Osteopathic Medicine	4598	118	87	1	2/1	$20,000 $20,000
*Ohio University College of Osteopathic Medicine	3569	57	44	14	1/2	$10,785 $15,279
*College of Osteopathic Medicine of Oklahoma State University	1927	57	31	13	1/4	$ 7,550 $18,660
Philadelphia College of Osteopathic Medicine	5,846	155	104	84	2/1	$21,000
Lake Erie College of Osteopathic Medicine	4128	74	41	44	3/15	$20,400 $20,400
*Texas College of Osteopathic Medicine	2219	70	44	8	12/1	$ 6,550 $19,550
*West Virginia School of Osteopathic Medicine	2423	38	27	20	2/1	$10,050 $25,900

* AACOMAS school

ARIZONA

Arizona College of Osteopathic Medicine of Midwestern University

19555 North 59th Avenue
Glendale, Arizona   85308

Phone: 800-458-6253

Application Filing		Accreditation
Earliest:	June 1	AOA
Latest:	February 1	
Fee:	$40	

Enrollment: 1996–97 First-Year Class

Men:	70	68%	Applied:	5400
Women:	33	32%	Enrolled:	103
Out of State:	87	84%		

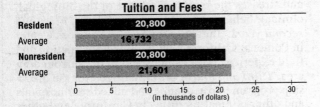

Tuition and Fees

Resident	20,800
Average	16,732
Nonresident	20,800
Average	21,601

(in thousands of dollars)

Introduction

Founded in 1995, this is the newest of the colleges of osteopathic medicine. With its sister college, the Chicago College of Osteopathic Medicine, it is part of Midwestern University. The school is located on a 122-acre site in Glendale, Arizona, a suburb of Phoenix. Midwestern University also includes a college of Pharmacy and a college of Allied Health Professions.

Admissions (AACOMAS)

Completion of a minimum of 3 years of college including the basic medical science courses plus 2 courses in English. Students are encouraged to take additional courses in the humanities, as well as the social and behavioral sciences. (The Admission Office is located at Midwestern University, 555 31st Street, Downers Grove, Illinois 60515).

Curriculum

Information not available.

Affiliated Teaching Hospitals

Information not available.

Housing

Information not available.

CALIFORNIA

Western University of Health Sciences

309 East College Plaza
Pomona, California   91766

Phone: 909-469-5200

Application Filing		Accreditation
Earliest:	June 1	AOA
Latest:	February 1	
Fee:	$50	

Enrollment: 1996–97 First-Year Class

Men:	393	62%	Applied:	3500
Women:	241	38%	Enrolled:	634
Out of State:	38	6%		

Tuition and Fees

Resident   n/av
Average

Nonresident   n/av
Average

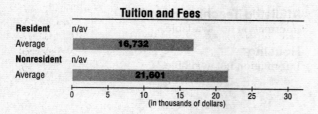

(in thousands of dollars)

Introduction

The College of Osteopathic Medicine of the Pacific was established in 1977. It is the only osteopathic medical school in the far West. It changed its name in 1996 to Western University of Health Sciences and is an independent, nonprofit institution, accredited by the state of California. In the vicinity of the college are many hospitals, clinics, colleges, and universities. Pomona is a multiethnic community in southern California known for its pleasant climate.

Admissions (AACOMAS)

Completion of a minimum of 3 years of college with a GPA of at least C+ (2.5); the MCAT is necessary. The basic premedical science courses plus 1 year of English and behavioral science are required. Students from all states are encouraged to apply.

Curriculum

4-year. In addition to the standard medical school curriculum, there is a strong emphasis on nutrition, prevention wellness, and osteopathic manipulative medicine. The curriculum is organized in semesters and stresses the interdependence of the biological, clinical, behavioral, and social sciences. *First and second years:* Taught in the Health Sciences Center in Pomona, California, with clinical instruction and field experiences on campus and in the surrounding area. *Third and fourth years:* Utilized for the clerkship program in osteopathic and mixed staff hospitals and other clinical facilities in California and other states throughout the country. The school also operates a family practice outpatient clinic in Pomona, which helps serve the health needs of the community and also provides clinical training for its students.

Affiliated Teaching Hospitals

The school is affiliated with many hospitals, physicians' offices, and ambulatory health care centers throughout the United States.

Housing

There is no on-campus housing. A housing referral system is available.

FLORIDA

Nova Southeastern University Health Professions Division College of Osteopathic Medicine

3200 South University Drive
Fort Lauderdale, Florida   33328

Phone: 954-723-1100

Application Filing		Accreditation
Earliest:	June 1	AOA
Latest:	February 1	
Fee:	$50	

Enrollment: 1996–97 First-Year Class

Men:	88	63%	Applied:	3300
Women:	52	37%	Enrolled:	140
Out of State:	60	43%		

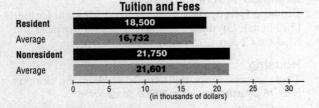

Tuition and Fees

Resident — 18,500
Average — 16,732
Nonresident — 21,750
Average — 21,601

(in thousands of dollars)

Introduction

Nova University was established in 1964. It is a private school offering both undergraduate and graduate degrees. The Health Professions Division was created when Nova University joined Southeastern University to become Nova Southeastern University. The College of Osteopathic Medicine is part of this division, which includes colleges of Pharmacy, Optometry, Allied Health, and Medical Sciences. In 1996 the Health Professions Divisions relocated from North Miami Beach to a 220-acre campus in Fort Lauderdale.

Admissions (AACOMAS)

The basic premedical science courses, plus courses in English composition and literature, a bachelor's degree, and the MCAT are required. Students are encouraged to take additional courses in behavioral sciences, cultural subjects, and the humanities.

Curriculum

4-year. *Phase I:* Two years are spent on campus and include the basic sciences and didactic clinical sciences. During this part of their training, students also are introduced to patient evaluation and the technology of medicine, and special emphasis is placed on manipulative medicine. *Phase II:* Students spend 22 months in clinical training, including teaching rotations in affiliated hospitals and experience in ambulatory care facilities. They then return to campus for a pre-internship seminar, just prior to graduation, in preparation for internship, residency, and practice. The curriculum emphasizes general practice and features training in ambulatory care, minority medicine, communication, and humanities.

Affiliated Teaching Hospitals

Twenty Florida hospitals and 16 other medical centers serve as teaching hospitals.

Housing

All students are required to secure their own housing accommodations. The school does have some limited on-campus housing facilities within a 2-block radius of the school.

ILLINOIS

Chicago College of Osteopathic Medicine Midwestern University

555 31st Street
Downers Grove, Illinois   60515

Phone: 630-969-4400   *Fax:* 630-971-6086

Application Filing	Accreditation
Earliest: June 1	AOA
Latest: February 1	
Fee: $40	

Enrollment: 1996–97 First-Year Class
Men:	94	61%	Applied:	5400
Women:	59	39%	Enrolled:	153
Out of State:	84	55%		

Tuition and Fees

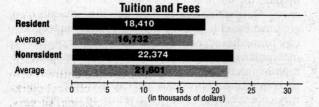

Resident 18,410
Average 16,732
Nonresident 22,374
Average 21,601

0 5 10 15 20 25 30
(in thousands of dollars)

Introduction
The Chicago College of Osteopathic Medicine originally opened in 1900. It later merged with another
osteopathic school, and in 1970 it assumed its present
name. The school later changed its name again by
adding Midwestern University when it expanded
beyond the osteopathic program. The basic sciences
are taught on the 103-acre Downers Grove Campus
in a western suburb of Chicago. In 1995, the Arizona
College of Osteopathic Medicine was founded as a
part of Midwestern University.

Admissions (AACOMAS)
Completion of a minimum of 3 years of college
(degree preferred), at least a B average, and the
MCAT are necessary. The basic premedical science
courses are required. A total of 153 students are
admitted each September. Approximately one half of
the class comes from Illinois.

Curriculum
Information not available.

Affiliated Teaching Hospitals
Chicago Osteopathic Hospital and Medical Center
(300 beds); Olympia Fields Osteopathic Hospital and
Medical Center (225 beds).

Housing
There are residence halls for 30 students on campus
plus 48 apartments for married students.

IOWA

University of Osteopathic Medicine and Health Sciences College of Osteopathic Medicine and Surgery

3200 Grand Avenue
Des Moines, Iowa   50312

Phone: 515-271-1400   *Fax:* 515-271-1545
E-mail: pglug@uomhs.edu

Application Filing	Accreditation
Earliest: June 1	AOA
Latest: April 1	
Fee: $50	

Enrollment: 1996–97 First-Year Class

Men:	132	64%	Applied:	4490
Women:	73	36%	Enrolled:	205
Out of State:	159	78%		

Tuition and Fees

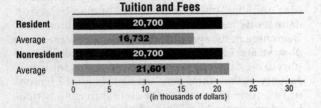

Resident	20,700
Average	16,732
Nonresident	20,700
Average	21,601

0   5   10   15   20   25   30
(in thousands of dollars)

Introduction

The University of Osteopathic Medicine was established in 1898. It is the second largest osteopathic school in the United States. The institution has undergone changes several times in name and location to accommodate expanding enrollment and programs of study. In 1972 the college relocated to its present 22-acre site in Des Moines, Iowa and in the 1980s the university enlarged by opening up a College of Podiatric Medicine and Surgery and a College of Health Sciences, which train physicians' assistants, physical therapists, and health care administrators.

Admissions (AACOMAS)

Minimum 3 years of college, bachelor's degree strongly preferred, at least a B– average, the MCAT. The basic premedical science courses plus 6 hours of English composition, speech, or language are required. Recommended courses include biochemistry, genetics, comparative anatomy, and psychology.

Curriculum

4-year. For the major part of the first year, students take core courses in the basic sciences. This is followed by the study of basic sciences and clinical medicine using an integrated organ system approach. The last half of the third year and the entire fourth year are devoted to preceptorships, clinical clerkships, and hospital clerkships in medicine, surgery, pediatrics, obstetrics-gynecology, and psychiatry. History and physical diagnosis are introduced in the first year. The principles, practices, and theory of osteopathic manipulative medicine are taught during the entire curriculum and are interwoven with the didactic, laboratory, and clerkship experiences.

Affiliated Teaching Hospitals

The university operates 5 clinics and is affiliated with selected rural and urban clinics throughout Iowa. Among the 18 affiliated hospitals are Des Moines General Hospital (270 beds).

Housing

The university maintains a minimal number of student housing units; however, students can obtain accommodations in private homes and nearby apartment complexes.

MAINE

University of New England College of Osteopathic Medicine

11 Hills Beach Road
Biddeford, Maine   04005

Phone: 207-283-0171
E-mail: msinke @mailbox.une.edu
WWW: http://www.une.edu

Application Filing		Accreditation
Earliest:	June 1	AOA
Latest:	January 1	
Fee:	$55	

Enrollment: 1996–97 First-Year Class

Men:	71	63%	Applied:	3186
Women:	41	37%	Enrolled:	112
Out of State:	1	1%		

Tuition and Fees

Resident	21,150
Average	16,732
Nonresident	21,150
Average	21,601

(in thousands of dollars) — scale 0 to 30

Introduction

The University of New England was established in 1953. It merged with St. Francis College of Osteopathic Medicine and opened in 1978. It is located in Biddeford on the southern coast of Maine. Its goal is to train family practice physicians who will provide health care in underserved areas in New England. Preventive medicine is strongly emphasized in addition to medical care.

Admissions (AACOMAS)

Minimum of 3 years of college, at least 2.7 GPA, total average MCAT score of 18 on the three science exams and at least "M" on the written essay.

Curriculum

4-year. The 2½ years on-campus portion of the program is primarily didactic. The first-year curriculum emphasizes instruction in the core basic sciences. In the second year and the first half of the third year, the curriculum shifts from the discipline focus to an integrated "body-system" approach, in which the impact of the various disciplines is integrated with the clinical sciences into each body system. To accomplish the college's specific purposes, the 2½ year curriculum places consistent emphasis on osteopathic principles and manipulative practice, human behavior, community health maintenance, and the humanities. Beginning in the spring of their first year, all students observe and later experience clinical practice through part-time clinical preceptorships. Beginning in January of their third year, students begin 17 months of full-time hospital-based clerkships and office-based preceptorships. This off-campus clinical training takes place in over 20 college affiliated community hospitals and medical centers throughout the Northeast. Consistent with the college's emphasis on health maintenance and family practice, several of the full-time clinical experiences are in ambulatory care clinics. Students have the option for 7 of the 17 months to self-select hospital rotations and sites and to submit these to the college for approval.

Affiliated Teaching Hospitals

Information not available.

Housing

A limited number of housing units are avaiable on campus.

MICHIGAN

Michigan State University College of Osteopathic Medicine

East Fee Hall
East Lansing, Michigan   48824

Phone: 517-353-7740   *Fax:* 517-355-3296

Application Filing   **Accreditation**
Earliest: June 1   AOA
Latest: December 1
Fee: $60

Enrollment: 1996–97 First-Year Class

Men:	70	56%	Applied:	3089
Women:	56	44%	Enrolled:	126
Out of State:	17	13%		

Tuition and Fees

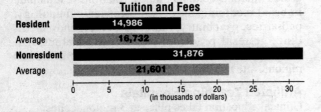

Resident	14,986
Average	16,732
Nonresident	31,876
Average	21,601

(in thousands of dollars)

Introduction

In 1855 Michigan State University was instituted. There are 11 undergraduate and 13 graduate schools. The school began as a private institution, the Michigan College of Osteopathic Medicine, in Pontiac. By an act of the Michigan legislature in 1969, it gained its current affiliation. The College of Osteopathic Medicine opened in 1971.

Admissions (AACOMAS)

Completion of the MCAT and a minimum of 3 years of college (but virtually all students have bachelor's degree by enrollment). The basic premedical science courses are required as well as 2 courses (9 credits) in English and in the behavioral sciences. Overall and science grade point averages must be no less than C+ (2.5). Suggested electives include biochemistry, anatomy, physiology, and histology.

Curriculum

4-year. Presents material in a coordinated manner so that students can better understand the basic processes of the human body, integrate a concept of the functions of bodily systems, and see their clinical applications. Clinical training is included at every level, progressing in difficulty, adding topical information and reinforcing concepts. The curriculum includes 3 semesters of an integrated basic sciences program, a study of individual body systems, and clinical clerkships, including ambulatory and inpatient care in community hospitals and health care agencies. The theories and applications of manipulative techniques are included at all levels of the curriculum.

Affiliated Teaching Hospitals

Several throughout the state, including many in the Detroit metropolitan area.

Housing

Some housing is available on campus and in the Lansing/East Lansing area.

MISSOURI

Kirksville College of Osteopathic Medicine

800 West Jefferson
Kirksville, Missouri 63501

Phone: 816-626-2354   *Fax:* 816-626-2969
E-mail: admissions@fileserver7,kcom.edu
WWW: http://www.kcom.edu

Application Filing		Accreditation
Earliest:	June 1	AOA
Latest:	February 1	
Fee:	$50	

Enrollment: 1996–97 First-Year Class

Men:	99	67%	Applied:	4577
Women:	48	33%	Enrolled:	147
Out of State:	125	85%		

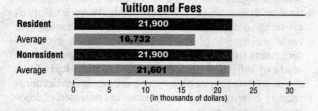

Tuition and Fees

Resident	21,900
Average	16,732
Nonresident	21,900
Average	21,601

(in thousands of dollars)

Introduction

The Kirksville College of Osteopathic Medicine was established in 1892. It was the first school of its type, originating as the American School of Osteopathy. The school's goal is the preparation of osteopathic physicians for primary care and specialty training. The school is located on a 60-acre campus in Kirksville, which is in northeastern Missouri.

Admissions (AACOMAS)

Completion of a minimum of 90 semester hours and the MCAT. The basic premedical science courses plus 1 year of English are required. Courses in biochemistry and comparative or human anatomy are recommended.

Curriculum

4-year. The goal is to prepare osteopathic physicians for primary care or specialty training. *First and second years:* Essentially consist of basic sciences with some clinical courses and training. *Third and fourth years:* Students conduct clinical rotations that include internal medicine, surgery, obstetrics/gynecology, pediatrics, psychiatry, radiology, emergency medicine, general practice, and required electives. Currently, students receive clinical training at 1 of 10 regional site training hospitals.

Affiliated Teaching Hospitals

Clinical education takes place at 3 regional sites.

Housing

There are 44 student apartments and private residences.

The University of Health Sciences College of Osteopathic Medicine

2105 Independence Boulevard
Kansas City, Missouri   64124

Phone: 800-234-4847   *Fax:* 816-283-2349

Application Filing
Earliest: June 1
Latest: February 1
Fee: $35

Accreditation
AOA

Enrollment: 1996–97 First-Year Class

Men: 165   75%   Applied: 4809
Women: 55   25%   Enrolled: 220
Out of State: 156   71%

Tuition and Fees

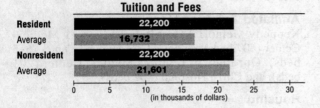

Resident	22,200
Average	16,732
Nonresident	22,200
Average	21,601

0   5   10   15   20   25   30
(in thousands of dollars)

Introduction

The Kansas City College of Osteopathic Medicine opened in 1916. In 1921 it moved to its present location. In 1970 the name of the college was changed to the Kansas City College of Osteopathic Medicine, and in 1980 it again changed to its present name, the University of Health Sciences College of Osteopathic Medicine.

Admissions

Completion of a baccalaureate degree with a GPA of at least 2.5 and the MCAT is advisable. The basic premedical science courses plus 1 year of English are required as well as comparative anatomy, genetics, and bacteriology.

Curriculum

4-year. *First year:* Emphasis is mainly on the basic science core curriculum; namely, gross anatomy, histology, biochemistry, physiology, neuroanatomy, and osteopathic principles and practice. *Second year:* An integrated basic and clinical sciences program, covering microbiology, pharmacology, human sexuality, medical ethics, osteopathic medicine and therapeutics, electrocardiography, obstetrics, medicine, otorhinolaryngology, pediatrics, surgery, cardiovascular medicine, radiology, medical jurisprudence, gerontology, opthalmalogy, neurology, anesthesiology, emergency medicine, oncology, and medical practice office management. *Third and fourth years:* Students begin 20 months of rotations and are required to complete rotations in general practice, rural general practice, psychiatry, pediatrics, obstetrics/gynecology, emergency medicine, internal medicine, surgery, and electives in other clinical areas.

Affiliated Teaching Hospitals

The college is affiliated with 26 hospitals providing access to more than 6590 beds.

Housing

Students must find their own housing.

NEW JERSEY

University of Medicine and Dentistry of New Jersey School of Osteopathic Medicine

1 Medical Center Drive
Stratford, New Jersey   08084

Phone: 609-566-6972   *Fax:* 609-566-6222

Application Filing		Accreditation
Earliest:	June 1	AOA
Latest:	February 1	
Fee:	$50	

Enrollment: 1996–97 First-Year Class

Men:	148	51%	Applied:	3211
Women:	142	49%	Enrolled:	290
Out of State:	30	10%		

Tuition and Fees

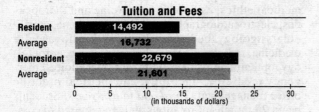

Resident	14,492
Average	16,732
Nonresident	22,679
Average	21,601

0   5   10   15   20   25   30
(in thousands of dollars)

Introduction

In 1976 the School of Osteopathic Medicine was founded as a division of the University of Medicine and Dentistry in New Jersey. The school is located in Stratford, in southern New Jersey, and within driving distance of both New York City and Philadelphia.

Admissions (AACOMAS)

Completion of the MCAT and a baccalaureate degree are necessary. The basic premedical science courses are required as is 1 year each of English, mathematics, and behavioral science.

Curriculum

4-year. Committed to an emphasis on primary patient care, the school provides a medical education that fully trains students in the principles of scientific medicine, while emphasizing the interrelation between structure and function in explaining the disease process.

Affiliated Teaching Hospitals

Kennedy Memorial Hospitals-University Medical Center (607 beds), Atlantic City Medical Center (615 beds), Our Lady of Lourdes Medical Center (201 beds), and Christ Hospital (402 beds).

Housing

Students are assisted in obtaining housing near the school.

NEW YORK

New York College of Osteopathic Medicine of New York Institute of Technology

Old Westbury, New York   11568

Phone: 516-626-6947   *Fax:* 516-626-6946

Application Filing
Earliest: June 1
Latest: February 1
Fee: $60

Accreditation
AOA

Enrollment: 1996–97 First-Year Class

Men:	118	58%	Applied:	4598
Women:	87	42%	Enrolled:	205
Out of State:	1	0%		

Tuition and Fees

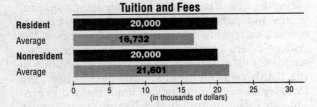

Resident	20,000
Average	16,732
Nonresident	20,000
Average	21,601

(in thousands of dollars)

Introduction

The New York Institute of Technology was created in 1955. It is a private school with 6 undergraduate and 6 graduate schools. As part of the New York Institute of Technology, the New York College of Osteopathic Medicine is the only school of osteopathic medicine in New York State. It is located on a scenic 700-acre campus on Long Island, about 25 miles east of New York City.

Admissions (AACOMAS)

Bachelor's degree, MCAT, and a GPA of 2.75.

Curriculum

4-year. Emphasizes needs and opportunities in primary health care and community health services, particularly health care problems of the inner city and smaller communities. The 2-year on-campus portion of the program consists primarily of didactic instruction in the basic and clinical sciences. The curriculum becomes progressively more and more clinical, with a program focusing on family practice and preventive health care constituting the last 2 years.

Affiliated Teaching Hospitals

Brookdale Hospital, Coney Island Hospital, Long Beach Memorial Hospital, Lutheran Medical Center, Jamaica Hospital, Methodist Hospital, and others.

Housing

No on-campus housing available.

OHIO

Ohio University College of Osteopathic Medicine

Grosvernor Hall
Athens, Ohio   45701

Phone: 614-593-4313
WWW: http://www.tcom.ohiou.edu/oucom

Application Filing		Accreditation
Earliest:	June 1	AOA
Latest:	January 1	
Fee:	$25	

Enrollment: 1996–97 First-Year Class

Men:	57	47%	Applied:	3569
Women:	44	36%	Enrolled:	121
Out of State:	14	12%		

Tuition and Fees

Resident	10,785
Average	16,732
Nonresident	15,279
Average	21,601

0   5   10   15   20   25   30
(in thousands of dollars)

Introduction

Ohio University was established in 1804. It is a public school with 9 undergraduate and 8 graduate schools. The College of Osteopathic Medicine was established in 1975. The school focuses on training in primary care including family medicine, internal medicine, and pediatrics. More than half its graduates practice primary care medicine.

Admissions (AACOMAS)

Completion of a baccalaureate degree and the MCAT are necessary. The basic premedical science courses plus 1 year each of English and behavioral science are required. Students with 3 years of exceptional college work are considered.

Curriculum

4-year. The focus of instruction is on the holistic approach to practicing primary care medicine, with the realization that even the medical specialist needs a firm understanding of these disciplines. The curriculum involves a combination of learning activities including case-based learning, computer-based programs, independent and group study, early clinical contact, and traditional lectures and laboratories. The college offers 2 curricular options to accommodate students with different learning styles. In addition to the traditional medical school curriculum, the Primary Care Continuum was implemented to provide specific training in the disciplines of family medicine, internal medicine, and pediatrics. Students are granted entrance to this program only after acceptance through our regular admission process.

Affiliated Teaching Hospitals

The school provides clinical training at hospitals that form regional training centers in 6 different areas of Ohio.

Housing

Student housing is available in residence halls, 2 married-student complexes, and off-campus apartments and houses.

OKLAHOMA

Oklahoma State University College of Osteopathic Medicine

1111 West 17th Street
Tulsa, Oklahoma   74107

Phone: 918-582-1972

Application Filing		Accreditation
Earliest:	June 1	AOA
Latest:	January 4	
Fee:	$25	

Enrollment: 1996–97 First-Year Class

Men:	57	65%	Applied:	1927
Women:	31	35%	Enrolled:	88
Out of State:	13	15%		

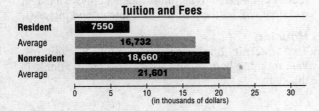

Tuition and Fees

Resident	7550
Average	16,732
Nonresident	18,660
Average	21,601

0 5 10 15 20 25 30
(in thousands of dollars)

Introduction

Oklahoma State University was established in 1890. It is a public school with 6 undergraduate schools, and 1 graduate school. The College of Osteopathic Medicine originally opened in 1972 and enrolled its first class in 1974, which graduated in 1977. That year the college moved to its permanent campus on the west bank of the Arkansas River, near downtown Tulsa. In 1988, the College of Osteopathic Medicine joined Oklahoma State University.

Admissions (AACOMAS)

Completion of 4 years of college, the MCAT, and at least a 3.0 grade point average and 2.75 science cumulative average are necessary. English and the basic premedical science courses are required plus 1 of the following courses: biochemistry, histology, embryology, comparative anatomy, cellular or molecular biology, or microbiology.

Curriculum

4-year. Divided into basic and clinical sciences, and emphasizes primary care. The program uses a coordinated, spiraling systems approach in which subject matter is continuously reintroduced in greater depth and complexity. *First year:* Concentrates on the basic sciences and preliminary clinical concepts. Preparation of the student for early patient contact requires a foundation in anatomy, physiology, behavioral science, techniques of physical examination, diagnosis and patient interview, and recognition of normal and abnormal patterns of physical conditions and disease. *Second year:* Emphasizes the interdisciplinary study of the structure and function of body systems. In addition, students are introduced to specialized clinical care and medical procedures related to each body system and receive continuing instruction in osteopathic principles and practices. *Third and fourth years:* Devoted exclusively to clinical rotations, where students work with patients under physician-faculty supervision. Students rotate through basic hospital services, including general medicine, surgery, obstetrics/gynecology, pediatrics, internal medicine, and emergency medicine. Other clinical training occurs at a small rural hospital, a primary care clinic, a psychiatric facility, a community health facility, and offices of private physicians. The curriculum is based on the semester system, with summers off, except the last year and one half, which is continuous.

Affiliated Teaching Hospitals

Tulsa Regional Medical Center (521 beds), Hillcrest Osteopathic Hospital (186 beds), Enid Regional Hospital (101 beds), and other hospitals in Missouri, Kansas, and Texas.

Housing

Information not available.

PENNSYLVANIA

Philadelphia College of Osteopathic Medicine

4170 City Avenue
Philadelphia, Pennsylvania   19131

Phone: 215-871-2711   *Fax:* 215-871-6719
E-mail: admissions@pcom.edu
WWW: http://www.pcom.edu

Application Filing	Accreditation
Earliest: June 1	AOA
Latest: February 1	
Fee: $50	

Enrollment: 1996–97 First-Year Class

Men:	155	60%	Applied:	5846
Women:	104	40%	Enrolled:	259
Out of State:	84	32%		

Tuition and Fees

Resident	21,000
Average	16,732
Nonresident	21,000
Average	21,601

0   5   10   15   20   25   30
(in thousands of dollars)

Introduction

The largest osteopathic college in the United States, the Philadelphia College of Osteopathic Medicine was established in 1899. The school has grown to be the hub of the Osteopathic Medical Center of Philadelphia and is a major health care complex.

Admissions

A bachelor's degree or 3 years of college work of exceptional quality, a minimum 2.5 average, the basic premedical science courses, and the MCAT are required. An early decision program is available.

Curriculum

4-year. A blend of classroom teaching, clinical experience, and research. The curriculum has been fine-tuned to assure that each student graduates with the broadest possible base of education that is relevant today and tomorrow. Specific areas of curriculum enhancement include primary care and the training of generalists throughout the 4-year program. The college is committed to helping students choose a career path that will let them fulfill their talents and interests.

Housing

Two fraternity houses accommodating 60 men, private rooming houses, and apartments are available in the vicinity.

Lake Erie College of Osteopathic Medicine

1858 West Grandview Boulevard
Erie, Pennsylvania   16509

Phone: 814-866-6641

Application Filing		Accreditation
Earliest:	June 1	AOA
Latest:	March 15	
Fee:	n/av	

Enrollment: 1996–97 First-Year Class

Men:	74	64%	Applied:	4128
Women:	41	36%	Enrolled:	115
Out of State:	44	38%		

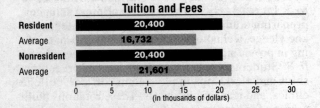

Tuition and Fees

Resident	20,400
Average	16,732
Nonresident	20,400
Average	21,601

0   5   10   15   20   25   30
(in thousands of dollars)

Introduction
This school was founded in 1992 with the goal of educating family physicians trained in osteopathic medicine as well as preparing those seeking careers in the specialties. It is located on a 75-acre site in Erie, the third largest city in Pennsylvania.

Admissions
Bachelor's degree or at least 96 credits, with minimum of 2.7 average. The basic premedical science courses and the MCAT are required.

Curriculum
4-year. Divided into 3 phases: introduction to the basic sciences, correlated system teaching (which incorporates basic and clinical sciences in the study of an organ system), and clinical experience. *Phase I:* During the first semester only, it consists of the basic science core curriculum, namely, gross anatomy, biochemistry, physiology, microbiology/immunology, embryology/histology, and medical ethics, with osteopathic principles/practices (OPP) and emergency medicine interwoven throughout. *Phase II:* Begins in the second semester of the freshman year and continues throughout the sophomore year. Emphasis at this point in the systems approach is on pathology, pharmacology, and neuroanatomy, along with concurrent integrated exposure to OPP and the relevant basic science/clinical aspects of these organ systems (dermal, neurosensory, musculoskeletal, cardiovascular, respiratory, reproductive, and gastrointestinal systems). Family medicine core courses, geriatric, human sexuality, pediatrics, and related disciplines are discussed when appropriate. *Phase III:* Begins with the junior year and involves primarily clinical experience. All students are required to complete rotations in internal medicine, rural general practice, psychiatry, pediatrics, obstetrics/gynecology, emergency medicine, internal medicine, surgery, and electives in other clinical areas.

Affiliated Teaching Hospitals
Information not available.

Housing
Information not available.

TEXAS

University of North Texas Health Science Center Texas College of Osteopathic Medicine at Fort Worth

3500 Camp Bowie Boulevard
Fort Worth, Texas 76107

Phone: 817-735-2000 *Fax:* 817-735-2225
WWW: http://www.hsc.unt.edu

Application Filing	Accreditation
Earliest: June 1	AOA
Latest: December 1	
Fee: $50	

Enrollment: 1996–97 First-Year Class

Men:	70	61%	Applied:	2219
Women:	44	39%	Enrolled:	114
Out of State:	8	7%		

Tuition and Fees

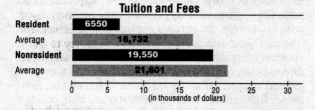

Resident	6550
Average	16,732
Nonresident	19,550
Average	21,601

(in thousands of dollars)

Introduction

The University of Texas system was created in 1950 and contains 4 different campuses. In 1970, the Texas College of Osteopathic Medicine was established. Students are encouraged to become family medicine or primary care physicians and to practice in communities where medical practice is most needed.

Admissions (AACOMAS)

Completion of baccalaureate degree with at least a B (3.0) average and the MCAT are necessary to be competitive. The basic premedical science courses plus 1 year of English are required.

Curriculum

4-year. *Semesters 1 and 2:* Devoted primarily to classroom and lab instruction in the basic sciences. At the same time, students are introduced to the clinical sciences through activities in the departments of family medicine and manipulative medicine. *Semesters 3 to 5:* Increasingly devoted to the clinical sciences, preparing students for the challenge of integrating knowledge, technology, sensitivity, and critical thinking in providing competent patient care. *Semesters 6 to 8:* Students rotate through a series of preceptorships and clerkships in physicians' offices, college clinics, and teaching hospitals. These rotations build a strong foundation for future success in any medical practice.

Affiliated Teaching Hospitals

Agreements were made with 20 Texas clinics and hospitals in the Fort Worth-Dallas Metropolitan Plan to provide 2500 patient care beds.

Housing

Apartments or rooms in private homes.

WEST VIRGINIA

West Virginia School of Osteopathic Medicine

400 North Lee Street
Lewisburg, West Virginia 24901

Phone: 304-645-6270
E-mail: gorby@mail.osteo.wvnet.edu

Application Filing		Accreditation
Earliest:	June 1	AOA
Latest:	February 1	
Fee:	$75	

Enrollment: 1996–97 First-Year Class

Men:	38	58%	Applied:	2423
Women:	27	42%	Enrolled:	65
Out of State:	20	31%		

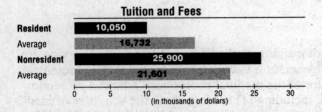

Tuition and Fees

Resident 10,050
Average 16,732
Nonresident 25,900
Average 21,601

0 5 10 15 20 25 30
(in thousands of dollars)

Introduction

The West Virginia School of Osteopathic Medicine was founded in 1974 as Greenbrier College of Osteopathic Medicine. It became part of the West Virginia system of higher education in 1976. Its 43-acre campus is located in rural Appalachia. Its focus is on training primary care physicians for service in rural communities of West Virginia.

Admissions (AACOMAS)

Completion of a minimum of 3 years of college, the MCAT, and at least a C+ average in the sciences are necessary. The basic premedical science courses plus 1 year of English are required. Additional courses in moelcular and organic biology are strongly recommended.

Curriculum

Consists of 3 phases. *Phase I:* Fundamentals of the biomedical sciences and osteopathic principles. In addition, courses of value to those planning careers in West Virginia, such as nutrition, geriatrics, community medicine, rural health care research, physical diagnosis and physicians skills are provided. *Phase II:* The presentation of organ systems, in which basic and clinical sciences are integrated in several courses that cover the major organ systems of body, and osteopathic principles. *Phase III:* Clinical education is provided giving students an opportunity to gain direct experience with patients at various settings, while assuming graduated responsibility.

Affiliated Teaching Hospitals

The college has contractual arrangements with off-campus hospitals and clinics that provide training in the clinical years.

Housing

There is no on-campus housing, but ample rentals are available in the immediate vicinity.

14 Medical Practice

Physician-patient relationship
Clinical skills
Diagnosing disease
Patient care
Assessing treatment
Accountability
Guidelines to practicing medicine
Teaching and research
Terminal illness and death
Types of practices
Professional hazards
Physician remuneration

Many years of study, a long interval of training, and a lifetime of dedicated service are required in order to become a good physician. It is therefore essential that a premedical student have an overview of the nature of the medical profession. This can be accomplished in a number of different ways, including (1) reading about the activities of medical students, physicians-in-training, and those in practice (see bibliography); (2) talking with medical students and doctors; and (3) performing volunteer work in a hospital.

This chapter seeks to supplement the aforementioned approaches by discussing the most basic elements of medical practice.

The practice of medicine is a combination of both science and art. The scientific component involves the application of technological modalities in solving clinical problems. This requires the judicious use of biochemical methods, biophysical imaging techniques, and therapeutic modalities—areas that have seen remarkable advances over the past decade. Competence in utilizing these areas, while essential, does not meet all the requirements of a good practitioner. What is needed, in addition to the aforementioned elements, is the ability to extract vital information from a mass of contradictory signs and computer-generated data in order to determine an appropriate course of action. This involves deciding whether to actively pursue a clinical clue or merely to continue observing as well as judging, if treating the condition involves a greater risk than not treating it at all. This combination of knowledge, judgment, and intuition is the key to the art of medicine.

Medical practice requires scientific knowledge, technical skill, and human understanding. The last quality involves treating the patient with tact and sympathy and realizing that a patient is a human being, not merely a collection of symptoms, damaged organs, and/or disturbed emotions. Rather, the patient is, at the same time, fearful and hopeful, and in need of relief, assistance, and reassurance. To meet this challenge, the physician must genuinely care for people.

PHYSICIAN-PATIENT RELATIONSHIP

As stated above, physicians must recognize that patients are not the equivalent of cases or diseases; they are individuals, whose problems often transcend the complaints they are verbalizing. They frequently are anxious and frightened when they visit their physicians and may try to convince themselves that their illness does not exist. They may even try unconsciously to divert attention from the real problem that they perceive to be threatening. At times, illness is used as a means to gain attention or as a way to extricate themselves from a difficult emotional situation. With this in mind, physicians need to view their clinical findings in a broader context involving not only the patient but the patient's family and social background.

Knowledge of the patient's origin, education, home, family, job, and goals is very desirable. It provides useful information that permits the physician to establish rapport with the patient and to develop a good insight into the patient's illness. Under these circumstances, mutual trust is developed and an open channel of communication is established.

The traditional one-on-one patient-physician relationship is changing due to the change in the setting in which medicine is practiced today. Frequently, when dealing with a serious illness, patient care involves a variety of allied health professionals, in addition to several medical specialists. A health team effort is therefore commonly mandated, which can prove especially beneficial if the primary care physician asserts a leadership position and maintains a special status in the patient's eyes. The primary care physician needs to retain the ultimate decision-making authority in the areas of diagnosis and treatment. This arrangement should also be in effect when medicine is practiced in a group setting, for it is the primary care physician who has an overview of the patient's problems and reaction to medications, as well as knowing the patient's response to his or her illness and to the challenges that must be faced.

The modern hospital can be an intimidating environment for most patients. Being confined to bed, surrounded by buttons, air jets, and lights, with one's body invaded by tubes and wires, visited randomly and at all hours of the day and night by members of the health care team—physicians, nurses, technicians, therapists, and aides—often stimulates a loss of a patient's sense of reality. This negative situation may be further reinforced by transporting the patient to X-ray departments or special testing and/or therapy facilities.

The primary care physician frequently serves as the pivotal link between the patient and reality. The stressful hospital situation can be somewhat ameliorated by a strong doctor-patient relationship.

There are a number of factors that lead to impersonalization of medical care. These include:

1. strong efforts to reduce the cost of health care;

2. heavy reliance on computerization and technological advances for diagnosis and treatment;

3. growth of health maintenance organizations (HMOs), which may not allow patients to select their physician;

4. need for more than one physician to be involved in the care of seriously ill patients;

5. increased mobility of physicians and patients;

6. increased frequency of litigation by patients to express their dissatisfaction with their physicians or treatment or results.

In the light of this medical climate, it is especially challenging for physicians to maintain a humanistic attitude. It is now even more essential that each patient, regardless of personal circumstances, be treated carefully and courteously. This means that the physician-patient relationship needs to be built on a foundation of respect, integrity, and compassion. The level of communication between both sides should allow the patient, to the fullest possible extent, to gain an understanding of the nature of the illness, the treatment protocol, and prognosis.

In dealing with patients, the physician should avoid being judgmental of their values and lifestyles unless it is medically relevant (for example, smoking and alcohol or substance abuse, which should be firmly discouraged). In the course of one's practice, every physician can anticipate meeting patients who evoke negative, as well as positive, emotional reactions. Physicians need to be aware of this possibility and should not allow their judgment or actions to interfere with their patients' best interests.

In order to treat a patient effectively, a good relationship between physician and patient must be established. This mainly depends on the empathetic response on the part of the physician and recognition of the physician's caring attitude by the patient.

CLINICAL SKILLS

The basic three-step approach used by physicians in diagnosing disease involves taking a patient's history, performing a physical examination, and ordering laboratory tests and/or imaging procedures. These steps are discussed in-depth below:

History Taking

All the facts in the patient's medical history should be noted in the written record. The history can be recorded in one of two ways: (1) it can be recorded in chronological order, in which case recent events should be emphasized most; or (2) if a problem-oriented approach is used, the problems that are clinically most pronounced should be noted first. The nature of the symptoms should be in the patient's own words. In eliciting the history, the physician needs to be careful to avoid suggesting answers in the course of guiding the patient through the interview. It is important that careful attention be given to all the details of the interview, no matter how minor, since a seemingly small detail may be important in making the diagnosis.

More than an organized listing of symptoms, a well-written history, elicited during the interview, should also reveal something about the patient, in addition to the nature of the patient's disease. This information may be extracted from facial expressions, voice inflections, and the attitude that is evident during the discussion of the illness. Taking a history is a challenge since patients are highly subjective in their presentation and may also be affected by their past experience. In addition, there is a fear of disability or even death, as the impact of illness on one's family inevitably influences a person's account of the problem. Unfortunately, language or sociological obstacles, as well as failing mental recall, can, in some cases, very significantly interfere with the patient giving an adequate history. In such cases, the physician may have to seek the help of an interpreter or a member of the patient's family in order to obtain an accurate history. The physician's skill, knowledge, patience, and experience will greatly influence the quality of the history taken.

Obtaining a family medical history can be very helpful in short-term care and preventive health. The process of history taking also serves to establish or strengthen the physician-patient relationship. Patients should be put at ease and should be allowed to express their thoughts. The confidential nature of the information should be emphasized.

Physical Examination

Physical signs are objective and verifiable evidence of disease. Their significance is enhanced when these signs confirm a structural or functional change indicated by the patient's history. On occasion, the physical signs may be the only evidence of disease, especially if the history is not informative.

The physical exam should be carried out methodically and thoroughly. While the focus of the exam may be on the diseased area or organ, in a new patient the exam should cover the entire body. The results should be recorded at the time they are obtained. Skill in this area is required and comes with time.

Laboratory Tests

The increase in the number, type, and availability of laboratory tests has resulted in the increased reliance on this approach for the solution of clinical problems. It is essential to bear in mind that laboratory tests are often believed by physicians to be the final authority, regardless of possible fallibility of the tests, the individuals handling or interpreting them, or of the instruments. Laboratory data cannot replace observation of the patient. Both the expense and possibilities of misinterpretation of the lab tests ordered should be taken into account by the physician. Laboratory tests are rarely done individually, but rather as batteries (24 up to 40). The various combinations of lab tests are frequently quite useful. The thoughtful use of screening tests should not be confused with indiscriminate lab testing. Screening tests are useful because they enable the physician to obtain a group of lab results conveniently, utilizing a single specimen of blood, at relatively low cost. Biochemical measurements, together with simple lab tests, such as blood counts, urine analyses, and sedimentation rate often provide the principle clue to the presence of a pathological process. The physician must be alert for abnormalities in screening test results that may not indicate significant disease. An isolated laboratory abnormality on an otherwise well patient should not provoke an in-depth medical workup. The lab test itself may bear repeating to see if the results are reproducible. The physician can then determine whether the results are significant. Clinical judgment will determine how to proceed if this occurs.

Imaging Techniques

Over the past quarter of a century, the use of imaging techniques as a diagnostic method has become well established. This includes ultrasonography, a method of examination using soundwaves to visualize internal organs; computerized axial tomography (CAT); magnetic resonance imaging (MRI); and position emission tomography (PET). This major new diagnostic approach has frequently replaced invasive techniques that require insertion into the body of tubes, wires, or catheters or surgical biopsy. The latter are frequently painful and at times quite risky to the patient. While very valuable, imaging technique results need validation and are often extremely expensive. Therefore, this approach should be used judiciously, but not as a supplement to invasive techniques.

DIAGNOSING DISEASE

Arriving at a diagnosis involves analysis and synthesis—two aspects of logic. The physician identifies all the problems raised after hearing the patient's complaints, performing a physical exam, and receiving lab findings. Most physicians try to place the medical problem they are dealing with into one of several syndromes. A syndrome is a group of symptoms associated with any disease process, which constitutes together a picture of the disease.

The syndrome incorporates a hypothesis concerning a tissue, organ, or organ system. For example, congestive heart failure will produce a wide variety of symptoms, all of which are connected to the single pathophysiological mechanism, namely inadequacy of the heart muscle. Similarly, identifying a syndrome usually narrows down the number of possibilities for an illness and suggests indicated clinical and lab studies.

Making a diagnosis is more difficult if one cannot categorize the patient's signs and symptoms. Nevertheless, the same logical approach, starting with the symptoms, proceeding to the physical findings, and lab results will usually lead to a diagnosis.

PATIENT CARE

This subject is initiated with the establishment of a personal relationship between the physician and patient. The effectiveness of therapeutic measures prescribed is enhanced in the presence of a sense of confidence and trust. Reassurance by the physician under these conditions may be all that is necessary to improve the patient's well-being. Similarly, for illnesses that are not easily treatable, a sense by the patient that the physician is doing everything possible is an essential therapeutic approach.

Clinical decision making should involve the patient, especially where quality of life issues are concerned. In such cases, a determination of what the patient values most should be made after lengthy conversation between physician and patient. When it is not medically possible to eliminate the disease and its consequences, improving the quality of life should of course be the treatment goal.

ASSESSING TREATMENT

Objective standards are usually used in judging the effectiveness of treatment. The patient measures the outcome in terms of relief of pain and preservation of or regaining lost function. Although subjective, a patient's state of health can be divided into a number of components: bodily comfort; physical, social, professional, and personal activities; sexual and cognitive functions; sleep; overall view of one's health; and general sense of well-being. Relative to these components, the patients' views of their disabilities can be obtained by verbal exchanges. Proper medical practice requires the consideration of both the objective and subjective aspects of treatment outcome.

Drug Therapy

New drugs are introduced every year. While it is hoped that they are significantly better than their predecessors, many have only a marginal advantage. With this in mind, a cautious approach should be used in dealing with a new medication, unless it is established with certainty to be a real advance. Otherwise, it is preferable to continue to use established drugs whose benefits and side-effects are known to the treating physician.

Over the next few decades, the practice of medicine will be greatly influenced by the health care needs of the elderly. It is estimated that the number of individuals over 65 will triple in the next 30 years. For this reason it is important for the physician to be familiar with the different responses of the elderly patient to disease. The physician must also be knowledgeable about common disorders that occur with aging and altered response of the elderly patient to medication.

Iatrogenic Disorders

These disorders refer to those generated by a testing or treatment modality and are not connected to the existing medical condition.

The judicious use of powerful medical tools requires that the physician consider their action, potential dangers, and costs. Every medical procedure carries certain risks; however, to benefit from the advances of modern medicine, reasonable risks need to be taken. Reasonable means considering both positive and negative aspects of a procedure and determining what is more desirable under the circumstances. Special attention must be given to the use of medications, which in some instances can generate more harm than good.

The physician's use of language and behavior can at times lead to needless anxiety if the patient is given a misleading impression of his or her condition. Being involved with treating the disease should not shift the physician's concern from the overall well-being and economic welfare of the patient.

ACCOUNTABILITY

Over the past several decades, there have been increased demands that physicians account for the way in which they practice by meeting certain federal and state standards. The hospitalization of patients whose care is funded by the government is subject to utilization review. This procedure requires the physician to defend the reason for the patient's hospital stay if it extends beyond the average standard. Elective surgery, in some cases, requires a second opinion. The purpose of these regulations is to try to limit the high cost of health care. Probably, all aspects of medical practice will in time be subjected to this type of review, which will profoundly alter medical practice.

Other approaches that may be used to judge continuing competence of physicians are an assessment of continuing education, auditing patients' records, reexamination for recertification, and time-limited certification as a prerequisite for relicensing. Such requirements clearly improve a physician's factual knowledge, but it is uncertain if they similarly effect the quality of practice.

GUIDELINES TO PRACTICING MEDICINE

Physicians have at their disposal a large number of diagnostic techniques and therapeutic modalities. The challenge is to select the most appropriate and cost-effective approach for the specific patient and that clinical condition. Formal clinical practice guidelines are being developed by government and professional organizations. These guidelines ensure that no patient, regardless of financial status, receives substandard care; protection is provided to the physician against inappropriate malpractice charges; and the insurance company is protected against excessive use of medical resources. There are, however, negative aspects to the use of guidelines. There may be major differences of opinion on the routine use of certain procedures, such as mammography. Guidelines, by being broadly applicable, cannot take into account the genetic and environmental effects on individuals. Therefore, the key is to utilize the guidelines as a meaningful framework while maintaining the flexibility to judge each case in the overall context of the reasonable standards set by knowledgeable clinicians. Under these circumstances, medicine will remain a learned profession rather than a mere technical vocation.

Cost Effectiveness in Medical Care

With the spiraling cost of health care, it is necessary to establish priorities as to how money is allocated. There is a greater emphasis today on the prevention of diseases. There is much that physicians can do to foster cost control but socioeconomic concerns should not interfere with the welfare of the patient.

TEACHING AND RESEARCH

It is obligatory for physicians to share their knowledge with colleagues, medical students, and members of the allied professions. Advances in medical knowledge depend on acquiring new information from various types of research, both basic and clinical. Publicizing this information can bring about improved medical care. Where appropriate, physicians should encourage participation in ethical clinical investigations.

TERMINAL ILLNESS AND DEATH

The most distressing problem facing a physician is that of the terminally ill patient. Great care needs to be taken in dealing with the variety of problems associated with this issue. These include what information should be given to the patient and the family and what steps should be taken to maintain life. These challenging problems do not have established answers, although ethical guidelines are available. It is hoped that senior medical staff and experts in medical ethics will provide junior personnel with appropriate assistance in this challenging area of medical practice.

TYPES OF PRACTICES

In the final year of postgraduate medical training (unless you are enrolled in the armed forces), planning ahead for opening a practice is essential. This involves determining the location as well as the nature of your practice. Many considerations are involved in both issues. They need to be carefully considered before making a final decision.

Location considerations include not only personal preferences regarding the type of community—rural or urban—but also how strong will be the demand for your services and for how long. In other words, a pediatrician obviously would not consider an area where the predominant population is made up of retirees. Even if you plan to join an older physician and ultimately take over his or her practice, you need to assess the likelihood of demand for your services down the line if the neighborhood changes.

As to the nature of your practice, it is important to determine if you prefer to start your own or work for others. There are several options in each of three major categories, solo, group and salaried practice. These will be explored below.

Solo Practitioners

Solo practitioners currently still remain the largest group of practicing physicians, but their numbers are diminishing as the health care system changes.

These physicians have direct contact with each one of their patients as the provider of professional services. In exchange for remuneration they are personally responsible for their patients' health.

There are several advantages to this traditional form of practice, particularly for primary care physicians, internists, pediatricians, and obstetricians/gynecologists. These include establishing long-term relationships, in most cases. (People do move out of the area or are dissatisfied and select someone else.) Another consideration is the independence that solo practice permits. Solo practitioners determine the location of their practice, arrange their office to their liking, hire the personnel they think they need and who they want to employ, select the laboratories that will perform their tests, set their own office hours, fees, and all the many other elements associated with a practice. To a large extent, therefore, they determine the extent of the success of their own practice.

On the negative side, there is the factor of uncertainty of how rapidly their practice will grow and how frequently they will get referrals from others; consequently, the rate of growth of their income will be unpredictable. Initially their income may be less than that of salaried practitioners whose expenses are paid for by their employers. Another major consideration is that solo practitioners assume full liability for the unavoidable overhead associated with such a practice. Another factor is the need to have coverage on days off or during vacations.

With the marked increase in paperwork required for Medicare, Medicaid, and insurance reimbursement, an additional heavy burden and expense has been placed on physicians. This issue adds to the already restricted autonomy of physicians due to federal, state, and insurance company regulations that evaluate the appropriateness of patient treatment and tests and set guidelines for the length of hospitalization.

There are a number of variations to solo practice that try to reduce some of its negative features. The following are some examples:

Solo-HMO Practice

Many established solo practitioners seeking to maintain this form of patient care that they have long been accustomed to, but realizing the changing situation in health care economics, have made a significant adjustment. They have decided to keep their solo practice, but at the same time be linked to an HMO accepting their lower levels of reimbursement and making up for it with a large volume of patients, for each of whom they receive a monthly stipend, if in a capitated HMO, or a reduced fee-for-service payment if in a noncapitated HMO.

Associateship

For younger physicians, establishing an expense-sharing relationship with another physician in the same specialty can be mutually rewarding. In such an arrangement both physicians agree to maintain their own solo practice and to share office expenses (rent, staff, etc.) in a proportionately acceptable way. The details of this relationship do not necessarily require a formal legal contract, but a written outline in the form of a memorandum of understanding should be signed by both associates. In the case of an association with a senior physician, the benefits for the younger practitioner being in practice with an established physician include an opportunity to obtain easier community recognition, a chance to learn the management aspects of a medical practice, a readily available consultant, and a way to keep operating costs down at a time when income levels are just building up. For the senior associate, such a relationship provides the benefit of having a covering physician readily available, providing an opportunity for more leisure time. It also lowers operating costs at a time when income may be declining, since it occurs in the last phase of professional life. Very often, an associateship can lead to a partnership; in such a case, a contract providing full details of the nature of the arrangement concerning the division of both income and expenses is essential.

Acquiring a Practice

Another way to establish a solo practice is to purchase one from a retiring or relocating physician. One can secure a practice in which the potential can be estimated based upon the practice's past performance. It is important to get an accurate assessment of the value of such a practice, which calls for an analysis of income, assets, and liabilities.

Group Practice

This is the second most popular form of practice. It is defined as three or more physicians, who provide medical care, jointly using the same facility and personnel and dividing the income as agreed to by the group. A group practice may be a corporation, a partnership, or an association of solo practitioners, but the majority of group practices are corporations. This arrangement provides a legal mechanism to protect the assets of the corporation from being seized in the event a member of the group is sued for malpractice and loses and cannot make full restitution from personal assets.

The number of group practices is increasing because they provide several advantages. They allow for a pooling of expenses for facilities, technical support services, and equipment, all of which come from a common revenue base. In other words, where the purchase of a piece of expensive equipment, such as an MRI machine, by an individual radiologist may well be prohibitive, a group can more easily afford it. This is because groups have the financial resources and space, and can use the equipment more fully to make it pay off. In addition, patient loads can be juggled easier so that, when one group member is occupied, another can be made available to the patient. The group members can easily schedule night coverage, vacation time, and emergency care.

Members of a group work shorter and more regular hours than solo practitioners. When a group has five or more members, income is on a par with that of physicians who are self-employed. In a successful group, a business manager may be hired to handle the many time-consuming bureaucratic aspects of an active practice and also supervise and coordinate personnel activities. Also, in a group practice, each physician has colleagues available to consult when necessary.

There are some negative aspects to group practice, such as the loss of independence by being a member of a group. Also, major business decisions regarding purchasing equipment, hiring or firing personnel, renovating, relocating, or expanding facilities require a consensus. For a group to practice successfully requires a compatibility of personalities and professional outlooks. Also, as implied above, in groups that are smaller than five—which is very common—income levels may well be lower than those of solo practitioners, since the number of patients may be restricted to space and personnel limitations.

As with most issues, therefore, there are both positive and negative sides to this type of professional practice. If you are considering it, you need to be cautious and thoroughly evaluate the nature of the practice and determine if you would be compatible with the group members. Certainly you should be the type of person who is a team player before you enter any group practice; however, the rewards of being a member of a successful group practice can readily outweigh its disadvantages.

Salaried Practitioners

These are physicians who work under contract for private hospitals, governmental institutions (hospitals, clinics, or agencies), commercial, industrial, or insurance companies or HMOs (see below), and receive a fixed remuneration for their services rendered over a given amount of time. This type of practice is especially appealing to those just beginning their practice. Over half begin this way and many move on to solo or group practices.

The advantages to those starting a medical practice as a salaried employee are clear. The principle reason given by many is to avoid the strain of having to cope with a relatively low income for many months when beginning a new solo practice and taking the gamble of succeeding, especially at a time when the new practitioner is perhaps still burdened by heavy student loans. It is extremely challenging under these conditions to have to sign an office lease, order furniture and equipment, engage a staff, and arrange for the many other requirements a new solo practice mandates.

A further element influencing a physician's career planning at an early stage is the knowledge that national economic trends, such as inflation and depression, as well as such issues as personal and professional contacts, can markedly impact on the degree of success in private practice. Achieving an active practice depends on more than one's technical skills as a physician.

Being a salaried physician is a means of avoiding the aforementioned risks while at the same time realizing many benefits. These include a secure position with reasonably good remuneration and an attractive benefit package that includes health care coverage (medical and dental for both physician and their family), paid vacations, holidays, sick leave, and shorter, defined working hours.

On the other hand, there are significant disadvantages to being a salaried practitioner, including a limit on one's income, which is generally less than that of successful solo practitioners (unless maintaining a limited outside practice is allowed). In addition, there is a loss of autonomy as a salaried practitioner. The latter includes having to respond to directives of the administration for whom one works and having to satisfy one's immediate supervisor. As a result of these liabilities, there is a marked tendency for physicians to undertake salaried appointments initially and, after a few years, move on to solo or group practices. Within six to eight years of beginning practice, therefore, the number of salaried physicians diminishes from well above half to under a third. In addition, the decline in the number of salaried employees varies for different specialties: Naturally, pathologists are 100% salaried with surgeons and psychiatrists being under 50%.

Health Maintenance Organization (HMO) Practitioners

Practitioners working for HMOs can be found in all of the employment options discussed above, depending on the organization's structure. Increasingly, HMOs are becoming a major source of employment for physicians and will undoubtedly become even more important as the health care system changes over the next several decades. Three types of arrangements are possible:

Staff Position
This is a salaried appointment under contract. It is a very common position for a new physician who intends, in a relatively short period of time, to go into solo practice or

join a group. It provides an opportunity to improve one's skills, develop self-confidence, and earn enough money to begin paying off debts. Physicians employed under such an arrangement do not share in the HMO's profits (or losses).

Group Member Position

In this case the physician members sign on as partners and as such have a direct interest in the success of the organization whose profits they share. This arrangement is an option for those physicians for whom salaried or solo practices are not attractive because they prefer fixed hours and wish to avoid all the other burdens that a private practice involves, even if it means possibly having a lower income.

Affiliated Position

This is an arrangement where physicians who belong to a group known as an Independent Practitioners Association (IPA) are contracted to serve a segment of an HMO's patient load. The primary activities of such physicians are outside of the HMO and not involved in the organization's business success.

Locum Tenens

After completing residency training, some physicians, albeit a minority, have opted to defer their decision for a while and have elected a more mobile form of practice. They have chosen to serve as substitutes in areas where there is a shortage of doctors. They are called *locum tenens*, the Latin name for place holder. They usually obtain their position through a placement agency, but some freelance. The *locum tenens* concept was developed to entice physicians to come to rural areas and to keep them there. They were used to substitute for physicians who wanted time off for vacations and continuing education, or who were ill. To replace them during such intervals, a network of temporary physicians was organized.

Currently, it is estimated that 12,000 physicians in every age group and specialty are working as *locum tenens*. While the majority of them are over 50 and semiretired, the fastest growing group are recent residency graduates. The reasons for engaging in this work are the desire to travel and the opportunity to explore a variety of practice opportunities. In addition, since this is a way to keep living expenses down, new physicians can use their savings to more rapidly pay off their medical school loans.

For some new practitioners this may prove to be a good transitional phase but they need to be aware of all of the ramifications. An assignment may last for a few days or several months and may vary from steady work in one area to practicing in widely separated locations. In addition, practitioners are responsible for their own health insurance. A major consideration is the impact of relocating one's family, both in physical and psychological terms, and it can prove costly in view of the need to store some belongings and ship others. Naturally, for single people, these problems are less troublesome.

There are currently about 25 agencies placing physicians, with CompHealth-Kron being the largest, but some prefer the freelance route. The key to success using this approach is to arrange a steady flow of assignments using an organized marketing plan. In addition to this substantial challenge, the freelancers must handle all the administrative details, such as obtaining and paying for medical licenses and malpractice insurance, travel and housing arrangements, etc., normally taken care of by the booking agency for a fee, which may be up to 40% of the client's income.

Practicing Abroad

Physicians seeking opportunities to serve overseas can contact the following sources for information.

National Council for International Health
1701 K Street NW Suite 600
Washington, DC 20006
(202) 833-5900

Health Volunteers Overseas
c/o Washington Station
P.O. Box 65157
Washington, DC 20035
(202) 296-0928

St. Joseph Medical Center
P.O. Box 1935
South Bend, Indiana 46634
(219) 237-7637

Volunteerism

Free clinics came into being in the 1960s. They primarily served the homeless and the underprivileged. While many still cater to indigent populations, numerous clinics serve working people who lack insurance coverage. What was originally begun as a fringe movement has evolved into a significant—if only partial—way to alleviate the health care crisis.

Free clinics provide physicians a chance to serve patients unencumbered by red tape and insurance regulations. They offer quality medical care that would otherwise not be available, because they operate on the principle that health care is a right and not a privilege. At most free clinics, part-time volunteer physicians (and medical students) offer out-patient primary care assisted by volunteer lay people. Administrative chores may be handled by salaried personnel and care is usually provided on the basis of genuine need. Many patients earn too much to qualify for public assistance, but too little to pay for medical benefits through insurance coverage.

To accommodate their working clientele, free clinics are usually open during the evenings. Most consist of an examining room, a small lab, and a dispensary, and can usually have some lab and X-ray work performed at local facilities. The sites of free clinics vary, some being in donated church basements; others in better facilities. In most cases, clinics need to be accessible to public transportation and an area considered safe by the volunteers. Since clinics usually do not receive governmental support, they are free from paper work and needed funds are supplied by grants, donations, and fund-raising events.

Physicians donate their time in varying amounts ranging from once a week to once every several months. Interns and residents—whose time is extremely limited—offer their services out of a desire to contribute to the welfare of the community. Some volunteer physicians are retirees.

Perhaps one of the considerations causing physicians to be reluctant to donate time is the malpractice liability issue. All states have Good Samaritan laws, but they vary, and not all offer free clinics immunity from negligence suits.

The high cost of prescription drugs presents a special problem: Free clinics try to secure samples donated by physicians or pharmaceutical companies or they distribute generic drugs that they purchase.

At this time free clinics offer a much-needed outlet for worthwhile services that the medical community can provide.

PROFESSIONAL HAZARDS _____

The practice of medicine, like other professions, has inherent occupational hazards, such as becoming infected with a bacterium or virus, and the very real risk of being sued for malpractice. Physicians take precautions for such problems by being careful in their management techniques and treatment and securing adequate liability insurance coverage. In addition, there is a more subtle way in which physicians can be severely impaired. In the intense drive to achieve professional success, they may ignore their own families, fail to form abiding personal friendships, never develop hobbies or find the time for relaxation and introspection. As in other professions, the obsession with success can lead to one becoming a workaholic and, in all too many cases, to the abuse of alcohol or drugs.

Work-related problems may stem from the combination of long working hours and the pursuit of excellence, causing physicians to lose sight of their own personal needs. They may repress and deny the strains, stresses, fatigue, and disappointments that are inevitable with the practice of medicine.

Patients can make enormous demands on their physicians, while the physicians themselves sometimes come to believe that they are invincible. This feeling is reinforced by the fact that they have successfully surmounted a vigorous and lengthy training regimen, replete with intense challenges and often demeaning activities. Further strengthening the all-powerful feeling is the success of becoming part of an elite group where their egos are enlarged by the adulation of patients, subordinates, and even colleagues. Maintaining this status demands enormous dedication and at times calls for others to "slow down and take it easy." Holding onto and even increasing one's monetary rewards can become a major driving force in professional life and being part of a "team" or medical group can increase the pressure for intensive activity.

After many years in active practice, physicians may find it difficult to retire; the respect and gratitude of patients can become an important element of their life. Retirement may therefore be delayed out of fear of boredom, the loss of personal satisfaction and financial rewards, or simply the fear of finding a new lifestyle. Physicians who continue to practice after their skills have begun to diminish risk making decisions that could be detrimental to themselves, their associates, and, most of all, their patients. However, with the changes in the practice of medicine today, more and more physicians are retiring at an early age rather than deal with the bureaucracy, mountains of paper work, and drop in income.

The changing climate in health care will have significant impact on the practice and rewards of the medical profession. It will challenge physicians to be even more alert to the potential dangers and require that they consider their own basic needs and periodically reevaluate the demands that they place on themselves and the toll that it takes.

PHYSICIAN REMUNERATION

It is thought by many that the recession of the 1980s contributed significantly to the substantial increase in the medical school applicant pool during the following decade. This is due to the perception that a career as a physician can ensure economic security.

The prospective physician needs to recognize that, while the income of physicians-in-training during post-graduate years has gone up over the past decade, in reality, other considerations come into play. New physicians starting their own practice need to be concerned with the unknown impact that the approaching changes in the health care system will have. They also need to take into consideration major overhead costs, such as those associated with purchasing medical equipment, malpractice insurance, office rental, employee salaries, etc. It is therefore more meaningful to deal with median net income, as shown in the accompanying graph. It demonstrates, over the past 25 years, a similar income pattern for each of the five-year periods, except at a higher overall level. We therefore find that there is a steep rise in income for the first dozen years. It rises less sharply over the next five years and peaks between 20 and 25 years, when the physician is about 50 years old. After a quarter of a century of practice, income gradually declines.

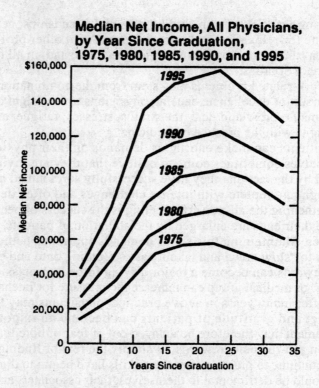

Median Net Income, All Physicians, by Year Since Graduation, 1975, 1980, 1985, 1990, and 1995

Remuneration in the Future

During the balance of this decade and into the early part of the next century, it is quite questionable if whether the pattern of the last 25 years as outlined above will be maintained. Indicators suggest that a leveling off or even possible decrease may be taking place from a peak median net annual income of nearly $150,000. This is particularly true for salaried physicians employed in group practices, hospitals, and health maintenance organizations. This potential trend reversal in the remuneration pattern will result from the steadily increasing power of managed care providers that are gaining dominance in a market containing an abundance of physicians who are seeking to tap into the patient pool.

Among physician employers, HMOs pay less since they feel they provide regular working hours and assume the expenses for office and malpractice insurance. Within this market, indications are that primary care physicians (family physicians, internists, and pediatricians) may be in a more favorable position in terms of remuneration. Their salaries may actually increase as a result of the fact that they are assuming the vital role of "gatekeeper" to the medical care establishment.

15 Physicians and Medicine in the Twenty-First Century

The challenge
Premedical education
Admission to medical school
Medical school education
Medical students
Medical practice
Specialists versus primary care physicians
Medical litigation crisis
Cybermedicine

THE CHALLENGE

The findings published in 1910 in the Flexner report served to revolutionize medical education in the United States. As this century nears its end, a new crisis seems to be looming. U.S. schools are producing some of the most technologically well-trained physicians in the world; nevertheless, critics argue that while our educational system is readily meeting the challenges of our technological advancement in medicine, it is failing in other respects. Physicians-in-training are being overwhelmed by the exploding volume of scientific knowledge and are not equipped to face the oncoming changing health care environment.

The planned reforms in the health care system will probably alter it dramatically and it is therefore essential that students be kept informed of the needs and opportunities that emerge. It is believed that one of the most significant needs will be for primary care physicians, and a surplus of specialists is predicted by the end of the century. Thus, health care reform is linked to medical education reform, because overreliance on specialists results in excessive costs and reduced access to health care. Additionally, market factors have not served to equalize distribution and specialists are less likely to practice in rural areas.

The decade between 1980 and 1990 saw a drop in the percentage of primary care physicians from 40% to about 30%. Some believe that medical education contributed to this downward trend, due to the fact that the first two years usually provides little clinical exposure and, in the last two years, student role models are subspecialists. In addition, many schools still do not require clerkships in family medicine. Some students are told by their teachers that general practice is not challenging enough. Others are dissuaded by the heavy debt loads that they have built up in medical school. Primary care is less remunerative than specialties; therefore, eliminating this debt is more difficult for a primary care physician than a specialist.

The response to demographic shifts in population has also been slow on the part of the medical education establishment. Minority groups are the fastest growing population segment, mandating an awareness of the impact of socioeconomic conditions that are specific to them. There is an increasing call for education in *population medicine,* considering the impact of social and economic factors on health. In addition, there is a belief that medical students are not taught disease prevention or how to encourage good health habits.

Preparing medical students to work in the new managed health care environment is another major challenge. In such settings, a health care team effort involves such allied health care professionals as physician assistants or advanced practice nurses, but this experience does not usually occur while one is a student.

There are those who feel that interpersonal and communication skills are not adequately emphasized during the educational phase. The educational system tends to diminish the students' sense of altruism during the course of their demanding education but some efforts to improve this situation have been initiated.

Educators argue that the curriculum is presently full and will become overloaded as biomedical information expands into new areas. Incorporating new information presents another challenge. Problem-based learning is an approach being tried in order to address this issue. The supporters of this educational method believe that the teaching under this system is more relevant and the students are more inclined to become lifelong learners. Many are using actors as standardized patients to present certain symptoms and thus better evaluate clinical competence. Increased use of computers can prove beneficial in the learning process.

Holding back better integration of the basic and clinical sciences is thought by some to be the timing of the USMLE, with Step 1 covering the basics and Step 2 the clinical sciences. Some have urged combining them, with both steps taken at the end of the medical education program, thus eliminating the focus of teaching solely for board preparation. Reforms that involve providing earlier clinical experience are difficult and costly to bring about. Translating sound ideas into practice presents major problems. In addition, central curriculum planning is frequently opposed at the departmental level.

There are those who call for reexamining the mission of medical schools, especially at state institutions. The reassessment can result in significant reforms.

Another problem is the lack of continuity between undergraduate and graduate education. Several schools are initiating programs that serve to combine both of these phases, with the usual aim being to encourage primary care.

More radical suggestions being heard are related to shortening medical education by accepting students into medical schools after their junior year in college and to eliminating the last year of medical school, which is in significant part devoted to securing a residency appointment. Thus, the undergraduate process would be reduced to six years, which is an option offered by a number of schools and is standard in Europe. Shortening the educational process would lower the debt obligations of medical students and, consequently, may reduce the pressures to seek training in higher paid subspecialties so as to wipe out such debt sooner and easier. This debt problem and its impact has prompted calls to make medical school tuition-free, an approach that in some quarters is being seriously considered. Supporters of this goal feel that it reinforces the concept that medicine is a profession with social obligations. Behind this approach is the desire to mandate that half of the residency appointments should be in primary care. Tuition relief, if elected, would be traded off by future professional choice limitation. There are even calls for a national program of mandatory service obligation. While it is quite unlikely that it will be introduced, some schools are requiring that their students perform community activities.

To graduate more socially responsible physicians, some schools are reviewing admission criteria and are looking beyond grades and MCAT scores to such factors as altruism and community involvement. To better judge this, some have appointed lay people to their admissions committee. One of the reasons for increasing minority representation is the fact that such students may be more responsive to community needs.

While medical schools can contribute to the increase in the number of primary care physicians, it is hoped that market forces will impact on this issue so that an overabundance of subspecialists will be translated into more primary care physicians.

An awareness of the future needs of society, which should be provided by medical schools, can influence residency choices. Health care reform may impact significantly on medical education. Schools will need to be offered the means of gaining a broad enough experience to train students to meet the needs of the coming century. Ideas for reforms are under active discussion and some have been made over the years. The prospects are favorable for significant progress in the foreseeable future.

While recognizing the need to develop a new type of physician, there is a realization that medical schools can't, on their own, generate more primary care M.D.s. The market forces seem now to be slowly reversing the equation, making subspecialists less in demand, while generalists are becoming more attractive. As the impact of these forces become known to medical students, their career goals may better fall in line with prospects for employment.

Medicine is a very dynamic profession. It changes not only as a result of advances in medical knowledge and technology, but also because of changes in the way medical care is offered. For the past number of years, health care has been the subject of a national debate. The reforms that will take place in the U.S. health system will significantly impact on all aspects of medicine including premedical education, admission to medical school, medical education, medical students, health care delivery, and physicians' specialties. The effect on each of these the components will be discussed in this chapter.

PREMEDICAL EDUCATION

Because the practice of medicine, as it has been evolving over the past decade, suggests that in the twenty-first century it will differ significantly from medical practice in the twentieth, it is reasonable to assume that premedical education goals will also need to be refocused appropriately. The basic learning goals to be emphasized in college are as follows:

1. Become familiar with the rapid advances in medicine that preclude the possibility of being able to rely indefinitely on knowledge solely gained in medical school and postgraduate training. One should pursue subjects of interest in either general or specialized areas for the sake of constantly acquiring more knowledge.

2. Develop skills in computer technology, especially with regard to communication skills. Accessing and sharing available information will be essential for making critical judgments.

ADMISSION TO MEDICAL SCHOOL

The AAMC's Council on General Professional Education of the Physician (GPEP), after a three-year study involving leading medical educators issued a report whose recommendations are believed to be of such import, that they could impact very significantly on the training of physicians for practice in the next century. The GPEP recommendations are relevant to both premedical and medical students. For those planning a medical career, the following recommendations are of special interest:

1. College faculties should require that the education of all students encompass broad study in the natural and social sciences and in humanities.

2. Medical schools should require only essential courses for admission; these should be part of the core curriculum that all college students must take.

3. Medical school admissions committees' practice of recommending additional courses beyond those required for admission should cease.

4. Medical schools should modify their admissions requirements, so that college students who apply and have successfully pursued a wide range of study may be viewed as highly as the students who have concentrated in the sciences.

5. Medical schools should devote more attention to selecting students who have the values and attitudes that are essential for members of a caring profession, who have critical analytical abilities, and who have the ability to learn independently.

Along with these recommendations, admissions criteria will be developed that are focused at increasing the proportion of students likely to enter primary care fields. Therefore, some priority will likely be given to women and married applicants and those from public colleges and rural backgrounds, as well as applicants with impressive evidence of community service.

MEDICAL SCHOOL EDUCATION

The AAMC's GPEP report was a comprehensive document that dealt with all aspects of medical education. As far as the curriculum is concerned, some of the recommendations by the panel of experts were:

1. Medical schools should develop procedures and adopt explicit criteria for the systematic evaluation of student performance.

2. Medical schools should emphasize the development of independent learning and problem-solving skills.

3. The level of skills and knowledge that a student should reach in order to enter graduate medical education (residency training) should be defined more clearly.

4. Medical schools should encourage their students to concentrate their elective programs on the advancement of their general professional education rather than on pursuit of a residency position.

5. Medical students' general professional education should include an emphasis on the physician's responsibility to work with individual patients and communities to promote health and prevent disease.

Obviously, each medical school will interpret these guidelines for curriculum changes according to its own philosophy of education. This will add greater variability to the learning experiences one can have at different institutions. It will obviously be another significant factor to consider when selecting a medical school.

Medical education will place less emphasis on mastery of content and greater emphasis on the learning process. The latter will include critical thinking, problem-solving skills, and the retrieval of information. In addition, attention will be focused on independent, self-directed learning skills. Medical school curricular time will increase for topics related to preventive medicine, public and community health, nutrition, geriatrics, behavioral sciences, and medical ethics. There will be greater educational opportunities in community health centers and out-patient clinics. Medical schools will place more emphasis on primary care and seek to channel a very substantial part of each graduating class into such residency programs. Thus, physician training will emphasize the health care needs of the community and nation, rather than being self-determined or determined by institutional agencies. Medical students will become better prepared for team-oriented practices.

MEDICAL STUDENTS

Medical students will probably consist of equal numbers of men and women. It is likely that, while in medical school, students will be provided with increased opportunities for community service. While financial aid will be available, it will be more difficult to obtain. Close to graduation, students may find reduced residency opportunities; after graduation, they will find that they will have to repay their student loans earlier, since deferral time will be reduced.

MEDICAL PRACTICE

The changes in the overall health care scene that have taken place in the 1980s and 1990s will have a profound impact on prospective medical students who will be the practitioners of the twenty-first century. These changes will be reflected in the three areas discussed separately below.

Physician Status

• In the twenty-first century most physicians will be salaried employees rather than fee-for-service practitioners. They will work in or for group practices, hospitals, insurance companies, medical schools, or health maintenance organizations (HMOs). Medical care will be provided to patients as a result of contractual agreements between business and governmental units and medical providing groups, with solo practitioners usually not having access to enrollees of such plans. As a result of this restructuring, competition will increase among individual health care providers.

• It is anticipated that there will be fewer specialists and a greater number of primary care physicians. Some subspecialists may have to retrain in order to also serve as primary care physicians.

• Practicing physicians will be held more accountable for their performance.

• Business managers will have more input into how medical services will be provided.

• On the positive side, there will be less paper work imposed on physicians and thus they will have more time to see patients. It is anticipated that primary care physicians will be reimbursed at a higher level while specialist remuneration will decrease. The working schedule of physicians will be more predictable. This will provide them with greater leisure time.

• Medical care in the next century will focus much more on prevention and patient education in order to both extend life and also reduce long-term medical costs. Physicians will experience reduced per-patient revenue, but with an increased number of patients having access to medical care, they will be forced to see more patients in order to maintain their income.

Physician-Patient Relationships

Today, the depersonalization of medical care due to the interference of administrative personnel has had a dehumanizing effect upon patients. The disease, rather than the patient, is being treated. A positive doctor-patient relationship can be restored by providing a more sympathetic and attentive attitude. Medical treatment is not always essential or even necessary, but the patient's psychological and emotional needs should always be addressed.

Physician Reimbursement

The focus in health care over the past several decades has changed from one aimed at increasing access to medical care to an emphasis on decreasing costs. Both public and private insurers have been seeking ways to significantly lower expenditures. Most current health care proposals have the following features in common. They would (1) insure access to health care of most, if not all, citizens, especially those in the central cities and rural areas (who are frequently uninsured); (2) establish cost controls; (3) establish defined criteria for quality; (4) require preventive care (such as immunizations, mammograms, etc.); and (5) introduce medical malpractice reform (see below).

Managed Care

Proposals for managed care fall into three major categories. The first is a national system (modeled on that in Canada) that is completely under government control. The second is diametrically opposite and is a "free market" approach, which allows the principle of supply and demand to control the health care system. The third, a middle of the road approach, is known as "play or pay." This involves businesses either purchasing insurance for their employees or paying into a health insurance pool for use in governmental pools.

All managed care is not government sponsored. Managed care is in effect, in the private sector, run by businesses that contract to provide comprehensive health care for their employees with group providers for specified time periods and preestablished costs for each employee. As a result, physicians have, in increasing numbers, become part of corporate medicine. They have been engaged as salaried employees of Health Maintenance Organizations (HMOs), which sometimes own hospitals. These organizations hospitalize patients much less frequently, and therefore are less expensive than traditional fee-for-service practitioners. HMOs have become increasingly successful. They have stimulated the formation of Independent Practice Associations (IPAs), in which groups of physicians treat patients in their own offices, and Preferred Provider Organizations (PPOs), which contract with companies to provide health care to employees.

Group providers seek to offer internally as much needed medical care as possible. Highly specialized care that the group cannot offer is supplied by outside specialists, who are reimbursed by the group. If the cost to the group at the end of the contract period is less than that guaranteed in the contract, the group will turn a profit. If the cost is more, it will incur a loss. In managed care under private control, physicians must make critical medical and ethical judgments about providing patients with access to diagnostic and therapeutic medical services. In contrast, in a fee-for-service relationship, the physician is paid to provide the patient with services that also necessitate making professional judgments about what medical tests and procedures are medically mandated, for it passes over into the area of "defensive" medicine.

All of these developments clearly indicate that increasing numbers of physicians will elect to become salaried employees rather than traditional fee-for-service doctors. The prediction has been made that more than 75% of newly graduated physicians will work this way by the end of the century.

SPECIALISTS VERSUS PRIMARY CARE PHYSICIANS

In the course of the past several decades, the number of specialists has increased dramatically. At the same time, the number of primary care physicians (general practitioners or family physicians) has declined substantially.

As noted above, primary care is becoming especially important as the health care system is being revamped. Because of the over-abundance of specialists, it is believed that health care is excessively expensive and less focused on prevention. The goal, therefore, is to establish a suitable balance between specialists and primary care physicians. To shift the trend away from specialization, there is a move on to restrict funding for subspecialization and to create incentives for those entering primary care.

Among the attractive features of primary care is the opportunity for treating patients of all ages. Another appealing element for a primary care physician is the wide variety of cases one is able to treat. A third feature is that of providing continuing care and the development of a special bond between the patient and the physician.

A survey of nearly 300 fourth year medical students was conducted to determine what factors played a role in choosing primary care careers. It was found that this group was more likely to be motivated by: (1) the opportunity to provide direct patient care in an ambulatory setting; (2) the fact that there is continuity of care; and (3) the possibility of being involved in the psychological aspects of medical care. Those electing high-tech specialties were more likely to be motivated by a desire for a large income, greater prestige, regular hours, and more leisure and family time. Furthermore, this study indicated that the significant factors involved in the choice did not include any of the following: student age; race; sex; marital status and level of indebtedness; concern about the increasing regulation of medical practice, malpractice, and health manpower reports; or the increasing number of elderly and chronically ill patients.

A developing challenge to primary care, whose impact can't as yet be measured, comes from proponents seeking to offer such care by nonphysician providers. Thus, primary care is currently available at offices where nurse practitioners, physician assistants, or other similar personnel work under the supervision of a physician. Their message to the public and the government is that there are less expensive alternatives available as sources of primary medical service. It remains to be seen how serious a threat this option will prove to be to primary care physicians.

MEDICAL LITIGATION CRISIS

The technological revolution in medicine, which has dramatically increased life expectancy, has raised patient expectations, in some cases unrealistically, resulting in an explosion of malpractice litigation. This in turn has caused insurance premiums to rise to such an extent as to motivate some doctors to curtail or even completely give up their practices. Others have taken up "defensive" medicine, which can result in overtesting and consequently contributes to the alarming increase in health care costs.

An unfortunate side effect of "litigation fever" has been a decrease in the production of vaccines because of a fear of lawsuits arising from adverse reactions. Pharmaceutical companies apparently prefer to give up this aspect of their business rather than risk the cost of litigation.

CYBERMEDICINE

The Internet is a conglomerate of computer networks that encircles the world. As of a few years ago there were upwards of 30,000 networks with about 5 million computers serving approximately 20 million users. The Internet or "information superhighway" is a spin-off from a project that was initiated in 1969 linking the computers of the government's military research centers to protect data in the event of a nuclear attack.

The public can access the Internet directly through universities, scientific organizations, and public libraries. The Internet is popular and busy because, for the most part, it is basically free. Your university or medical school is most likely to have an account and be on line.

Using your own home computer you need a modem to access the Internet over your phone line and a communications program to communicate with the computer at the other end of the line. Using a university account has a major disadvantage for it requires technical skill to work through a maze without the help of a customer service department. Time has to be invested to learn how to proceed and find what you are looking for; nevertheless, there is a substantial savings using a university account rather than a commercial one.

On the other hand, if you feel overwhelmed by such chores you have the option of gaining Internet access through a commercial company (such as America Online, Compuserve, Prodigy, etc.). You may also use an ISP (Internet Service Provider), which is a company that provides direct access to the Internet for a low monthly fee. It is important to learn which features you will have access to and how much it will cost. This should be weighed against your specific needs and budget limitations. Once you have adjusted to the Internet and find it essential, you may decide to move over to a university account and drastically lower your costs.

While the Internet is expanding, its basic types of services are:

1. **E-Mail.** With this system, you prepare a communication using a text editor, and then send it to an e-mail address, which is in the form of a code, containing the symbol @. To the left of the symbol is the recipient's name or assigned code number, and on the right are letters and numbers separated by dots. These serve

to identify the recipient's department and institution ("domains"). The last three letters indicate the type of institution (such as educational, edu.; commercial, com.; governmental, gov., etc.) (A two-letter overseas code may be used instead of the three-letter institutional code when appropriate.)

Dialing your Internet account via a local phone number permits you to send your message locally, cross-country, or overseas, at no extra cost. It should be noted that with e-mail you lose the privacy provided by the postal service, but you gain in speed and delivery reliability.

2. **Internet "chat."** This is similar to e-mail, but involves "talking" to the recipient by typing messages back and forth. It provides instant access and prompt response but requires some degree of rapid typing skill. Internet books provide pointers on "computer-etiquette."

3. **Projecting.** There are networks that enable you to link up with "news-groups" and provide access to mailing lists of computerized meetings.

After mastering e-mail and news-groups technique, the basis has been set to move out and access computers located in distant places with the assistance of available commercial services, such as Gopher, Tel-net, ftp (file transfer protocol), etc.

For the medical student, the Internet provides a means for a break from the isolation of study and tension of exams and rounds. It allows one to communicate with old or new friends by e-mail or "chatting."

The Internet provides students with the ability to access numerous medical information sites and, as computer skills improve, more medical students and physicians will take advantage of it and benefit from it.

PART TWO

DENTISTRY

DENTISTRY

16 Dentistry as a Career

Why study dentistry?
The need for dentists
Today's trends in dentistry
Dental specialties
Is dentistry for you?
Dentistry as an alternative to medicine

Dentistry is a profession dealing with the prevention, diagnosis, and treatment of oral diseases and disorders, with primary emphasis on the health of teeth and gums. In a sense, dentistry is a medical subspecialty. Good oral health is critical to human psychological and physical well-being since the state of the teeth affect speech and expression, and, also, systemic diseases frequently manifest themselves in the oral cavity.

There are more than 140,000 active dentists in the United States; most of them are in private practice with the remainder working as salaried professionals. Of those in private practice, 80% are general practitioners who are contributing to the improvement of their communities' health standards and are rewarded by having favorable working conditions and ample financial remuneration.

Many thousands of dentists hold positions as commissioned officers in the armed forces. Others are employed by the Veterans Administration and in public health dentistry at the state or local level. There are also several thousand full- or part-time teachers, administrators, and investigators in dental schools and in dental research laboratories.

WHY STUDY DENTISTRY?

Dentistry provides young men and women of talent and dedication with an opportunity for a lifetime of professional satisfaction. The following are some of the attractive attributes of the dental profession:

1. It provides a strong sense of inner satisfaction derived from the knowledge that one is contributing to the physical well-being of one's patients.

2. It provides a personal feeling of achievement that comes from the successful application of one's judgmental and manual skills in resolving problems.

3. It provides an opportunity for group leadership as the head of a dental care team, making use of one's managerial and organizational skills.

4. It provides a basis for economic security and long-term financial stability.

5. It provides an opportunity to gain status in the community and thereby serve one's neighbors outside of one's professional capacity.

THE NEED FOR DENTISTS

The demands for dental care by the public have increased annually. The three factors responsible for this situation are greater affluence, better education, and increased population growth. (Nevertheless, only about 50% of the general population sees a dentist with any regularity.) The response to the demand for increased dental care has been an increase in the number of patients handled by dentists. Nevertheless, it should be realized that the demand for dental services tends to fluctuate with changes in economic conditions. In any case, the national need for dental care will not only be maintained, but will probably be increased, thus suggesting a bright future for most prospective members of the dental profession.

A note of caution is necessary, for in a recent report on employment prospects for dentists, the U.S. Department of Labor has said: "employment prospects to grow about as fast as average. . . . Increasingly abundant supply of practitioners will make it more difficult to start a practice. Competition for patients is likely to be intense in some localities, which could adversely affect earnings."

TODAY'S TRENDS IN DENTISTRY

Over the past several decades a gradual reevaluation of both the philosophy and the practice of dentistry has taken place. Whereas around World War II it was estimated that half of all Americans over 65 had lost all their teeth, by the end of this century, this figure for the same age group will have been reduced dramatically. The reason for this is that there has been a profound improvement in the oral health of recent generations of Americans caused by water fluoridation and the associated change in the role of dentistry, from one of treatment to one of prevention of tooth decay and gum diseases.

In terms of dental practice, an arsenal of new tools, techniques, drugs, and restorative materials has been developed over the past 30 years. These have dramatically expanded and improved the dentist's capacity for providing care in all areas. Among these developments are: (1) the high-speed air drill that minimizes the pain, time, and noise associated with drilling; (2) a variety of materials, both metal and plastic, that can now make up crowns and bridges; (3) plastic sealants that can be applied as a coating film over children's teeth to prevent decay-causing bacteria from attacking them for up to two years; (4) an alternative to bridges and dentures whereby one or more teeth can be set over metal implants inserted into the jaw bone; (5) a new technique called bonding in which a composite material that is undetectable can be glued onto the tooth, enabling chipped teeth to be repaired, spaces between teeth to be filled, and worn-down teeth to be restored, all with aesthetically appealing results.

Advances have also been made in diagnostic techniques, and research is continuing with the focus on preventive dentistry. The prospects for better oral health, therefore, are much higher, provided that increasing numbers of people practice good oral hygiene and avail themselves regularly of competent dental care.

Another major change that may be in the offing is the way dental services will be delivered. The traditional approach since the development of modern dentistry has been to have services provided by the individual practitioner. During the last decade groups of specialists in a particular specialty area have joined together to utilize a common facility on a rotation basis, thereby cutting down significantly on operating expenses. Thus group practices devoted exclusively to endodontics, for example, have developed.

Since about 1977, multipractitioner dental clinics, that is, clinics that offer primarily general but also specialty services, have sprung up in department stores and shopping centers. It is estimated that currently there are at least 500 such facilities in the United States. Their expansion from only a handful in 1978 has primarily been stimulated by legal decisions allowing dentists to advertise. Other contributing factors are the high cost of quality dental care at private offices and the unequal distribution of dentists in some areas.

In 1979, about 125 million Americans spent more than $13 billion for dental treatment, 90% of which was provided by individual practitioners. Some estimates predict that by the year 2000 only 10% of dental care will be provided by small-office dentists. While this may well be an exaggeration, it is certain that the trend is away from private care and toward multipractitioner clinics. This will have enormous implications both for patients and for dentists already in practice and those planning careers in dentistry. The new approach to dental care delivery holds the promise of offering less expensive and more convenient quality care. Whether it will do so in reality remains to be seen.

DENTAL SPECIALTIES

With advances in a variety of dental techniques and with the current focus on preventive and restorative dentistry, the need for special expertise in the various branches of dentistry has significantly increased. While general practitioners have training in and frequently do work in specialty areas, there are currently about 16,500 dentists whose practice is limited exclusively to one specialty. These dentists have had from one to four years of additional training (depending on the specialty), during which time their diagnostic and operative skills were further developed to achieve a superior degree of competence.

The following eight areas of specialization are recognized by the American Dental Association. (They are listed in order of the number of practitioners in each specialty.)

Orthodontics

This specialty has about 6,500 practitioners. It is concerned with correcting irregular and abnormal dental development. Orthodontic procedures are applicable to patients in any age group, but treatment is more easily and effectively achieved on youngsters. The goal is not only to improve appearance, but to correct the functioning of the teeth by altering the bite. Correcting a bad bite, or malocclusion, will aid in eating and speaking, and will prevent eventual loosening or even loss of teeth, in addition to having a positive cosmetic effect. A bad bite is generally the result of an incorrect relationship that developed during childhood between jaw shape and teeth size. It may also result from habits such as thumb-sucking, nail-biting, or night grinding. Since teeth are moved to improper positions by forces that are out of balance in the mouth, they can be moved back by opposing forces. This is done by the use of various fixed orthodontic appliances such as metal braces, rubber bands, or plastic brackets. Removable appliances may also be used on occasion.

Oral Surgery

There are more than 3,600 practitioners in this specialty. They use surgical procedures to deal with defects and diseases of the entire maxillofacial region—the middle and lower face. Their work encompasses the jaws, cheekbones, and other skeletal elements and their surrounding structures. In addition, the oral surgeon diagnoses and treats injuries, deformities, and growths in and around the jaw. When a tooth (or teeth) must be extracted, the procedure is usually carried out in an oral surgeon's office. Another common surgical procedure is apicoectomy, or surgical removal of a tooth's root tip. Reemplanting teeth knocked out in an accident and treating simple or compound jaw fractures are types of traumatic-injury treatments requiring an oral surgeon's skills.

Periodontics

This specialty has about 2,000 practitioners. It is concerned with the diagnosis and treatment of diseases affecting the periodontal tissues that support the teeth, namely the gum, periodontal membrane, and surrounding bone. These diseases are very insidious and become increasingly prevalent with age. The earlier treatment is instituted, the more likely it is that teeth loss can be prevented. Periodontal diseases are diagnosed by several procedures; probing the depth of the space around a tooth, comparing bone level as reflected in X-rays taken at two different dates, and examining for tooth mobility. Slight or somewhat moderate disease can be readily treated by scaling—the removal of plaque or tartar, or root planing—a fine smoothing of the surface of the root. More advanced cases require curettage—scraping of the tissues lining the infected tooth pocket. In severe cases, surgical intervention to expose teeth, or even bone grafting, may be necessary. Various splinting techniques that join loose teeth to firm ones are also utilized.

Pedodontics

The specialty also has about 2,000 practitioners. It is concerned with the treatment of children, adolescents, and young adults exclusively. Pedodontists are in a sense equivalent to pediatricians. In their special facilities and in the approach they use, they strive to establish in the child a positive attitude towards dentistry and a disposition to develop good oral hygiene habits. It is essential to maintain the health of the primary ("baby") teeth for, if decay sets in or premature loss occurs, the health and shape of the permanent teeth could be adversely affected. Also, the overall health of a child will be influenced by the condition of the primary teeth. Undetected decaying teeth can cause poor eating and chewing habits and thereby influence the overall state of a child's health.

Endodontics

There are about 1,000 specialists in the field. It deals with the diagnosis and treatment of diseases of the pulp (nerve) of the tooth. With the current emphasis on saving teeth and utilizing extraction only as a last resort, root canal therapy is a vitally important dental specialty. A tooth needs endodontic treatment if the nerve has been damaged by decay, infection, irritation, or trauma. In such cases, the endodontist cleans out the nerve canal(s), removing the degenerated pulp. When the tooth is asymptomatic and has stabilized, the canal(s) can be filled. The complexity of the treatment is determined by how many canals the tooth may have. Also, a live (vital) tooth is more readily treated than a dead (non-vital) tooth, especially if the latter has abscessed.

Prosthodontics

There are about 750 dentists in this field. Only several decades ago it was a common assumption that as one grew older, teeth would have to be lost, and a partial or even full set of dentures was thought to be unavoidable. While the current philosophy is that with good oral hygiene and prompt and competent treatment extraction can be minimized, there are nevertheless patients who will lose teeth and require a replacement for them. Replacement of even a single (non-wisdom) tooth is desirable, since if it is not replaced the teeth on either side of the gap may move. To replace missing or extracted teeth, a fixed or removable bridge can be attached to one or both adjacent teeth, or, in some situations, removable partial or full dentures may be required.

Oral Pathology

There are currently about 100 specialists in oral pathology. They are concerned with diseases of the mouth, studying their causes, processes, and effects. Essentially a diagnostician, an oral pathologist usually serves as a consultant to other specialists, as well as a teacher of dental students.

Dental Public Health

This field also has about 100 specialists. They are involved in promoting the oral health of communities by stimulating development of programs that aid in the prevention and control of dental diseases. Such specialists also gather and analyze data that are useful in determining the effectiveness of the oral health methods being used in a community.

IS DENTISTRY FOR YOU? _____

In evaluating whether dentistry is a suitable career for you, consider the following:

1. Do you possess the attributes that are prerequisites for dentistry?
2. Do you have adequate native manual dexterity?
3. Does your family support you in choosing dentistry as a career?
4. Do your teachers and faculty advisor feel that dentistry is a desirable career for you?
5. After speaking with and observing one or more dentists at work, do you find their profession attractive?

6. After visiting a dental school and/or clinic and speaking with administrators, faculty, and students, are you still strongly in favor of pursuing a dental career?

DENTISTRY AS AN ALTERNATIVE TO MEDICINE

Dentistry offers an attractive alternative career for *borderline* premedical and preosteopathic juniors. In such circumstances you should carefully evaluate whether dentistry is of sufficient interest to you as an alternative career. If this is the case, you should consider applying for admission to both medical and dental schools simultaneously at the end of your junior year in college (although obviously not to both types of schools at the same university). This can be done because admission requirements are almost identical and the medical and dental aptitude tests are very similar. Students who apply to medical and dental schools should inform their preprofessional advisory office of this fact so that appropriate evaluations can be prepared.

Trying to gain admission to dental school with the intent of using this as an avenue or lever to get into medical school, however, is self-defeating. Medical schools will not be favorably impressed by an applicant who is taking a valuable dental class place and is obviously using it primarily to aid his or her transfer from one professional school to another. When such a student lacks a genuine interest in dentistry, he or she may also end up wasting time and money in dental school.

If you fail to gain admission to medical school and did not apply to dental school in your junior year, you can consider doing so in the senior year or even later. Dental school admission committees are well aware that premedical or former premedical students will also apply for admission to dental school. While they naturally prefer "straight" predental majors, they know that many able and successful practicing dentists were former premedical students.

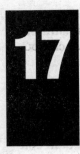

17 Preparing for and Applying to Dental School

Educational preparation
Application procedures
Admissions criteria

EDUCATIONAL PREPARATION

The discussion in Chapter 2 concerning high school and college education is generally applicable to predental students and should be reviewed.

High School

While in high school, you should acquire a broad liberal arts education and at the same time demonstrate that you have a genuine interest and good ability in the sciences, especially biology. Taking an advanced course in biology (if available) and/or undertaking a special science project may be particularly useful. In addition, completing a course in art, sculpture, mechanical drawing, or machine shop work will help determine and improve your manual dexterity. Active participation in a variety of extracurricular activities, such as a dramatic society or sports team, will assist you in judging your interest in and ability to work with people.

Undergraduate Studies

The criteria for selecting a college noted on page 11 are fully applicable to predental students.

The overwhelming majority of students entering dental school have completed four years of college. Thus you should plan your program on this basis (unless you have valid reasons for applying earlier). There is no specific required major for predental students, although most quite naturally select biology or chemistry. It is essential that your college studies:

1. include the minimum science course requirements, namely, inorganic chemistry—1 year, biology—1 year, physics—1 year, and organic chemistry—1 year;

2. demonstrate that you have solid abilities in the sciences by satisfactorily completing the aforementioned required courses and any science electives you take;

3. provide you with a well-rounded background in the social sciences and humanities by completing courses in English composition, history, and psychology;

4. reinforce your manual dexterity by taking courses that require use of your hands (such as art, sculpture, drafting). If this is not possible, then an extracurricular program involving such activities as model building, chalk carving, or playing a musical instrument can substitute for formal experience.

APPLICATION PROCEDURES

General Considerations

The initial step in the application process is to select the schools to which you will seek admission. The selection process should take into consideration the following:

1. *School requirements.* Dental schools have varying requirements for organic chemistry, elective science courses, and even some nonscience courses. School catalogs should be consulted to ensure that you will be able to meet all the requirements prior to enrolling.

2. *Financial status.* The cost of dental education is high. The best means of keeping costs down is to attend a state school in the state where you are a legal resident. Also, transportation costs will be less if you go to school as close to your permanent home as possible.

3. *School curriculum.* There are different perspectives in dental education as reflected in the various types of curricula currently in use. These are defined in Chapter 22, and the individual school curriculum is identified as part of the profiles given for each dental school in that chapter.

4. *Alumni admission ratio.* Admissions Committees give careful consideration to the undergraduate school the applicant attends, and this can influence the chance of acceptance. By applying to schools that have consistently accepted a significant number of students from your college, you will automatically improve your chances.

5. *Admissions criteria.* The four factors determining admission are academic performance (both overall and in science), recommendations, DAT scores, and interview performance. Schools place varying degrees of emphasis on these factors, as shown in Tables 17.1 and 17.2. By applying to schools where your weaknesses may be less significant, you can possibly improve your chances for admission. As to the total number of schools to which one should apply, this depends on your basic admission potential (academic average and DAT scores) and the amount of money you are prepared to spend as part of the admissions process. It should be realized that being called for out-of-town interviews can substantially increase the costs of applying. Generally, the number of applications can vary from 5 to 15 for A to C students, respectively.

How to Apply

There are two methods of applying: either directly to the school or through an application service. In the former case, the application must be secured from the dental school and the applicant will have to have all transcripts and recommendations sent to each dental school he or she is applying to. When applying to one of the 50 (out of 54) schools participating in the American Association of Dental Schools Application Service (AADSAS), the Application Booklet of the AADSAS must be used. This can be secured from your predental advisor or from AADSAS, 1625 Massachusetts Avenue, NW, Washington, DC 20036.

As part of the AADSAS application, an essay dealing with your career motivation is expected. A sample essay is reproduced on the following page, to give you an idea of what may be submitted.

In addition to the completed Application Booklet, AADSAS receives copies of all transcripts and the processing fee ($95.00 for the first school and $15.00 for each additional school). AADSAS processes the information provided, computes GPAs, and sends a screening copy to the applicant for approval or correction. AADSAS then sends each of the dental schools selected a copy of the approved screening copy and copies of transcripts. Also, the applicant is sent a confirmation copy. Thus only one set of transcripts is needed when applying through AADSAS, but letters of recommendation and photographs must be sent directly to each of the schools. The school usually will have its own application fee that may be required either at the time you apply through AADSAS or at a later date.

Sample Essay for AADSAS Application

My interest in dentistry is the result of the inspiration of two people: my maternal grandfather and my family dentist. My late grandfather lived in our home and thus was personally aware of my ability, already as a child, to assemble kits and, more generally, to fix things around the house. He graduated from the New York School of Mechanical Dentistry in 1941, and understandably channeled my interest toward the dental profession.

When I entered college, I enrolled as a pre-dentistry major. Nevertheless, I wanted to be certain that dentistry was the profession to which I wanted to devote my life. My family dentist allowed me to watch him at work. He patiently explained to me the basic problem of each patient and how he went about treating it. Each patient required a different type of therapy and the variety of cases thoroughly fascinated me.

My reason for preferring dentistry above any other health profession is that the former allows me more eye contact and friendliness between doctor and patient. A good dentist must be concerned with more than just the patient's oral health; he must consider the patient's physical appearance, comfort, and ability to properly maneuver his teeth. The teenager's teeth must be straightened for esthetic reasons. The older patient must be fitted with dentures that will serve him well in both speech and mastication. And the young child whose permanent teeth are now appearing must be observed, to prevent the development of speech impediments, as a result of abnormal tooth growth.

The first year of college represented, for me, an induction period in my academic growth. Since I entered college on early admission at the age of 16, I have gotten progressively better adjusted to the work load. This change is reflected in my gradually improving index. The transition from only three years of high school (which I finished with a 94 average) to the more intense pressure and heavier workload, on the college level, explains my unimpressive performance in my freshman year. This is despite the fact that I was as conscientious then as I am now and as I have always been.

Besides understating my scholastic potential, my college transcript cannot reflect my interest in a highly specialized area of chemistry. During the Spring Semester of 1990, I presented a seminar on catenanes and knots (i.e., cyclic molecules that are mechanically linked or interlocked), which have been shown to be the basis of certain viral infections and cancers. I am currently investigating the possible role of catenanes in oral pathology.

As a result of my consistently improving academic performance, I was named to the Dean's list with high honor at my college. In an effort to gain experience toward my intended profession, I worked at a local dental hospital in New York, during the 1991–92 academic year. The preceding year, I worked as a volunteer dental assistant at a dental clinic affiliated with a New York dental school. I am currently volunteering at another local dental clinic, while completing my undergraduate studies. My extensive dental exposure and academic work has provided me with both the motivation and background to successfully complete a program of dental studies and develop into a competent and empathic practitioner.

ADMISSIONS CRITERIA

Aside from the applicant's personal qualifications as reflected in the grade point average, DAT scores, recommendations, and interview rating, the most important factor in determining admission to dental school is the number of people making up the pool of applicants from which the entering class is selected. Therefore this consideration will be discussed first and then the personal attributes next.

Applicant Pool

In 1992 there were 6,108 applicants for admission to dental schools in the United States. Of these, approximately 4,072 were admitted to the freshman class, giving about a 1.3:1 applicant/acceptance ratio. Each of the applicants filed an average of 6 applications to secure a place.

The number of dental school applicants has tended to follow a pattern of cycles. During the post-World War II period (1945–57) there was an abundance of applicants.

From 1958 to 1963 there was a sharp decline. Subsequently, from 1964 to 1974 a steady increase in the applicant pool was recorded. Since 1974, there has been a dramatic decrease (about 50%) in the number of male applicants. This has been reflected in the change in the applicant/acceptance ratios from 3.0:1 to 1.2:1 over the past five years. It seems likely that at least for the immediate future the favorable acceptance ratio (from the applicant's point of view) will be maintained since the number of first-year places is projected to remain basically unchanged.

Grade Point Average (GPA)

The applicant's overall and science grade point averages (especially at a school where grade inflation is not a factor) along with the DAT scores (see below) will provide admissions committees with the screening factors necessary to determine if an interview should be granted. Obviously the college's reputation is an important consideration in assessing the credibility of the applicant's GPA. For the 1994–95 class, the mean GPA was 3.19 (and the mean science GPA was 3.09).

DAT Scores

As indicated in Table 17.1, most dental schools place considerable emphasis on the DAT scores. However, the importance of the individual subtest scores varies considerably, as shown in Table 17.2.

The DAT is designed to predict capabilities in two areas, academic and manual. Thus in addition to the nine subtest scores, average scores are reported in both of these categories. The academic average represents the average of all but the two perception ability test (PAT) scores, while the manual ability is summarized by the average of the two- and three-dimensional PAT scores. Table 17.2 suggests that more importance is given to the academic average than to the PAT average.

Recommendations

These are usually provided by a committee and/or the predental advisor. The recommendations may be submitted in the form of a letter incorporating faculty comments and/or an evaluation form. This material serves to provide a personalized evaluation that makes your transcript more meaningful. Recommendations can serve to enhance your chances for admission by bringing to the admissions committee's attention information about your personality, motivation, and innate abilities, as well as clarifying any uncertain aspects relative to your credentials.

Letters of recommendation from former employers (especially dentists, research laboratories, and/or dental clinics) can provide useful information to the admissions committee. However, personal recommendations from your family dentist or religious leader are not especially meaningful.

Interview

Most dental schools require a personal interview as part of the admission procedure. Being granted one implies that the school is seriously considering your application. The interview provides an opportunity for you to "sell yourself" as well as to explain any discrepancies or weaknesses, and to elaborate on your strengths. The discussion of "The Interview" in Chapter 3 is, for the most part, relevant to predental students as well and should be reviewed.

Table 17.1. THE IMPORTANCE GIVEN TO VARIOUS SOURCES OF INFORMATION CONCERNING THE DENTAL SCHOOL APPLICANT
(10 = MOST, 1 = LEAST)

School	Science GPA	Non-Science GPA	General GPA	Interview	Recom-mendations†	Manual Dexterity Test
Univ of Alabama	8	8	8	8	5	3
Univ of the Pacific	10	8	8	10	10	na
Univ of California—San Francisco	9	8	10	9	8	6
Univ of California—Los Angeles	10	8	9	na	7	8
Univ of Southern California	10	8	9	10	10	na
Loma Linda Univ	10	na	8	5	2	na
Univ of Colorado	10	7	9	10	7	6
Univ of Connecticut	1	3	2	1	2	na
Howard Univ	9	7	9	na	8	na
Univ of Florida	10	7	8	10	8	na
Medical College of Georgia	na	na	na	na	na	na
Northwestern Univ	10	8	10	9	7	na
Southern Illinois Univ	10	8	8	10	10	na
Univ of Illinois	10	10	10	9	10	10
Indiana Univ	10	9	10	8	7	na
Univ of Iowa	10	8	10	8	8	na
Univ of Kentucky	8	8	6	8	6	4
Univ of Louisville	8	na	10	9	5	na
Louisiana State Univ	10	8	10	10	8	9
Univ of Maryland	10	na	10	8	7	na
Harvard Univ	10	na	10	10	7	na
Boston Univ	10	9	9	10	10	9
Tufts Univ	10	8	10	10	8	na
Univ of Detroit—Mercy	10	5	9	10	7	na
Univ of Michigan	8	na	10	4	3	na
Univ of Minnesota	10	7	10	na	9	na
Univ of Mississippi	10	7	9	8	6	na
Univ of Missouri—Kansas City	10	7	10	8	7	na
Creighton Univ	7	2	10	5	5	8
Univ of Nebraska	10	8	10	10	2	5
Univ of Dentistry, New Jersey	10	8	10	10	10	8
Columbia Univ	7	7	7	8	7	na
New York Univ	9	8	10	10	9	na
SUNY, Stony Brook	10	8	9	10	9	9
SUNY, Buffalo	9	6	9	9	7	na
Univ of North Carolina	9	7	7	9	7	na
Ohio State Univ	9	5	8	6	6	na
Case Western Univ	8	7	7	10	7	na
Univ of Oklahoma	9	9	10	10	6	na
Oregon Health Sciences Univ	10	9	9	8	6	na
Temple Univ	10	6	10	10	9	9
Univ of Pennsylvania	9	8	10	10	9	5
Univ of Pittsburgh	10	9	9	10	10	na
Medical Univ of South Carolina	10	6	9	8	6	9
Meharry Medical College	10	na	10	9	9	8
Univ of Tennessee	10	2	6	10	5	na
Baylor College of Dentistry	10	na	10	10	5	na
Univ of Texas—Houston	10	na	9	8	6	na
Univ of Texas—San Antonio	10	na	10	6	3	na
Virginia Commonwealth Univ	10	8	9	10	10	na
Univ of Washington—Seattle	10	na	6	8	7	8
West Virginia Univ	10	9	10	10	9	na
Marquette Univ	10	5	10	5	3	3
Univ of Puerto Rico	na	na	10	8	na	na

† Recommendations include letters of recommendation in general.

Table 17.1. THE IMPORTANCE GIVEN TO VARIOUS SOURCES OF INFORMATION CONCERNING THE DENTAL SCHOOL APPLICANT (Continued)
(10 = MOST, 1 = LEAST)

School	Science GPA	Non-Science GPA	General GPA	Interview	Recommendations	Manual Dexterity Test
Median	10	8	9	9	7	8
Nonzero entries used in calculation	52	42	53	50	52	18
McGill Univ	8	na	9	7	4	9
Univ of Saskatchewan	9	na	9	3	1	na
Univ of Alberta	10	na	10	3	na	na
Univ of British Columbia	na	na	10	8	2	9
Univ of Manitoba	7	2	7	7	na	10
Dalhousie Univ	2	2	2	2	0	na
Univ of Toronto	na	na	10	na	5	na
Univ of Western Ontario	1	na	na	na	na	na
Univ of Montreal	10	na	10	10	na	na
Univ of Laval	10	na	9	na	na	8
Median	9	2	9	7	2	9
Nonzero entries used in calculation	8	2	9	7	5	4

Source: American Dental Association, Survey Center, 1995–96 *Survey of Predoctoral Dental Educational Institutions.* Data reprinted with permission.

Table 17.2. THE IMPORTANCE GIVEN TO DENTAL ADMISSION TEST SCORES
(10 = MOST, 1 = LEAST)

School	Academic Average	PAT	Science	Quantitative Reasoning	Reading Comprehension	Biology	General Chemistry	Organic Chemistry
Univ of Alabama	8	8	8	5	5	8	8	8
Univ of the Pacific	10	10	10	8	10	10	10	10
Univ of California—San Francisco	10	6	9	7	8	7	6	5
Univ of California—Los Angeles	10	8	10	5	7	6	5	7
Univ of Southern California	10	10	9	9	9	9	na	4
Loma Linda Univ	1	9	7	na	6	3	5	7
Univ of Colorado	10	9	8	4	9	5	8	7
Univ of Connecticut	2	6	1	3	5	4	8	8
Howard Univ	10	10	10	5	9	7	5	6
Univ of Florida	10	10	7	1	9	7	5	na
Medical College of Georgia	na	na	na	na	na	na	na	na
Northwestern Univ	10	8	9	7	8	8	8	8
Southern Illinois Univ	10	10	8	8	8	8	8	10
Univ of Illinois	10	10	10	10	10	10	10	9
Indiana Univ	10	10	10	9	9	9	9	10
Univ of Iowa	10	7	10	8	8	10	10	8
Univ of Kentucky	8	8	8	8	8	8	8	8
Univ of Louisville	6	6	5	5	6	5	5	5
Louisiana State Univ	10	9	9	8	10	9	8	7
Univ of Maryland	10	6	10	6	6	8	7	9
Harvard Univ	10	4	10	4	9	9	9	9
Boston Univ	10	8	10	9	9	9	9	9

Table 17.2. THE IMPORTANCE GIVEN TO DENTAL ADMISSION TEST SCORES (Continued)
(10 = MOST, 1 = LEAST)

School	Academic Average	PAT	Science	Quanti-tative Reasoning†	Reading Compre-hension	Biology	General Chemistry	Organic Chemistry††
Tufts Univ	10	10	10	6	6	6	6	6
Univ of Detroit—Mercy	9	7	9	6	10	10	8	8
Univ of Michigan	9	5	2	na	7	6	na	1
Univ of Minnesota	10	7	10	9	9	9	9	9
Univ of Mississippi	7	6	5	5	5	5	5	5
Univ of Missouri— Kansas City	7	7	7	na	8	7	7	7
Creighton Univ	9	8	7	1	6	6	3	4
Univ of Nebraska	10	10	8	5	7	10	8	10
Univ of Dentistry, New Jersey	10	8	10	7	8	10	10	10
Columbia Univ	10	4	8	8	8	7	6	8
New York Univ	9	8	6	7	10	5	3	4
SUNY, Stony Brook	9	8	10	8	8	8	8	8
SUNY, Buffalo	9	9	6	5	7	5	5	5
Univ of North Carolina	8	7	9	7	6	9	9	9
Ohio State Univ	8	9	8	5	7	9	8	8
Case Western Univ	10	9	8	7	8	8	8	8
Univ of Oklahoma	8	8	7	7	8	6	6	6
Oregon Health Sciences Univ	9	5	8	5	8	7	7	7
Temple Univ	10	10	10	8	9	10	8	10
Univ of Pennsylvania	10	4	9	7	8	7	7	7
Univ of Pittsburgh	10	10	10	8	8	8	9	9
Medical Univ of South Carolina	10	9	8	6	6	6	6	7
Meharry Medical College	10	10	10	10	10	8	6	5
Univ of Tennessee	10	8	8	5	5	10	10	10
Baylor College of Dentistry	8	9	5	5	8	8	8	7
Univ of Texas—Houston	10	10	9	6	10	6	6	6
Univ of Texas—San Antonio	10	10	na	na	na	na	na	na
Virginia Commonwealth Univ	10	10	10	8	8	10	8	10
Univ of Washington—Seattle	8	8	8	8	6	6	6	6
West Virginia Univ	10	10	9	8	9	9	8	9
Marquette Univ	10	10	5	5	6	5	4	6
Univ of Puerto Rico	9	7	na	na	na	na	na	na
Median	10	8	9	7	8	8	8	8
Nonzero entries used in calculations	53	53	51	48	51	51	49	51
Univ of Saskatchewan	na	2	na	5	5	na	na	
Univ of Alberta	na	3	na	3	3	na	na	
Univ of British Columbia	10	9	na	9	na	na	na	
Univ of Manitoba	7	7	7	7	5	1	1	
Dalhousie Univ	na	2	2	2	2	na	na	
Univ of Toronto	10	na	na	na	na	na	na	
Univ of Western Ontario	na	5	na	5	5	5	5	
McGill University	10	7	7	9	5	7	7	
Univ of Montreal	na	10	na	10	na	na	na	
Univ of Laval	10	8	5	8	na	na	na	
Median	10	7	6	7	5	5	5	
Nonzero entries used in calculations	5	9	4	9	6	3	3	

†   For the Canadian DAT, this refers to the chalk carving scale.
††   The Canadian DAT does not include an organic chemistry subtest.

Source: American Dental Association, Survey Center, 1995–96 *Survey of Predoctoral Dental Educational Institutions.*
         Data reprinted with permission.

18 The Dental Admission Test (DAT)

Importance of the DAT
Contents of the DAT
Preparing for the DAT
Sample DAT questions
Scoring of the DAT
Canadian DAT

This test is conducted two times a year (October and April) and is sponsored by the Division of Educational Measurements, American Dental Association, 211 East Chicago Avenue, Chicago, IL 60611. Students planning to enter in the fall of the following year should take the examination in the preceding April or October. The choice between these two dates is dependent on your state of preparedness (since admission announcements are not made before December 1). If you plan to use the summer to study, the DAT should be taken in October; otherwise, it should be taken earlier and gotten out of the way (as well as ensure an opportunity to repeat it if necessary).

An application for the DAT can be obtained from the Division of Educational Measurements at the address above, or from the predental advisor. The application should include a recent photo and the $75 fee. This fee covers the cost of sending five official transcripts of scores to selected dental schools, as well as a copy for the applicant and the predental advisor, and DAT preparation materials. Additional official transcripts of scores can be sent if requested. The charge is $2 each if ordered at the time of applying and $5 each if requested later.

Testing centers for the Saturday administration are located in one or more cities in each state, as well as in the District of Columbia. Sunday (or Monday) administrations are provided in about 10 states and require a letter from a religious leader confirming the applicant's affiliation with a Sabbath-observing religious group. Foreign testing centers are set up as needed, but require special arrangements. The fee for a test administered in a foreign country is $25.

IMPORTANCE OF THE DAT

About six weeks after taking the DAT, each applicant will receive a personal copy of the scores (with an explanation of them) at the permanent address listed on the original application form. DAT scores are based on the number of correct answers recorded. The scores are reported to the dental schools requested by the applicant as standard scores rather than raw scores. The conversion of raw scores to standard scores is based on the distribution of applicant performances. Scores used in the testing program range from 1 to 30. There is no passing or failing score, but a standard score of 15 signifies average performance on a national basis.

By the use of standard rather than raw scores it is possible to compare the performance of one applicant with the performance of all applicants. Also, since the DAT is designed to predict performance in both academic and technical areas, two average scores are included in the test report—the academic average and the Perceptual Ability Test (PAT) average. The former is an average of quantitative reasoning, verbal reasoning, reading comprehension, biology, and inorganic and organic chemistry test scores; the latter is an average of the two- and three-dimensional Perceptual Ability Test scores.

Dental schools place varying degrees of emphasis on the two average scores and the individual subtest scores (see Tables 17.1 and 17.2). In any case the DAT scores are not taken out of context, but rather they represent one of the four major elements considered by admissions committees. The other elements are the grade point and science averages, letters of recommendation and evaluations, and the dental school interview. Good DAT scores will reinforce a strong applicant's chances for admission and help a weak candidate get in-depth consideration and possibly an interview. Poor DAT scores will raise doubts about a strong candidate's true abilities and serve to defeat a weak candidate's chances completely.

CONTENTS OF THE DAT

There are four examinations included in the Dental Admission Testing Program. The entire program requires one half day for administration. The examinations included are:

I.   Survey of Natural Sciences

BIOLOGY—Origin of Life. Cell Metabolism (including photosynthesis). Enzymology. Thermodynamics. Organelle Structure and Function. Biological Organization and Relationship of Major Taxa (monera, angiosperms, arthropods, chordates, etc.) using the five-kingdom system. Structure and function of the following vertebrate systems: integumentary, skeletal, muscular, circulatory, immunological, digestive, respiratory, urinary, nervous, endocrine, and reproductive. Fertilization, Descriptive Embryology, and Developmental Mechanics. Mendelian Inheritance, Chromosomal Genetics, Meiosis, Molecular and Human Genetics. Natural Selection, Population Genetics, Speciation, Population and Community Ecology, Animal Behavior (including social behavior).

GENERAL CHEMISTRY—Stoichiometry (percent of composition, empirical formulas from percent of composition, balancing equations, weight/weight, weight/volume, density problems). Gases (kinetic molecular theory of gases, Graham's, Dalton's, Boyle's, Charles', and ideal gas laws). Liquids and Solids. Solutions (colligative properties, concentration calculations). Acids and Bases. Chemical Equilibrium (molecular, acid/base, precipitation, equilibria calculations). Thermodynamics and Thermochemistry (laws of thermodynamics, Hess's law, spontaneity prediction). Chemical Kinetics (rate laws, activation energy, half life). Oxidation-Reduction Reactions (balancing equations, determination of oxidation numbers, electro-chemical concepts and calculations). Atomic and Molecular Structure (electron configuration, orbital types, Lewis-Dot diagrams, atomic theories, molecular geometry, bond types, quantum mechanics). Periodic Properties (include categories of nonmetals, transition metals, and non-transition metals). Nuclear Reactions.

ORGANIC CHEMISTRY—Bonding (atomic orbitals, molecular orbitals, hybridization, Lewis structures, bond angles, bond lengths). Mechanisms (energetics, structure & stability of intermediates: S_N1, S_N2, elimination, addition, free radical and substitution mechanisms. Chemical & Physical Properties of Molecules (stability, solubility, polarity, inter- and intra-molecular forces: separation techniques). Organic Analysis (introductory infrared and H NMR spectroscopy, simple chemical tests). Stereochemistry (conformational analysis, optical activity, chirality, chiral centers, places of symmetry, enantiomers, diastereomers, meso compounds). Nomenclature (IUPAC rules, identification of functional groups in molecules). Reaction of the Major Functional Groups (prediction of reaction products and important mechanistic generalties). Acid-Base Chemistry (resonance effects, inductive effects, prediction of products and equilibria). Aromatic (concept of aromaticity, electrophilic aromatic substitution). Synthesis (identification of the product of, or the reagents used in, a simple sequence of reactions).

II.   Reading Comprehension
Ability to read, organize, and remember new information in dental and basic sciences. Ability to comprehend thoroughly when studying scientific information. Reading materials are typical of materials encountered in the first year of dental school and require no prior knowledge of the topic other than a basic undergraduate preparation in science. The Reading Comprehension test will contain three reading passages.

III.   Quantitative Reasoning
Algebraic Equations, Fractions, Conversions (pounds and ounces; inches and feet), Percentage, Exponential Notation, Probability and Statistics, Geometry, Trigonometry, and Applied Mathematics Problems.

IV.   Perceptual Ability
Angle Discrimination, Form Development, Block Counting, Orthographic Projections, and Object Visualization.

(*Reprinted with permission of the American Dental Association.)

PREPARING FOR THE DAT

To do well on the DAT you should start preparing for the test two to three months prior to the test date. Preparation should be done on a regular basis, devoting a set number of hours each week exclusively to reviewing the necessary material. A study plan that takes into consideration your strong and weak areas of knowledge should be thoughtfully prepared prior to initiating your study program. Special emphasis should be placed on learning facts that are organized around principles and concepts, rather than on isolated details, since the former will be retained longer. Frequent review at regular intervals will be of special help in retaining details that are not of primary importance. Study and review sessions should be terminated as soon as signs of mental fatigue become evident.

Since the DAT is a multiple-choice test, some general considerations may prove helpful. Too much should not be read into a question; it is best to take the questions at face value. Avoid the impulse to change answers when some uncertainty develops. Look for the general principle involved in the question and try to recall specific details you have memorized.

When taking the DAT make certain that you:

1. have a good night's sleep before the day of the exam. Also, try to relax between the various parts of the exam;

2. avoid taking medications that will inhibit your performance (such as antihistamines or tranquilizers);

3. use regular reading glasses rather than contact lenses;

4. carefully read all directions before you start to answer the questions;

5. answer the questions in the exact manner and the exact place specified;

6. concentrate exclusively on the question under consideration;

7. determine how much time you have for each question (divide the number of questions in the subtest by the time allotted for that subtest);

8. respond first to all questions you are sure of the answers to;

9. next, answer those questions that require guessing (since the test score is based on the total number of questions answered correctly);

10. finally, answer questions that are time consuming. (Coding these and "guessing" questions for identification at the outset may save time later.)

The exam will usually begin at 8:00 A.M. and will last until 1:30 P.M. For individual tests the time limit is indicated on the cover of each of the four exam booklets.

The Survey of Natural Sciences and the Perceptual Ability tests are administered first. The Reading Comprehension and the Quantitative Reasoning tests are administered after a 15-minute break. A confidential biographical questionnaire accompanies the test and is used for studies on test validity and test usage.

The test scores for the DAT are reported to the dental schools upon the written request of the test candidates in terms of standard scores rather than raw scores. Through the use of standard scores it is possible to compare the performance of one applicant with the performance of all applicants on any or all of the topics included in the DAT.

SAMPLE DAT QUESTIONS

The following are examples of typical DAT questions covering all four categories on this examination:

PART 1 Survey of Natural Sciences

100 QUESTIONS; TIME LIMIT: 90 minutes

Biology (40 questions on test)

1. Exocytosis occurs when this organelle's membrane fuses with the plasma membrane.
    A. Secretory vesicle
    B. Nucleus
    C. Mitochondrion
    D. Ribosome
    E. Golgi body

2. NAD and FAD are important molecules in living systems because they
    A. cause the synthesis of ATP from ADP and phosphate.
    B. serve as oxidation-reduction coenzymes.
    C. can reduce the activation energy of a biological reaction.
    D. control the level of acetyl Co-A in the cell.
    E. are essential reactants in those reactions called dehydration reactions.

3. The addition of potassium iodide as a nutritional supplement to common table salt would most directly affect the function of which of these glands?
    A. Thyroid
    B. Sweat glands
    C. Adrenal cortex
    D. Kidneys
    E. Parathyroid

4. The outer layer of cells, the ectoderm, in a developing embryo gives rise to the
    A. muscle system.
    B. reproductive system.
    C. circulatory system.
    D. skeletal system.
    E. nervous system.

5. Removal of the gallbladder makes it more difficult to digest foods high in
    A. carbohydrates.
    B. nucleic acids.
    C. proteins.
    D. fats.
    E. vitamins.

Inorganic Chemistry (30 questions on test)

6. Supercooled water at –10°C can spontaneously warm to 0°C in a perfectly insulated container. This is possible because
   A. supercooled materials do not obey energy conservation laws.
   B. supercooled water needs less energy for change of temperature than ordinary water.
   C. a small amount of energy is given to the surroundings.
   D. some of the water freezes and this provides energy.
   E. ice is unusual in that it is less dense than liquid water.

7. How many grams of NaOH (40.0 g/mol) are required to make 250 ml of a 0.500 M solution?
   A. $(250)(0.500)$

   B. $\dfrac{(250)(500)}{1000}$

   C. $\dfrac{(250)(0.500)(40.0)}{1000}$

   D. $\dfrac{1000}{(250)(0.500)(40.0)}$

   E. $(250)(0.500)(40.0)$

8. What is the percentage of oxygen by weight in $Zn(H_2PO_4)_2$ (259g/mol)?
   A. 53.3%
   B. 24.7%
   C. 39.5%
   D. 6.18%
   E. 49.4%

9. At 0°C and 1.0 atmosphere pressure (STP) 22.0 grams of gas occupies 11.2 liters. The gas could be which of the following?
   A. $CO_2 = 44$g/mol
   B. $CO = 28$g/mol
   C. $NH_3 = 17$g/mol
   D. $CH_4 = 16$g/mol
   E. $C_4H_{10} = 58$g/mol

10. When the following equation is properly balanced, the coefficient of H_2O is
    $$Mg_3N_2 + H_2O \rightarrow Mg(OH)_2 + NH_3$$
    A. 9
    B. 6
    C. 4
    D. 3
    E. 2

Organic Chemistry (30 questions on test)

11. In the reaction, CH_3—⬡=CH_2 + HCl → the major product is
(with Cl on ring)

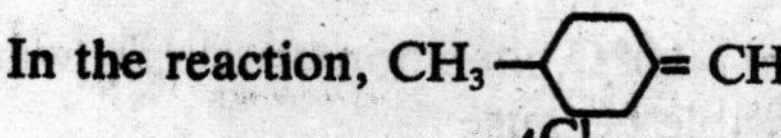

A. 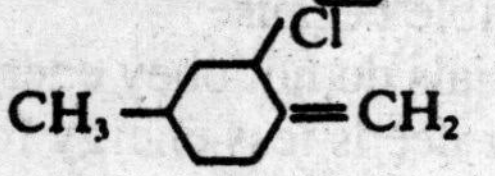 CH_3—⬡=CH_2

B. 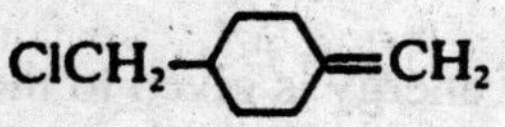 $ClCH_2$—⬡=CH_2

C. 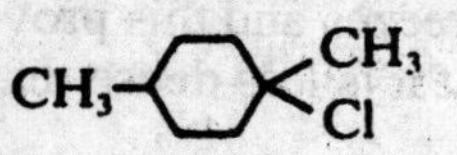 CH_3—⬡ with CH_3 and Cl

D. 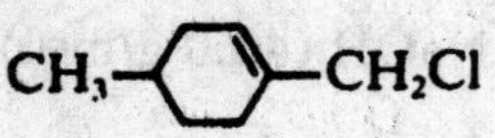 CH_3—⬡—CH_2Cl

E. 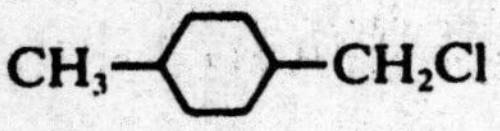 CH_3—⬡—CH_2Cl

12. Which reaction below is a possible termination step in the free radical chlorination of $CH_3CH_2CH_2CH_3$ by Cl_2?

A. $CH_3CH_2CH_2CH_3 + Cl \rightarrow CH_3CH_2\overset{\cdot}{C}HCH_3 + HCl$
B. $CL_2 \rightarrow Cl\cdot + Cl\cdot$
C. $CH_3CH_2CH_2CH_2\cdot + Cl\cdot \rightarrow CH_3CH_2CH_2CH_2Cl$
D. $CH_3CH_2CH_2CH_3 + Cl\cdot \rightarrow CH_3CH_2CH_2CH_2\cdot + HCl$
E. $CH_3CH_2\overset{\cdot}{C}HCH_3 + CL_2 \rightarrow CH_3CH_2CHCH_3 + Cl\cdot$

13. Which is the correct structure of *para*-aminobenzoic acid, PABA, a common ingredient in sunscreens?

A. 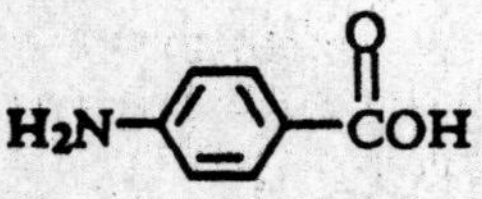 H_2N—⬡—COH (with =O on carbonyl)

B. 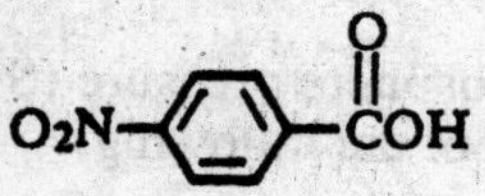 O_2N—⬡—COH (with =O on carbonyl)

C. 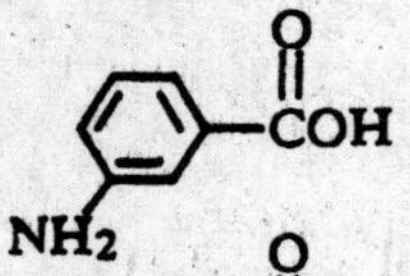 ⬡—COH (with =O), NH_2 meta

D. 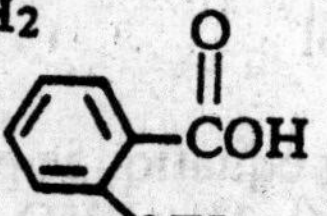 ⬡—COH (with =O), NH_2 ortho

E. 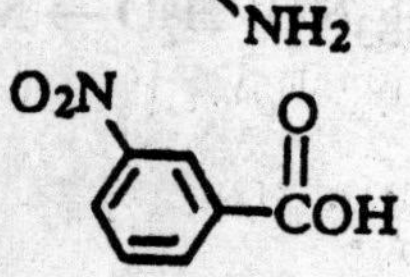 O_2N—⬡—COH (with =O)

14. What is the product of the following reaction?

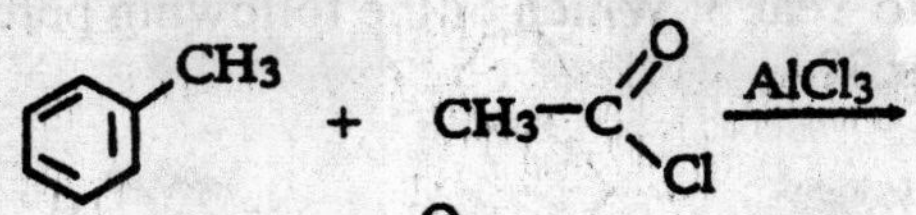

A.

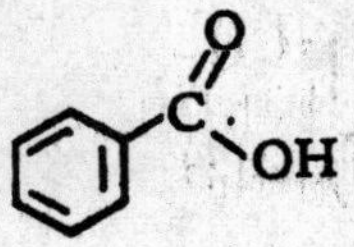

B.

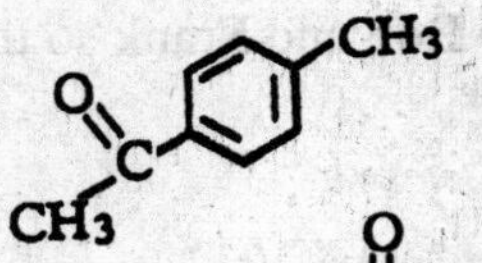

C.

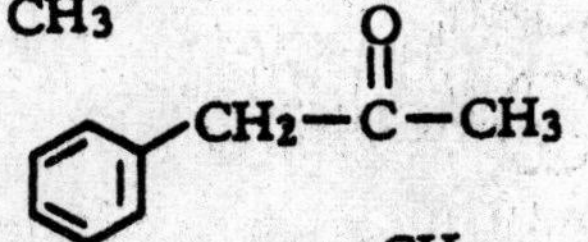

D.

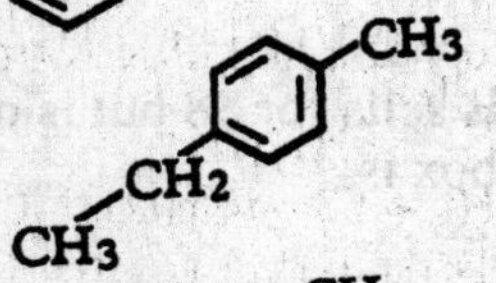

E.

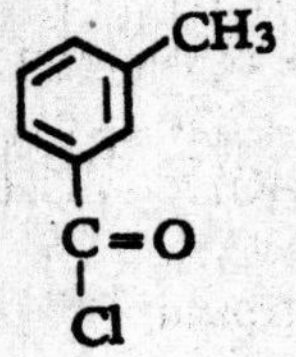

15. The IUPAC name for the compound shown below is:

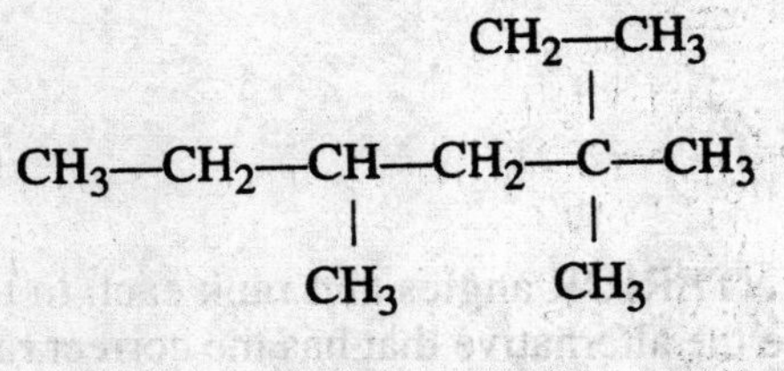

A. 3,5-Dimethyl-3-ethylhexane
B. 4,4-Dimethyl-2-ethylhexane
C. Trimethylheptane
D. 3,3,5-Trimethylheptane
E. 3,5-Trimethylheptane

PART 2 Quantitative Reasoning

16. $1/4 + 2/5 - 1/6 = ?$
    A. $-1/60$
    B. $2/15$
    C. $29/60$
    D. $8/15$
    E. $49/60$

17. A person's earnings increased by 10% from Year 1 to Year 2, and decreased 10% from Year 2 to Year 3. Which of the following percentages represents the change from Year 1 to Year 3?

    A. +20
    B. +1
    C. 0
    D. −1
    E. −11

18. $180 is to be shared by Bob and Frank so that Frank gets 25% more than Bob. How much does Bob get?

    A. $72
    B. $80
    C. $100
    D. $108
    E. $144

19. A box of clarinet reeds sells for $8 but is on sale at 25% off. If there is a sales tax of 6%, the total cost of one box is

    A. $5.52
    B. $5.65
    C. $6
    D. $6.36
    E. $6.48

20. $42\text{-}1/6 = 0.1x$ What is x?

    A. 7
    B. 25.2
    C. 70
    D. 252
    E. 2520

PART 3 Perceptual Ability

21. Examine the four INTERIOR angles and rank each in terms of degrees from SMALL TO LARGE. Choose the alternative that has the correct ranking.

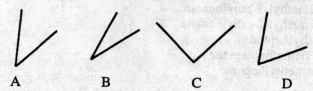

    A   B   C   D

ALTERNATIVES

    (A) A—B—C—D
    (B) B—A—D—C
    (C) A—C—B—D
    (D) C—D—A—B

22. The pictures that follow are top, front, and end views of various solid objects. The views are without perspective. That is, the points in the viewed surface are viewed along parallel lines of vision. The projection of the object looking DOWN on it is shown in the upper left-hand corner (TOP VIEW). The projection looking at the object from the FRONT is shown in the lower left-hand corner (FRONT VIEW). The projection looking at the object from the END is shown in the lower right-hand corner (END VIEW). These views are ALWAYS in the same positions and are labeled accordingly.

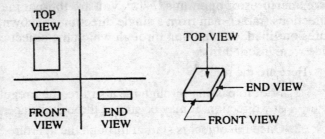

If there were a hole in the block, the views would look like this:

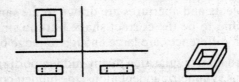

Note that lines that cannot be seen on the surface in some particular view are DOT-TED in that view.

In the problems that follow, two views will be shown, with four alternatives to complete the set. You are to select the correct one and mark its number on the answer sheet.

EXAMPLE: Choose the correct END VIEW.

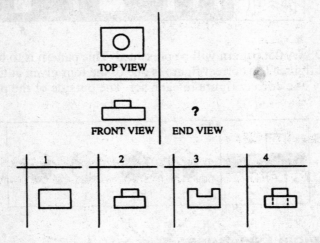

23–25. This group of cubes has been made by cementing together cubes of the same size. After being cemented together, each group was PAINTED ON ALL EXPOSED SIDES EXCEPT THE BOTTOM ON WHICH IT IS RESTING.

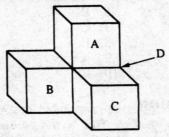

In the figure how many cubes have

23. two of their exposed sides painted?
24. four of their exposed sides painted?
25. five of their exposed sides painted?

26.   This visualization test consists of a number of items similar to the following sample. A three-dimensional object is shown at the left. This is followed by outlines of five apertures or openings. *First*, you are to imagine how the object looks from *all* directions (rather than from a single direction as shown). *Then*, pick from the five apertures outlined, the opening through which the object could pass directly if the proper side were inserted first.

Here are the rules:

1. Prior to passing through the aperture, the irregular solid object may be turned in any direction. It may be started through the aperture on a side not shown.

2. Once the object is started through the aperture, it may not be twisted or turned. It must pass completely through the opening. The opening is always the exact shape of the appropriate external outline of the object.

3. Both objects and apertures are drawn to the same scale. Thus it is possible for an opening to be the correct shape but too small for the object. In all cases, however, differences are large enough to judge by eye.

4. There are no irregularities in any hidden portion of the object. However, if the figure has symmetric indentations, the hidden portion is symmetric with the part shown.

5. For each object there is only one correct aperture.

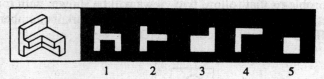

27.   A flat pattern will be presented. This pattern is to be folded into a three-dimensional figure. The correct figure is one of the four given at the right of the pattern. There is only one correct figure in each set. The outside of the pattern is what is seen at the left.

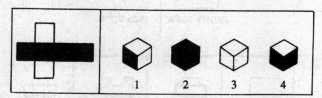

Answers to Sample Questions
Part 1   Survey of Natural Science

BIOLOGY	INORGANIC CHEMISTRY	ORGANIC CHEMISTRY
1. **A**	6. **D**	11. **C**
2. **B**	7. **C**	12. **C**
3. **A**	8. **E**	13. **A**
4. **E**	9. **A**	14. **B**
5. **D**	10. **B**	15. **D**

Part 2   Quantitative Reasoning

16. **C**
17. **D**
18. **B**
19. **D**
20. **E**

Part 3 Perceptual Ability

21. **B**
22. **B**
23. **A**
24. **B**
25. **A**
26. **C**
27. **D**

Explanation of Perceptual Ability Questions

21.   The correct ranking of the angles from small to large is B-A-D-C; therefore, alternative **B** is correct.

22.   The front view shows that there is a smaller block on the base and that there is no hole. The top view shows that the block is round and in the center of the base. The answer, therefore, must be **B**.

23–25. We are determining the number of exposed and painted sides for each of the four cubes. A cube by definition has six sides. Because the bottom of these four cubes are unpainted, there can be a maximum of five painted sides. In addition, where cubes are cemented together, the number of possible unpainted sides is diminished.

Cube A has five painted sides: its bottom is unpainted and is glued to the top of cube D, thus answering question 25.

Cubes B and C each have four painted sides, because their bottoms are unpainted and one of their sides is cemented to cube D. This answers question 24.

Cube D, which is hidden below cube A and behind cube C, has two painted sides. Its bottom (all the cubes) is unpainted, and two of its sides and its top are cemented to cubes A, B, and C, respectively. This answers question 23.

26.   The correct answer is **C** since the object would pass through this aperture if the side at the left were introduced first.

27.   One of the figures (A,B,C,D) can be formed from the flat pattern at the left. The only figure that corresponds to the pattern is D. If the shaded surfaces are looked at as the sides of the box, then all four sides must be shaded, while the top and bottom are white.

SCORING OF THE DAT

DAT test scores are determined on the basis of the number of correct answers on your scoring sheet. Thus, there is no penalty for guessing wrong, and you should record an answer to every question rather than leave any blank.

The comparison of raw scores to standard scores is based on distribution of the performances of all those who took the exam. A standard score of 15 is considered average, within the program range of 1 to 30. As with comparable aptitude tests, there is no passing or failing grade. Examinees will receive a copy of their test scores as well as a detailed explanation of their meaning.

CANADIAN DAT

A Canadian Dental Aptitude Test has been developed by the Canadian Dental Association and the Association of Canadian Faculties. For information on this test contact the Canadian Dental Association (l' Association Dental Canadienne), 1815 Alta Vista Drive, Ottawa, Ontario K1G 3Y6.

Opportunities in Dentistry for Women and Minorities

Doors are opening for women
Minorities in dentistry

DOORS ARE OPENING FOR WOMEN

In many respects the United States is clearly a world leader in matters of progress. Yet the number of women in professional life in this country is disproportionate to the population as a whole. Less than 10% of the dentists here are women. This figure stands in marked contrast to that of Russia or Finland, where about 80% of the dentists are women. It is also very different from other nations, such as Greece, France, Sweden, and Holland, where 25% to 50% of the dentists are women.

While the reasons for the sparsity of women dentists in this country are not positively known, one of the significant factors probably has been the belief that the profession is too physically demanding for women. While this widely held assumption is questionable to begin with, it has lost any possible validity in light of the drastic change in dentistry from a two-hand, stand-up profession to a four-hand, sit-down one.

Over the past decade, whatever barriers may have existed to prevent women from entering the field of dentistry have certainly fallen. This is evident from the dental school enrollment figures for women, which show a 400% increase since 1970. Women have responded to favorable opportunities in dentistry. Thus, even though the pool of

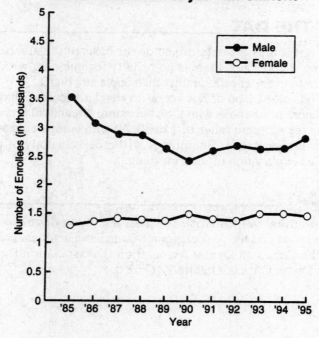

Comparison of Male and Female Dental School First-year Enrollment

male applicants has been decreasing, the pool of female applicants has held constant or increased somewhat over the past five years. Concomitantly, the same is true for the number of first-year males and females enrolled over this time period (see following graph). For 1995, the number of women enrolled was 1,483 out of 1,995, or 29%. This percentage is almost identical with that of women enrolled in the past five years. No evidence of sex bias is suggested from the application data of the past five years. Thus it is clear that motivated and qualified women can readily find a place in dental school. The profession is receptive to their admittance and it is likely that women will play a significant role in oral health care in the years to come.

MINORITIES IN DENTISTRY

While there has been a substantial decrease in the total applicant pool to dental school, the minority applicant pool, on the other hand, has increased. Thus, for 1995–96, a total of 5,423 out of 16,552 or about 32.8% of all students enrolled in dental schools in the United States were minority group members. The breakdown among minority groups for first-year enrollees is 24% Asian, 4.9% Hispanic, 5.9% African-American, and 0.6% Native American. Within these four groups, the enrollment of the first three has gone down a little over the past year and that of Asian students has increased slightly. This suggests that minority enrollment may be leveling off. The minority enrollment for freshmen for 1996–97 in each of the dental schools is given in Table 19.1.

Minority Recruitment in Dental Schools

To help improve the proportion of minority students represented in the dental schools, special recruitment and retention efforts are employed by many schools. The following are some of the approaches used by dental schools to enhance recruitment and retention of minority and disadvantaged students.

1. Recruitment extends into high schools and community centers, using seminars and workshops to inform prospective students of the opportunities that are available.

2. Contacts are developed and maintained with prospective applicants by means of college campus visits and communicating with predental advisors and other relevant faculty members.

3. In some cases application fees are waived.

4. Prematriculation orientation programs are frequently offered for from two to ten weeks during the summer. As part of such a program, learning skills, test-taking methods, and training to improve study habits and note-taking abilities may be offered.

5. Prematriculation summer programs in dental anatomy, histology, or biochemistry are offered by some schools to lighten the freshman-year load.

6. Students may be assigned special faculty and/or upper-class student advisors. Personal professional counseling may also be offered.

7. Students may be provided with tutorial assistance when necessary.

8. Students may be permitted to extend their educational program to five instead of four years, thereby lightening their load each semester by one or two courses.

9. Individual teaching utilizing audiovisual learning modules may be offered.

10. Special scholarship and loan funds may be provided.

Table 19.1. FIRST-YEAR DENTAL SCHOOL MINORITY ENROLLMENT

Dental School	African Amer. Men	African Amer. Women	Hispanic Men	Hispanic Women	Native Amer. Men	Native Amer. Women	Asian Men	Asian Women	Combined Men	Combined Women	Total
Univ of Alabama	0	2	0	1	0	0	3	4	3	7	10
Univ of the Pacific	1	0	0	1	0	0	21	28	22	29	51
Univ of California—San Francisco	2	1	7	4	0	0	15	29	24	34	58
Univ of California—Los Angeles	0	1	4	2	0	0	37	24	41	27	68
Univ of Southern California	3	2	3	1	0	0	57	20	63	23	86
Loma Linda Univ	0	2	3	2	1	2	27	14	31	20	51
Univ of Colorado	0	0	3	0	0	0	2	1	5	1	6
Univ of Connecticut	1	1	0	1	0	0	3	0	4	2	6
Howard Univ	24	30	2	0	0	0	2	5	28	35	63
Univ of Florida	4	2	8	5	0	0	4	5	16	12	28
Medical College of Georgia	2	3	0	0	0	0	1	3	3	6	9
Northwestern Univ	0	0	1	0	1	0	25	16	27	16	43
Southern Illinois Univ	2	1	1	0	1	0	1	3	5	4	9
Univ of Illinois	0	0	2	1	0	0	11	4	13	5	18
Indiana Univ	3	1	0	0	1	0	3	7	7	8	15
Univ of Iowa	2	2	4	1	2	0	1	2	9	5	14
Univ of Kentucky	2	1	0	0	0	0	2	1	4	2	6
Univ of Louisville	1	2	2	0	0	0	1	3	4	5	9
Louisiana State Univ	1	1	0	0	0	0	2	1	3	2	5
Univ of Maryland	4	6	2	1	1	0	13	11	20	18	38
Harvard Univ	1	0	1	0	0	0	5	10	7	10	17
Boston Univ	0	4	3	3	0	0	29	9	32	16	48
Tufts Univ	0	0	2	1	0	0	50	33	52	34	86
Univ of Detroit—Mercy	3	1	0	0	0	0	3	4	6	5	11
Univ of Michigan	2	10	3	3	0	0	11	14	16	27	43
Univ of Minnesota	0	0	0	0	0	0	6	0	6	0	6
Univ of Mississippi	0	2	0	0	0	0	0	0	0	2	2
Univ of Missouri—Kansas City	2	3	1	0	1	0	7	3	11	6	17
Creighton Univ	2	0	0	0	2	0	5	4	9	4	13
Univ of Nebraska	0	0	0	2	1	0	1	0	2	2	4
Univ of Medicine & Dentistry of New Jersey	4	8	0	5	1	0	8	5	13	18	31
Columbia Univ	0	2	0	1	0	0	29	23	29	26	55
New York Univ	3	0	4	2	0	1	54	38	61	41	102
SUNY, Stony Brook	0	0	0	0	0	0	2	6	2	6	8
SUNY, Buffalo	0	0	0	0	0	0	8	5	8	5	13
Univ of North Carolina	2	3	0	2	0	1	2	0	4	6	10
Ohio State Univ	0	0	0	0	0	0	15	4	15	4	19
Case Western Reserve Univ	0	0	0	0	0	0	10	8	10	8	18
Univ of Oklahoma	0	0	1	0	4	1	4	1	9	2	11
Oregon Health Sciences Univ	0	0	0	1	0	0	5	4	5	5	10
Temple Univ	4	4	8	1	1	0	16	12	29	17	46
Univ of Pennsylvania	1	1	3	1	0	0	13	8	17	10	27
Univ of Pittsburgh	4	2	2	2	0	0	5	7	11	11	22
Medical Univ of South Carolina	2	1	0	0	0	1	2	2	4	4	8
Meharry Medical College	18	30	0	1	1	0	3	0	22	31	53

Table 19.1. FIRST-YEAR DENTAL SCHOOL MINORITY ENROLLMENT (Continued)

Dental School	African Amer.		Hispanic		Native Amer.		Asian		Combined		Total
	Men	Women	Men	Women	Men	Women	Men	Women	Men	Women	
Univ of Tennessee	3	2	1	0	0	0	3	3	7	5	12
Baylor College of Dentistry	2	5	4	0	0	1	14	12	20	18	38
Univ of Texas— Houston	0	1	3	3	0	0	13	9	16	13	29
Univ of Texas— San Antonio	2	2	11	9	2	0	6	8	21	19	40
Virginia Commonwealth Univ	2	0	0	0	0	0	12	7	14	7	21
Univ of Washington— Seattle	0	0	3	0	1	0	6	11	10	11	21
West Virginia Univ	0	0	1	0	0	0	1	1	2	1	3
Marquette Univ	3	0	5	5	0	0	10	2	18	7	25
Univ of Puerto Rico	0	0	25	22	0	0	0	0	25	22	47
Median by Sex	2	2	3	2	1	1	6	6			
Total by Sex	112	140	122	84	19	7	589	424	842	655	1497
Total	252		206		26		1013				

Source: American Dental Association, Survey Center, 1995–96 *Survey of Predoctoral Dental Educational Institutions.*
Data reprinted with permission.

20 Financing Your Dental Education

The current financial aid crisis
Scholarships and loans

The total cost of a dental education depends on a number of factors, such as: (1) whether the dental school is a public or private institution; (2) whether the student is a state resident; (3) whether the student is single or married; (4) the location of the school; and (5) the student's lifestyle. Obviously, there can be wide differences in total costs. For most students, selecting a school involves not only its reputation, location, and educational program, but, first and foremost, its costs. A reliable estimate of costs for the freshman year can be readily ascertained by examining the last two columns of Table 22.1 in Chapter 22 and then multiplying by four to get an estimate of the total costs for all four years.

THE CURRENT FINANCIAL AID CRISIS

Most students applying to dental school can expect to incur high educational costs. Moreover, with the inflation rate slowly continuing to escalate, these costs can be expected to continue to rise. Unfortunately, while costs are rising dramatically, federal aid, which is the major source of scholarships and loans awarded to students in the health professions, is being cut back. This has had a strong negative impact on prospective applicants and their families and may be one of the most significant factors in the decline in the applicant pool.

SCHOLARSHIPS AND LOANS

The major portion of financial support that is made available to dental students is provided, either directly or indirectly, by the federal government. These funds are channeled through such programs as:

1. Scholarships for Health Professions Students of Exceptional Financial Need

2. Armed Forces Health Professions Scholarship Programs

3. National Health Corps Scholarship Program

These three scholarship programs and loan programs are discussed in Chapter 9. Financial aid officers at the dental schools should be consulted regarding these and all other forms of support.

There are also regional groups that provide support for students living in certain states. These are:

Western Interstate Commission for Higher Education (WICHE)

Students who are residents of western states that do not have dental schools (Alaska, Arizona, Hawaii, Montana, Nevada, Utah, and Wyoming) may apply to the WICHE Student Exchange Programs. The home state contributes a support fee to the dental school to offset part of the educational costs of its resident. The student then has to pay resident's tuition at a public or reduced tuition at a private school. For more information, contact The Professional Student Exchange Program, Western Interstate Commission for Higher Education, PO Box 9752, Boulder, CO 80301-9752.

Southern Regional Education Board (SREB)

Students who are residents of southern states (Alabama, Arkansas, North Carolina, and Tennessee) some of which do not have dental schools, are eligible to participate in SREB's Regional Contract Program. Each home state contributes a fixed fee, while the student pays the resident's tuition at a public school and receives a reduction in tuition at a private school. For more information contact: Ann H. Creech, Southern Regional Education Board, 592 Tenth Street NW, Atlanta, GA 30318-5790, Phone: (404) 875-9211.

United Student Aid Funds

This fund endorses loans up to $5,000 per year for a total of $15,000 for all guaranteed loan programs. Repayment begins ten months after leaving school, with interest not exceeding 7%. For additional information contact: USA Funds Endorsement Center, 1100 USA Parkway, Fishers, IN 46038.

Two restricted sources of financial aid are:

American Fund for Dental Health Minority Scholarship Program

This program provides recipients with scholarships of up to $2,000 per year for the first two years of dental school. One must be accepted by a dental school and be a member of an underrepresented minority (African-American, Native American, Mexican-American, or Puerto Rican) to apply. For information contact: American Fund for Dental Health, 211 East Chicago Avenue, Suite 1630, Chicago, IL 60611.

Dentistry Canada Fund

This program provides information concerning scholarships and loans. For information contact: Dentistry Canada Fund, 1815 promenade Alta Vista Drive, Ottawa, ON, Canada, K1G 3Y6.

Financial aid on a state level is also available for some state residents. These sources are listed below by state.

Indiana
Student Loan Fund Program
Indiana Dental Association
PO Box 2467
Indianapolis, IN 46202-2467

Kansas
Loan Fund
Kansas State Dental Auxiliary
School of Dentistry
University of Missouri at Kansas City
Kansas City, MO 64108

Louisiana
Dental Student Loan Fund
Women's Auxiliary to the Louisiana Dental Association
10 Stilt Street
New Orleans, LA 70124

Minnesota
Student Loan Fund
Minnesota State Dental Association
2236 Marshall Avenue
St. Paul, MN 55104

Loan Funds
School of Dentistry
University of Minnesota
Washington Avenue and Union Street, S.E.
Minneapolis, MN 55455

New Mexico
Student Loan Fund
New Mexico Dental Association
2917 Santa Cruz Avenue, S.E.
Albuquerque, NM 87106

Virginia
Rural Scholarship/Loan
Virginia Commonwealth University
520 North 12th Street, Room 309
Richmond, VA 23298

West Virginia
Dental School General Loan Fund
School of Dentistry
West Virginia University
Morgantown, WV 26506

21 Dental Education

Dental curriculum
Other educational programs
Postgraduate training

DENTAL CURRICULUM

Dental schools are located within or close to medical and hospital facilities. The traditional four-year program of studies corresponds to that of medicine and consists of two preclinical years of basic sciences and two years of clinical study. The basic sciences (anatomy, physiology, biochemistry, etc.) are taken by dental students in some schools together with medical students; in others, instruction is given exclusively in dental school. While most work consists of lecture and laboratory experiments, preclinical study also includes learning the basic techniques of dental restoration and treatment through practice on inanimate models.

The two clinical years are spent treating patients having a variety of oral diseases and disorders, while working under the supervision of clinical instructors. A variety of clinical procedures and dental care for special patients (for example, the old and infirm) are mastered during this period. Making use of dental auxiliary personnel is outlined.

Beginning in the 1960s, the traditional curriculum in dentistry underwent change; the nature of this change was two fold. First there was a new approach that involved integration of the basic and clinical sciences with emphasis on relevance, and thus students were introduced to the patient earlier. Also, greater emphasis was placed on preventive dentistry, public health dentistry, practice management, and hospital dentistry. The curricula of almost all dental schools have been updated to a greater or lesser extent along these lines.

A second major change that was attempted was the shortening of the curriculum to three years. This experiment, however, appears not to have been successful and, as of this time, all dental schools have a four-year program leading to the D.D.S. or D.M.D. degree except the University of the Pacific, which has a three-year program, and Harvard, which has a five-year program.

To provide an insight into the various dental school courses and the approximate amount of time devoted to each, a summary is presented in Table 21.1.

Table 21.1
DENTAL SCHOOL COURSES AND HOURS ALLOTTED

Course	Average number of hours
Basic Sciences	
Anatomy (gross)	200
Anatomy (histology, general and oral)	135
Biochemistry	100
Microbiology	100
Pathology (general and oral)	185
Pharmacology	75
Physiology	100
subtotal	895
Clinical Sciences	
Anesthesiology	50
Auxiliary Utilization	140
Dental Materials	70
Diagnosis	120
Emergency Treatment	50
Endodontics	150
Hospital Dentistry	40
Nutrition	25
Occlusion	115
Operative Dentistry	475
Oral Surgery	140
Orthodontics	125
Pedodontics	150
Periodontics	220
Physical Evaluation	60
Prosthodontics (fixed and removable)	800
Special Care	70
Tooth Morphology	85
subtotal	2885
Total hours of training	3780

A sample breakdown of the major courses by year is shown in Table 22.2. Schools will allot varying amounts of time to the different courses and some courses may appear under different titles.

Table 21.2
MAJOR COURSES IN THE DENTAL CURRICULUM—BY YEAR

First Year	Second Year	Third Year	Fourth Year
Biochemistry	Endodontics	Endodontics	Endodontics
Dental Anatomy	Complete Dentures	Crown and Bridge	Oral Surgery
Dental Materials	Removable Prosthodontics	Operative Dentistry	Operative Dentistry
Gross Anatomy	Pathology	Pharmacology	Periodontics
Histology	Partial Dentures	Oral Diagnosis	Partial Dentures
Physiology	Operative Dentistry	Periodontics	Pedodontics
Microbiology			

To clarify the nature of the major courses taken in dental school, a brief description of their content follows. (Courses are listed alphabetically.)

Biochemistry
The course covers the biochemical processes that occur at the cellular and subcellular levels, and with tissue and organ metabolism and function. Emphasis is placed on the molecular basis of oral and other human disease.

Complete Dentures
Both the theoretical and practical aspects related to the construction of complete dentures are considered during this second-year course. A complete denture is constructed for a mannequin.

Crown and Bridge (Fixed Prosthodontics)
This course extends over the last three years. In the second year the student is introduced to the principles and basic techniques of fixed prosthodontics. Included are such topics as articulation, tooth preparation, impressions, working cast construction, waxing, casting, soldering, and finishing. The third year focuses on the research aspects, evaluating comparative studies of materials and techniques used in prosthodontics. The fourth year is devoted to seminars on current problems in the field and to clinical procedures for more complex problems.

Dental Anatomy
This freshman course deals with the anatomical structure, individual characteristics, and the functional arrangement of teeth and their development.

Dental Materials
This first-year course serves to introduce the student to the basic principles and properties of materials used in dental treatment. Experience to gain and improve manipulative skills with selected materials is provided.

Endodontics
This subject is usually taught starting in the sophomore year. The differential diagnosis of dental pain is taught. Emphasis is placed on the technique used for preparing access cavities, preparing the root canal, obliterating the canal space, and utilizing endodontic instruments. The periodontal diseases and the use of surgical techniques in their treatment are discussed. The fourth year emphasizes clinical work such as surgical treatment of pathological disorders of tissues and all phases of root canal therapy.

Gross Anatomy
The goal of this course is to familiarize the student with the anatomical basis for the study of the basic sciences and the clinical practice of dentistry. Emphasis is placed on the functional significance of various organ systems and regions by means of integrating the lectures and laboratory sessions. The latter use predissected cadavers, skeletons, models, X-rays, and movies.

Histology
A study of the microscopic structure of tissues with special reference to the morphology of the oral cavity, particularly the teeth. Both light and electron microscopic levels of organization of tissues are analyzed.

Microbiology
The course introduces the student to bacteriology, virology, parasitology, immunology, and mycology as related to the oral cavity. The student learns the microbial diagnostic techniques and studies the bacteria of the nasopharynx and the processes of antibiotic resistance.

Operative Dentistry
In the second year, the basic concepts and procedures of tooth restoration are presented. Cavity preparation and restoration are taught in the laboratory. All types of cavities and

the use of various restorative materials are covered. An anatomical mannequin is used to obtain experience. After a transition period from mannequin to patient, students are provided with an opportunity, over the last two years, to apply their theoretical knowledge in the clinic under supervision. Lectures, demonstrations, and seminars provide the opportunity to evaluate progress and receive individual guidance.

Oral Diagnosis

This course extends over the last two years. In the third year, students are taught how to take a history and carry out a clinical examination in light of the patient's complaint. The course serves to correlate the basic and clinical information by focusing on diseases and abnormalities of the oral cavity. Clinical work involving oral diagnosis is required. The fourth year consists of a seminar course devoted to diagnosis and treatment planning of specially selected cases.

Oral Surgery

Having had courses in anesthesiology, radiology, and exodontics in the first through third years, the student is prepared for this fourth-year course in oral surgery. The course is devoted to the diagnosis and surgical treatment of diseases, injuries, and defects of the jaws and related structures.

Partial Dentures

The student is taught partial denture concepts and techniques. Technical experience is gained by fabricating dentures, using a mannequin as a patient.

Pathology

Taught during the second and third years, this course stresses the recognition and treatment of oral diseases based on their clinical characteristics and an understanding of the disease process.

Pharmacology

Taught in the second or third year, this course aims to acquaint students with drugs currently in use, and to prepare them for the rational application of the drugs in dental practice.

Physiology

Taught in the first year, the course deals first with cell physiology and then with the function of the organ system. The physiological basis of dentistry and its application to clinical practice are emphasized.

Pedodontics

This subject is taught from the second to the fourth years. In the second year, the emphasis is on the procedures used with children of primary and mixed dentition ages, related to child management, oral pathology, preventive orthodontics, and operative techniques. The laboratory deals with restorative dentistry in the primary dentition. In the third year, the lectures deal with the procedures utilized, etiology, prognosis, and treatment of the dental problems of children. Supervised clinical experience is provided to learn the art of teaching dental hygiene to children and to develop the skills to diagnose and treat them. The fourth year is a continuation of the third year course.

Periodontics

This subject is usually taught during the last two years. The course includes a study of periodontal diseases, incorporating clinical and histopathological findings, etiological factors, and methods of prevention. The techniques of periodontal therapy are taught and clinical experience is provided.

OTHER EDUCATIONAL PROGRAMS

A small number of students enter dental school prior to completion of their undergraduate studies. In many such cases a bachelor's degree can be earned while completing the dental curriculum, but only if the college at which the individual did undergraduate work offers such a program and awards the degree independently.

Some schools provide the opportunity for selected students to earn their dental degree together with one of the following advanced degrees:

Master of Science (M.S.)

This degree is usually offered in oral biology or a basic science. It usually requires about one additional year of study.

Masters in Public Health (M.P.H.)

This is a program designed for those especially interested in dental public health. It requires from one summer to one year of additional study.

Doctor of Philosophy (Ph.D.)

This degree is usually awarded for work completed in one of the basic sciences. It requires at least two additional years of study and is designed for those planning careers in academic dentistry.

Table 21.3

DENTAL SCHOOLS PROVIDING OPPORTUNITIES TO EARN OTHER DEGREES CONCURRENTLY

MS	MPH	PhD
Alabama	Alabama	Alabama
California, Los Angeles	California, Los Angeles	California, Los Angeles
California, San Francisco	Connecticut	Case Western Reserve
Case Western Reserve	Columbia	Connecticut
Columbia	Harvard	Harvard
Illinois	Illinois	Illinois
Louisville	Loma Linda	Iowa
Medical College of Georgia	North Carolina	Loma Linda
Medical College of Virginia	Northwestern	Maryland
Ohio State		Medical College of Georgia
Oregon		Medical College of Virginia
Pennsylvania		New Jersey
Tennessee		North Carolina
Washington		Northwestern
West Virginia		Pennsylvania
		South Carolina
		Southern California
		SUNY, Buffalo
		Tennessee
		Texas, San Antonio
		Washington
		West Virginia

POSTGRADUATE TRAINING

There are eight dental specialties that are recognized by the American Dental Association. Becoming a specialist usually requires from one to four additional years of training beyond the dental degree and, in most instances, practical experience in the field.

Specialty training is offered at some dental schools and at many hospitals and medical centers. Further information on institutions offering postgraduate training can be secured from: The Commission on Dental Accreditation, American Dental Association, 211 East Chicago Avenue, Chicago, IL 60611.

Dental Schools

The dental scene in a nutshell
In-depth dental school profiles

This chapter consists of two components: a table and school profiles. Table 22.1 in "The Dental Scene in a Nutshell" provides numerical data dealing with various items and serves as a quick source of information and a means for comparing elements of various schools. The "In-Depth Dental School Profiles" offer detailed information that distinguishes the individual schools.

THE DENTAL SCENE IN A NUTSHELL

Table 22.1, Basic Data on the Dental Schools, contains the kind of data that should be useful in helping you decide which schools to apply to. At a glance you can see and compare application data, admission statistics, academic statistics, and expenses.

Please note that while the information in this table is as up to date and accurate as possible, it is recommended that you check with the individual dental schools before applying.

How To Use This Table

The following list explains the column headings in Table 22.1.

Application Fee
In many cases, this fee is required only at the time of final application. The preliminary application is usually the AADSAS application, for which a fee is paid when submitting the form.

Earliest and Latest Filling Dates
These are usually firm dates.

Number of Applicants
This column gives an idea of how many applications were received for the 1996–97 class.

Entering Class
The columns indicate the men, women, minority, and out-of-state students who enrolled in the 1996–97 entering class.* The ratio of the total number of men and women accepted to the total number of applicants gives an indication of the competitive nature of admissions at each school.

Two Years College
This shows the relative chances of a second-year student gaining admission.

Three Years College
This shows the relative chances of a third-year student gaining admission.

*Where data for 1996–97 were unavailable, those for 1995–96 were used. Such cases are identified by # after the school name.

Mean Total GPA

The mean grade point average. It is usually somewhat lower for residents.

Mean Science GPA

The mean science grade point average. It also is usually somewhat lower for residents.

DAT Academic Average

The mean academic average test score for entering first-year students.

DAT PAT Average

The mean perceptual ability test score for entering first-year students. This and the preceding score can serve as a guide for the standards and competitive nature of each school.

Tuition

1996–97 tuition costs (annual) for first-year students, unless otherwise indicated.

Other

This estimate covers fees, books, instruments, and other supplies and materials for the first year.

Table 22.1 BASIC DATA ON THE DENTAL SCHOOLS (1996–97 ACADEMIC YEAR)

| School | Application Data | | | Admission Statistics | | | |
| | Fee | Filling Dates | | Number of Applicants | Entering Class | | |
		Earliest	Latest		Men	Women	Minority
ALABAMA							
*University of Alabama School of Dentistry	$25	6/1	1/15	685	41	14	5
CALIFORNIA							
*Loma Linda University School of Dentistry	$ 0	6/1	12/15	1524	64	21	52
*University of California—Los Angeles School of Dentistry	$75	5/1	1/1	1470	53	44	4
*University of California—San Francisco, School of Dentistry#	$40	6/1	1/1	833	51	31	14
*University of Southern California School of Dentistry	$55	7/1	4/1	2061	98	45	n/app
*University of the Pacific School of Dentistry	$50	6/20	3/1	2284	93	43	44
COLORADO							
*University of Colorado School of Dentistry#	$50	6/1	1/1	880	29	7	3
CONNECTICUT							
*University of Connecticut School of Dental Medicine	$60	7/1	4/1	1200	24	20	5
DISTRICT OF COLUMBIA							
*Howard University College of Dentistry	$25	6/1	4/1	1407	34	50	52
FLORIDA							
*University of Florida School of Dentistry	$20	6/1	10/15	768	51	27	22
Nova Southeastern University College of Dental Medicine#	$50	6/1	4/1	n/app	n/app	n/app	n/app
GEORGIA							
Medical College of Georgia School of Dentistry	$ 0	7/1	11/1	213	37	19	7
ILLINOIS							
*Northwestern University Dental School	$45	6/1	2/1	2320	51	25	1

*   AADSAS school
#   1995–96 data
n/app   not applicable

Academic Statistics			Admission Statistics				Expenses	
Entering Class			Accepted Out-of State Applicants		Entering Class			
Out-of-State	Percent with		Mean Total GPA	Mean Science GPA	DAT Academic Average	DAT PAT Average	Tuition Res/Nonres	Other
	Two Years College	Three Years College						
1	0	.04	3.3	3.1	17	17	$ 5,163 $15,489	$ 3,300
n/app	0	2.0	3.1	3.0	17	17	$22,380 $22,380	$ 7,210
2	0	9	3.4	3.3	21	19	$ 8,509 $21,033	$29,542
4	0	1	3.4	3.3	11	10.0	$ 0 $ 8,394	$20,000
75	12	23	3.3	3.3	18	17	$33,363 $33,363	$ 9,700
35	4	3	3.1	2.9	19	18	$38,456 $38,456	$11,829
11	0	2	3.3	3.3	17.8	17.7	$ 6,980 $23,259	$20,200
21	0	2	3.4	3.0	19	17	$10,750 $22,150	$14,000
82	2	10	2.8	2.7	15	14	$12,500 $12,500	$ 6,967
5	0	6.4	3.3	3.2	18	18	$ 7,749 $16,751	$ 9,500
n/app	n/app	n/app	n/app	n/app	n/app	n/app	$25,000 $25,000	$ 3,100
0	5	90	3.3	3.3	19	19	$24,894 $24,894	$20,892
1	0	3	3.3	3.2	17	17	$ 5,292 $18,261	$ 4,409

Table 22.1. BASIC DATA ON THE DENTAL SCHOOLS (1996–97 ACADEMIC YEAR)—CONTINUED

School	Application Data			Admission Statistics			
		Filling Dates				Entering Class	
	Fee	Earliest	Latest	Number of Applicants	Men	Women	Minority
*Southern Illinois University School of Dental Medicine	$20	7/1	3/1	758	38	12	6
*University of Illinois at Chicago College of Dentistry#	$30	7/1	3/1	1339	39	25	3
INDIANA							
*Indiana University School of Dentistry	$30	6/1	2/1	1123	66	34	3
IOWA							
*University of Iowa College of Dentistry	$20	6/1	1/1	1037	46	28	15
KENTUCKY							
*University of Kentucky College of Dentistry	$25	6/1	1/1	1102	27	25	9
*University of Louisville School of Dentistry	$10	6/1	2/1	1651	44	28	7
LOUISIANA							
*Louisiana State University School of Dentistry	$50	10/1	2/28	165	33	23	8
MARYLAND							
*University of Maryland Baltimore College of Dental Surgery	$50	6/1	2/15	1915	57	41	37
MASSACHUSETTS							
*Boston University Medical Center, School of Dental Medicine	$50	6/1	3/1	2646	57	34	42
*Harvard School of Dental Medicine	$50	7/1	1/1	800	12	18	17
*Tufts University School of Dental Medicine	$50	7/1	3/1	2647	89	59	59
MICHIGAN							
*University of Detroit Mercy School of Dentistry	$35	5/1	3/1	1384	48	26	13
*University of Michigan School of Dentistry	$50	5/1	2/1	1448	53	48	38

*	AADSAS school
#	1995–96 data
n/av	data not available

Academic Statistics			Admission Statistics				Expenses	
Entering Class			Accepted Out-of State Applicants		Entering Class			
Out-of-State	Percent with		Mean Total GPA	Mean Science GPA	DAT Academic Average	DAT PAT Average	Tuition Res/Nonres	Other
	Two Years College	Three Years College						
1	0	18	3.1	3.0	17	17.8	$ 5,682 $17,046	$ 7,648
1	6	27	3.2	3.0	17	17	$ 7,050 $20,280	$18,766
40	0	2	3.2	3.1	17.3	17	$ 9,860 $21,120	$ 5,800
18	0	4	3.3	3.2	18	17	$ 5,632 $17,496	$ 7,312
16	0	11	3.2	3.0	17	16	$ 6,765 $17,045	$ 5,703
26	0	6	3.3	3.1	16	16	$ 6,630 $16,910	$ 3,100
8	0	10	3.3	3.2	17	16	$ 5,736 n/av	$ 4,990
40	n/av	7	3.2	3.1	18	17	$ 9,631 $20,715	$ 6,238
78	2	14	3.2	3.1	17	18	$29,500 $29,500	$21,859
27	n/av	n/av	3.5	3.5	22	18	$24,150 $24,150	$15,031
114	1	2	3.2	3.1	18	17	$26,600 $26,600	$ 6,500
20	4.3	19	3.2	3.2	18	17	$20,500 $20,500	$ 4,580
40	0	9	3.4	3.0	18	17	$13,184 $23,862	$ 1,920

Table 22.1. BASIC DATA ON THE DENTAL SCHOOLS (1996–97 ACADEMIC YEAR)—CONTINUED

| School | Application Data | | | Admission Statistics | | | |
| | | Filling Dates | | | Entering Class | | |
	Fee	Earliest	Latest	Number of Applicants	Men	Women	Minority
MINNESOTA							
*University of Minnesota School of Dentistry	$50	6/1	3/1	948	57	29	8
MISSISSIPPI							
*University of Mississippi School of Dentistry	$25	7/1	12/1	134	22	9	0
MISSOURI							
*University of Missouri-Kansas City School of Dentistry	$25	6/1	1/1	1019	36	22	10
NEBRASKA							
*Creighton University School of Dentistry	$35	7/1	3/1	1979	57	27	6
*University of Nebraska Medical Center College of Dentistry#	$25	7/1	2/1	652	36	7	3
NEW JERSEY							
*New Jersey Dental School University of Medicine and Dentistry of New Jersey	$125	6/1	2/1	1145	39	36	17
NEW YORK							
*Columbia University School of Dental and Oral Surgery	$50	7/1	3/1	1808	45	25	10
*New York University College of Dentistry	$35	7/1	6/1	2395	123	79	80
*State University of New York at Buffalo, School of Dental Medicine#	$50	7/1	2/15	857	59	26	0
*State University of New York at Stony Brook, School of Dental Medicine	$75	7/1	1/15	800	17	15	0
NORTH CAROLINA							
*University of North Carolina School of Dentistry	$60	6/15	11/1	922	34	42	7

*   AADSAS school

\#   1995–96 data

Academic Statistics			Admission Statistics				Expenses	
Entering Class			Accepted Out-of State Applicants		Entering Class			
Out-of-State	Percent with		Mean Total GPA	Mean Science GPA	DAT Academic Average	DAT PAT Average	Tuition Res/Nonres	Other
	Two Years College	Three Years College						
29	0	7	3.3	3.4	18	18	$ 9,466 $13,968	$ 3,947
0	0	3	3.5	3.4	16	16	$ 4,400 $10,400	$ 3,502
29	9	6	3.3	3.2	17	17	$12,160 $24,461	$ 7,123
73	0	12	3.3	3.1	18	18	$19,578 $19,578	$ 3,810
8	0	8	3.5	3.4	17	17	$ 9,350 $21,550	$17,900
10	0	3	3.1	3.0	17	16	$14,492 $22,672	$ 5,672
46	0	1	3.0	3.0	21	18	$25,070 $25,070	$ 5,957
94	0	12	3.3	3.0	18.2	16	$32,950 $32,950	$ 4,841
6	0	4	3.2	3.2	18	18	$10,840 $21,940	$ 1,740
0	0	0	3.3	3.3	18	16	$10,840 $21,680	$ 1,348
12	0	6.6	3.3	3.3	18	17	$ 4,584 $27,748	$ 2,890

Table 22.1. BASIC DATA ON THE DENTAL SCHOOLS (1996–97 ACADEMIC YEAR)—CONTINUED

School	Application Data			Admission Statistics			
		Filling Dates			Entering Class		
	Fee	Earliest	Latest	Number of Applicants	Men	Women	Minority
OHIO							
*Case Western Reserve University School of Dentistry	$35	6/1	3/1	2201	43	19	17
*Ohio State University College of Dentistry	$125	7/1	2/1	1125	66	32	23
OKLAHOMA							
*University of Oklahoma College of Dentistry	$50	7/1	12/1	713	38	16	16
OREGON							
*Oregon Health Science University, School of Dentistry	$40	7/1	11/1	996	53	17	8
PENNSYLVANIA							
*Temple University School of Dentistry	$30	7/30	4/1	2384	85	34	14
*University of Pennsylvania School of Dental Medicine	$45	6/1	2/1	1642	45	47	35
*University of Pittsburgh School of Dental Medicine	$35	6/1	2/1	1576	50	31	14
SOUTH CAROLINA							
*Medical University of South Carolina College of Dental Medicine	$45	6/1	12/1	726	39	16	3
TENNESSEE							
*Meharry Medical College School of Dentistry#	$25	6/1	4/1	1089	21	26	41
*University of Tennessee College of Dentistry	$50	6/1	12/31	250	62	18	8
TEXAS							
*Baylor College of Dentistry	$35	6/1	11/1	1470	35	22	5
*University of Texas Health Science Center Houston Dental Branch#	$35	4/15	11/1	814	38	23	7
University of Texas Health Science Center San Antonio Dental School	$45	4/15	11/1	846	60	30	30

*   AADSAS school
\#   1995–96 data
n/av data not available

Academic Statistics			Admission Statistics				Expenses	
Entering Class			Accepted Out-of State Applicants		Entering Class			
Out-of-State	Percent with		Mean Total GPA	Mean Science GPA	DAT Academic Average	DAT PAT Average	Tuition Res/Nonres	Other
	Two Years College	Three Years College						
4	1	6	3.1	3.0	18	17	$23,900 $23,900	$ 6,271
15	2	10	3.4	3.2	17	17	$ 8,586 $25,104	$ 4,725
12	2	17	3.3	3.2	17	17	$ 6,260 $15,534	$ 5,953
20	0	2	3.4	3.5	18	19	$ 8,850 $18,336	$ 6,123
71	n/av	n/av	3.0	3.0	18.2	18	$18,328 $26,000	$ 7,103
72	0	0.3	3.3	3.1	19	17	$30,100 $30,100	$17,050
25	n/av	14	3.0	3.0	15	15	$17,630 $25,400	$12,000
8	0	0.6	3.1	n/av	17	17	$ 6,403 $18,607	$ 6,038
39	0	3	2.8	2.6	15	14	$16,500 n/av	$14,100
6	0	39	3.23	3.13	16.9	16.5	$ 5,744 $13,454	$ 9,056
6	0	3	3.2	3.1	17	16	$ 5,400 $16,200	$ 6,000
3	0	3	3.3	3.1	16	16	$ 5,400 $16,200	$16,100
4	1	9	3.4	3.3	18	18	$ 5,400 $16,200	$ 2,700

Table 22.1. BASIC DATA ON THE DENTAL SCHOOLS (1996–97 ACADEMIC YEAR)—CONTINUED

| School | Application Data | | | Admission Statistics | | | |
| | | Filling Dates | | | Entering Class | | |
	Fee	Earliest	Latest	Number of Applicants	Men	Women	Minority
VIRGINIA							
*Virginia Commonwealth University Medical College of Virginia School of Dentistry	$50	5/1	1/1	1370	52	28	19
WASHINGTON							
*University of Washington School of Dentistry	$35	7/1	12/1	1018	36	18	6
WEST VIRGINIA							
*West Virginia University School of Dentistry	$45	7/1	3/1	1187	32	9	4
WISCONSIN							
*Marquette University School of Dentistry	$25	7/15	4/1	2017	52	23	26
CANADA							
*Dalhousie University Faculty of Dentistry	$55	10/1	12/1	224	121	103	0
*McGill University Faculty of Dentistry	$60	7/1	12/1	252	10	15	0
Université de Montréal Faculté de Médecine Dentaire	$55	3/1	3/1	541	40	45	0
Université Laval Faculté Médecine Dentaire	$55	9/1	4/15	393	26	20	0
University of Alberta Faculty of Dentistry	$60	7/1	11/1	303	20	12	n/av
University of British Columbia Faculty of Dentistry	$50	8/15	12/15	263	14	23	0
University of Manitoba Faculty of Dentistry#	$55	11/1	1/24	223	17	8	0
*University of Saskatchewan College of Dentistry#	$ 0	9/1	1/1	165	12	9	0
*University of Toronto Faculty of Dentistry	$100	8/15	2/1	627	37	28	0
University of Western Ontario Faculty of Dentistry	$50	10/1	12/1	599	31	17	8

*   AADSAS school
\#   1995–96 data
n/av   data not available

Academic Statistics			Admission Statistics				Expenses	
Entering Class			Accepted Out-of State Applicants		Entering Class			
Out-[1] of- State	Percent with		Mean Total GPA	Mean Science GPA	DAT Academic Average	DAT PAT Average	Tuition Res/Nonres	Other
	Two Years College	Three Years College						
20	0	0	3.4	3.3	18	18	$ 8,698 $20,136	$ 2,605
9	0	2	3.5	3.4	20	20	$ 8,172 $20,584	$ 4,688
21	n/av	2	3.5	3.2	17	17	$ 4,806 $12,954	$ 6,058
1	0	18	3.3	3.2	17	16.1	$26,995 $26,995	$20,930
0	63	94	3.7	3.7	19	18	$ 5,755 $ 8,455	$ 4,804
4	24	16	3.5	n/av	19.8	18.4	$ 1,669 $ 7,459	$ 360
n/av	48	52	n/av	n/av	n/av	n/av	$ 3,000 n/av	$ 6,800
n/av	4.4	13.0	86	88	n/av	18.9	$ 3,000 n/av	$ 5,600
n/av	33	37	8.1	8.1	n/av	19.1	$ 5,874 $11,746	$ 7,997
3	0	100	3.6	n/av	21	19	$ 3,937 n/av	$ 6,276
11	2	8	n/av	n/av	18.3	19	$ 4,162 $ 4,162	$ 8,642
n/av	9	6	3.3	n/av	n/av	n/av	$ 4,673 $ 4,673	$ 7,124
1	22	39	n/av	n/av	n/av	n/av	$ 8,037 $ 8,037	$ 4,945
3	29	71	86	n/av	n/av	n/av	$ 8,037 $23,037	$ 6,474

[1]   For Canadian schools "Out-of-State" means "Out-of-Province."

IN-DEPTH DENTAL SCHOOL PROFILES _____

The dental school profiles consist of in-depth descriptions of the 54 accredited U.S. dental schools and the 10 Canadian dental schools. The profiles include an introductory paragraph, admission procedures and requirements, curriculum, grading and promotion policies, facilities, and special features as described below.

Capsule

Each profile is preceded by a capsule featuring the essential information that defines each school. It includes communication addresses and numbers; facts on application deadlines, accreditation, and degrees; enrollment figures and test scores; and a graphic display of tuition, broken out by residents and nonresidents as compared with average nationwide costs.

Introduction

The background of the dental school as well as the parent institution (if any) is described in this section.

Admissions

Although the minimum requirement for most U.S. schools is at least three years (90 semester hours) of undergraduate study at an accredited college or university, the percentage of those accepted with only this background is quite small. Most students hold a baccalaureate degree at the time they begin their dental school studies. (Some Canadian schools have a one- or two-year college prerequisite.) *The DAT is required for admission by essentially all U.S. schools* (but not by those in Canada). The basic or minimum predental science course requirements referred to in this section consist of one year each of biology, inorganic chemistry, organic chemistry, and physics along with their appropriate laboratory work. Any additional required or recommended courses are indicated. Most other required courses include those covered by any regular general education program at an undergraduate college. An interview may or may not be required but it is given only at the invitation of the school. Since residence is in some cases a significant element in the admission process, the general policy is noted. (For an overall picture of this factor, see Table 22.1, which lists the number of nonresidents accepted.)

Transfer and Advanced Standing

The level to which transfer is possible varies from school to school. Foreign dental school graduates may be accepted at some undergraduate level at institutions that grant advanced standing (usually only into the second year).

Curriculum

The curriculum is described as to length and type. The classifications used are: *traditional* (basic science taught during the first two years, although some clinical exposure may be provided. Last two years consist of clerkships in major and minor clinical specialties with little or no time allotted for electives); *diagonal curriculum* (phases in clinical experience to significant extent beginning in the first year, but the bulk of the clinics are still scheduled for the last two years); *flexible curriculum* (no rigid course curriculum and students complete the program in varying amounts of time).

Grading Policy

Where known, the grading policy is described. These policies may be different in the basic and clinical sciences.

Facilities

The facilities utilized both in the basic sciences and for clinical training are described.

Special Features

Other degree programs or special programs for recruiting and retaining disadvantaged students are described in this section.

ALABAMA

University of Alabama School of Dentistry

1919 Seventh Avenue, South
University Station
Birmingham, Alabama 35294

Phone: 205-934-3387   *Fax:* 205-975-5364

Application Filing		**Accreditation**
Earliest:	June 1	CDA
Latest:	January 15	
Fee:	$25	**Degrees Granted**
AADSAS:	yes	DMD, DMD-MS, DMD-PhD

Enrollment: 1996–97 First-Year Class

Men:	41	75%	*Mean*	
Women:	14	25%	total GPA:	3.3
Minorities:	3	5%	science GPA:	3.1
Out of State:	1	2%		
With 2 years of college:	0%		*Average*	
With 3 years of college:	4%		DAT academic:	17
			DAT-PAT:	17

Tuition

Resident	5163
Average	13,560
Nonresident	15,489
Average	18,855

(in thousands of dollars) — scale 0 5 10 15 20 25 30 35

Percentage receiving financial aid: 71%

Introduction

The University of Alabama was first established in 1831. After the Civil War, the school was rebuilt and reopened in 1869. In 1969 the University of Alabama system was established, and included 3 universities. The Birmingham campus of the University of Alabama holds the Medical Center, the University College, and the Graduate School. The 2 other campuses are located in Tuscaloosa and Huntsville. The School of Dentistry is part of the Medical Center at Birmingham, and was established in 1945. It admitted its first class of students in 1948. In addition to offering a program leading to the DMD degree, the School of Dentistry has accredited programs in all the specialties as well as in dental hygiene and dental assisting. This school pioneered the development of "four-handed dentistry" and the expanded utilization of trained auxiliary personnel.

Admissions (AADSAS)

In addition to the basic predental science courses, 1 year of mathematics and English and 1 additional biology course are required. Recommended electives may be from biology (embryology, genetics, comparative anatomy, cell physiology), chemistry (quantitative analysis, physical chemistry), calculus, literature, foreign languages, business, art, and sculpting. Preference is given to residents of Alabama and neighboring states. *Transfer and advanced standing:* Transfer to the third-year class only; no advanced standing for graduates of foreign schools of dentistry.

Curriculum

4-year traditional. The curriculum incorporates innovative interdisciplinary programs that emphasize the application of the basic sciences to various clinical problems. Initial clinical experience is provided during the latter part of the first year, at intervals during the second year, and intensively during the third and fourth years. Elective programs are offered to fourth-year students.

Facilities

The School of Dentistry Building is located within the medical facilities campus in downtown Birmingham. Off-campus clinical experience is also provided at a hospital for the mentally ill and at a geriatric setting.

Special Features

A program exists that is designed to interest, recruit, and retain minority students and women. Programs leading to the DMD-MS or PhD in one of the basic sciences are available.

CALIFORNIA

Loma Linda University School of Dentistry

Loma Linda, California 92350

Phone: 909-824-4621

Application Filing		Accreditation
Earliest:	June 1	CDA
Latest:	December 15	
Fee:	n/av	**Degrees Granted**
AADSAS:	yes	DDS, DDS-PhD

Enrollment: 1996–97 First-Year Class

Men:	64	75%	*Mean*		
Women:	21	25%	total GPA:	3.1
Minorities:	44	52%	science GPA:	3
Out of State:	n/av	n/av		
With 2 years of college:	0%	*Average*		
With 3 years of college:	2%	DAT academic:	17
			DAT-PAT:	17

Tuition

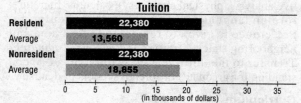

Resident	22,380
Average	13,560
Nonresident	22,380
Average	18,855

0 5 10 15 20 25 30 35
(in thousands of dollars)

Percentage receiving financial aid: 81%

Introduction

In 1905 Seventh-Day Adventists established Loma Linda University. In 1953 the School of Dentistry at Loma Linda University was founded. Located 16 miles east of Los Angeles, the university consists of 7 health science schools including schools of Dentistry, Medicine, Pharmacy, Nursing, Health-Related Professions, and a Graduate School. Besides offering a DDS program, the school has advanced educational programs in a variety of specialties and also offers a BS in dental hygiene. An International Dental Program trains dentists from other countries according to the standards of American dental medicine.

Admissions (AADSAS)

In addition to the basic predental science courses (which are required), 1 year of English, a management course, and upper level biological science courses are recommended. A minimum GPA of 2.7 is required.

Curriculum

4-year traditional. The courses in anatomy have clinical applications, and the laboratories in physiology, biochemistry, and pharmacology are based on problem-oriented case presentations. Clinical experience begins with the second year. Electives are available during all 4 years.

Facilities

The school is located on the university's campus in Loma Linda along with the university's other health profession training schools.

Special Features

Remedial and tutorial programs are available for all students. Placement services for locating and evaluating practice opportunities are available at no cost to the student. Outreach programs are carried out for underserved population groups locally, in Mexico, and other foreign countries.

University of California— Los Angeles School of Dentistry

Center for Health Sciences
Los Angeles, California 90095

Phone: 310-206-1718   *Fax:* 310-206-5539

Application Filing		Accreditation
Earliest:	May 1	CDA
Latest:	January 1	
Fee:	$75	**Degrees Granted**
AADSAS:	yes	DDS, DDS-MS

Enrollment: 1996–97 First-Year Class

Men:	53	55%	*Mean*	
Women:	44	45%	total GPA:	3.4
Minorities:	4	4%	science GPA:	3.3
Out of State:	2	2%		
With 2 years of college:	0%		*Average*	
With 3 years of college:	9%		DAT academic:	21
			DAT-PAT:	19

Tuition

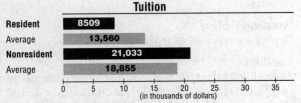

Resident	8509
Average	13,560
Nonresident	21,033
Average	18,855

0 5 10 15 20 25 30 35
(in thousands of dollars)

Percentage receiving financial aid: 87%

Introduction

The University of California at Los Angeles, an undergraduate and a graduate school, was established in 1919. In 1960 the University of California Los Angeles School of Dentistry was founded. The initial class was enrolled in 1965. The school is located in the Center of Health Sciences on the UCLA campus in west Los Angeles, along with the schools of Medicine, Nursing, and Public Health. The school has expanded by developing postdoctoral programs, establishing a research institute, organizing a satellite clinic in Venice, California, and collaborating with adjacent colleges in training dental hygienists and dental assistants.

Admissions (AADSAS)

In addition to the minimum predental science courses, courses in English and introductory psychology are required. There are no residency restrictions. Minority and underprivileged students are encouraged to apply. *Transfer and advanced standing:* Not available.

Curriculum

4-year. In addition to the basic sciences, students are trained in the use of clinical preventive measures during the first year. They are also exposed to an integrated basic-clinical sciences program section on oral biology that begins in the first year and continues into the third. Clinical experience in comprehensive patient care begins in the first year. Mandatory selectives are offered in the fourth year.

Grading Policy

The grading system used is a modification of the Pass/Not Pass rating system.

Facilities

The Dental School Building is located in the Center for Health Sciences on the UCLA campus. Off-campus clinical instruction is also provided.

Special Features

A combined DDS-MS program requires 1 additional year to complete.

University of California— San Francisco School of Dentistry

513 Parnassus Avenue
San Francisco, California   94143

Phone: 415-476-2737

Application Filing		Accreditation
Earliest:	June 1	CDA
Latest:	January 1	
Fee:	$90	**Degrees Granted**
AADSAS:	yes	DDS

Enrollment: 1996–97 First-Year Class

Men:	51	62%	*Mean*
Women:	31	38%	total GPA: 3.4
Minorities:	11	14%	science GPA: 3.3
Out of State:	4	5%	
With 2 years of college:		0%	*Average*
With 3 years of college:		1%	DAT academic: 10.6
			DAT-PAT: 10

Tuition

Resident	0
Average	13,560
Nonresident	8394
Average	18,855

(in thousands of dollars): 0, 5, 10, 15, 20, 25, 30, 35

Percentage receiving financial aid: 83%

Above data applies to 1995-96 academic year.

Introduction

The San Francisco campus of the University of California is dedicated to the health sciences only, and consists of schools of Dentistry, Medicine, Nursing, and Pharmacy, and their teaching hospitals. No undergraduate degrees can be obtained there. The University of California in San Francisco was established in 1873; the School of Dentistry was founded in 1881. In addition to offering a DDS degree, the School of Dentistry has a graduate program leading to a PhD in oral biology and postgraduate programs in various specialties as well as classes in dental hygiene.

Admissions (AADSAS)

Two semesters of psychology are required. A minimum GPA of 2.4 for residents and 2.8 for nonresidents is also required. Strong priority is given to California residents, but serious consideration will be given to a small number of outstanding non-California residents.

Curriculum

As early as the first year the basic sciences are supplemented by orientation to clinical practice, participation in community clinical activities, and research projects.

Grading Policy

Grades are reported as letter grades.

Facilities

The school is part of the health science campus. In addition to its own facilities, 2 community dental clinics, affiliated hospitals, and schools contribute to providing additional opportunities for clinical experience.

Special Features

Student Academic Services has been established to provide equal educational opportunities for academically qualified underrepresented minority students and students in need of assistance due to socioeconomic circumstances. A joint DDS-MD oral and maxillofacial program is sponsored by the schools of Dentistry and Medicine. Applicants must hold the DDS degree from an accredited school and must be accepted into the UCSF School of Dentistry's oral and maxillofacial surgery program before seeking admission to the School of Medicine.

University of Southern California School of Dentistry

Room 203, University Park—MC 0641
Los Angeles, California   90089

Phone: 213-740-2841   *Fax:* 213-740-8109
E-mail: scdental@hsc.edu
WWW: http://www.usc.edu

Application Filing		Accreditation	
Earliest:	July 1	CDA	
Latest:	April 1		
Fee:	$55	**Degrees Granted**	
AADSAS:	yes	DDS	

Enrollment: 1996–97 First-Year Class

Men:	98	69%	*Mean*	
Women:	45	31%	total GPA:	3.3
Minorities:	n/av	n/av	science GPA:	3.3
Out of State:	75	52%		
With 2 years of college:		12%	*Average*	
With 3 years of college:		23%	DAT academic:	18
			DAT-PAT:	17

Tuition

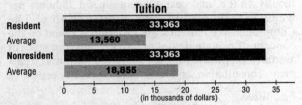

Resident	33,363
Average	13,560
Nonresident	33,363
Average	18,855

0   5   10   15   20   25   30   35
(in thousands of dollars)

Percentage receiving financial aid: 90%

Introduction

Established in 1880, the University of Southern California is a private school. The University of Southern California School of Dentistry was founded in 1897. The goal of the school is the education of highly trained general practitioners. Its faculty have contributed significantly to advances in dental medicine, particularly in the area of the use of semi-precious metal alloys and tooth restorative materials. The school offers a DDS and BS in dental hygiene.

Admissions (AADSAS)

The school requires the basic predental science courses and 1 year of English composition, as well as 1 year of philosophy, history, or fine arts. Nonresidents are evaluated and selected based on the same criteria as California residents. A personal interview may be required. *Transfer and advanced standing:* Transfers from American and Canadian schools may be considered on a space-available basis.

Curriculum

3–4 years diagonal. Patient treatment is a dominant theme in the dental curriculum and begins during the first trimester. It increases until the fourth year when it occupies the student's total efforts. Honors and elective programs are also available, and research in the biomedical and dental sciences is encouraged.

Facilities

The school is located on the USC campus and is housed in the Norris Dental Science Center. Other teaching resources include affiliated hospitals and a mobile clinic.

Special Features

An Office of Admissions coordinates all recruitment and retention programs. This office also coordinates other student services, including tutorial, financial aid, and job placement.

University of the Pacific School of Dentistry

2155 Webster Street
San Francisco, California   94115

Phone: 415-929-6495   *Fax:* 415-929-6654

Application Filing		Accreditation
Earliest:	June 20	CDA
Latest:	March 1	
Fee:	$50	**Degrees Granted**
AADSAS:	yes	DDS

Enrollment: 1996–97 First-Year Class

Men:	93	68%	*Mean*
Women:	43	32%	total GPA: 3.1
Minorities:	60	44%	science GPA: 2.9
Out of State:	35	26%	
With 2 years of college:		4%	*Average*
With 3 years of college:		3%	DAT academic: 19
			DAT-PAT: 18

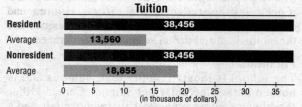

Tuition

Resident	38,456
Average	13,560
Nonresident	38,456
Average	18,855

(in thousands of dollars)

Percentage receiving financial aid: 85%

Introduction

In 1962 the College of Physicians and Surgeons merged with the University of the Pacific, which was established in 1851, thereby creating the University of the Pacific School of Dentistry. The University of the Pacific is located in Stockton and includes 8 undergraduate and 1 graduate schools. The school is located in the heart of San Francisco in a 9-story building, completed in 1967, which was designed for both teaching and research. Equipment and facilities have been updated as needed.

Admissions (AADSAS)

One year of English is required, plus the predental sciences courses. First consideration is given to applicants who have or will attain a baccalaureate degree prior to matriculation, have a GPA of 3.0 or above and DAT scores of 16 or better, and have financial resources adequate to meet the cost of dental education and living expenses. Established review procedures ensure applicants an equal opportunity to be considered for admission. The Admissions Committee has a firm policy of not discriminating against any applicant because of age, creed, handicap, national or ethnic origin, marital status, race, color, or sex. *Transfer and advanced standing:* Rarely possible.

Curriculum

Four academic/three calendar year (12 consecutive quarters), accelerated learning program. Biomedical sciences and preventive and community services instruction is presented throughout the curriculum. During the first year, students are introduced to comprehensive patient care and preclinical techniques. During the second year, 18 hours per week are devoted to providing comprehensive dental care under the supervision of a multidisciplinary teaching faculty. In the final year, students spend 35 hours per week in school and community clinics. The Comprehensive Patient Care Program is based on the concept of private dental practice where the student assumes responsibility for assigned patients' treatment, consultation, and referral for specialty care.

Facilities

The school is located on the university's San Francisco campus in the prestigious Pacific Heights neighborhood. It has a major extended campus, the Union City Dental Clinic. Through the extramural clinic program, students provide dental care, under faculty supervision, in selected northern California community clinics that resemble private practice settings.

Special Features

The school has an affirmative action program with regard to admission of qualified ethnic minorities, females, and members of underrepresented groups.

COLORADO

University of Colorado School of Dentistry

4200 East Ninth Avenue, Box AD 95
Denver, Colorado   80262

Phone: 303-270-8891

Application Filing		**Accreditation**
Earliest:	June 1	CDA
Latest:	March 1	
Fee:	$50	**Degrees Granted**
AADSAS:	yes	DDS

Enrollment: 1996–97 First-Year Class

Men:	29	81%	*Mean*
Women:	7	19%	total GPA: 3.3
Minorities:	1	3%	science GPA: 3.3
Out of State:	11	31%	
With 2 years of college:		0%	*Average*
With 3 years of college:		2%	DAT academic: 17.8
			DAT-PAT: 17.7

Tuition

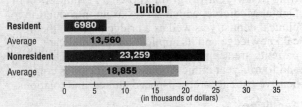

Resident	6980
Average	13,560
Nonresident	23,259
Average	18,855

0   5   10   15   20   25   30   35
(in thousands of dollars)

Percentage receiving financial aid: **92%**

Above data applies to 1995-96 academic year.

Introduction

The University of Colorado public system was founded in 1876. The School of Medicine at the University of Colorado was formerly at the Boulder campus, but later moved to the Denver campus, which was established in 1912 and merged with the Denver and Gross College of Medicine. The School of Dentistry at the University of Colorado opened in 1973. In addition to granting a DDS degree, the School of Dentistry offers a BS degree in dental hygiene and a postgraduate residency in general dentistry.

Admissions (AADSAS)

The basic predental science courses, 2 semesters of humanities, and 1 semester of English composition are required. Preference is given to state residents and applicants from western states under the WICHE agreement. Nonresidents are considered. *Transfer and advanced standing:* This is considered on an individual basis.

Curriculum

4-year traditional. Certain electives in the clinical sciences and research are offered in the last 2 years. Clinical experience begins in the sophomore year and continues as increasing levels of competence are acquired. Behavioral sciences, business administration, history, and ethics are incorporated into the curriculum.

Facilities

The school building was occupied in 1976 and contains the clinic, oral surgery suite, classrooms, laboratories, and offices. Certain facilities are available at the University of Colorado Medical School.

CONNECTICUT

University of Connecticut School of Dental Medicine

263 Farmington Avenue
Farmington, Connecticut   06030

Phone: 800-679-2175   *Fax:* 860-679-1899
E-mail: thibodean@nso.uchc.edu

Application Filing		**Accreditation**
Earliest:	July 1	CDA
Latest:	April 1	
Fee:	$60	**Degrees Granted**
AADSAS:	yes	DMD, DMD-PhD

Enrollment: 1996–97 First-Year Class

			Mean	
Men:	24	55%		
Women:	20	45%	total GPA:	3.4
Minorities:	2	5%	science GPA:	3
Out of State:	21	48%		
With 2 years of college:		0%	*Average*	
With 3 years of college:		2%	DAT academic:	19
			DAT-PAT:	17

Tuition

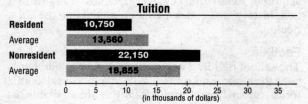

Resident	10,750
Average	13,560
Nonresident	22,150
Average	18,855

0   5   10   15   20   25   30   35
(in thousands of dollars)

Percentage receiving financial aid: 87%

Introduction

The University of Connecticut is a public institution that was originally founded in 1881. The Health Center at the University of Connecticut, established in the 1960s, encompasses the School of Dental Medicine, the School of Medicine, and the John Dempsey Hospital. This dental school is the only public one in New England. The university's main campus is located in Storrs, while the Health Center is situated in a wooded suburban campus in Farmington.

Admissions (AADSAS)

The basic predental courses are required. Students should have a strong facility in English and should be able to handle quantitative concepts. Credits in behavioral sciences and upper division biology courses are desirable. *Transfer and advanced standing:* Students from United States, Canadian, and foreign dental schools may apply for advanced standing.

Curriculum

4-year diagonal. During the first 2 years, students take an integrated course of study in the basic sciences that takes place in multidisciplinary laboratories. Simultaneously, students devote gradually increasing time to a 4-year program known as Foundation of Dental Medicine, which serves as an introduction to clinical dentistry as well as a bridge between theoretical knowledge and its application to dental care. First patients are seen during the second year. The third- and fourth-year clinical component includes comprehensive patient care, self-paced clinics, and rotations.

Facilities

The school is part of the University of Connecticut Health Center. A satellite clinic is located in the Burgdorf Health Center in Hartford.

Special Features

A combined DMD-PhD program is offered, which takes about 2 additional years to complete.

DISTRICT OF COLUMBIA

Howard University College of Dentistry

600 W Street, N.W.
Washington, DC   20059

Phone: 202-806-0400   *Fax:* 202-806-0354

Application Filing		Accreditation	
Earliest:	June 1	CDA	
Latest:	April 1		
Fee:	$25	**Degrees Granted**	
AADSAS:	yes	DDS	

Enrollment: 1996–97 First-Year Class

Men:	34	40%	*Mean*	
Women:	50	60%	total GPA:	2.8
Minorities:	44	52%	science GPA:	2.7
Out of State:	82	98%		
With 2 years of college:	2%		*Average*	
With 3 years of college:	10%		DAT academic:	15
			DAT-PAT:	14

Tuition

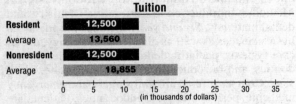

Resident	12,500
Average	13,560
Nonresident	12,500
Average	18,855

0   5   10   15   20   25   30   35
(in thousands of dollars)

Percentage receiving financial aid: 77%

Introduction

In 1867 Howard University was established as the largest private, primarily African-American school. Fourteen years later, the College of Dentistry was established. It is the fifth oldest dental school in the United States. The Center for Health Sciences of the University includes colleges of Medicine, Nursing, Pharmacy, and Allied Health Sciences. The 89-acre campus is 5 minutes from downtown Washington, D.C.

Admissions (AADSAS)

The basic predental courses and a year of English are required. Recommended electives are French or German, history, psychology, sociology, economics, humanities, behavioral sciences, and biostatistics. The GPA should be more than 2.5. Citizenship is not considered a requirement for admission, nor is residence within the District of Columbia. *Transfer and advanced standing:* Transfer from American schools is possible.

Curriculum

4-year traditional. Clinical experience begins in the second year. Basic and clinical sciences are integrated. Special features of the curriculum involve a program for the chronically ill and aged that takes dental care to the home- and institution-bound patient.

Facilities

The college is housed in a 5-story complex containing classrooms, clinics, laboratories, offices, research facilities, a learning resources area, and convertible clinic-laboratories. Programs are also conducted at the university hospital, as well as other affiliated hospitals.

Special Features

Many of the school's activities are devoted to the education of minorities, the educationally disadvantaged, and women. This commitment involves a prematriculation and a postmatriculation academic program. Several community-based programs and patient services are offered by the college and other affiliated hospitals.

FLORIDA

Nova Southeastern University College of Dental Medicine

3200 South University Drive
Ft. Lauderdale, Florida   33328

Phone: 954-723-1000

Application Filing		Accreditation
Earliest:	June 1	CDA
Latest:	April 1	
Fee:	$50	**Degrees Granted**
AADSAS:	yes	DMD

Enrollment: 1996–97 First-Year Class

Men:	n/av	n/av	*Mean*
Women:	n/av	n/av	total GPA:	n/av
Minorities:	n/av	n/av	science GPA:	n/av
Out of State:	n/av	n/av	
With 2 years of college:	n/av	*Average*
With 3 years of college:	n/av	DAT academic:	n/av
		DAT-PAT:	n/av

Tuition

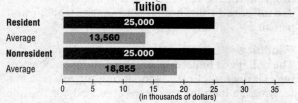

Resident	25,000
Average	13,560
Nonresident	25.000
Average	18,855

0   5   10   15   20   25   30   35
(in thousands of dollars)

Percentage receiving financial aid: n/av

n/av = not available

Introduction

Nova Southeastern University is the largest independent institution of higher learning in the state of Florida. It resulted from the merger of Nova University and Southeastern University. The College of Dental Medicine is the newest of the 6 schools in the Health Professions Division and was established in 1996. The other health profession schools are the colleges of Osteopathic Medicine, Pharmacy, Optometry, and Allied Health and Medical Sciences.

Admissions (AADSAS)

A minimum of 90 semester hours are required and no more than 60 will be accepted from a community or junior college in meeting this prerequisite. The basic predental science courses are also necessary. Zoology or microbiology can be substituted for general biology. The required science courses must be completed with a C (2.0) or better grade. Courses in English composition and literature are also required. The overall GPA of the applicant should be C+ (2.5) or better. *Transfer and advanced standing:* Information not available.

Curriculum

4-year traditional. *First year:* Includes the basic sciences and an Introduction to Pedodontics/Oral Medicine, Introduction to Restorative Dentistry, and dental materials. *Second year:* Includes the advanced basic sciences as well as diagnostic radiology, dental care systems, pediatric dentistry, endodontics, orthodontics, and Introduction to Clinical Practice. *Third year:* Courses offered are oral surgery and emergency medicine, periodontics, and endodontics. Patient care and patient behavioral techniques are taught. Twenty weeks of clinical practice are required followed by courses in oral medicine, periodontics, practice management and community dentistry. *Fourth year:* Forty weeks will be devoted to expanding clinical expertise in patient care. Community health-based programs for the care of aging population and disabled children will be conducted in various affiliated hospitals and clinical facilities.

Facilities

Plans are being made for construction of a 3-story 60,000 square foot building that is scheduled for completion in August 1997.

Special Features

The College of Dental Medicine encourages the application of qualified minority applicants and is committed to a policy of nondiscrimination.

University of Florida College of Dentistry

P.O. Box 100405
Gainesville, Florida   32610

Phone: 352-392-4866   *Fax:* 352-846-0311
E-mail: bennett@dental.ufl.edu na

Application Filing			**Accreditation**
Earliest:	June 1		CDA
Latest:	October 15		
Fee:	$20		**Degrees Granted**
AADSAS:	yes		DMD

Enrollment: 1996–97 First-Year Class

Men:	51	65%	*Mean*
Women:	27	35%	total GPA:	3.3
Minorities:	17	22%	science GPA:	3.2
Out of State:	5	6%	
With 2 years of college:	0%	*Average*
With 3 years of college:	6%	DAT academic:	18
			DAT-PAT:	18

Tuition

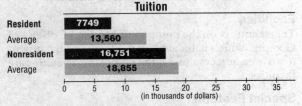

Resident	7749
Average	13,560
Nonresident	16,751
Average	18,855

0   5   10   15   20   25   30   35
(in thousands of dollars)

Percentage receiving financial aid: 95%

Introduction

The University of Florida was established in 1853 and has 14 undergraduate schools and 17 graduate schools. The University of Florida Health Science Center was founded in 1956 and the College of Dentistry admitted its first student in 1972. The Health Science Center, besides a College of Dentistry, includes colleges of Medicine, Nursing, Pharmacy, Veterinary Medicine, and Health-Related Professions.

Admissions (AADSAS)

The basic predental courses are required, and courses in biochemistry, microbiology, and immunology are recommended. Applicants with an overall B+ average as a minimum will receive strongest consideration for admission. A limited number of nonresidents are admitted. *Transfer and advanced standing:* Limited numbers are admitted.

Curriculum

4-year. Consists of 2 components: (a) core courses that are required of all, and (b) elective courses that are optional. The latter may include a research project. Basic sciences, correlated dental sciences, dental didactic activities, and dental clinical activities are presented in both the core and the electives.

Facilities

The college, with its 11-story dental clinical-science building, is an integral part of the J. Hillis Miller Health Center located on the university campus.

GEORGIA

Medical College of Georgia School of Dentistry

1459 Laney Walker Boulevard
Augusta, Georgia   30912

Phone: 706-721-3587   *Fax:* 706-721-6276
E-mail: ossas@mail.mcg.edu
WWW: http://www.mcg.edu/SOD/html#admisssions

Application Filing		Accreditation
Earliest:	July 1	CDA
Latest:	November 1	
Fee:	n/av	**Degrees Granted**
AADSAS:	no	DMD, DMD-PhD

Enrollment: 1996–97 First-Year Class

Men:	37	66%	*Mean*	
Women:	19	34%	total GPA:	3.3
Minorities:	4	7%	science GPA:	3.2
Out of State:	1	2%		
With 2 years of college:	0%		*Average*	
With 3 years of college:	3%		DAT academic:	17
			DAT-PAT:	17

Tuition

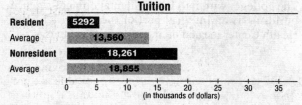

Resident	5292
Average	13,560
Nonresident	18,261
Average	18,855

0   5   10   15   20   25   30   35
(in thousands of dollars)

Percentage receiving financial aid: 86%

Introduction

In 1828 the Medical College of Georgia was established and in 1965 the School of Dentistry was founded. It offers a DMD program and its modern facilities are located in Augusta. The Medical College of Georgia also has schools of Medicine, Nursing, Allied Health, and Graduate Studies. The School of Dentistry has made significant contributions to research in the field.

Admissions

Completion of a minimum of 90 quarter hours of college level work, the basic predental courses, and 2 courses in English are required. A course in biochemistry is recommended. Preference is given to Georgia residents. *Transfer and advanced standing:* Students are not accepted.

Curriculum

4-year flexible. Elementary clinical treatment of patients begins in the first year, including restorative dentistry in the third quarter. Conversely, some basic science courses are not completed until the senior year. Treatment of patients is carried out in a system of comprehensive care, rather than in block assignments, so as to simulate private practice of general dentistry.

Facilities

The school is on the campus of Medical College of Georgia, which is located on the fringe of the downtown area adjacent to a large complex of health-care facilities.

Special Features

A combined DMD-PhD program is offered, requiring 2 additional years of study. Minority students who have been accepted but have recognizable deficiencies can attend a special presession. Students may be provided with tutors, special curricular loads, and self-paced learning packages, if they encounter academic difficulties.

Northwestern University Dental School

240 East Huron, Suite 3415
Chicago, Illinois   60611

Phone: 312-503-8334   *Fax:* 312-503-2499
E-mail: b-witt@nwu.edu
WWW: http://www.nwy.nuds.edu

Application Filing		Accreditation	
Earliest:	June 1	CDA	
Latest:	February 1		
Fee:	$45	**Degrees Granted**	
AADSAS:	yes	DDS, DDS-MS, DDS-PhD	

Enrollment: 1996–97 First-Year Class

			Mean	
Men:	51	67%		
Women:	25	33%	total GPA:	3.3
Minorities:	1	1%	science GPA:	3.3
Out of State:	66	87%		
With 2 years of college:	0%		*Average*	
With 3 years of college:	5%		DAT academic:	19
			DAT-PAT:	19

Tuition

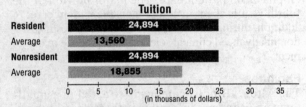

Resident	24,894
Average	13,560
Nonresident	24,894
Average	18,855

0   5   10   15   20   25   30   35
(in thousands of dollars)

Percentage receiving financial aid: 83%

Introduction

Northwestern University is an independent liberal arts school that was established in 1851. The dental school was originally a private school established in 1887 in Chicago, and in 1891 became part of Northwestern University. It is located on the Chicago campus near Lake Michigan. During its formative years, the dental school was led by Dr. G. U. Black, who was instrumental in its formation and is credited with being responsible for the evolution of dentistry from an apprenticeship occupation to a science-based profession. The school's educational program rests on a combination of the traditional and the innovative.

Admissions (AADSAS)

The basic predental science courses plus 1 year of English are required. There is no residency requirement. *Transfer:* May be granted under special circumstances.

Curriculum

4-year flexible. The dental school places strong emphasis on basic and behavioral sciences while primarily focusing on clinical education. Basic science courses are taught in the first and second years through lectures, laboratory experiences, and seminars. Relationships between basic and behavioral sciences and clinical dentistry are emphasized throughout the curriculum. Students are introduced to patient care in the second trimester of the sophomore year through a Sophomore-Senior Match program. Students obtain clinical competence through a combination of assigned clinical rotations and comprehensive patient care. An innovative 3-track curriculum enables students to build a concentration of courses in an area of particular interest to them. Two nonclinical tracks are available for students interested in pursuing research or learning more about practice management. There are also honors programs in orthodontics and implants.

Facilities

The dental school, with approximately 350 DDS and 50 postgraduate students, is in the Gold Coast area of Chicago. The ultramodern Health Science Building houses 283 operatories, fully equipped lecture halls, the junior-senior laboratories, an instrument sterilization facility, and a central laboratory employing professional dental technicians. Also available are preclinical technique labs with 77 dental patient simulator units.

Special Features

Students may participate in extramural clinical experiences, including geriatric programs in metropolitan area nursing homes, the inner city Boy's Club, and a summer program in Colorado working with migrant farmers and their families. The Saturday Morning People's Clinic is a student-run, volunteer program for children of low-income families. Students in all 4 dental school classes participate according to their abilities and expertise.

Southern Illinois University School of Dental Medicine

Building 273
2800 College Avenue, Room 2300
Alton, Illinois   62002

Phone: 618-474-7170   *Fax:* 618-474-7150

Application Filing		Accreditation
Earliest:	July 1	CDA
Latest:	March 1	
Fee:	$20	**Degrees Granted**
AADSAS:	yes	DMD

Enrollment: 1996–97 First-Year Class

Men:	38	76%	*Mean*
Women:	12	24%	total GPA: 3.2
Minorities:	3	6%	science GPA: 3.1
Out of State:	1	2%	
With 2 years of college:		0%	*Average*
With 3 years of college:		18%	DAT academic: 17
			DAT-PAT: 17.8

Tuition

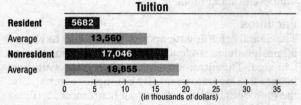

Resident	5682
Average	13,560
Nonresident	17,046
Average	18,855

0 5 10 15 20 25 30 35
(in thousands of dollars)

Percentage receiving financial aid: 86%

Introduction

The Southern Illinois University system is one of 2 university systems in Illinois. There are 2 campuses in the system, 1 in Carbondale, and 1 in Edwardsville. The School of Dental Medicine, which was established in 1969, is located in Alton, Illinois, near both Edwardsville and St. Louis. The unique location of the school places it within the urban environment of metropolitan St. Louis and rural southern Illinois.

Admissions (AADSAS)

The basic predental school courses plus 1 year of English are required. Priority is given to state residents. *Transfer and advanced standing:* An applicant accepted for admission to the first-year class who has advanced training in any discipline listed in the curriculum may request advanced placement.

Curriculum

4-year. The first and second year of the curriculum present to the student biomedical information on the human organism and information necessary to recognize the disease states in humans. In addition, these 2 years are preparation time for clinical dentistry. The students are first involved in direct patient treatment during the second semester of the second year. Year 3 consists of clinical sciences instruction, application-type courses in biomedical sciences, and increasing emphasis on patient care. The major portion of the fourth year is spent in comprehensive patient care; in addition, during this time, the student receives instruction in advanced clinical sciences and practice management.

Facilities

The Alton, Illinois, campus is situated in a small-town environment just minutes from downtown St. Louis, Missouri. The campus includes 22 buildings and a modern, state-of-the art dental clinic. Training is also available in hospital programs, private practices, and community health centers.

Special Features

The school actively encourages applications from persons in those segments of society currently underrepresented in the dental profession.

University of Illinois at Chicago College of Dentistry

801 South Paulina Street
Chicago, Illinois   60612

Phone: 312-996-1020

Application Filing		**Accreditation**
Earliest:	July 1	CDA
Latest:	March 1	
Fee:	$30	**Degrees Granted**
AADSAS:	yes	DDS, DDS-MS, DDS-PhD

Enrollment: 1996–97 First-Year Class

Men:	39	61%	*Mean*	
Women:	25	39%	total GPA:	3.2
Minorities:	2	3%	science GPA:	3
Out of State:	1	2%		
With 2 years of college:	6%		*Average*	
With 3 years of college:	27%		DAT academic:	17
			DAT-PAT:	17

Tuition

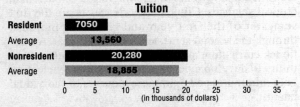

Resident	7050
Average	13,560
Nonresident	20,280
Average	18,855

0   5   10   15   20   25   30   35
(in thousands of dollars)

Percentage receiving financial aid: 80%

Above data applies to 1995-96 academic year.

Introduction

The University of Illinois, a public system that was founded in 1867, is an undergraduate and graduate educational institution. The 2 main campuses are located in Chicago and Urbana-Champaign. The College of Dentistry was originally established in 1898 as the Columbian Dental College and later joined the University of Illinois in 1913. It is located on the University of Illinois Chicago campus. In addition to a DDS degree, it offers postgraduate programs in a variety of specialties as well as MS-PhD degrees through the Graduate College. Other health care institutions associated with the university are colleges of Medicine, Nursing, Pharmacy, Associated Health Professions, and a School of Public Health.

Admissions (AADSAS)

The basic predental science courses plus 1 year of English are required. It is recommended that electives be chosen from the social sciences and humanities, and include at least 1 foreign language. Students interested in practicing in a rural community are encouraged to apply. A minimum GPA of 2.25 is necessary. Very high priority is given to residents. *Transfer and advanced standing:* Students from other U.S. and Canadian dental schools are considered for advanced standing.

Curriculum

4-year traditional. Students are introduced to clinical experience in the first year. From then on, clinical emphasis increases, the fourth year comprising clinical practice almost exclusively.

Facilities

The college is located in the Health Sciences Center of the University of Illinois at Chicago.

Special Features

A combined DDS-MS program, which can usually be completed within the basic 4-year period, is offered. A DDS-PhD program is offered, but requires an additional 2 or 3 years.

INDIANA

Indiana University School of Dentistry

1121 West Michigan Street
Indianapolis, Indiana 46202

Phone: 317-274-8173   *Fax:* 317-274-2419
E-mail: ckacus@iusd,iupui.edu www.iusd,iupui.edu
WWW: http://www.iusd.iupui.edu

Application Filing		Accreditation
Earliest:	June 1	CDA
Latest:	February 1	
Fee:	$30	**Degrees Granted**
AADSAS:	yes	DDS, DDS-PhD

Enrollment: 1996–97 First-Year Class

Men:	66	66%	*Mean*	
Women:	34	34%	total GPA:	3.2
Minorities:	3	3%	science GPA:	3.1
Out of State:	40	40%		
With 2 years of college:	0%		*Average*	
With 3 years of college:	2%		DAT academic:	17.3
			DAT-PAT:	17

Tuition

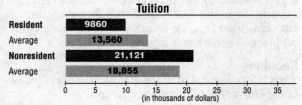

Resident	9860
Average	13,560
Nonresident	21,121
Average	18,855

0   5   10   15   20   25   30   35
(in thousands of dollars)

Percentage receiving financial aid: 88%

Introduction

The Indianapolis campus of Indiana University, established in 1946, is governed by Indiana-Purdue University. The Indiana University School of Dentistry was originally established as the Indiana Dental College in 1879. In 1925 the Dental College joined the university's Medical Center, which includes a medical school, School of Nursing, and a complex of hospitals. Aside from the DDS, the School of Dentistry offers a PhD degree in most departments and has programs in dental hygiene, dental assisting, and dental laboratory technology.

Admissions (AADSAS)

The basic predental science courses as well as courses in English composition, interpersonal communications/speech, and psychology are required. One-semester courses in anatomy (with lab), physiology (with lab), and biochemistry lectures are also required. Minimum GPA for residents is 2.5 and for nonresidents is 2.7.

Curriculum

4-year traditional. Special clinical correlation lectures are scheduled to achieve an integration of basic and clinical sciences. Clinical experiences begin the first semester of the first year and gradually increase through the second semester of the third year. A multitrack curriculum allows the fourth-year student flexibility to develop a personalized program by electing both intramural and extramural courses of individual interest.

Facilities

The school is an integral part of Indiana University's Medical Center. Dental students rotate through hospital-based programs in oral and maxillofacial surgery and pediatric dentistry. They have an opportunity to treat patients who are mentally and physically disabled or medically compromised. Extensive clinical preparation in all disciplines of dentistry is offered throughout the 4-year program.

Special Features

Following admission, an effort is made to assist any student needing financial, academic, or other types of counseling to ensure satisfactory progress toward graduation.

IOWA

University of Iowa College of Dentistry

Dental Building
Iowa City, Iowa   52242

Phone: 319-335-7157   *Fax:* 319-335-7155
E-mail: claine-brown@uiowa.edu
WWW: http://www.uiowa.edu

Application Filing			Accreditation	
Earliest:	June 1		CDA	
Latest:	January 1			
Fee:	$20		**Degrees Granted**	
AADSAS:	yes		DDS	

Enrollment: 1996–97 First-Year Class

Men:	46	62%	*Mean*	
Women:	28	38%	total GPA:	3.1
Minorities:	11	15%	science GPA:	3.2
Out of State:	18	24%		
With 2 years of college:	0%		*Average*	
With 3 years of college:	4%		DAT academic:	18
			DAT-PAT:	17

Tuition

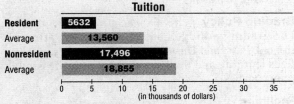

Resident	5632
Average	13,560
Nonresident	17,496
Average	18,855

0   5   10   15   20   25   30   35
(in thousands of dollars)

Percentage receiving financial aid: 93%

Introduction

The University of Iowa was established in 1847 and offers both undergraduate and graduate degrees. The University of Iowa College of Dentistry, established in 1900, is located on the 900-acre campus, through which the Iowa River passes. The school offers postgraduate programs in all dental specialties and master's and PhD degrees, including the NIH-funded Dental Scientist Program.

Admissions (AADSAS)

The applicant's background should include at least 3 years of college work incorporating the basic predental science courses and the English composition, rhetoric, and speech requirements for a bachelor's degree. *Transfer and advanced standing:* All applicants must apply through AADSAS for the first year.

Curriculum

4-year. To achieve a close correlation of the basic sciences with clinical disciplines, students are introduced to clinical situations during the first year. The second-year program continues the basic sciences and technical courses, plus definitive clinical patient treatment. Third-year students rotate through a series of clinical clerkships in each of 8 clinical disciplines. Seniors are involved in the delivery of comprehensive dental care under conditions closely approximating those in private practice.

Facilities

The Dental Science Building is part of the university's health sciences campus, which includes the colleges of Dentistry, Medicine, Nursing, and Pharmacy.

Special Features

The Educational Opportunity Program is available to persons of all races and ethnic backgrounds. It provides both financial and academic assistance to a limited number of students who have experienced environmental, economic, or academic hardships that cause them to compete for admission at a disadvantage because their grade point average and DAT scores do not reflect true ability. Program eligibility must be formally requested by the applicant.

KENTUCKY

University of Kentucky College of Dentistry

800 Rose Street
Medical Center
Lexington, Kentucky   40536

Phone: 606-323-7071   *Fax:* 606-323-1042

Application Filing		Accreditation
Earliest:	June 1	CDA
Latest:	January 1	
Fee:	$25	**Degrees Granted**
AADSAS:	yes	DMD

Enrollment: 1996–97 First-Year Class

Men:	27	52%	*Mean*	
Women:	25	48%	total GPA:	3.2
Minorities:	5	9%	science GPA:	3
Out of State:	16	31%		
With 2 years of college:	0%		*Average*	
With 3 years of college:	11%		DAT academic:	17
			DAT-PAT:	16

Tuition

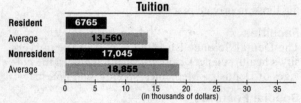

Resident: 6765
Average: 13,560
Nonresident: 17,045
Average: 18,855

(in thousands of dollars)

Percentage receiving financial aid: 88%

Introduction

The University of Kentucky was established in 1865, and has 13 undergraduate and 1 graduate school. The University of Kentucky College of Dentistry was founded in 1962. Postdoctoral programs are offered in most specialties and the school also has strong research and continuing education programs. The College of Dentistry is located in an attractive suburban setting in Lexington.

Admissions (AADSAS)

The UK College of Dentistry seeks to enroll students whose backgrounds, personalities, and motivations indicate that they will make the best possible future dental practioners. As a state institution, the college gives preference to qualified applicants who are residents of Kentucky; however, a limited number of highly qualified out-of-state applicants are considered each year and such candidates are encouraged to apply.

Curriculum

The curriculum is based on a diagonal plan. Basic science courses are taught along with clinical applications throughout the 4-year program, with clinical work intensifying in the third and fourth years. Clinical experiences begin during the fall of the first year and continue as students gain further competence in delivering dental care to patients.

Grading Policy

The grading policy is based on a 3-tier rating of Honors, Pass, and Unsatisfactory. This policy emphasizes learning and the development of professional competencies.

Facilities

The College of Dentistry is an integral part of the University of Kentucky, the Commonwealth's flagship university. The 6-story dentistry building is linked to the University of Kentucky Albert B. Chandler Medical Center, which includes the five colleges—Dentistry, Medicine, Nursing, Pharmacy, and Allied Health—and the university's teaching hospital. The main UK campus is across the street, and downtown Lexington is a 10-minute bus ride away.

Special Features

Financial assistance is available, and the college has a full-time director of this program. Personal and career counseling are also an integral part of the curriculum. Entering students are assigned an advisor who works with them throughout their dental education. Tutorial support services are readily obtained for students needing assistance in developing study skills or mastering content/skill areas.

University of Louisville School of Dentistry

Health Sciences Center
Louisville, Kentucky 40292

Phone: 502-852-5081 *Fax:* 502-852-1210
E-mail: slkenn01
WWW: http://www.ULKYVM.Louisville.edu

Application Filing		Accreditation	
Earliest:	June 1	CDA	
Latest:	February 1		
Fee:	$10	**Degrees Granted**	
AADSAS:	yes	DMD	

Enrollment: 1996–97 First-Year Class

Men:	44	61%	*Mean*	
Women:	28	39%	total GPA:	3.3
Minorities:	5	7%	science GPA:	3.1
Out of State:	26	36%		
With 2 years of college:	0%		*Average*	
With 3 years of college:	6%		DAT academic:	16
			DAT-PAT:	16

Tuition

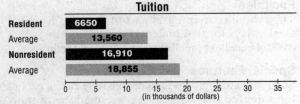

Resident	6650
Average	13,560
Nonresident	16,910
Average	18,855

0 5 10 15 20 25 30 35
(in thousands of dollars)

Percentage receiving financial aid: 96%

Introduction

The University of Louisville was established in 1798. The University of Louisville School of Dentistry was founded in 1887. In addition to the School of Dentistry, other components located in the Health Science Center are the schools of Medicine, Nursing, and Allied Health. Graduates of the school enter general practice or continue their education in a dental specialty of interest.

Admissions (AADSAS)

Applicants are encouraged to have earned 90 semester hours, including 32 credits of science or health-related coursework. The basic predental science courses best meet this requirement. A very limited number of well-qualified out-of-state residents are accepted. *Transfer and advanced standing:* In exceptional situations only.

Curriculum

4-year traditional. The basic and clinical sciences are integrated. Patient contact is initiated in the first year. The majority of electives are usually taken in the fourth year.

Grading Policy

Most grading is by letter grades, but several courses are offered, especially in the clinical program, on a Pass/Fail basis.

Facilities

The school occupies a new building in the Health Sciences Center located in downtown Louisville. The physical plant and all equipment are the most advanced available. Some off-campus programs are also available.

Special Features

An extensive support system of faculty advising, clinical monitoring, and student tutoring serves the needs of all dental students. Counseling services and assistance in developing study skills are also available.

LOUISIANA

Louisiana State University School of Dentistry

1100 Florida Avenue, Building 101
New Orleans, Louisiana   70119

Phone: 504-619-8579   *Fax:* 504-619-8740
E-mail: jweir3lsusd.lsumc.edu

Application Filing		Accreditation	
Earliest:	October 1	CDA	
Latest:	February 28		
Fee:	$50	**Degrees Granted**	
AADSAS:	yes	DDS	

Enrollment: 1996–97 First-Year Class

Men:	33	59%	*Mean*	
Women:	23	41%	total GPA:	3.3
Minorities:	4	8%	science GPA:	3.2
Out of State:	8	14%		
With 2 years of college:	0%		*Average*	
With 3 years of college:	10%		DAT academic:	17
			DAT-PAT:	16

Tuition

Resident	5736
Average	13,560
Nonresident	n/av
Average	18,855

0   5   10   15   20   25   30   35
(in thousands of dollars)

Percentage receiving financial aid: 82%

n/av = not available

Introduction
The Louisiana State University System was created in 1860. The Louisiana State University School of Dentistry was founded in 1968 and is part of the Louisiana State University Medical Center. The teaching facilities in the basic and clinical sciences were dedicated in 1972. In addition to its DDS program, the School of Dentistry provides educational opportunities on the postgraduate level and programs in dental hygiene and dental laboratory technology.

Admissions
The basic predental science courses plus 9 semester hours of English are required. Additional courses in comparative anatomy, histology, and biochemistry are recommended. Priority is given to state residents. A few out-of-state residents may be accepted. *Transfer and advanced standing:* Available.

Curriculum
4-year diagonal. The basic, clinical, and social science courses are presented individually and then interrelated by the free use of correlation courses. As the emphasis on basis and preclinical sciences decreases from year one to year four, the students' exposure to the clinical sciences increases.

Facilities
The school is an integral part of the LSU Medical Center. It is located in dental school buildings that contain excellent preclinical and clinical facilities.

Special Features
Students entering without a degree may earn a bachelor's degree if arrangements are made with their undergraduate school.

MARYLAND

University of Maryland Baltimore College of Dental Surgery

666 West Baltimore Street
Baltimore, Maryland   21201-1586

Phone: 410-706-7472   *Fax:* 410-706-0945
E-mail: wing001@dental3,umabnet.ab.und.edu

Application Filing		Accreditation	
Earliest:	June 1	CDA	
Latest:	February 15		
Fee:	$50	**Degrees Granted**	
AADSAS:	yes	DDS, DDS-PhD	

Enrollment: 1996–97 First-Year Class

Men:	57	41%	*Mean*		
Women:	41	42%	total GPA:	3.2	
Minorities:	36	37%	science GPA:	3.1	
Out of State:	40	41%			
With 2 years of college:		0%	*Average*		
With 3 years of college:		.7%	DAT academic:	18	
			DAT-PAT:	17	

Tuition

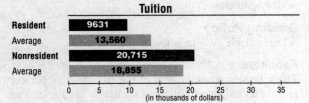

Resident	9631
Average	13,560
Nonresident	20,715
Average	18,855

0   5   10   15   20   25   30   35
(in thousands of dollars)

Percentage receiving financial aid: 63%

Introduction

The University of Maryland System is a public system that was created in 1807. The Baltimore County campus became part of the state university system in 1963. Established in 1840, the dental school at the University of Maryland was the first dental college to exist in the world. The Baltimore College of Dental Surgery is located in the same 32-acre urban campus in downtown Baltimore, as are the schools of Medicine, Pharmacy, Nursing, and Allied Health Professions, as well as Law and Social Work. In 1983 a Center for the Study of Human Performance in Dentistry was established at the school.

Admissions (AADSAS)

Minimum requirements are 8 credits of inorganic chemistry, general biology, organic chemistry, physics, and 6 credits of English. Applicants presenting the minimum science requirements should show better than average performance in these courses. Both science and nonscience majors are encouraged to apply. Nonresidents should have a minimum science GPA of 3.2 and DAT of 18. *Transfer and advanced standing:* Students from other U.S. or Canadian schools may be admitted with advanced standing.

Curriculum

4-year. Integration of biological and clinical sciences takes place by the use of the curriculum unit, "conjoint sciences." Preclinical technical courses employ simulators for realism. Elective basic science courses or clinical clerkship programs may be taken in the senior year. Students are required to complete a research project (essay or table clinic) to fulfill their requirements for graduation.

Facilities

Each student has an individual space during preclinical laboratory instruction and an individual operatory in the clinical years. Training is also provided in affiliated hospitals.

Special Features

Research experience is available at the student's option. A combined DDS-PhD program is also available for qualified applicants. Tutors and a special program are available for those in need of academic assistance while in attendance.

MASSACHUSETTS

Boston University Goldman School of Dental Medicine

100 East Newton Street
Boston, Massachusetts 02118

Phone: 617-638-4787   *Fax:* 617-638-4798
E-mail: busdnadmit@aik.com
WWW: http://www.dental.bu.edu/

Application Filing		Accreditation	
Earliest:	June 1	CDA	
Latest:	March 1		
Fee:	$50	**Degrees Granted**	
AADSAS:	yes	DMD	

Enrollment: 1996–97 First-Year Class

Men:	57	63%	*Mean*
Women:	34	37%	total GPA: 3.1
Minorities:	38	42%	science GPA: 3.1
Out of State:	78	86%	
With 2 years of college:	2%		*Average*
With 3 years of college:	14%		DAT academic: 17
			DAT-PAT: 18

Tuition

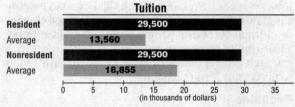

Resident	29,500
Average	13,560
Nonresident	29,500
Average	18,855

(in thousands of dollars)

Percentage receiving financial aid: 53%

Introduction

Boston University has been a private school since 1839. As part of Boston University's Medical Center, the Goldman School of Dental Medicine was established in 1963. Also included in Boston University's Medical Center are the School of Medicine, the University Hospital, the Humphrey Cancer Research Center, and the Cardiovascular Institute.

Admissions (AADSAS)

The basic predental sciences plus 2 years of English and 1 year of mathematics are recommended. Two courses in psychology, sociology or anthropology, and economics are strongly recommended. There are no geographical restrictions on attendance. *Transfer and advanced standing:* Students from other U.S., Canadian, and foreign dental schools are considered for advanced standing.

Curriculum

The DMD program requires 4 years of didactic and clinical study. Students integrate a comprehensive understanding of the science of dentistry with an ability to apply clinical judgment and technique. Courses build a foundation of knowledge and teach the analytical skills needed to apply the knowledge. In addition to required courses and clinical rotations, interested students may choose such electives as hospital dentistry, general anesthesia, otolarynology, and senior seminars.

Grading Policy

A letter grade system is used.

Facilities

The school is a component of the BU Medical Center and its teaching and clinical facilities are located in Boston's south end, along the Charles River. Facilities of affiliated institutions and community-based clinics are also utilized.

Special Features

The APEX Program offers students the opportunity to function as dental interns in affiliated dental practices. This exposure helps prepare students for managing a dental practice.

Harvard School of Dental Medicine

188 Longwood Avenue
Boston, Massachusetts   02115

Phone: 617-432-1443
E-mail: hsdnaoos@warren.med.harvard.edu
WWW: http://www.med.harvard.edu

Application Filing		Accreditation	
Earliest:	July 1	CDA	
Latest:	January 1		
Fee:	$50	**Degrees Granted**	
AADSAS:	yes	DMD, MMSc	

Enrollment: 1996–97 First-Year Class

Men:	12	40%	*Mean*		
Women:	18	60%	total GPA:	3.5	
Minorities:	5	17%	science GPA:	3.5	
Out of State:	27	90%			
With 2 years of college:		n/av	*Average*		
With 3 years of college:		n/av	DAT academic:	22	
			DAT-PAT:	18	

Tuition

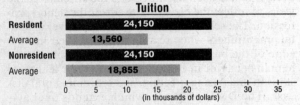

Resident	24,150
Average	13,560
Nonresident	24,150
Average	18,855

0   5   10   15   20   25   30   35
(in thousands of dollars)

Percentage receiving financial aid: 70%

Introduction

Harvard College was established in 1636. Harvard University has 10 graduate schools that were founded later. The Harvard School of Dental Medicine was established in 1867. In 1940 the school was reorganized and given its present name with the aim of placing greater emphasis on the biological base of oral medicine and to institute multidisciplinary programs of dental research.

Admissions (AADSAS)

The basic predental science courses plus 1 year each of calculus and English are required. It is also recommended that 2 or 3 additional advanced science courses be taken, such as biochemistry, physiology, or genetics. There are no specific GPA, DAT, or residency requirements. *Transfer and advanced standing:* Students are not accepted.

Curriculum

4-year program leading to DMD. Dentistry is considered a specialty of medicine. Basic sciences are learned during the first 2 years, by case method, with the medical students in small tutorial groups. Students are also instructed in oral and dental health sciences, doctor/patient relationships, and introductory clinical medicine. The third year is spent mastering the didactic and clinical skills of general dentistry in comprehensive care clinics. During the fourth year students practice dentistry at selected Harvard-affiliated institutions in required and elective externships. Students are also required to perform a research project culminating in a written thesis and oral or poster presentation.

Grading Policy

The Honors/Pass/Fail system is used.

Facilities

Training is obtained at the dental school and the medical school as well as at Harvard-affiliated institutions including Forsyth Dental Center, Massachusetts General Hospital, Children's Hospital, several VA Medical Centers, other Harvard schools, and the Massachusetts Institute of Technology.

Special Features

Students spend the first 2 years in the "New Pathway Curriculum" at Harvard Medical School and continue problem-based learning during their clinical training in dentistry. Externships during the fourth year enable the student to practice dentistry in alternative clinical settings, including dental schools and hospitals in the United States or in foreign countries.

Tufts University School of Dental Medicine

One Kneeland Street
Boston, Massachusetts 02111

Phone: 617-636-6639
E-mail: jenlewis@infonet.tufts.edu

Application Filing		Accreditation	
Earliest:	July 1	CDA	
Latest:	March 1		
Fee:	$50	**Degrees Granted**	
AADSAS:	yes	DMD	

Enrollment: 1996–97 First-Year Class

Men:	89	60%	*Mean*	
Women:	59	40%	total GPA:	3.2
Minorities:	87	59%	science GPA:	3.1
Out of State:	114	77%		
With 2 years of college:	1%		*Average*	
With 3 years of college:	2%		DAT academic:	18
			DAT-PAT:	17

Tuition

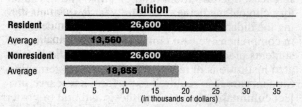

Resident	26,600
Average	13,560
Nonresident	26,600
Average	18,855

0 5 10 15 20 25 30 35
(in thousands of dollars)

Percentage receiving financial aid: 78%

Introduction

Tufts University has 2 undergraduate, and 9 graduate schools. It was originally established in 1852. The School of Dental Medicine was founded in 1868 as the Boston Dental College, which in 1889 joined with Tufts College. The Medical Center includes, in addition to the dental school, the School of Medicine, Sackler School of Graduate Medical Sciences, the School of Veterinary Medicine, and other institutions. In addition to the DMD degree, it offers graduate training in many dental specialties.

Admissions (AADSAS)

The basic predental science courses (but only 1 semester of organic chemistry) plus 1 year of English are required. Courses in histology, comparative anatomy, genetics, biochemistry, physiology, general psychology, mathematics, economics, statistics, and an anthropology course are recommended. A minimum GPA of 3.0 and DAT of 16 are preferred. *Transfer and advanced standing:* Students from other U.S. and foreign dental schools may be considered for advanced standing.

Curriculum

4-year. The curriculum of the School of Dental Medicine has been designed and modified over the years to reflect the changing needs of the dental profession. The school's primary goal is to develop dental practitioners who are able to utilize their knowledge of the basic principles of human biology and human behavior in conjunction with their technical skills in diagnosing, treating, and preventing oral disease. The DMD program, which extends over a 4-year period, consists of a series of didactic, laboratory, and clinical experiences, all of which are programmed to result in the logical development of concepts and skills.

Facilities

The school is located in the Tufts Dental Health Science Building, a 10-story structure located in midtown Boston in the Tufts-New England Medical Center.

Special Features

The school encourages applications by women and minorities.

MICHIGAN

University of Detroit Mercy School of Dentistry

2985 East Jefferson Avenue
Detroit, Michigan   48207

Phone: 313-446-1858   *Fax:* 313-446-1839

Application Filing		Accreditation	
Earliest:	May 1	CDA	
Latest:	March 1		
Fee:	$35	**Degrees Granted**	
AADSAS:	yes	DDS	

Enrollment: 1996–97 First-Year Class

Men:	48	65%	*Mean*	
Women:	26	35%	total GPA:	3.2
Minorities:	10	13%	science GPA:	3.2
Out of State:	20	27%		
With 2 years of college:		4%	*Average*	
With 3 years of college:		19%	DAT academic:	18
			DAT-PAT:	17

Tuition

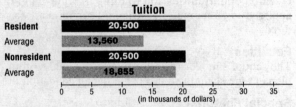

Resident	20,500
Average	13,560
Nonresident	20,500
Average	18,855

0   5   10   15   20   25   30   35
(in thousands of dollars)

Percentage receiving financial aid: 83%

Introduction

Originally established in 1877 as Detroit College, the University of Detroit Mercy is associated with the Jesuits and Sisters of Mercy. It has both undergraduate and graduate programs. The dental school was established in 1932. In 1981 the school opened up a Dental Service at Detroit Receiving Hospital, where students had an opportunity for clinical training. In 1997 the school expects to relocate to a new facility in northwest Detroit that will allow for state-of-the-art teaching and patient care. In addition to a DDS degree, the school offers postgraduates studies and a dental hygiene program.

Admissions (AADSAS)

The basic predental science courses plus a course in English are required. Recommended courses include comparative anatomy, histology, biochemistry, and psychology. No priority is given to state residents. *Transfer and advanced standing:* Foreign dental graduates as well as those attending U.S. and Canadian schools are considered.

Curriculum

4-year traditional. Clinical experience begins on a limited basis during the first year and extends through the second year. Approximately one half the time during the last 2 years is devoted to clinical dentistry, which is taught principally by a combination of the "block system" and comprehensive patient care method.

Facilities

The school is located in downtown Detroit and contains well-equipped dental clinics and laboratories. It has embarked on the construction of a new dental teaching and patient care facility located in northwest Detroit. Clinical facilities will consist of 147 fully equipped dental units. In addition, dental students provide patient care at the University of Detroit Mercy, Dental Service at Detroit Receiving Hospital located in the Detroit Medical Care Center. Students also rotate on assignments through various satellite clinics and participate in programs in local nursing homes, providing care utilizing portable equipment.

Special Features

Women and members of minority groups are encouraged to apply.

University of Michigan School of Dentistry

1234 Dental Building
Ann Arbor, Michigan 48109

Phone: 313-763-3316
WWW: http://www.dent.umich.edu

Application Filing		Accreditation	
Earliest:	May 1	CDA	
Latest:	February 1		
Fee:	$50	**Degrees Granted**	
AADSAS:	yes	DDS	

Enrollment: 1996–97 First-Year Class

Men:	53	52%	*Mean*
Women:	48	48%	total GPA: 3.4
Minorities:	38	38%	science GPA: 3
Out of State:	40	40%	
With 2 years of college:	0%	*Average*	
With 3 years of college:	9%	DAT academic: 18
		DAT-PAT: 17

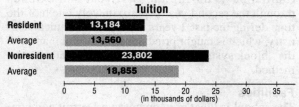

Tuition

Resident	13,184
Average	13,560
Nonresident	23,802
Average	18,855

(in thousands of dollars)

Percentage receiving financial aid: 75%

Introduction
The University of Michigan System was founded in 1817. The University of Michigan at Ann Arbor is on the main campus, which was founded that same year. Other campuses of the university are located in Dearborn and Flint. Aside from the DDS degree program, the dental school offers programs leading to specialty certification and a master of science degree, as well as dental hygiene and continuing education courses.

Admissions (AADSAS)
The basic predental science courses plus a year of English composition are required. Biochemistry and comparative anatomy courses are highly recommended, and exposure to non-science courses is encouraged. While preference is given to Michigan residents, 36% of the class are nonresidents. *Transfer and advanced standing:* Possible within the first 2 years.

Curriculum
4-year stepped, trimester-based. Clinical training emphasizing comprehensive patient care begins in the first year and is closely integrated with supporting basic science and preclinical courses. Student research opportunities and training in wide-ranging application of computer-assisted information are featured.

Facilities
The school's modern quarters were designed to complement the changing concepts in dental education.

Special Features
Substantial research facilities, faculty, and activities in basic and applied sciences are features of the school. Women, veterans, and minority group members are encouraged to apply. A summer enrichment program for entering students and students who apply to dental school is offered. Academic counseling and tutorial assistance are available.

University of Minnesota School of Dentistry

515 S.E. Delaware Street
Minneapolis, Minnesota 55455

Phone: 612-624-6960   *Fax:* 612-626-2654
E-mail: bolan005@maroon.tc.umn.edu

Application Filing		Accreditation	
Earliest:	June 1	CDA	
Latest:	March 1		
Fee:	$50	**Degrees Granted**	
AADSAS:	yes	DDS	

Enrollment: 1996–97 First-Year Class

Men:	57	66%	*Mean*	
Women:	29	34%	total GPA:	3.3
Minorities:	7	8%	science GPA:	3.4
Out of State:	29	34%		
With 2 years of college:	0%		*Average*	
With 3 years of college:	7%		DAT academic:	18
			DAT-PAT:	18

Tuition

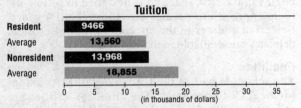

Resident	9466
Average	13,560
Nonresident	13,968
Average	18,855

0   5   10   15   20   25   30   35
(in thousands of dollars)

Percentage receiving financial aid: 73%

Introduction

The University of Minnesota was established in 1851 and took over the Minnesota College Hospital in 1888, establishing its own Department of Medicine. The Dental School, originally a part of this department, became separated in 1892, and in 1932 became known as the School of Dentistry. The school is a component of the University Health Center, which also contains schools of Medicine, Pharmacy, Nursing, and Public Health. The School of Dentistry offers postgraduate training in the dental specialties and has a dental hygiene program.

Admissions (AADSAS)

The basic predental science courses and 1 year of English, 1 course in psychology, and mathematics (at least through college algebra) are required. Other recommended courses include speech, art (such as basic drawing and sculpturing), cell biology, histology, gross anatomy, and biochemistry. Strong preference is given to Minnesota residents, but residents from Montana, North and South Dakota, Manitoba, and Wisconsin also are given special consideration. *Transfer and advanced standing:* Opportunities are extremely limited.

Curriculum

4-year. The basic sciences are taught throughout the first 3 years. Integration is accomplished by offering clinically oriented phases of the basic sciences. The students begin their clinical experience in oral radiology and occlusion during the first year in school. Some electives are offered during the second year, but most are taken during the last year.

Facilities

The school is part of the University Health Center. Its facilities are located in an up-to-date health science building. Off-campus facilities of the Hennepin County Medical Center and VA Hospital are also utilized.

Special Features

Academic counseling and tutorial assistance are available to students in need.

MISSISSIPPI

University of Mississippi School of Dentistry

2500 North State Street
Jackson, Mississippi 39216

Phone: 601-984-6009   *Fax:* 601-984-6014
E-mail: brownjc@fiona.umsmed.edu

Application Filing		Accreditation	
Earliest:	July 1	CDA	
Latest:	December 1		
Fee:	$25	**Degrees Granted**	
AADSAS:	yes	DMD	

Enrollment: 1996–97 First-Year Class

Men:	22	71%	*Mean*	
Women:	9	29%	total GPA:	3.5
Minorities:	0	0%	science GPA:	3.4
Out of State:	0	0%		
With 2 years of college:		0%	*Average*	
With 3 years of college:		3%	DAT academic:	16
			DAT-PAT:	16

Tuition

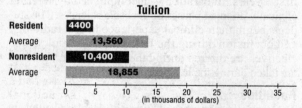

Resident	4400
Average	13,560
Nonresident	10,400
Average	18,855

0   5   10   15   20   25   30   35
(in thousands of dollars)

Percentage receiving financial aid: 89%

Introduction

The University of Mississippi is a public school that was established in 1844. The University of Mississippi School of Dentistry, located in the Medical Center, enrolled its first class in 1975. In addition to the School of Dentistry, the University of Mississippi Medical Center contains the schools of Medicine, Nursing, and Health-Related Professions, Graduate Studies in the Medical Sciences, and the University Hospital. The goal of the school is to train general dentists to practice in Mississippi.

Admissions

The basic predental science courses plus 2 years of English, 1 year each of mathematics and behavioral sciences, and 1 semester of advanced biology or chemistry are required. Recommended courses include biochemistry, comparative anatomy, histology, cell biology, humanities, communication, and a foreign language. Currently, only legal Mississippi residents are admitted. *Transfer and advanced standing:* Only a few students are admitted with advanced standing.

Curriculum

4-year traditional. A systems approach to a problem-oriented curriculum is used. Clinical experience begins in the first year and is designed to follow the team approach to patient care through all 4 years. Selective courses in the specialty areas of clinical dentistry are available in the last year.

Facilities

The school is part of the University of Mississippi Medical Center campus. The clinical facilities are self-contained in the dental school building.

Special Features

By making proper arrangements, students entering without a degree may earn their bachelor's degree while completing the dental program.

MISSOURI

University of Missouri—Kansas City School of Dentistry

650 East 25th Street
Kansas City, Missouri   64108

Phone: 816-235-2080   *Fax:* 816-235-2157

Application Filing		Accreditation	
Earliest:	June 1	CDA	
Latest:	January 1		
Fee:	$25	**Degrees Granted**	
AADSAS:	yes	DDS	

Enrollment: 1996–97 First-Year Class

Men:	36	62%	*Mean*	
Women:	22	38%	total GPA:	3.3
Minorities:	6	10%	science GPA:	3.2
Out of State:	29	50%		
With 2 years of college:	9%		*Average*	
With 3 years of college:	6%		DAT academic:	17
			DAT-PAT:	17

Tuition

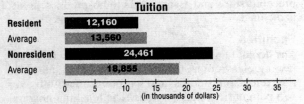

Resident	12,160
Average	13,560
Nonresident	24,461
Average	18,855

0   5   10   15   20   25   30   35
(in thousands of dollars)

Percentage receiving financial aid: 83%

Introduction

The University of Missouri system is public with 4 campuses. Besides Kansas City, campuses are located in Columbia, Rolla, and St. Louis. In 1919 the Kansas City Dental College joined the Western Dental College to become the Kansas City Western Dental College. In 1941 the name changed to the School of Dentistry of the University of Kansas City. The school did not become part of the state university system till 1963. In addition to the DDS degree, the School of Dentistry offers a postdoctoral program leading to a Dental Specialty Certificate and BS in dental hygiene.

Admissions (AADSAS)

A minimum of 2 years of predental education is required as well as attainment of other academic and nonacademic criteria. *Transfer and advanced standing:* Students wishing to transfer from another dental school are considered, assuming availability of positions in the appropriate class.

Curriculum

4-year; 8 semesters plus 2 summer terms (13 weeks each). Emphasis is on preventive and comprehensive dentistry. The student is introduced to clinical procedures during the first year and progresses to the comprehensive treatment of patients during the third and fourth years in a team clinical setting.

Facilities

The school is located in midtown Kansas City. It maintains affiliations with 6 hospitals in the area. It has 2 dental production laboratories in-house and a full-service library with an extensive instructional materials component.

Special Features

A wide range of personal and/or academic assistance, such as tutoring and counseling, is available as needed.

NEBRASKA

Creighton University School of Dentistry

2500 California Street
Omaha, Nebraska   68178

Phone: 402-280-2965   *Fax:* 402-280-5094
E-mail: fayer@bluejay.creighton.edu
WWW: http://www.creighton.edu

Application Filing		Accreditation	
Earliest:	July 1	CDA	
Latest:	March 1		
Fee:	$35	**Degrees Granted**	
AADSAS:	yes	DDS	

Enrollment: 1996–97 First-Year Class

Men:	57	68%	*Mean*
Women:	27	32%	total GPA:	3.3
Minorities:	5	6%	science GPA:	3.1
Out of State:	73	87%	
With 2 years of college:		0%	*Average*
With 3 years of college:		12%	DAT academic:	18
			DAT-PAT:	18

Tuition

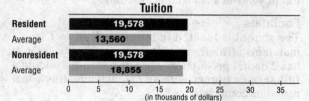

Resident	19,578
Average	13,560
Nonresident	19,578
Average	18,855

0   5   10   15   20   25   30   35
(in thousands of dollars)

Percentage receiving financial aid: 92%

Introduction

Creighton University, a private Catholic school, was established in 1878 but its health science programs did not begin until much later. The Creighton University School of Dentistry was created in 1905. The present dental facility was completed in 1977. In addition to its DDS program, the School of Dentistry, in cooperation with several local junior colleges, is involved in the training of dental auxiliaries. Creighton also has schools of Medicine, Pharmacy, Nursing, and Allied Health Professions.

Admissions (AADSAS)

The basic predental science courses plus 1 year of English are required. Recommended courses include psychology, modern languages, history, speech, economics, and comparative anatomy. The school has admission agreements with Idaho, New Mexico, Utah, and Wyoming. *Transfer and advanced standing:* Students from other U.S. and Canadian dental schools are considered for advanced standing.

Curriculum

4-year traditional. Basic and clinical sciences are coordinated by the Department of Oral Biology. Clinical experience begins in the second year. A variety of electives are available in the fourth year. Off-campus clinical opportunities include private practice preceptorships and assignments to hospitals, schools, and clinics.

Facilities

The dental facility is a modern, 3-level structure containing classrooms, teaching and research laboratories, television studios, and various clinics with over 175 patient treatment stations. The teaching hospital offers additional clinical facilities.

Special Features

Financial assistance to minority, disadvantaged, and other traditionally underrepresented students in addition to that available to all students varies from year to year.

University of Nebraska Medical Center College of Dentistry

40th and Holdrege Streets
Lincoln, Nebraska   68583

Phone: 402-472-1363

Application Filing		**Accreditation**
Earliest:	July 1	CDA
Latest:	February 1	
Fee:	$25	**Degrees Granted**
AADSAS:	yes	DDS

Enrollment: 1996–97 First-Year Class

Men:	36	84%	*Mean*
Women:	7	16%	total GPA: 3.5
Minorities:	1	3%	science GPA: 3.4
Out of State:	8	19%	
With 2 years of college:	0%		*Average*
With 3 years of college:	8%		DAT academic: 17
			DAT-PAT: 17

Tuition

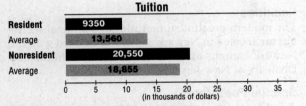

Resident	9350
Average	13,560
Nonresident	20,550
Average	18,855

0   5   10   15   20   25   30   35
(in thousands of dollars)

Percentage receiving financial aid: 73%

Above data applies to 1995–96 academic year.

Introduction

The University of Nebraska system was founded in 1869, and has campuses in Kearney, Lincoln, and Omaha. The Lincoln Dental College was established in 1899. Less than 20 years later it became a part of the University of Nebraska system and is known as the University of Nebraska College of Dentistry. The school is located on the Lincoln campus. Postgraduate programs are offered in many specialties and a graduate program that leads to the MS degree is available.

Admissions (AADSAS)

The basic predental science courses plus 1 year of English are required. The college has no specific requirements regarding the absolute minimal scholastic average or DAT scores. Priority is given to applicants from Nebraska, North Dakota, and Wyoming. *Transfer and advanced standing:* Transfer is possible but advanced standing is not.

Curriculum

4-year traditional. The basic sciences are taught by the team method. Students are introduced to clinical observation and personal participation during the first year. Patients are assigned and clinical activity is amplified in the sophomore year. Integration of the basic and clinical sciences is emphasized. Electives may be taken during the senior year. Off-campus clinical experience is possible.

Facilities

Modern preclinical and clinical facilities exist in Lincoln. Hospital affiliations provide opportunities for additional clinical experience. A learning center is available in association with the school library.

Special Features

Counseling is accessible to underrepresented minority applicants.

NEW JERSEY

New Jersey Dental School University of Medicine and Dentistry

110 Bergen Street
Newark, New Jersey   07103

Phone: 201-982-5063
E-mail: lamettjw@umdnj.edu

Application Filing		Accreditation	
Earliest:	June 1	CDA	
Latest:	February 1		
Fee:	$125	**Degrees Granted**	
AADSAS:	yes	DMD, DMD-PhD	

Enrollment: 1996–97 First-Year Class

Men:	39	52%	*Mean*	
Women:	36	48%	total GPA:	3.1
Minorities:	13	17%	science GPA:	3.1
Out of State:	10	0%		
With 2 years of college:		0%	*Average*	
With 3 years of college:		3%	DAT academic:	17
			DAT-PAT:	16

Tuition

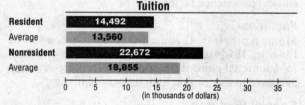

Resident	14,492
Average	13,560
Nonresident	22,672
Average	18,855

0   5   10   15   20   25   30   35
(in thousands of dollars)

Percentage receiving financial aid: 92%

Introduction

The New Jersey Dental School at the University of Medicine and Dentistry opened in 1956. It became part of the University of Medicine and Dentistry of New Jersey in 1970. In addition to a DMD degree, the school offers graduate dental education specialty programs leading toward a certificate. Also offered are programs in advance education in general dentistry, a general practice residency, and a fellowship in oral medicine.

Admissions (AADSAS)

The basic predental science courses and 1 year of English are required. A strong background in the natural and biological sciences is necessary. Preference is given to state residents. *Transfer and advanced standing:* Considered only on a space available basis.

Curriculum

4-year flexible. Some basic science instruction continues beyond the second year. Clinical activity begins with an introduction to clinical dentistry in the first year. In the next year students are rotated through clinical departments in a structured manner. During the last year a student may select a portion of his or her program from clinical courses or research.

Facilities

The modern preclinical facilities and clinical facilities are located in Newark and are associated with the Newark campus of the University of Medicine and Dentistry of New Jersey.

Special Features

A Students for Dentistry Program, consisting of 8 weeks of academic work, was established to aid in the recruitment and preparation of disadvantaged students for dental school.

NEW YORK

Columbia University School of Dental and Oral Surgery

630 West 168 Street
New York, New York 10032

Phone: 212-305-3478 *Fax:* 212-305-1034
E-mail: emw5@columbia.edu

Application Filing		Accreditation
Earliest:	July 1	CDA
Latest:	March 1	
Fee:	$50	**Degrees Granted**
AADSAS:	yes	DDS, DDS-MPH

Enrollment: 1996–97 First-Year Class

Men:	45	64%	*Mean*	
Women:	25	36%	total GPA:	3
Minorities:	7	10%	science GPA:	3
Out of State:	46	66%		
With 2 years of college:	0%		*Average*	
With 3 years of college:	1%		DAT academic:	21
			DAT-PAT:	18

Tuition

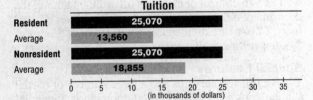

Resident	25,070
Average	13,560
Nonresident	25,070
Average	18,855

0 5 10 15 20 25 30 35
(in thousands of dollars)

Percentage receiving financial aid: 96%

Introduction

Founded in 1754, Columbia University is a private higher educational system. In 1852 the School of Dental and Oral Surgery was established, and in 1923 it merged with the dental school at Columbia University, the New York Postgraduate School of Dentistry, and the New York School of Dental Hygiene, to become the Columbia University School of Dental and Oral Surgery that exists today. The school has, in addition to its DDS program, postdoctoral and continuing education programs.

Admissions (AADSAS)

The basic predental science courses plus 1 additional year of English composition and literature are required. Courses in chemistry, biochemistry, mathematics, foreign languages, sociology, history, and the fine industrial arts are recommended. There is no residency requirement.

Curriculum

4-year traditional. Emphasis is placed on an understanding of broad biomedical principles integrated with clinical dentistry. Initially, students are exposed to the full spectrum of dental problems as observers; subsequently, they are introduced to surgical and manipulative procedures and to methods of diagnosis and prevention. Clinical training is broad in scope. All basic science courses are taken jointly with the medical students of the College of Physicians and Surgeons, during years one and two.

Facilities

The school is an integral part of the Columbia Presbyterian Medical Center within which it occupies 3 floors. These house clinics, research facilities, faculty offices, and student facilities.

Special Features

A combined DDS-MPH is available to selected students, as well as the possibility of completing an MA in research and educational administration.

New York University College of Dentistry

David B. Kriser Dental Center
345 East 24 Street
New York, New York   10010

Phone: 212-998-9818   *Fax:* 212-995-4240
E-mail: bellm@nyudent2.nyu.edu
WWW: http://www.nyu.dent.edu

Application Filing		Accreditation	
Earliest:	open	CDA	
Latest:	open		
Fee:	$35	**Degrees Granted**	
AADSAS:	yes	DDS	

Enrollment: 1996–97 First-Year Class

Men:	123	61%	*Mean*	
Women:	79	39%	total GPA:	3.3
Minorities:	80	40%	science GPA:	3
Out of State:	108	53%		
With 2 years of college:		0%	*Average*	
With 3 years of college:		6%	DAT academic:	18.1
			DAT-PAT:	16.5

Tuition

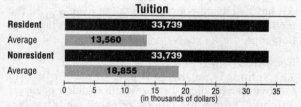

Resident	33,739
Average	13,560
Nonresident	33,739
Average	18,855

(in thousands of dollars)

Percentage receiving financial aid: 93%

Introduction

New York University opened in 1831. It is a private school with 7 undergraduate and 7 graduate schools. In 1865 the New York University College of Dentistry was established. In addition to the DDS degree, it offers bachelor's and associate degrees in dental hygiene and has a dental assistant training program as well as postgraduate and specialty training. There is also a continuing dental education program, an advanced standing program for foreign trained dentists, a program for advanced study in dentistry, dental specialties for international graduates, and an MS degree program in oral biology.

Admissions (AADSAS)

Students with a GPA of 3.5 or higher may be admitted with 90 credits including all prerequisite courses. A BA or BS degree is required from an approved college or university. Graduate dentists from foreign dental schools may qualify for our Advanced Standing Program for Foreign-Trained Dentists. This is a three-year program that culminates in a DDS degree from NYUCD. Out-of-state residents are admitted. *Transfer and advanced standing:* Students who have completed graduate-level courses in the basic sciences or preclinical courses may be admitted with advanced standing.

Curriculum

4-year continuum leading to a DDS. All core subjects are completed in the first 3 years of study. Students have 3 full years of clinical experiences. Emphasis is on clinical practice and research. An innovative fourth year is spent in a Comprehensive Care and Applied Practice Administration group practice in which the senior student spends the entire year in a private officelike setting.

Facilities

The Kriser Dental Center comprises 2 contiguous 11-story buildings. The Weissman Clinical Science Building and the Schwartz Hall of Dental Sciences house all the basic science and research departments as well as 576 clinical operatories (distributed among the departments) devoted to the various disciplines of dentistry. Classes are divided into small learning groups of 8 or fewer for closely supervised proactive instruction.

Special Features

Twelve full scholarships and a large number of partial scholarships are awarded based upon merit. Financial aid (loans and NYU grant scholarships) is available for those who demonstrate need. Early applications are recommended for those who seek financial aid and all types of scholarships.

State University of New York at Buffalo
School of Dental Medicine

Farber Hall
3435 Main Street
Buffalo, New York 14214-3008

Phone: 716-829-2839

Application Filing		Accreditation
Earliest:	July 1	CDA
Latest:	February 15	
Fee:	$50	**Degrees Granted**
AADSAS:	yes	DDS, DDS-PhD

Enrollment: 1996–97 First-Year Class

Men:	59	69%	*Mean*	
Women:	26	31%	total GPA:	3.2
Minorities:	0	0%	science GPA:	3.2
Out of State:	5	6%		
With 2 years of college:		0%	*Average*	
With 3 years of college:		4%	DAT academic:	18
			DAT-PAT:	18

Tuition

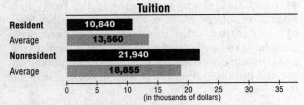

Resident	10,840
Average	13,560
Nonresident	21,940
Average	18,855

(in thousands of dollars)

Percentage receiving financial aid: n/av

Introduction

As 1 of 2 public university systems in the state, the State University of New York was founded in 1948. The State University of New York at Buffalo was created in 1846. In 1962 the Buffalo campus joined the state university system. The School of Dental Medicine was created in 1892 and is now part of the Health Science Center, which includes schools of Medicine, Nursing, Biomedical Sciences, and Health-Related Professions.

Admissions (AADSAS)

The basic predental courses are required. Courses in microbiology, biochemistry, physiology, computer science, and statistics are recommended. DATs should be taken no later than October of the year before the applicant wishes to matriculate. Preference is given to New York State residents. Applicants are strongly encouraged to seek a clinical experience in dentistry prior to applying. Students from other dental schools may be considered for transfer with advanced standing into the second year program.

Curriculum

4-year. Clinical science studies begin in the first year; students start to provide patient care in the second semester of the freshman year. Integration of the basic and clinical sciences is accomplished in all the clinical courses but is particularly emphasized in such courses as oral biology, oral diagnosis, and oral pathology. In the senior year, students take elective courses in area(s) of their choice.

Facilities

The School of Dental Medicine is one of 5 schools that compose the Health Science Center. In the summer of 1986 the school was moved to new facilities in the renovated Squire Hall. They include 325 dental units for instructional purposes, new preclinical laboratories, and new basic science and clinical science research facilities. It is one of the most modern facilities of its kind in the country.

Special Features

Modest class size (86 students) and modern patient care facility. Easy patient access to school clinics. Extensive student summer research program in both basic sciences and clinical sciences.

State University of New York at Stony Brook School of Dental Medicine

Rockland Hall
Stony Brook, New York   11794

Phone: 516-632-8780   *Fax:* 516-632-9105
E-mail: suny@stonybrookschoolofdentalmed

Application Filing		Accreditation	
Earliest:	July 1	CDA	
Latest:	January 15		
Fee:	$75	**Degrees Granted**	
AADSAS:	yes	DDS	

Enrollment: 1996–97 First-Year Class

Men:	17	53%	*Mean*	
Women:	15	47%	total GPA:	3.3
Minorities:	0	0%	science GPA:	3.3
Out of State:	0	0%		
With 2 years of college:		0%	*Average*	
With 3 years of college:		18%	DAT academic:	18
			DAT-PAT:	16

Tuition

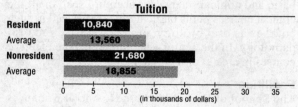

Resident	10,840
Average	13,560
Nonresident	21,680
Average	18,855

0   5   10   15   20   25   30   35
(in thousands of dollars)

Percentage receiving financial aid: 100%

Introduction

Stony Brook, established in 1957, is 1 of the 4 universities in the state education system. The School of Dental Medicine was founded in 1973 and is located 60 miles east of New York City on the north shore of Long Island. The school is a component of the Health Sciences Center, which also includes schools of Medicine, Nursing, Health Technology, and Social Welfare. The school offers postgraduate dental programs in orthodontics, periodontics, an advanced education in general dentistry program, and a program for dental care for the developmentally disabled.

Admissions (AADSAS)

All applicants are required to complete the appropriate predental science courses prior to admission to the school. One year of mathematics (preferably calculus or statistics), and 1 year of social and behavioral sciences are strongly recommended. Strong preference is given to New York State residents. *Transfer and advanced standing:* Students from other U.S. and Canadian dental schools, as well as holders of a PhD in one of the basic sciences, may be considered for advanced standing.

Curriculum

4-year. Clinical science begins in the first year. Emphasis is placed on the restorative dental procedures by early introduction of students to patient care. Integration of basic and clinical sciences is emphasized and is especially evident in the courses in oral biology and oral pathology. Elective courses are available in the fourth year.

Facilities

The school is 1 of 5 making up the Health Sciences Center. Clinical campus-affiliated hospitals are the Long Island Jewish Medical Center, the Northport VA Hospital, and the Nassau County Medical Center.

Special Features

The school encourages applications from individuals from those groups that have been underrepresented in the dental profession in the past or that have been socioeconomically deprived.

NORTH CAROLINA

University of North Carolina School of Dentistry

105 Brauer Hall, 211H
Chapel Hill, North Carolina   27511

Phone: 919-966-4565   *Fax:* 919-966-7007
E-mail: wtrapp.dentce@mhs.unc.edu
WWW: http://www.dent.unc.edu

Application Filing		Accreditation	
Earliest:	June 15	CDA	
Latest:	November 1		
Fee:	$60	**Degrees Granted**	
AADSAS:	yes	DDS, DDS-PhD, DDS-MPH	

Enrollment: 1996–97 First-Year Class

Men:	34	45%	*Mean*		
Women:	42	55%	total GPA:	3.3	
Minorities:	5	7%	science GPA:	3.3	
Out of State:	12	16%			
With 2 years of college:	0%		*Average*		
With 3 years of college:	7%		DAT academic:	18	
			DAT-PAT:	17	

Tuition

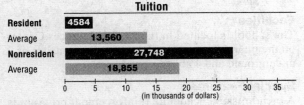

Resident	4584
Average	13,560
Nonresident	27,748
Average	18,855

0   5   10   15   20   25   30   35
(in thousands of dollars)

Percentage receiving financial aid: 85%

Introduction

The University of North Carolina system was founded in 1931 and has campuses in Asheville, Chapel Hill, Greensboro, and Wilmington. The University of North Carolina at Chapel Hill was the first state university created in the United States when it was established in 1789. In 1949 the School of Dentistry was created and is considered a part of the Division of Health Affairs. Other schools in the division include the schools of Nursing, Pharmacy, and Public Health. The School of Dentistry offers graduate training in many disciplines and a master's degree in dental hygiene, which prepares graduates for teaching careers.

Admissions (AADSAS)

The basic predental science courses plus 2 semesters of English are required. Students should complete the regular 4-year curriculum leading to the AB or BS degree. Students not pursuing a degree should complete at least 3 years of accredited college courses (96 semester hours or 144 quarter hours). A maximum of 64 semester hours credit will be accepted from a 2-year community college, and all additional coursework must be completed at a 4-year institution. Foreign trained dentists must enter as first-year students and must submit acceptable scores on the Test of English as a Foreign Language (TOEFL), satisfactory scores on the DAT, and/or acceptable scores on Part I of the National Board Dental Examination. *Transfer and advanced standing:* Transfers are considered on an individual basis. Factors considered will be prior academic record and background, available space in the class, consistency between the curriculum of the 2 schools, and residency status.

Curriculum

The goal is to produce dental practitioners qualified to enter general practice, and provide advanced educational programs, research, teaching and/or public service. The first year is highlighted by basic science and dental science courses with participation in preventive patient care activities. During the remaining years, primary emphasis is on the management and delivery of comprehensive care for a family of assigned patients. Patient care activities are supplemented by didactic experiences and numerous enrichment opportunities such as electives, externships, and research.

Grading Policy

The traditional letter grading system is used, but some courses are graded Pass/Fail.

Facilities

The school consists of the original dental school building, Braver Hall, and a dental research center. A basic science building and the Division of Health Sciences provide direct support to the programs. A Learning Resources Center is also available. A new clinical facility is under construction.

Special Features

Both DDS-MPH and DDS-PhD degrees are offered and require additional time.

OHIO

Case Western Reserve University School of Dentistry

2123 Abingdon Road
Cleveland, Ohio   44106

Phone: 216-368-2460   *Fax:* 216-368-3204
E-mail: dad4@po.cwru.edu

Application Filing		Accreditation	
Earliest:	June 1	CDA	
Latest:	March 1		
Fee:	$35	**Degrees Granted**	
AADSAS:	yes	DDS, DDS-MBA	

Enrollment: 1996–97 First-Year Class

Men:	43	63%	*Mean*	
Women:	19	31%	total GPA:	3.1
Minorities:	11	17%	science GPA:	3
Out of State:	4	6%		
With 2 years of college:	1%		*Average*	
With 3 years of college:	6%		DAT academic:	18
			DAT-PAT:	17

Tuition

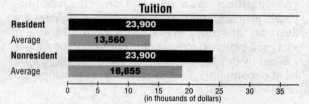

Resident	23,900
Average	13,560
Nonresident	23,900
Average	18,855

0   5   10   15   20   25   30   35
(in thousands of dollars)

Percentage receiving financial aid: 85%

Introduction

Case Western Reserve University was established in 1826. It is a private school with 4 undergraduate and 7 graduate schools. The Case Western Reserve University School of Dentistry was established in 1892 as the dental department of the university. In 1969 the school's facilities were relocated to the Health Sciences Center of the university. Included in the center are the schools of Medicine and Nursing, and University Hospitals of Cleveland.

Admissions (AADSAS)

The basic predental science courses plus 1 year each of English and mathematics are required. Recommended courses include comparative anatomy, developmental biology, genetics, cell biology, and/or biochemistry. A substantial number of out-of-state residents are admitted. *Transfer and advanced standing:* Students from other U.S. dental schools may be admitted with advanced standing.

Curriculum

4-year traditional. Clinical experience is introduced early in the program. Recent curriculum innovations include an integrative experience in preclinical procedures basic to restorative dentistry, and experience in the use of dental auxiliaries and in the comprehensive care concept. A number of multidisciplinary subjects are taught.

Facilities

The school is located in the Health Sciences Center on the main campus. The dental facility consists of 2 underground and 4 aboveground levels.

Special Features

A preadmission academic reinforcement program is available for minority students.

Ohio State University College of Dentistry

305 West 12th Avenue
Columbus, Ohio   43210

Phone: 614-292-3361   *Fax:* 614-292-7619
E-mail: Rowland.3@osu.edu

Application Filing			Accreditation	
Earliest:	July 1		CDA	
Latest:	February 1			
Fee:	$125		**Degrees Granted**	
AADSAS:	yes		DDS, DDS-MS	

Enrollment: 1996–97 First-Year Class

Men:	66	67%	*Mean*	
Women:	32	33%	total GPA:	3.4
Minorities:	23	23%	science GPA:	3.2
Out of State:	15	15%		
With 2 years of college:	2%		*Average*	
With 3 years of college:	10%		DAT academic:	17
			DAT-PAT:	17

Tuition

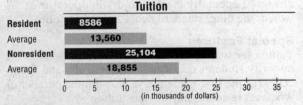

Resident	8586
Average	13,560
Nonresident	25,104
Average	18,855

0   5   10   15   20   25   30   35
(in thousands of dollars)

Percentage receiving financial aid: 90%

Introduction

The Ohio State University system was established in 1870; the Columbus campus was created in the same year. In 1925 the Ohio State University College of Dentistry moved to Columbus after its beginning as part of Ohio Medical University in 1890. Ohio Medical University joined the Starling Medical College in 1906 and became a component of Ohio State in 1914. The College of Dentistry is located in the Health Sciences Center, which also includes the College of Medicine and Biological Sciences and School of Nursing and Allied Health Sciences.

Admissions (AADSAS)

The basic predental science courses and 1 year of English composition or literature are required. A minimum of 20 documented hours of observation in a general dental office is required. *Transfer and advanced standing:* Students from other U.S. schools may be admitted with advanced standing.

Curriculum

4-year traditional. Clinical experience begins after the first year and a half. The basic and clinical sciences are integrated during both coursework and practice sessions. Ten percent of the senior year must be devoted to electives. Off-campus clinical experience is available at hospitals and clinics.

Facilities

The school is located in the Health Sciences Center on the main campus in a 5-story building. Dental clinics are also located in University and Children's Hospitals and in Nisonger Center. City Health Department clinics, VA hospitals, and state institutions also offer facilities for student training.

Special Features

Tutorial and financial assistance are available to qualified women, minorities, and disadvantaged students. A combined DDS-MS degree is offered, but requires additional time.

OKLAHOMA

University of Oklahoma College of Dentistry

P.O. Box 26901
Oklahoma City, Oklahoma   73190

Phone: 405-271-3530   *Fax:* 405-271-3423
E-mail: kevin-avery@uokhsc.edu

Application Filing
Earliest: July 1
Latest: December 1
Fee: $50
AADSAS: yes

Accreditation
CDA

Degrees Granted
DDS

Enrollment: 1996–97 First-Year Class

Men:	38	70%	*Mean*
Women:	16	30%	total GPA: 3.3
Minorities:	9	16%	science GPA: 3.2
Out of State:	12	22%	
With 2 years of college:		2%	*Average*
With 3 years of college:		17%	DAT academic: 17
			DAT-PAT: 17

Tuition

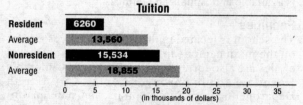

Resident	6260
Average	13,560
Nonresident	15,534
Average	18,855

0   5   10   15   20   25   30   35
(in thousands of dollars)

Percentage receiving financial aid: 82%

Introduction
In 1890 the University of Oklahoma was established. It contains 9 undergraduate and graduate schools. The College of Dentistry is part of the Health Sciences Center, which includes colleges of Medicine, Nursing, Pharmacy, Allied Health, Public Health, and a Graduate College. The dental school offers graduate programs in orthodontics and periodontics.

Admissions (AADSAS)
The basic predental science courses plus 1 year of English composition or literature are required. Preference is given to Oklahoma residents.

Curriculum
4-year traditional. Clinical experience in prevention, oral diagnosis, and simple treatment begins during the first year and increases thereafter. Basic sciences are taught by joint departments of the dental and medical schools. During the fourth year students may choose courses of special interest from a wide range of electives. Honors programs are available for out-standing proficiency.

Facilities
A 5-floor school building houses 5 general practice clinics, 3 specialty clinics, and 180 operatories, as well as the other standard dental school facilities.

Special Features
Tuition fee waiver scholarships are available to some minority students qualifying academically and financially for the first academic year. A limited number of Arkansas residents pay in-state tuition.

OREGON

Oregon Health Sciences University School of Dentistry

Sam Jackson Park
611 S. W. Campus Drive
Portland, Oregon   97201

Phone: 503-494-8825   *Fax:* 503-494-4666
E-mail: cromkyn@ohsu.edu
WWW: http://www.ohsu.edu/sod

Application Filing		Accreditation	
Earliest:	July 1	CDA	
Latest:	November 1		
Fee:	$40	**Degrees Granted**	
AADSAS:	yes	DMD, DMD-MS	

Enrollment: 1996–97 First-Year Class

Men:	53	76%	*Mean*	
Women:	17	24%	total GPA:	3.2
Minorities:	6	8%	science GPA:	3.5
Out of State:	20	29%		
With 2 years of college:	0%		*Average*	
With 3 years of college:	2%		DAT academic:	18
			DAT-PAT:	19

Tuition

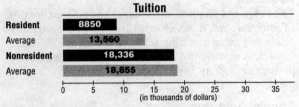

Resident	8850
Average	13,560
Nonresident	18,336
Average	18,855

0   5   10   15   20   25   30   35
(in thousands of dollars)

Percentage receiving financial aid: 73%

Introduction

This dental school was established in 1898. In 1945 the Oregon University School of Dentistry was incorporated into the Oregon state system for higher education and in 1974 it became part of the Oregon Health Science University, which also includes the School of Medicine and School of Nursing. The School of Dentistry is located on a 116-acre campus in the wooded hills of southwest Portland.

Admissions (AADSAS)

The basic predental science courses plus English are required. Applicants from Oregon, from states certified under the WICHE program, and from the remaining states and Canada are eligible for consideration in the priority order listed. *Transfer:* Only at the beginning of the second year if there is space available in the class.

Curriculum

4-year traditional. Students see their first patient during their freshman year in the preventive dentistry course. Some subjects are organized into conjoint courses, taught cooperatively by separate departments. Correlation and application of the biological and clinical sciences are emphasized.

Facilities

As a part of the Oregon Health Sciences University, the dental school building houses classrooms, a modern clinic containing 200 dental work stations, and individual X-ray rooms.

Special Features

A Disadvantaged Student Recruitment Program is in effect and a tutorial program is also available. A fifth-year fellowship program with a stipend is available in a private practice setting.

PENNSYLVANIA

Temple University School of Dentistry

3223 North Broad Street
Philadelphia, Pennsylvania   19140

Phone: 215-707-2801   *Fax:* 215-707-5461

Application Filing		Accreditation
Earliest:	July 30	CDA
Latest:	April 1	
Fee:	$30	**Degrees Granted**
AADSAS:	yes	DMD, DMD-MBA

Enrollment: 1996–97 First-Year Class

Men:	85	71%	*Mean*
Women:	34	29%	total GPA: 3
Minorities:	17	14%	science GPA: 3
Out of State:	71	60%	
With 2 years of college:	n/av		*Average*
With 3 years of college:	n/av		DAT academic: 18.2
			DAT-PAT: 18

Tuition

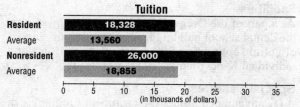

Resident	18,328
Average	13,560
Nonresident	26,000
Average	18,855

0   5   10   15   20   25   30   35
(in thousands of dollars)

Percentage receiving financial aid: 94%

Introduction

Temple University was established in 1884. It belongs to the Commonwealth System of Higher Education in Pennsylvania. The School of Dentistry was established in 1863 as the Philadelphia Dental College. It joined Temple University in 1907 and is part of the Health Sciences Center, which includes schools of Medicine, Pharmacy, and Allied Health, and the University Hospital. The School of Dentistry offers programs in continuing education.

Admissions (AADSAS)

The basic predental science courses and 1 year of English are required. Where time permits, the following science courses are recommended: histology, biochemistry, mammalian anatomy, physiology, and microbiology. Applications from minority students are encouraged. *Transfer and advanced standing:* Under exceptional circumstances, students from U.S. and Canadian schools are considered as transfers.

Curriculum

4-year. Some flexibility has been introduced into the curriculum, permitting students to progress at their own pace in the clinic. It is possible for students to gain additional experience in subjects in which they have special interest. The School of Dentistry and the School of Business and Management at Temple offer a program leading to the DMD and MBA dual degrees.

Facilities

The school is situated in a densely populated section of Philadelphia. It has close affiliations with area hospitals and other teaching units of the Health Sciences Center. A new dental school building has been completed, providing very modern facilities and equipment.

Special Features

Tutorial assistance and academic advising are available. The School of Dentistry includes 5 specialty programs, in addition to an advanced education general dentistry program. Temple's Infectious Disease Clinic offers an educational experience in the management of HIV-positive patients. Luxury housing is available at affordable cost.

University of Pennsylvania School of Dental Medicine

4001 West Spruce Street
Philadelphia, Pennsylvania   19104

Phone: 215-898-8943   *Fax:* 215-898-5243

Application Filing		**Accreditation**
Earliest:	June 1	CDA
Latest:	February 1	
Fee:	$45	**Degrees Granted**
AADSAS:	yes	DMD

Enrollment: 1996–97 First-Year Class

Men:	45	49%	*Mean*	
Women:	47	51%	total GPA:	3.3
Minorities:	32	35%	science GPA:	3.1
Out of State:	72	78%		
With 2 years of college:		0%	*Average*	
With 3 years of college:		0%	DAT academic:	19
			DAT-PAT:	17

Tuition

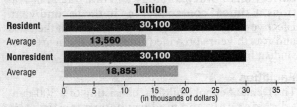

Resident	30,100
Average	13,560
Nonresident	30,100
Average	18,855

0   5   10   15   20   25   30   35
(in thousands of dollars)

Percentage receiving financial aid: 73%

Introduction

The University of Pennsylvania was established in 1740 as a private institution. The University of Pennsylvania School of Dental Medicine was created in 1878. Originally known as the Thomas W. Evans Museum and Dental Institute, it became the School of Dental Medicine in 1964. It is located on the west end of the 250-acre university campus in central Philadelphia, making it accessible to the many educational and cultural facilities in this city.

Admissions (AADSAS)

The basic predental science courses plus 1 semester of mathematics (calculus preferred) and 1 year of English are required. Courses in biochemistry, physiology, and microbiology are recommended. *Transfer and advanced standing:* Students from other U.S. dental schools may be admitted with advanced standing into the third year only.

Curriculum

4-year. Clinical experience begins with Preventive Dentistry Education in the first year and increases thereafter. Elective time is available in the second and third years. Fourth-year students spend 6 weeks gaining additional medical skills at selected hospitals.

Grading Policy

The A, B, C, I evaluation system is used.

Facilities

The school is located on the university campus. Facilities include microbiological testing, the laboratory microcomputer center, implant dentistry center, and general dentistry clinic.

Special Features

Qualified students are invited to participate in the ongoing programs of the Center for Oral Health Research, periodontical diseases research center, center for research in oral biology, and the clinical research center.

University of Pittsburgh School of Dental Medicine

3501 Terrace Street
Pittsburgh, Pennsylvania   15261

Phone: 412-648-8424   *Fax:* 412-648-9571
E-mail: stj+@Pitt.edu
WWW: http://www.pitt.edu/pittdent

Application Filing			Accreditation	
Earliest:	June 1		CDA	
Latest:	February 1			
Fee:	$35		**Degrees Granted**	
AADSAS:	yes		DMD	

Enrollment: 1996–97 First-Year Class

Men:	50	62%	*Mean*	
Women:	31	38%	total GPA:	3
Minorities:	11	14%	science GPA:	3
Out of State:	25	31%		
With 2 years of college:	n/av		*Average*	
With 3 years of college:	14%		DAT academic:	15
			DAT-PAT:	15

Tuition

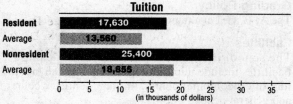

Resident	17,630
Average	13,560
Nonresident	25,400
Average	18,655

(in thousands of dollars)

Percentage receiving financial aid: 81%

Introduction

The University of Pittsburgh was established in 1787 and has campuses in Pittsburgh, Bradford, Greensburg, and Johnstown. In 1896 the School of Dental Medicine was founded. It is part of the university health complex, the other components being the schools of Medicine, Pharmacy, Nursing, Health-Related Professions, Public Health, and their affiliated hospitals. The School of Dental Medicine offers graduate programs in advanced education in general dentistry and many specialties as well as a dental hygiene program.

Admissions (AADSAS)

The basic predental science courses plus 1 year of English are required. Recommended courses include mathematics, statistics, psychology, and sociology. *Transfer and advanced standing:* Possible if space available.

Curriculum

4-year. Instruction in the biological and technological principles provides a basis for the clinical prevention of oral disease, the maintenance of oral health, and correction of oral pathology and oral-facial deviations. Clinical contact begins in the second year. Elective programs, or selective research, in the third and fourth years provide in-depth study in areas of student interest.

Facilities

The Dental School Building, consisting of a 300-dental chair clinic and modern lecture facilities, is located in the city's Oakland district within the University Health Complex. An audiovisual instructional resource center, consisting of individual stations, is available for study.

Special Features

Postgraduate specialty programs are available in each of the dental areas.

SOUTH CAROLINA

Medical University of South Carolina College of Dental Medicine

171 Ashley Avenue
Charleston, South Carolina   29425

Phone: 803-792-2344   *Fax:* 803-792-1376
E-mail: javedt@musc.edu

Application Filing		Accreditation
Earliest:	June 1	CDA
Latest:	December 1	
Fee:	$45	**Degrees Granted**
AADSAS:	yes	DMD, DMD-PhD

Enrollment: 1996–97 First-Year Class

Men:	39	71%	*Mean*
Women:	16	29%	total GPA: 3.1
Minorities:	2	3%	science GPA: n/av
Out of State:	8	15%	
With 2 years of college:		0%	*Average*
With 3 years of college:		1%	DAT academic: 17
			DAT-PAT: 17

Tuition

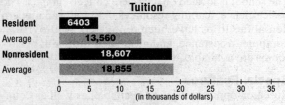

Resident	6403
Average	13,560
Nonresident	18,607
Average	18,855

0   5   10   15   20   25   30   35
(in thousands of dollars)

Percentage receiving financial aid: 87%

Introduction

The College of Dental Medicine, opened in 1967, is part of the Medical University of South Carolina, which was established in 1824. The dental school offers a general practice residency as well as graduate programs in advanced education in general dentistry and in a number of specialties.

Admissions (AADSAS)

A minimum of 3 years of college work (90 semester hours), including the basic predental science courses plus a science elective, and 1 year of English and mathematics is required. *Transfer and advanced standing:* Rarely possible.

Curriculum

4-year. The focus of the curriculum is to produce clinicians able to practice dentistry with an understanding of biological principles. The first 2 years include basic science courses and preclinical dental courses, with some clinical observation and experience. The final 2 years concentrate on clinical practice. During the fourth year, the student will be assigned rotations at various facilities, thereby experiencing dentistry as it is practiced throughout the state.

Facilities

The school is located in the Basic Science-Dental Building of the Medical University complex. Dental students also participate in programs at other South Carolina facilities.

TENNESSEE

Meharry Medical College School of Dentistry

1005 18th Avenue North
Nashville, Tennessee   37208

Phone: 615-327-6223

Application Filing		Accreditation	
Earliest:	June 1	CDA	
Latest:	April 1		
Fee:	$25	**Degrees Granted**	
AADSAS:	yes	DDS	

Enrollment: 1996–97 First-Year Class

Men:	21	45%	*Mean*	
Women:	26	55%	total GPA:	2.8
Minorities:	19	41%	science GPA:	2.6
Out of State:	39	83%		
With 2 years of college:		0%	*Average*	
With 3 years of college:		3%	DAT academic:	15
			DAT-PAT:	14

Tuition

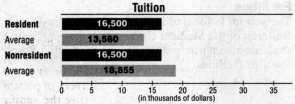

Resident	16,500
Average	13,560
Nonresident	16,500
Average	18,855

0   5   10   15   20   25   30   35
(in thousands of dollars)

Percentage receiving financial aid: n/av

Above data applies to 1995–96 academic year.

Introduction

Meharry Medical College was founded in 1876. In 1886 the School of Dentistry was established. It is located near the center of Nashville. Three other academic divisions are part of the college: the schools of Medicine, Graduate Studies and Research, and Allied Health.

Admissions (AADSAS)

The basic predental science courses and 1 year of English composition are required. Recommended courses include those in engineering, design, human psychology, and sociology. State residents and students from states with which the school has admission agreements are given priority. *Transfer and advanced standing:* Students from other U.S. and Canadian dental schools can apply for advanced standing.

Curriculum

4-year flexible. The first year concentrates on the basic sciences. The middle years concentrate on a mixture of basic and clinical courses, and the last year largely on clinical courses. Integration of basic and clinical sciences is achieved by multidisciplinary councils and didactic/clinical hospital dentistry experiences.

Facilities

The school is located on a 24-acre college campus. The basic science, learning resources, hospital, and modern dental facilities have been renovated. Audiovisual, computer assistance, and group and individual study rooms are available.

Special Features

Research opportunities are available, as well as counseling.

University of Tennessee College of Dentistry

875 Union Avenue
Memphis, Tennessee 38163

Phone: 901-448-6200   *Fax:* 901-448-7104
E-mail: p.dowdle@utmem.dent.edu

Application Filing		Accreditation	
Earliest:	June 1	CDA	
Latest:	December 31		
Fee:	$50	**Degrees Granted**	
AADSAS:	yes	DDS, DDS-MS, DDS-PhD	

Enrollment: 1996–97 First-Year Class

Men:	62	78%	*Mean*	
Women:	18	23%	total GPA:	3.2
Minorities:	6	8%	science GPA:	3.1
Out of State:	6	8%		
With 2 years of college:	0%		*Average*	
With 3 years of college:	39%		DAT academic:	16.9
			DAT-PAT:	16.5

Tuition

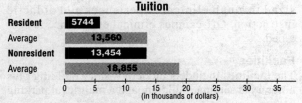

Resident	5744
Average	13,560
Nonresident	13,454
Average	18,855

(in thousands of dollars)

Percentage receiving financial aid: 89%

Introduction

The University of Tennessee system was established in 1794 with campuses in Chattanooga, Martin, and Knoxville. The University of Tennessee at Memphis was established in 1911 and the Health Sciences Center is located there. The College of Dentistry is a component of this center. It offers a general practice residency program as well as graduate programs in advanced education in general dentistry and a variety of specialties.

Admissions

The basic predental science courses plus 1 year of English composition are required. Additional course-work in biology and chemistry is recommended. Qualified Tennesseans are given first priority, and a number of Arkansas students are also accepted under a formal agreement. A few additional out-of-state students may be accepted if they possess superior qualifications. *Transfer and advanced standing:* Transfer students with advanced standing from ADA-accredited schools may be accepted where strong similarities exist between the curricula of the institutions. Students requesting transfer must be independently evaluated by a faculty board appointed from the various departments for proper placement in the curriculum.

Curriculum

4-year traditional. Selected segments of the basic and clinical sciences are presented by an interdisciplinary, team-teaching approach. Students are oriented to clinical activities in the first year. Delivery of patient care begins in the second year. During the senior year, 100 clock hours of electives from special clinical projects, lectures, and research projects are available to students.

Facilities

The college is located on the Health Sciences Center campus and has a modern clinical facility. Off-campus clinics are also used.

Special Features

The school encourages applications from minority and disadvantaged students.

TEXAS

Baylor University
Baylor College of Dentistry

P.O. Box 660677
Dallas, Texas 75246

Phone: 214-828-8230

Application Filing		Accreditation	
Earliest:	June 1	CDA	
Latest:	November 1		
Fee:	$35	**Degrees Granted**	
AADSAS:	yes	DDS	

Enrollment: 1996–97 First-Year Class

Men:	35	61%	*Mean*	
Women:	22	39%	total GPA:	3.2
Minorities:	3	5%	science GPA:	3.1
Out of State:	6	11%		
With 2 years of college:	0%		*Average*	
With 3 years of college:	3%		DAT academic:	17
			DAT-PAT:	16

Tuition

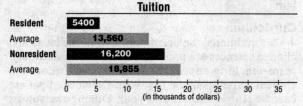

Resident	5400
Average	13,560
Nonresident	16,200
Average	18,855

0 5 10 15 20 25 30 35
(in thousands of dollars)

Percentage receiving financial aid: 91%

Introduction

Baylor University was established in 1845 and has 7 undergraduate and 9 graduate schools. The Baylor College of Dentistry is located in the Baylor University Medical Center in Dallas' metropolitan area. The school opened in 1905 as the State Dental College and joined the university system in 1918. Its status changed in 1971 when it became a private, nonprofit, nonsecterian corporation under its present name. Graduate programs are offered in a large number of specialties and a continuing educational program is also available as is a BS in dental hygiene.

Admissions (AADSAS)

The basic predental science courses and 1 year of English are required. Recommended courses include embryology, psychology, sociology, bookkeeping, speech, foreign languages, reading improvement, and mechanical drawing. Strong priority is given to state residents.

Curriculum

4-year traditional. First- and second-year students devote their time primarily to the basic biological and dental science courses. Starting with the second year, the various subdisciplines of dentistry are emphasized through clinical experiences and didactic instruction. Off-campus clinical experience is provided.

Facilities

The facilities include a modern 7-story building plus a library, a seminar building, and a multilevel parking garage.

University of Texas Houston Dental Branch Health Science Center

6516 John Freeman Avenue
Houston, Texas   77225

Phone: 713-792-4151

Application Filing		Accreditation
Earliest:	April 15	CDA
Latest:	November 1	
Fee:	$35	**Degrees Granted**
AADSAS:	no	DDS

Enrollment: 1996–97 First-Year Class

Men:	38	62%	*Mean*	
Women:	23	38%	total GPA:	3.3
Minorities:	4	7%	science GPA:	3.1
Out of State:	3	5%		
With 2 years of college:		0%	*Average*	
With 3 years of college:		3%	DAT academic:	16
			DAT-PAT:	16

Tuition

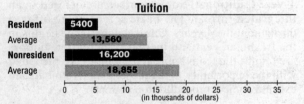

Resident	5400
Average	13,560
Nonresident	16,200
Average	18,855

0   5   10   15   20   25   30   35
(in thousands of dollars)

Percentage receiving financial aid: 86%

Above data applies to 1995-96 academic year.

Introduction

The University of Texas system was established in 1950 with campuses located in Arlington, Austin, El Paso, and San Antonio. The Houston Dental Branch was founded in 1905 as the Texas Dental College and later became part of the University of Texas Health Science Center at Houston. This center includes the Medical School, the Graduate School of Biomedical Sciences, School of Nursing, and the Speech and Hearing Institute. The Dental Branch offers graduate and postgraduate dental programs and a program in continuing education as well as one in dental hygiene.

Admissions

A minimum of 2 years of college (60 semester hours) plus the basic predental science courses and 1 year of English is required. High priority is given to state residents. *Transfer and advanced standing:* Students from other U.S., Canadian, and foreign dental schools may apply.

Curriculum

4-year. The curriculum consists of basic science, preclinical, clinical, behavioral science, and elective instruction. The didactic material is presented in lectures, seminars, problem-based learning sessions, and laboratories. The clinical portion begins with Introduction to the Clinic and continues with patient treatment that is focused on completing patient needs in a timely manner based on a well-developed treatment plan. Students are mentored by academic advisers and clincial facilitators. Overall management of the clinical curriculum is through a fully computerized clinical information system. Each class of 60 progresses through the curriculum together. The Dental Branch also has programs in all 8 of the dental specialties and dental hygiene.

Facilities

The school is located in the Texas Medical Center and is housed in a self-contained, 6-floor building. Preclinical training is carried out in multidisciplinary laboratories provided with closed-circuit television facilities. Clinical activities are performed in individualized clinical cubicles. Extramural rotations are an integral part of clinical training.

University of Texas San Antonio Dental School Health Science Center

Dental School
7703 Floyd Curl Drive
San Antonio, Texas   78284

Phone: 210-567-3181   *Fax:* 210-567-6271
E-mail: carr@uthscsa

Application Filing		Accreditation	
Earliest:	April 15	CDA	
Latest:	November 1		
Fee:	$45	**Degrees Granted**	
AADSAS:	no	DDS, DDS-PhD	

Enrollment: 1996–97 First-Year Class

Men:	60	67%	*Mean*		
Women:	30	33%	total GPA:	3.4	
Minorities:	27	30%	science GPA:	3.3	
Out of State:	4	4%			
With 2 years of college:		1%	*Average*		
With 3 years of college:		9%	DAT academic:	18	
			DAT-PAT:	18	

Tuition

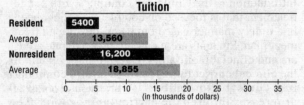

Resident	5400
Average	13,560
Nonresident	16,200
Average	18,855

0   5   10   15   20   25   30   35
(in thousands of dollars)

Percentage receiving financial aid: 90%

Introduction

The University of Texas at San Antonio was established in 1883 and became part of the University of Texas system in 1969. The Dental School is located in the Health Science Center, whose other components are the Medical School, schools of Nursing and Allied Health Sciences, and the Graduate School of Biomedical Sciences. The Dental School provides graduate education in many specialties as well as general dentistry. The programs in dental hygiene and dental laboratory technology offered by the School of Allied Sciences are housed in the Dental School Building.

Admissions

The basic predental science courses, 1 year of English, and 1 additional year of biology are required. Recommended courses include conversational Spanish and those that will assist in the development of manual skills (such as sculpting, typing, etc.) Strong preference is given to legal residents of Texas. *Transfer and advanced standing:* Students from other U.S., Canadian, and foreign dental schools may apply for advanced standing.

Curriculum

4-year traditional. Some courses are offered in an integrated format. The basic sciences are offered throughout the 4 years. Clinical experience begins in the freshman year and increases thereafter. Juniors are taught the team approach. Seniors are provided with the opportunity to diagnose, plan treatment, and execute clinical procedures on patients.

Grading Policy

A letter grade system is used.

Facilities

The school building is designed to facilitate the educational process. It provides an individual cubicle for each lower-level student in multidiscipline laboratories and a fully equipped clinical cubicle for upper-level students. Off-campus facilities are also used.

Special Features

A combined DDS-PhD program is offered with the Graduate school of Biomedical Sciences.

VIRGINIA

Virginia Commonwealth University
Medical College of Virginia

School of Dentistry
P.O. Box 566
Richmond, Virginia   23298

Phone: 804-786-9196

Application Filing		Accreditation	
Earliest:	May 1	CDA	
Latest:	January 1		
Fee:	$50	**Degrees Granted**	
AADSAS:	yes	DDS, DDS-MS, DDS-PhD	

Enrollment: 1996–97 First-Year Class

Men:	52	65%	*Mean*	
Women:	28	35%	total GPA:	3.4
Minorities:	15	19%	science GPA:	3.4
Out of State:	20	25%		
With 2 years of college:	0%		*Average*	
With 3 years of college:	0%		DAT academic:	18
			DAT-PAT:	17

Tuition

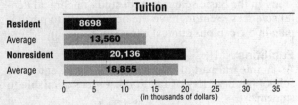

Resident	8698
Average	13,560
Nonresident	20,136
Average	18,855

0   5   10   15   20   25   30   35
(in thousands of dollars)

Percentage receiving financial aid: 91%

Introduction
Virginia Commonwealth University was established in 1838. The School of Dentistry was founded in 1893 as a division of the University College of Medicine. It is the only dental school in Virginia. The school is located on the Health Sciences campus, which includes schools of Medicine, Nursing, Pharmacy, Allied Health, and basic sciences. In addition to postgraduate programs in many specialties, the school offers a general practice residency and advanced education in dentistry programs.

Admissions (AADSAS)
The basic predental science courses plus courses in English are required. Courses in general microbiology, biochemistry, and behavioral sciences as well as courses involving psychomotor skills are recommended. The school accepts both state residents and nonresidents. *Transfer and advanced standing:* Students from other U.S. dental schools may apply for advanced standing.

Curriculum
4-year. The subject matter of the curriculum is divided into the basic, clinical, and social sciences. The basic sciences, including preclinical didactic and laboratory preparation and comprehensive patient care, begin in the second year. The social sciences cover such topics as dental health needs, health care delivery systems, and practice management. Elective courses are offered in the senior year.

Facilities
The facilities of the school are housed in 2 modern buildings, containing clinical facilities, classrooms/laboratories, group and individual study areas, department offices, and a closed-circuit color television studio. Dormitories, athletic facilities, and a student center are located on campus.

Special Features
Combined DDS-MS and DDS-PhD programs are offered. They require additional time beyond the 4-year DDS program.

WASHINGTON

University of Washington School of Dentistry

Health Science Building SC-62
Seattle, Washington   98195

Phone: 206-543-5840   *Fax:* 206-616-2612
E-mail: evrgeen@washington.edu
WWW: http://www.dental.wa.edu

Application Filing		Accreditation	
Earliest:	July 1	CDA	
Latest:	December 1		
Fee:	$35	**Degrees Granted**	
AADSAS:	yes	DDS	

Enrollment: 1996–97 First-Year Class

Men:	36	67%	*Mean*	
Women:	18	33%	total GPA:	3.5
Minorities:	3	6%	science GPA:	3.4
Out of State:	9	17%		
With 2 years of college:	0%		*Average*	
With 3 years of college:	2%		DAT academic:	20
			DAT-PAT:	20

Tuition

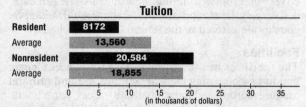

Resident	8172
Average	13,560
Nonresident	20,584
Average	18,855

0   5   10   15   20   25   30   35
(in thousands of dollars)

Percentage receiving financial aid: n/av

Introduction

The University of Washington was established in 1861. There are 17 undergraduate schools and 1 graduate school. The University of Washington School of Dentistry was founded in 1945 and is now located on the 700-acre main campus. The School of Dentistry is part of the Warren G. Magnuson Health Science Center, whose other components are the schools of Medicine, Nursing, Pharmacy, Public Health, and Community Medicine. In addition to the DDS degree, the school offers a BS in dental hygiene, an MS in dentistry, and graduate training in a variety of specialties leading to a certificate of proficiency.

Admissions (AADSAS)

One year of biology or zoology, 1 year of general physics, 1 semester/2 quarters of inorganic and organic chemistry, and 1 semester/2 quarters of general biochemistry are required. Entering classes are 75% Washington State residents; students from foreign countries are rarely admitted. While a majority of the entering class have completed an undergraduate degree, applicants who have at least 3 years of college coursework are considered. *Transfer and advanced standing:* Advanced standing or transfer students are rarely accepted.

Curriculum

4-year. Strong emphasis is placed on integrating study in the basic sciences with study in clinical dental sciences. Seniors have the opportunity to participate in off-campus clinical experiences.

Facilities

As an integral part of the Health Sciences Center, the school has a variety of facility resources available to students.

Special Features

Students with special backgrounds can utilize the diverse resources of the Health Sciences Center to plan joint MS and/or PhD programs.

WEST VIRGINIA

West Virginia University School of Dentistry

Medical Center
Morgantown, West Virginia 26506

Phone: 304-293-6646   *Fax:* 304-293-2859
E-mail: sprice@wvuvphs.hsc.wvu.edu

Application Filing		Accreditation	
Earliest:	July 1	CDA	
Latest:	March 1		
Fee:	$45	**Degrees Granted**	
AADSAS:	yes	DDS, DDS-MS, DDS-PhD	

Enrollment: 1996–97 First-Year Class

Men:	32	78%	*Mean*	
Women:	9	22%	total GPA:	3.5
Minorities:	2	4%	science GPA:	3.2
Out of State:	21	51%		
With 2 years of college:		0%	*Average*	
With 3 years of college:		42%	DAT academic:	17
			DAT-PAT:	17

Tuition

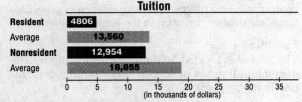

Resident	4806
Average	13,560
Nonresident	12,954
Average	18,855

(in thousands of dollars)

Percentage receiving financial aid: 81%

Introduction

West Virginia University was established in 1867. The West Virginia University School of Dentistry was opened in 1957 and is part of the Robert C. Byrd Health Sciences Center. The School of Dentistry offers, in addition to the DDS degree, a BS and MS in dental hygiene and graduate training in a number of specialties. Continuing education courses for dentists and auxiliaries are available as is an advanced education in general dentistry program.

Admissions (AADSAS)

The basic predental science courses and 1 year of English composition and rhetoric are required. Preference is given to state residents. Nonresidents should have at least a GPA of 3.0 and DAT scores of 15-15. *Transfer and advanced standing:* Opportunities are limited.

Curriculum

4-year flexible. Clinical observation begins during the first semester of the second year. A transition to hands-on assisting assignments occurs in the second semester of the second year. Clinical experience begins during the summer of the second year. The fourth year provides an option of 3 basic tracts: basic biological science, general practice, and a specific clinical tract. Students pursuing an approved tract must take at least 3 hours of electives each semester and must register for clinical courses. Off-campus clinical experience is completed in the fourth year.

Facilities

The school is part of the WVU Health Sciences Center. It has modern, fully equipped teaching and clinical facilities.

Special Features

Combined DDS-MS and DDS-PhD programs are available on an individual basis. They require several years of study in addition to time needed for the dental curriculum.

WISCONSIN

Marquette University School of Dentistry

604 North 16th Street
Milwaukee, Wisconsin   53233

Phone: 414-288-3532   *Fax:* 414-288-3586
E-mail: trec@caries.dental.mu.edu
WWW: http://www.ldental.mu.edu

Application Filing		Accreditation	
Earliest:	July 15	CDA	
Latest:	April 1		
Fee:	$25	**Degrees Granted**	
AADSAS:	yes	DDS	

Enrollment: 1996–97 First-Year Class

Men:	52	69%	*Mean*	
Women:	23	31%	total GPA:	3.1
Minorities:	20	26%	science GPA:	3.2
Out of State:	1	1%		
With 2 years of college:		0%	*Average*	
With 3 years of college:		18%	DAT academic:	17
			DAT-PAT:	16.1

Tuition

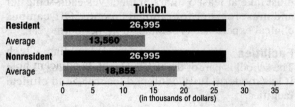

Resident	26,995
Average	13,560
Nonresident	26,995
Average	18,855

0   5   10   15   20   25   30   35
(in thousands of dollars)

Percentage receiving financial aid: 99%

Introduction

Marquette University was founded in 1881. The Marquette University School of Dentistry was created in 1907 when Milwaukee Medical College merged with Marquette College and formed Marquette University. Graduate programs leading to an MS degree are offered in several specialties. Continuing education courses are available in all phases of dentistry through the year.

Admissions (AADSAS)

The basic predental science courses and 1 year of English are required, and additional courses in biology and biochemistry are strongly recommended. *Transfer and advanced standing:* Students from other U.S. and Canadian dental schools and foreign dental school graduates can apply for advanced standing only into the second year.

Curriculum

4-year traditional. A diagonal format allows the presentation of the basic science courses throughout the 4-year curriculum. Clinical experience commences early in the freshman year and expands to a strong junior-senior clinical program. Collaborative, interdepartmental coverage of selected topics has been used for the integration of relevant basic and clinical science topics. Elective courses are available in the senior year and off-campus experience is possible. Graduate courses are open to top senior students.

Facilities

The school is located on the university campus. The dental building has undergone extensive modernization in recent years.

Special Features

A combined BS/DDS program is available on an individual basis, and a DDS+ program encompassing graduate courses in both dental and nondental fields exists.

CANADA

Dalhousie University Faculty of Dentistry

5981 University Avenue
Halifax, Nova Scotia   B3H 3J5

Phone: 902-494-2274   *Fax:* 902-494-2527
E-mail: j.roski@dal.ca

Application Filing		Accreditation
Earliest:	October 1	CDA
Latest:	December 1	
Fee:	$55	**Degrees Granted**
AADSAS:	no	DDS

Enrollment: 1996–97 First-Year Class

Men:	121	54%	*Mean*	
Women:	103	46%	total GPA:	3.7
Minorities:	0	0%	science GPA:	3.7
Out of Province:	0	0%		
With 2 years of college:		63%	*Average*	
With 3 years of college:		94%	DAT academic:	19
			DAT-PAT:	18

Tuition

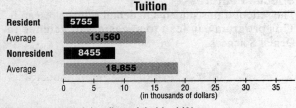

Resident 5755
Average 13,560
Nonresident 8455
Average 18,855

(in thousands of dollars)

Percentage receiving financial aid: 44%

Averages are for U.S. schools

Introduction

Dalhousie University, in Nova Scotia, was established in 1818. It is a public, nonsectarian school. The Faculty of Dentistry opened in 1912. Through its Alumni Affair Development, the school provides continuing education courses for dentists and dental hygienists.

Admissions

A minimum of 10 credits of university study, as well as basic predental science courses including biochemistry, microbiology, and vertebrate physiology, plus 1 writing course and 2 credits from the humanities and/or social sciences, are required. Preference is given to students from the Atlantic Provinces of Canada. The Canadian Dental Association's Dental Aptitude Test must also be completed prior to the December 1 application deadline. *Transfer and advanced standing:* Not possible.

Curriculum

Integration of dental, biological, and behavioral sciences is emphasized throughout the 4 years. Didactic and laboratory classes comprise most of the first 2 years, with patient care introduced late in the first year and continued through the second year. The clinically oriented disciplines and total patient care are emphasized during the third and fourth years, respectively. Selective study programs are required during the fourth year.

Facilities

All subjects are taught in the Dental Building, which has ample and modern facilities. Three adjacent hospitals provide additional clinical facilities.

Special Features

A limited number of student research fellowships are available on an irregular basis each summer.

McGill University Faculty of Dentistry

3640 University Street
Montreal, Québec   H3A 2B2

Phone: 514-398-7227   *Fax:* 514-398-8900
E-mail: hogan@medcor.mcgill.ca

Application Filing		Accreditation	
Earliest:	July 1	CDA	
Latest:	December 1		
Fee:	$60	**Degrees Granted**	
AADSAS:	yes	DDS	

Enrollment: 1996–97 First-Year Class

Men:	10	40%	*Mean*	
Women:	15	60%	total GPA:	3.5
Minorities:	0	0%	science GPA:	n/av
Out of Province:	4	16%		
With 2 years of college:		24%	*Average*	
With 3 years of college:		16%	DAT academic:	19.8
			DAT-PAT:	18.4

Tuition

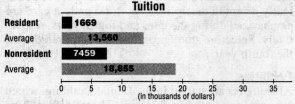

Resident	1669
Average	13,560
Nonresident	7459
Average	18,855

0   5   10   15   20   25   30   35
(in thousands of dollars)

Percentage receiving financial aid: n/av

Averages are for U.S. schools

Introduction

McGill University was established in 1821 and is a public school. It has 11 undergraduate schools and 17 graduate schools. The school offers masters programs in oral biology as well as in maxillofacial surgery.

Admissions (AADSAS)

The basic predental science courses plus 1 year each of mathematics, as well as half-year university-level courses in cell biology, and molecular biology are required. (A full-year course in biochemistry may be substituted for the courses in cell and molecular biology.) Very strong preference is given to provincial residents. *Transfer and advanced standing:* Not available.

Curriculum

Basic sciences are taught in the first 3 years of the program. Introduction to clinical experience begins in the first year, and the integration of basic sciences into clinical dentistry occurs in the second year.

Facilities

The faculty is located in downtown Montreal. The preclinical training is provided on the McGill campus and the clinical training takes place in the McCall Dental Clinic of Montreal General Hospital and other teaching hospitals.

Special Features

The school trains students in dental science research. This program can lead to a masters of science in Dental Sciences.

Université de Montréal
Faculté de Médecine Dentaire

C.P. 6128, Succursale A
Montréal, Québec   H3C 3T5

Phone: 514-343-6005   *Fax:* 514-343-2233
E-mail: heliep@medent.umontreal.ca

Application Filing		Accreditation	
Earliest:	March 1	CDA	
Latest:	March 1		
Fee:	$55	**Degrees Granted**	
AADSAS:	no	DMD	

Enrollment: 1996–97 First-Year Class

Men:	40	47%	*Mean*	
Women:	45	53%	total GPA:	n/av
Minorities:	0	0%	science GPA:	n/av
Out of Province:	n/av			
With 2 years of college:		48%	*Average*	
With 3 years of college:		52%	DAT academic:	n/av
			DAT-PAT:	n/av

Tuition

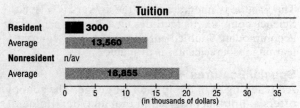

Resident	3000
Average	13,560
Nonresident	n/av
Average	18,855

0   5   10   15   20   25   30   35
(in thousands of dollars)

Percentage receiving financial aid: n/av

Averages are for U.S. schools

Introduction

The Université de Montréal was established in 1878 and is the largest university in North America. It conducts its classes in French. The Université de Montréal Faculté de Médecine Dentaire was established in 1904. Postgraduate programs are offered in a variety of specialties, some of which lead to masters degrees or certificates.

Admissions

The basic predental science courses plus 3 semesters of mathematics, physics, chemistry, and biology, as well as 4 semesters of philosophy and French, are required. All candidates must be Canadian citizens or permanent residents. Strong preference is given to provincial residents. Instruction is given in French.

Curriculum

Coverage of the basic sciences takes place during the first 2 years, and clinical training is secured during the last 2 years. Avenues are provided to permit continuous integration between the 2 segments. In addition to required course work, seniors must spend a full week in a hospital to become familiarized with dental surgery and another 2 weeks in pedodontics.

Facilities

The Faculté is located in the main building of the university and occupies the street and second-floor levels of the east end. Students have access to university audiovisual and computer facilities.

Special Features

All teaching is in the French language. Joint postgraduate programs in the biomedical sciences are offered in association with the medical faculty.

Laval University
Faculté de Médecine Dentaire
Sainte-Foy, Québec   G1K 7P4

Phone: 418-656-2120

Application Filing		**Accreditation**
Earliest:	September 1	CDA
Latest:	April 15	
Fee:	$55	**Degrees Granted**
AADSAS:	no	DMD

Enrollment: 1996–97 First-Year Class

Men:	26	57%	*Mean*	
Women:	20	43%	total GPA:	88
Minorities:	0	0%	science GPA:	86
Out of Province:	5	11%		
With 2 years of college:		4%	*Average*	
With 3 years of college:		13%	DAT academic:	n/av
			DAT-PAT:	18.9

Tuition

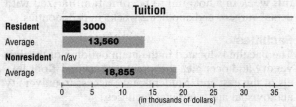

Resident	3000
Average	13,560
Nonresident	n/av
Average	18,855

0   5   10   15   20   25   30   35
(in thousands of dollars)

Percentage receiving financial aid: n/av

Averages are for U.S. schools

Introduction
Laval University was established in 1852 and is the oldest university in North America. It conducts its classes in French. The Université Laval Ecole Médecine Dentaire was founded in 1969. The school also offers a diploma program in oral and in maxillo-facial surgery.

Admissions
The basic predental science courses plus 1 semester of English, 4 semesters of French, and 3 semesters of mathematics are required. Only residents of Quebec are accepted. *Transfer and advanced standing:* Students from other Canadian dental schools can apply for advanced standing.

Curriculum
4-year nontraditional. The first 2 years are devoted to the basic and preclinical sciences. The last 2 years are devoted almost entirely to clinical work. Elective specialization is possible in the senior year. Electives in hospital dentistry, public health, and basic research are available. Self-pacing is possible in a few courses.

Facilities
The Faculté is integrated into the university's Health Science complex. Its facilities have been expanded to accommodate doubled enrollment. A well-equipped learning resource center is available.

Special Features
All teaching is in the French language. The school offers a diploma program in oral and maxillofacial surgery.

University of Alberta Faculty of Medicine and Oral Health Sciences

Room 3032, Dental/Pharmacy Building
Edmonton, Alberta   T6G 2N8

Phone: 403-492-2945
E-mail: eleanor.mcisaac@ualberta.ca

Application Filing			Accreditation
Earliest:	July 1		CDA
Latest:	November 1		
Fee:	$60		**Degrees Granted**
AADSAS:	no		DDS

Enrollment: 1996–97 First-Year Class

Men:	20	63%	*Mean*	
Women:	12	38%	total GPA:	8.1
Minorities:	32	n/av	science GPA:	8.1
Out of Province:	n/av			
With 2 years of college:		33%	*Average*	
With 3 years of college:		37%	DAT academic:	n/av
			DAT-PAT:	19.1

Tuition

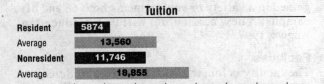

Resident	5874
Average	13,560
Nonresident	11,746
Average	18,855

(in thousands of dollars)

Percentage receiving financial aid: 13%

Averages are for U.S. schools

Introduction

The University of Alberta was established in 1906. It is a public institution with both undergraduate and graduate schools. The University of Alberta Faculty of Dentistry has both Canadian and American Dental Association approval. The school is located on the North Saskatchewan River. It offers dental hygiene and graduate studies programs. Senior students gain experience in treating underprivileged people by service in Northern Alberta.

Admissions

The basic predental science courses, statistics, and 1 English course are required. Recommended electives include psychology and genetics. High priority is given to provincial residents, but candidates from other provinces and other countries are admitted. Although it is not necessary to complete requirements for a degree prior to applying, it is to the student's advantage to register in a degree program for preprofessional study. *Transfer and advanced standing:* Not possible.

Curriculum

The course of study lasts 4 years. The first 3 years contain 3 terms: 15 weeks, 15 weeks, and 10 weeks. *First year:* Consists of basic science courses with an introduction to dental sciences in the third term. *Second and third years:* Discipline-oriented programs with the final year emphasizing total patient care.

Facilities

The dental facilities are housed in the Dental Pharmacy Center. The students also rotate through the University Hospital, the Geriatric Youville Hospital, and Northern Alberta Clinics.

Special Features

Limited research opportunities are available through employment as summer research assistants.

University of British Columbia Faculty of Dentistry

Room 350, 2194 Health Sciences Mall
Vancouver, British Columbia   V6T 1Z3

Phone: 604-822-3416   *Fax:* 604-822-4532

Application Filing		Accreditation	
Earliest:	August 15	CDA	
Latest:	December 15		
Fee:	$50	**Degrees Granted**	
AADSAS:	no	DMD, DMD-MS, MSc, DMD-PhD	

Enrollment: 1996–97 First-Year Class

Men:	14	38%	*Mean*		
Women:	23	62%	total GPA:	3.6	
Minorities:	0	0%	science GPA:	n/av	
Out of Province:	3	8%			
With 2 years of college:		0%	*Average*		
With 3 years of college:		100%	DAT academic:	21	
			DAT-PAT:	19	

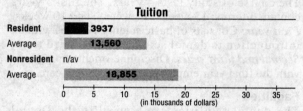

Tuition

Resident — 3937
Average — 13,560
Nonresident — n/av
Average — 18,855

(in thousands of dollars)

Percentage receiving financial aid: 60%

Averages are for U.S. schools

Introduction
The University of British Columbia was founded in 1908. It is supported by the province and offers both undergraduate and graduate programs. The University of British Columbia Faculty of Dentistry first opened in 1964. It is a part of the Health Science Center, which includes the faculties of Medicine and Pharmaceutical Sciences, and schools of Nursing, Rehabilitation Medicine, and others. The school is located on a 1,000-acre site on the Point-Grey Peninsula at the west end of Vancouver.

Admissions
The basic predental science courses plus 1 year each of English, biochemistry, and mathematics are required, and electives in the social sciences and humanities are recommended. Preparatory study for entry must comprise at least 3 years at the college or university level. An overall GPA of 2.8 (70%) is also required. Very strong preference is given to provincial residents. *Transfer and advanced standing:* If space is available.

Curriculum
Students are given clinic exposure early in their program, and actual clinical instruction begins during the second half of the second year. Clinical experience is gained in a variety of environments both on and off campus. A new curriculum will be introduced in August, 1997.

Facilities
The faculty is located within the Health Sciences Center on the university campus. The facilities of community health clinics and other health care units are also utilized.

Special Features
Combined DMD-MSc and DMD-PhD programs are available.

University of Manitoba Faculty of Dentistry

780 Bannatyne Avenue, Room D-113
Winnipeg, Manitoba   R3T 2N2

Phone: 204-474-8815

Application Filing		Accreditation
Earliest:	November 1	CDA
Latest:	January 24	
Fee:	$55	**Degrees Granted**
AADSAS:	no	DMD

Enrollment: 1996–97 First-Year Class

			Mean	
Men:	17	68%	total GPA:	n/av
Women:	8	32%	science GPA:	n/av
Minorities:	0	0%		
Out of Province:	11	44%	*Average*	
With 2 years of college:		2%	DAT academic:	18
With 3 years of college:		8%	DAT-PAT:	19

Tuition

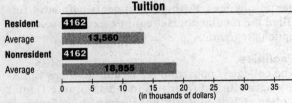

Resident	4162
Average	13,560
Nonresident	4162
Average	18,855

0   5   10   15   20   25   30   35
(in thousands of dollars)

Percentage receiving financial aid: 48%

Above data applies to 1995–96 academic year

Averages are for U.S. schools

Introduction

In 1957 the University of Manitoba Faculty of Dentistry was established. The school offers specialty training programs in clinical areas and a 2-year dental hygiene program as well as continuing education programs. An opportunity exists for securing masters and PhD degrees in oral biology.

Admissions

The basic predental science courses and 1 year each of mathematics and biochemistry plus 5 electives are required. Very high priority is given to provincial residents. *Transfer and advanced standing:* Students from other Canadian, U.S., and foreign dental schools may apply for advanced standing.

Curriculum

The basic sciences are taught primarily in the first 2 years. Clinical experience begins in the second term of the second year. There are no electives; however, all senior students are required to spend 4 weeks in a rural community clinic and 4 weeks in a teaching hospital.

Grading Policy

Letter grades are used in the didactic portion of the curriculum and Pass/Fail in the clinical segment.

Facilities

The faculty is located on the health science campus in downtown Winnipeg. Additional space is devoted to dental teaching and service in the Health Sciences Center, a consortium of 4 hospitals.

Special Features

A limited number of undergraduate students are employed in research laboratories during the summer months.

University of Saskatchewan College of Dentistry

Room B526, Health Science Building
Saskatoon, Saskatchewan   S7N 0W0

Phone: 306-966-5119

Application Filing

Earliest:	September 1
Latest:	January 1
Fee:	n/av
AADSAS:	yes

Accreditation

CDA

Degrees Granted

DMD

Enrollment: 1996–97 First-Year Class

Men:	12	57%	*Mean*		
Women:	9	43%	total GPA:	3.3
Minorities:	0	0%	science GPA:	n/av
Out of Province:	n/av			
With 2 years of college:		9%	*Average*	
With 3 years of college:		6%	DAT academic:	n/av
			DAT-PAT:	n/av

Tuition

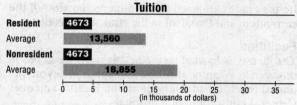

Resident	4673
Average	13,560
Nonresident	4673
Average	18,855

(in thousands of dollars)

Percentage receiving financial aid: n/av

Averages are for U.S. schools

Introduction

The University of Saskatchewan was established in 1907. It is a public school with both undergraduate and graduate schools. In 1965 the University of Saskatchewan College of Dentistry was established. Continuing education courses are offered by the College of Dentistry. The colleges of Medicine, Dentistry, and Nursing are housed in a common Health Sciences building.

Admissions (AADSAS)

A predental year of studies, including the basic science courses, at the University of Saskatchewan is required. Also required is a course in psychology, sociology, philosophy, or anthropology. High priority is given to provincial residents. *Transfer and advanced standing:* Graduates of foreign dental schools may apply for advanced standing, and may be admitted if space is available.

Curriculum

5-year. The curriculum is diagonal. Clinical exposure begins in the first year with an introduction to clinical dentistry and restorative dentistry. Positive efforts are made at all levels to closely integrate the basic and dental sciences. Fifth-year students who have fulfilled the regular course requirements can select an option program.

Facilities

The college is housed in the Health Sciences Building with clinical facilities in the adjoining Dental College Clinical Building. Hospital experience is acquired at the Royal University Hospital Dental Department.

Special Features

Fifth year students who meet all their requirements by the end of the first term may take optional courses in one or more departments at the college or at another teaching or service institution.

University of Toronto Faculty of Dentistry

124 Edward Street
Toronto, Ontario   M5G 1G6

Phone: 416-979-4901   *Fax:* 416-979-4936
E-mail: ahaldane@dental.utoronto.ca
WWW: http://www.utoronto.ca/dentistry

Application Filing		Accreditation	
Earliest:	August 15	CDA	
Latest:	February 1		
Fee:	$100	**Degrees Granted**	
AADSAS:	yes	DDS, DDS-PhD	

Enrollment: 1996–97 First-Year Class

Men:	37	13%	*Mean*
Women:	28	43%	total GPA: n/av
Minorities:	0	0%	science GPA: n/av
Out of Province:	1	2%	
With 2 years of college:		22%	*Average*
With 3 years of college:		39%	DAT academic: n/av
			DAT-PAT: n/av

Tuition

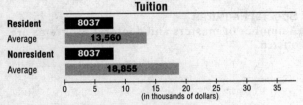

Resident	8037
Average	13,560
Nonresident	8037
Average	18,855

(in thousands of dollars)

Percentage receiving financial aid: n/av

Averages are for U.S. schools

Introduction

The University of Toronto was established in 1827. It contains 9 undergraduate and 1 graduate school. The school was founded in 1875, and in 1888 it became affiliated with the University of Toronto and was accredited to award the DDS degree.

Admissions (AADSAS)

Applicants must have completed 2 years of university before entry to the DDS program. This undergraduate program must have comprised at least 10 courses, with acceptable courses in the basic predental sciences. A minimum cumulative GPA of 2.7 is expected. It is important that applicants select courses that will provide them with an educational background in keeping with their own interests and possible future employment opportunities. It is strongly suggested that applicants include courses in English, humanities, social sciences, and advanced biology. *Transfer:* For nonresidents of Canada the government of Ontario has made it possible for a limited number to apply to the DDS program. A person is eligible to apply if he/she can enter or is already in Canada with a student visa (or equivalent immigration authorization) or is already enrolled in a foreign dental school and may wish to transfer. *Advanced standing:* To be eligible, applicants must (1) meet all academic and English facility requirements for admission to the first year of the DDS program; (2) hold a dental degree from an accredited foreign university; and (3) have successfully completed the written examination and Clinical Examinations I and II of the Canadian National Dental Examining Board Examinations. Space permitting, once these criteria have been met, the applicant will be considered for admission to the second year. *Special applicants* who have had extensive previous work experience in areas acceptable but not necessarily related to dentistry, and a minimum of 2 years of university, and who can demonstrate their ability to successfully complete the dental program without having completed all of the prerequisites, are eligible to apply.

Curriculum

The dental program is designed to unify the basic and clinical sciences, as it is believed that scientific and professional development cannot be sharply differentiated, but should proceed concurrently throughout the program. From the first year, with an emphasis on sciences basic to dentistry, the instruction shifts gradually to a clinically oriented program by the fourth year.

Facilities

The facility has been completely renovated and expanded, making it one of the most modern in North America. New modern research laboratories, clinics, offices and ancillary services enable the faculty to provide the best possible climate for teaching and research.

Special Features

A DDS-PhD program is offered jointly with the School of General Studies.

University of Western Ontario Faculty of Dentistry

1151 Richmond Street
London, Ontario   N6A 5C1

Phone: 519-661-3330
E-mail: denmpa@uwoadmin.uwo.ca

Application Filing		Accreditation	
Earliest:	October 1	CDA	
Latest:	December 1		
Fee:	$50	**Degrees Granted**	
AADSAS:	no	DDS	

Enrollment: 1996–97 First-Year Class

Men:	31	65%	*Mean*		
Women:	17	35%	total GPA:		86
Minorities:	4	8%	science GPA:		n/av
Out of Province:	3	6%			
With 2 years of college:		29%	*Average*		
With 3 years of college:		71%	DAT academic:		n/av
			DAT-PAT:		n/av

Tuition

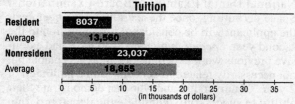

Resident	8037
Average	13,560
Nonresident	23,037
Average	18,855

0   5   10   15   20   25   30   35
(in thousands of dollars)

Percentage receiving financial aid: 63%

Averages are for U.S. schools

Introduction

The University of Western Ontario was chartered in 1878. It is a public school with 14 undergraduate and 4 graduate schools. The school offers, besides its DDS degree, 2 graduate programs leading to specialist certification and a 3-year masters program in orthodontics and oral biology.

Admissions

Requirements include successful completion of a second-year program at an Ontario university, or an equivalent second year at another university, provided that the program has included a minimum of 4 honors courses or equivalent within the first 10 courses completed. All applicants must have successfully completed the basic predental science courses. *Transfer and advanced standing:* Transfer is possible into the second year, if a position is available.

Curriculum

4-year traditional. The first 2 years provide exposure to the basic sciences. Clinical exposure is introduced to a limited extent during this period. During the last 2 years, major emphasis is placed on clinical studies.

Facilities

Teaching takes place at the Dental Science Building.

Special Features

A number of masters and doctoral programs are offered.

APPENDIX A

A SELF-ASSESSMENT ADMISSION PROFILE _____

As discussed in Chapter 3, admission to medical or dental school is dependent upon a multiplicity of factors. Some of the specific data associated with admissions criteria are known to you (such as the quality of your GPA, science cumulative average, etc.), while others are either unknown or unpredictable at this time (such as recommendations or aptitude test scores). Nevertheless, of the ten major admission requirements, most can be quantified with adequate accuracy so as to allow you to formulate a reasonably accurate assessment of your admission chances. More importantly, completing an assessment profile will serve to identify your strengths and weaknesses and thus provide you with information as to which of the areas need improvement. (It will, in addition, identify what assets you should, if possible, emphasize about yourself at an interview and in your AMCAS application essay.)

Success with the use of this profile requires accuracy and as much completeness as possible. In dealing with criteria where data are uncertain, you should make a realistic estimate based on the information currently at your disposal. You may, after completion of the assessment profile, wish to review its content, conclusions, and recommendations with your school's Prehealth Professions Advisor in order to validate your facts, assumptions, and interpretation.

Each of the admission criteria listed in the profile will be discussed briefly. (A fuller treatment is given in Chapter 3.)

1. *College attended.* The established admission "track" record to medical and dental schools by students from your own college is the major consideration for this category. A *superior* rating would be used if most applicants from your school succeed in gaining admission, whereas *weak* would reflect the opposite position, and *adequate*, about a 50% acceptance rate. Taking the exact acceptance rate for the most recent year available into consideration will help you identify where in each box to place your mark (such as at the left, right, or middle of the appropriate box).

2. *Grade point average (GPA).* Your current GPA should be plotted on the profile by using the following rating scheme:

	Superior	Adequate	Weak
Medical	4.0–3.5	3.4–3.2	3.1–2.5
Dental	4.0–3.3	3.2–2.8	2.7–2.0

You should determine where to place your rating in each box by noting the consistency of your level of academic performance. Thus, a 3.5 GPA representing a 3.5 for each of approximately three years would merit the rating sign being placed at the right end of the *superior* box. However, a 3.5 GPA resulting the sum of 4.0, 3.5, and 3.0 for each year respectively over a three-year period would mandate that the marker be placed near the left end of the *adequate* box. Placing the marker at the beginning of the superior box, as in the first case, would be misleading, since a downward trend in a GPA suggests an inability to sustain academic work at a superior level over a long course, assuming no mitigating circumstances exist. If such circumstances exist, they should be noted under "Comments."

3. *Science cumulative average.* This should be determined by the sum of your biology, chemistry, physics, and mathematics (B, C, P, M) grades over the length of your college stay (bearing in mind the credit value for each course).

The same considerations applicable to your GPA are relevant to your science cum as noted in item 2 above. Thus, the consistency of your science courses performance should be considered in determining your rating in this category.

4. *MCAT or DAT scores*. Where these are known, your rating can be determined by using the following scheme (given as total exam score range):

	Superior	Adequate	Weak
*Medical	30–45	25–29	1–24
Dental	20–30	15–19	1–14

*These figures represent total scores for the Verbal Reasoning, Physical Sciences, and Biological Sciences subtests of the MCAT (see Chapter 4).

This determination is usually available to college juniors, most of whom take the appropriate aptitude exam in April. For lowerclassmen or juniors who plan to take the fall exam, a rough estimate of one's possible aptitude test performance can be attempted by using your SAT I or ACT scores as a reference source. Thus, an average performance on either of these tests can be reflected as an average potential performance on the MCAT or DAT. This should be taken as a working hypothesis subject to revision when the results are in. But for those with average or below average SAT I or ACT scores, this would suggest that a meaningful effort be directed to obtain a more impressive result on the Medical or Dental Aptitude Test.

5. *Recommendations*. Most schools request that students waive their legal right to see letters of recommendation sent out in their behalf. Thus, rating this factor with certainty is impossible. However, you may be able to make a realistic approximation for this category through *discreet* inquiry of a member of your Prehealth Advisory Committee with whom you may have an especially friendly relationship. You should not seek to find out your specific ranking or rating, but rather merely to ascertain whether you can expect your candidacy for admission to professional school to secure either strong, modest, or weak support from the committee.

6. *Extracurricular activities*. Your rating in this category should be obtained after first itemizing your activities and then comparing them with some of your fellow students who are also applying to medical or dental school. On this basis, you can judge if your participation is well above average and thus superior, or well below average or weak, or simply average and therefore adequate.

7. *Professional exposure*. The nature and extent of your professional exposure to medicine or dentistry will determine your rating in this category. Thus, a physician's assistant or former army medical corpsman will gain an especially strong rating. On the other hand, one whose exposure is limited to a discussion with his family physician or dentist should gain only a very modest rating.

8. *Achievements*. By identifying special accomplishments that are of an academic or a nonacademic nature, you will be able to assess if your credentials will stand out from among the multitude of applications received by the professional schools. You can then rate yourself accordingly.

9. *Personal attributes*. This criterion refers to qualities such as appearance, personality, capacity for critical judgment under stress and for perseverance under pressure, level of maturity, innate flexibility of character, etc. These factors will be relevant to your performance at an interview. The conclusions about your own characteristics should be based on evidence that can be exemplified. Your prior history as to your performance at interviews is very relevant in assessing

your rating on this important issue. Thus, individuals who are endowed with innate personal charm and an attractive physical appearance and who are good conversationalists have an enhanced potential for interview success and should rate themselves accordingly.

When you have completed the rating segment of the profile, you are in a position to arrive at an overall assessment of your admission potential, draw conclusions, and draft recommendations on areas where you need to improve.

Your overall assessment should be established by noting where the majority of criteria ratings have been placed. A distribution weighted to the left, where placement of ratings predominates in the superior and adequate categories, should be considered as indicating a good likelihood to achieve success in gaining admission. If the distribution is, however, weighted to the right, the reverse may be true, and an intense remediation effort in appropriate areas is called for.

In drawing your conclusions, you should bear in mind that the criteria are *not* of equal importance—the first five carry greater weight than the last four and your conclusions should be formulated appropriately.

Self-assessment Admission Profile

Name: _____   Date: _____

College: _____   Class: _____

Admission Criteria	Superior	Adequate	Weak	Comments
1. College attended				
2. GPA				
3. Science cumulative average				
4. MCAT or DAT scores				
5. Recommendations				
6. Extracurricular activities				
7. Professional exposure				
8. Achievements				
9. Personal attributes				

n.a.—adequate information is not available on this issue.

Comments:

_____

_____

_____

_____

Overall rating and conclusions:

_____

_____

Recommendations:

1. _____

2. _____

3. _____

APPENDIX B

MEDICAL SCHOOL APPLICATION FORMS

For many students, a major obstacle to admission can be that of successfully completing the application forms. Many of the forms are lengthy and all should be completed when you are relaxed, not rushed. Read all instructions carefully and answer all questions completely. Don't jeopardize your chances for admission by submitting an incomplete application form. Type all your answers neatly and be sure to review your application before sending it off. If the appearance of your application is in question, obtain a new one and fill it out more carefully. For additional information on applications, read Chapter 3.

Note: You must obtain the current application forms from the schools directly or through one of the application services (AMCAS, AACOMAS, AADSAS). Do not use these sample forms as your final application. They will not be accepted by the schools.

This appendix contains two application forms. Medical schools that do not subscribe to AMCAS have their own application forms; an example is the New York University form, which is shown on page 559. All osteopathic medical schools belong to AACOMAS, which has its own standard application form (see page 563). This application is very similar to the one used by AMCAS. Almost all dental schools belong to AADSAS. Nonsubscribing dental schools have their own application forms.

NEW YORK UNIVERSITY SCHOOL OF MEDICINE
A private university in the public service

APPLICATION FOR ADMISSION IN SEPTEMBER, 1997

OPTIONAL

A 2″x2″ passport-type photograph is required at the time of interview for purposes of identification and recall. You may enclose it with your application if you wish.

Name _____ Sex _____
            Last   First   Middle

Home Address _____

_____ Zip Code _____

Telephone (Please Include Area Code) _____

Mailing Address _____

_____ Zip Code _____

Telephone (Please Include Area Code) _____

Where should your mail be sent during the winter holidays? Give dates _____

_____

Date of Birth _____ Place of Birth _____ Citizenship _____

Social Security No. _____

Have you applied previously to the NYU School of Medicine? _____ Year _____

Have you attended another medical school? _____ If so, when and where? _____

This application is for admission to the
☐ First Year
☐ Second Year
☐ Third Year

The closing date for applications to the First Year Class is December 1, 1996. The closing date for transfer applications is May 1, 1997.

Name of parents or nearest living relatives _____

Address _____

Parents' occupations _____ (If retired or deceased, former occupation)

How many brothers and sisters in your family? _____

Your high school _____ City and State _____ Year of Graduation _____

RECORD OF COLLEGES ATTENDED

Please include *all* undergraduate and graduate level work, including summer school. Indicate any degree toward which you are now working, and date expected.

Name of College (and branch, if any)	Dates of Attendance	Field of Major Study	Degree	Mo/Yr

Has your education been continuous except for the standard vacations? _____

If not, or if not now in college, describe what you have done while out of school or since graduation.

Please account, chronologically, for all periods of time _____

_____

College academic honors _____

Extracurricular and summer activities, including employment _____

_____

_____

_____

_____

_____

_____

APPLICANT'S SUMMARY OF COLLEGE COURSES

Please list *all* courses taken and grades received.

Please specify *all* advanced standing credits you received upon entering college.

Prerequisite Course Work	College	Course Title	Semester Hours†	Grade
English*				
Physics*				
Inorganic Chemistry*				
Organic Chemistry *				
General Biology or Zoology*				
Additional Sciences and Mathematics				
Humanities, Social Sciences and Foreign Languages				

(Use additional page if necessary.)

* Six semester hours minimum. If these course requirements have not yet been met, please indicate in the grade column when they will be completed (Mo/Yr).

† or equivalent (indicate unit used)

If there is any information you wish to bring to the attention of the Admissions Committee regarding a physical or emotional condition or a family problem which you feel may have affected your scholastic performance, please indicate below or on a separate sheet.

_____

_____

_____

_____

_____

The Medical College Admission Test is a requirement for admission. Please state, in the left column below, dates (Mo/Yr) when the test was or will be taken and/or repeated. You may enter your scaled scores if you know them.

Date	Verbal Reasoning	Physical Sciences	Writing Sample	Biological Sciences

In the space below or on an accompanying sheet of paper please explain the key motivational factors in your decision to apply to medical school. Please feel free to supply any other information you would like to bring to the attention of the Committee on Admissions. Send completed application, completed statistical form, self-addressed acknowledgement card, $65 application fee made payable to NYU School of Medicine* and photograph (optional) to: _Committee on Admissions, New York University School of Medicine, P.O. Box 1924, New York, NY 10016._

*Applicants from Canada should submit their fee through a postal money order in U.S. funds rather than by personal check.

_____

_____

_____

_____

_____

_____

_____

_____

_____

_____

_____

_____

_____

Signature _____ **Date** _____

☐ If you plan to file an application for the
M.D.-Ph.D. Program please check here.

252 NYUMC 4/94

62-1/D NYUMC (V, XIV, XLII) Rev. 4/94

AACOMAS Application for the 1997 Entering Class
See AACOMAS Instruction Booklet before completing this form.

1.   **SSN** |_|_|_|_|_|_|_|_|_| **2. Name** _____
                                                              last   first   middle

3.   **Do you have educational materials under another name?**   Yes [   ]   No [   ]   **If yes, indicate name** _____

4.   **Preferred Mailing Address** _____
                                                                    street   city

      _____ **Telephone** _____
                        state   zip code   area code   number

5.   **Permanent and/or Legal Residence** _____
                                                                    street   city   township

      _____ **Telephone** _____
              county   state   zip code   area code   number

6.   **Are you a U.S. Citizen?**   Yes [   ]   No [   ]   **If No, what is your residency status?**   Temporary [   ]   Permanent [   ]

7.   **Sex***   Male [   ]   Female [   ]   **8. Birth Date*** |_|_|_|_|_|_|
                                                                       mo.   day   yr.

9.   **How do you**   [   ] 1. Black (non Hispanic)   Hispanic (choose only one)   [   ] 8. Asian or Pacific Islander
      describe yourself?* [   ] 2. American Indian or Alaskan Native   [   ] 4. Mexican American or Chicano   [   ] 9. Other _____
                              [   ] 3. White (non Hispanic)   [   ] 5. Puerto Rican (Mainland)
                                                                      [   ] 6. Puerto Rican (Commonwealth)
                                                                      [   ] 7. Other Hispanic _____

10.   **Parent/Guardian**   Name   Living   State of   Education/College
                                                     Yes No   Occupation   Residence   or highest level

      Father   _____ [   ][   ] _____
      Mother   _____ [   ][   ] _____
      Guardian _____ [   ][   ] _____

11.   **Secondary School** _____
                                        name   city   state   year of graduation

12.   **A. All Undergraduate Colleges Attended** (list in chronological order)

		Dates of Attendance	Check if Summer Only		
Institution	Campus/Location/State			Major	Degree Granted or Expected (with date)
_____	_____	19 ___ to 19 ___	[ ]	_____	_____
_____	_____	19 ___ to 19 ___	[ ]	_____	_____
_____	_____	19 ___ to 19 ___	[ ]	_____	_____
_____	_____	19 ___ to 19 ___	[ ]	_____	_____
_____	_____	19 ___ to 19 ___	[ ]	_____	_____
_____	_____	19 ___ to 19 ___	[ ]	_____	_____

      B. All Graduate or Professional Schools Attended

_____	_____	19 ___ to 19 ___	[ ]	_____	_____
_____	_____	19 ___ to 19 ___	[ ]	_____	_____
_____	_____	19 ___ to 19 ___	[ ]	_____	_____

13.   **Have you had any U.S. military experience?**   Yes [   ]   No [   ]   **Was your discharge dishonorable?**   Yes [   ]   No [   ]

* See Instruction Booklet for non-discrimination policy statement.   **DO NOT TYPE OUTSIDE THE BORDER**

                                                                             FOR OFFICE USE ONLY |_|_|_|_|_|_|

DO NOT TYPE OUTSIDE OF BORDER

ACADEMIC RECORD

SSN | | | | | | | | | |

Name _____

Last   First   Middle   Suffix

College	Location	Year	Term	Number	Course Name	Type	Academic Status	Subject	Semester Hours	AACOMAS Grade	Actual Grade	AACOMAS Use	

DO NOT TYPE BELOW BORDER   **FOR OFFICIAL USE ONLY.** _____

College	Location	Year	Term	Number	Course Name	Type	Academic Status	Subject	Semester Hours	AACOMAS Grade	Actual Grade	AACOMAS Use		

MCAT INFORMATION

Test Scores (New Format, April 1991 or Later, Only)				
Date	Verbal	Phys Sci	Writing	Biology

How many times have you taken the MCAT test? ☐

If you plan to take or retake the MCAT — enter date. ☐ ☐
mo.   yr.

ACADEMIC RECORD

SSN | | | | | | | | |

Name _____

Last   First   Middle   Suffix

College	Location	Year	Term	Number	Course Name	Type	Academic Status	Subject	Semester Hours	AACOMAS Grade	Actual Grade	AACOMAS Use		

DO NOT TYPE BELOW BORDER

ACADEMIC RECORD

SSN |__|__|__|__|__|__|__|__|__| Name _____
                                              Last   *First*   *Middle*   *Suffix*

College	Location	Year	Term	Number	Course Name	Type	Academic Status	Subject	Semester Hours	AACOMAS Grade	Actual Grade	AACOMAS Use	

DO NOT TYPE BELOW BORDER

14. **List employment in chronological order since your graduation, beginning with your current position:**

Title or Description   Dates   Level of Responsibility

> ### It is imperative that you answer questions 15-19 (see page 5 of the Instruction Booklet
> ### If the answer to questions 16-18 is yes, or if 19 is "F", please explain fully in Personal Comments

15. **Have you ever matriculated in or attended any medical school as a candidate for the M.D. or D.O. degree?**........... Yes [   ]   No [   ]
16. **Were you ever the recipient of any action for unacceptable academic performance or conduct violations (e.g. dismissal, suspension, disqualification, etc.) by any college or school?** ....Yes [   ]   No [   ]
     If yes, Were you ever denied readmission?   Yes [   ]   No [   ]
17. **Have you ever been convicted of or have pending a misdemeanor or felony (exclude parking violations)?** .... Yes [   ]   No [   ]
18. **Is a family member a D.O.?** (if yes, list up to three codes from the Instruction Booklet Page 4)................... Yes [   ] [   ] [   ]   No [   ]
19. **How did you first learn about osteopathic medicine?** (choose only one) .... A) Pre-professional advisor_____ B) D.O. _____
    C) Representative from an osteopathic college _____ D) Recruitment Mailing _____ E) AACOM _____ F) Other (please specify) _____

PERSONAL COMMENTS (see AACOMAS Instruction Booklet before completing)

I authorize AACOMAS to release the following information to pre-professional health advisors to assist those advisors in counseling students: my name; the osteopathic medical school at which I matriculate; my state or country of legal residence, as stated in my application materials; my undergraduate institution; and my degree date from that institution... Yes [   ]   No [   ]

I have read and understand the instructions and other information in the AACOMAS Instruction Booklet, including the statement above. I certify that the information submitted in these application materials is complete and correct to the best of my knowledge. I agree that this information may be used by the AACOM and its member institutions for research and development purposes aimed at improving osteopathic medical education and admissions programs.

Date _____ Signature _____

AMERICAN ASSOCIATION OF COLLEGES OF OSTEOPATHIC MEDICINE
6110 EXECUTIVE BLVD., SUITE 405, ROCKVILLE, MD 20852

APPENDIX C

SAMPLE ESSAYS FOR AMCAS APPLICATION _____

Most U.S. medical and osteopathic schools make use of the application services, AMCAS and AACOMAS, respectively. The major component of the application used by these services, as well as the dental service (AADSAS), is the blank page allotted for a personal statement or essay (see Chapter 3). This is a valuable opportunity that can impact very significantly on one's admission potential. Appendix C contains ten sample conventional essays. These, like the two presented in Chapter 3, were written by applicants seeking admission to professional schools. (To avoid any possibility of identifying the writers of these essays, specific names are not used.) These essays are included to give a prospective applicant an insight into the different approaches that can be used. Some are general essays covering personal characteristics, education, relevant experience, and motivation. Other essays are more focused on aspects of the applicant's background. These essays should provide helpful ideas on how to approach the important part of the application process—the essay.

Essay 1

I have elected to apply to medical school because I believe that this unique profession will provide me with a lifetime of personal satisfaction. Moreover, I am convinced that I possess the basic attributes that are essential for those who seek to enter this demanding field. I know that I have the intellectual potential, especially in the sciences, as well as the temperament and drive necessary to meet the challenge that the lifelong study of medicine requires.

I enrolled at _____ University after successfully completing a demanding high school (graduating eighth of 85). I chose _____ because of its reputation for providing both a well-rounded education and a strong science background. I elected to major in general science to obtain the broad base of knowledge that would serve as a solid foundation for my future professional school studies. Aside from the required premedical curriculum, I have taken courses ranging from astronomy to computers, with a concentration in the biological sciences. My educational goal was not grade-oriented, but directed to securing the best grasp of the material. I feel that my academic average, while satisfactory, does not accurately reflect my academic potential, which I feel is significantly higher. I also sought an education that would incorporate non-science courses to the extent possible and I participated in a wide variety of extracurricular activities.

I am patient, self-disciplined, and caring. I like to accept a challenge and I then apply my talents to successfully achieve the realistic goals I set. In the field of experimental medicine, I spent two summers at _____ Hospital. I was engaged in research projects concerned with drug blood levels using various analytical tools, and also did a time-action study to determine the feasibility of laboratory computerization. In my free time, I organized my own band and succeeded in winning several talent contests, as well as being hired to play at a variety of social affairs. Both of these efforts involved assuming responsibilities, demonstrating initiative and leadership capacity, and having good interpersonal ability.

My hospital experience served to convince me of the genuineness of my feeling of empathy for those in need of healing or relief from pain. It also convinced me of the need to keep the patient in proper focus, since technological advances, although most valuable, can tend to impede the establishment of good physician-patient relationships.

While I am not certain at this time in what area of medicine I will find my place, I believe my talents will enable me to contribute to the welfare of those I will serve. I sincerely hope I will be granted the opportunity to pursue my professional goals.

Essay 2

My career goal to become a physician is long-standing and deep-rooted. Two of the major drives to attain my professional goal include a broad educational involvement and interest in the sciences and a unique set of life experiences over the past five years that have crystallized my aspirations.

Supplementing this application are transcripts reflecting my scientific exposure. However, what is most significant regarding my career decision is my personal experience. Always athletic, I sustained a sports-related accident at the age of seventeen, and became a patient in a hospital, where surgery and several months of rehabilitation were required. My complete recovery was due to the medical expertise and compassion of my physician, and the patience and support of my physical therapist. I learned a great deal, not only about my medical condition in particular, but also about being a patient and how important an understanding physician is to the healing process. Since then, I have developed a firm conviction that those practicing the healing arts not only restore the body, but give people hope to overcome many of the hardships related to illness.

Due to my experience as a patient, I was removed from familiar surroundings and forced to contend with difficult situations. At nineteen, I again found myself in an unfamiliar setting. This time, it was for a year and a half of college studies overseas. Relocating to a foreign country for an extended period had a strong impact on my individual growth and helped develop my sense of identity and responsibility. I improved my capacity to cope with change, the unknown, and multicultural environments. The ability to adapt, to overcome adversity, and to welcome new and formidable tasks, are skills I will bring with me to the medical profession.

During my college studies abroad, I was fortunate to have a premedical placement in a local hospital. There, I was exposed to the unpredictable and challenging activities of an emergency room. In addition, my school provided me with a type of "settlement house" placement, working with underprivileged, immigrant children. These placements allowed me to learn more about the interrelationship between poverty and the poor utilization of health service.

A constant source of inspiration has come from living in a cohesive, civic-minded community with numerous practicing physicians. I have been impressed with the communal and charitable roles played by the physicians my family knows. Several of these physicians have been especially supportive in my pursuits and have become role models whom I would hope to emulate in the future.

The attainment of a black belt from a prestigious karate school is among the many skills that I have mastered. To achieve this required many years of study, practice, and commitment to a discipline. Training others to master the art of self-defense, while teaching them diligence and perseverance, has solidified these qualities within myself.

My cumulative college index for my studies both in the United States and abroad was 3.9, demonstrating my ability to be scholastically consistent and outstanding in varied academic settings. Throughout my college years, I have been involved in numerous communication arts and educational seminars, such as: Dramatic Society, Speech Club, and preparing instructional/cultural workshops for high school and college students. Upon graduation from college this past June, I accepted a position furnishing outreach services to the homebound elderly. I also plan to take graduate courses in medical ethics.

To me, medicine is unique for its restorative potentials made possible through a combination of advanced technologies and human compassion. I am deeply committed to seeking a career in medicine, and believe that I have the capabilities to succeed.

Essay 3

"Please doctor help me!" an elderly woman called out anxiously, while lying on a stretcher in the emergency room at _____ Hospital. "I am not yet a doctor; just try to relax and I will get help right away," I responded.

Before my hospital exposure as a volunteer in the emergency room, I was attracted to a medical career because of the intellectual life that it offers. This appeal was stimulated by my long-standing insatiable scientific curiosity. I am strongly motivated to learn about science in general and medicine in particular. My academic record demonstrates that I have an ability to meet the demanding challenges that medical school presents. My GPA rose rapidly from 2.98, which I received in my first semester of freshman year, to the 3.48 that I have now (which includes the 3.93 that I received in the first semester of junior year). I anticipate that I will apply to medical school with a GPA that will exceed 3.50.

A physician needs a great deal more than academic competence. With the enormous advances in recent years in diagnostic technology, the patient is no longer the spokesman for his or her body. Although diseases can be detected earlier and therefore treated more effectively as a result of advances in modern medicine, there has been a tendency for the physician to become more impersonal. I believe the greatest challenge facing a medical practitioner today is to develop an approach that will prevent technology from coming between himself or herself and the patient. Lewis Thomas, in his book, *The Youngest Science,* writes, "Doctors the critics say, are applied scientists, concerned only with the disease at hand but never with the patient as an individual, whole person." If this is true it is quite disturbing because I feel that a good doctor-patient rapport can have a positive impact on a patient's treatment and recovery. A physician must be a confidant, gaining the trust of those he or she is treating. I would seek to utilize the tools of modern medicine to supplement, but not replace, an empathizing approach to human suffering and anxiety.

The issue that I am concerned about in the future is how I will react to the ethical challenges that face a medical practitioner today. I am especially interested in the discipline of medical ethics, and I am pleased to see that the subject has been included in the medical school curriculum. I am confident that further training in this area will prepare me to meet these challenges.

One reason why I want a career in medicine is that, as a physician, I will be able to provide care for those who need it. When the elderly woman in the emergency room at _____ Hospital cried for help, I had a strong desire to alleviate her suffering. Considering my innate love of science and my academic achievements in college, I am confident that I will succeed and become a credit to the medical profession.

Essay 4

Contemplating what the future holds for a prospective physician in the twenty-first century would suggest the probability of changes in the practice of medicine. While medicine will continue to make significant advances, increased government regulation will impose bureaucratic hardships and technological breakthroughs will increase the pressures toward depersonalization of medical practice. Prospective physicians (as myself) will, therefore, be required to possess the innate personal characteristics that will enable us to accept a sense of gratification for services rendered as a significant measure of compensation for the difficulties that we will have to accept.

In the limited free time available to me, I involved myself in various communal and charitable endeavors, which brought me into contact with the youth and elderly, infirm, indigent, and handicapped. I not only served personally but was motivated to stimulate others to do so and thereby helped improve the life of those less fortunate than myself. By being a service-oriented individual, I hope that my years as a physician will allow me to alleviate the pain of my fellow man and offer the ailing comfort and support during their trying times.

Medicine also offers its professionals a chance to unravel the mysteries of the human being. Its focus on man as a primary subject of study has long intrigued me and it will undoubtedly continue to grant me intellectual stimulation in future years. A summer of research experience in an honors program, an intense emergency medical training course, and acting as a volunteer in the Emergency Room of a local hospital have sparked my interests, and I look forward to contributing my own insights and skills to this ever progressing science.

As a health-care professional entrusted with life and death decisions, a physician must possess the highest intellectual capabilities. My academic career has been characterized by superlatives, and I am confident that this pattern will continue. My selection as salutatorian of my elementary school class and valedictorian of my high school class (with the simultaneous reception of a Governor's Scholarship Award) confirmed that I had the capabilities for superior academic achievement. Excelling in my scholastic studies during my college career in both the science and nonscience courses has reinforced this conviction.

Medicine is both the art and science of healing. As my extracurricular activities and scholastic achievements indicate, I realize the vital importance of both aspects. My background and education have instilled in me the ethical concepts and sense of dedication that the medical professional demands. By becoming a physician qualified to practice in the twenty-first century, I will be afforded the privilege of sharing in the effort to improve the quality of life of my fellow human beings and, simultaneously, the quality of my own life will be more meaningful.

Essay 5

While at Yale I have become interested in a career in medicine through my studies and extracurricular activities. Before coming to college I was interested in science and was considering a career in scientific research. In the last three years my attention has become focused on medicine, as I feel this profession offers the best opportunity to pursue my interests in a way that will be beneficial and useful to others.

For three years I have worked in the astronomy department on a variety of research projects. I helped compile the most recent versions of the Yale Bright Star Catalogue and the Yale Parallax Catalogue. These projects allowed me to get a taste of scientific research. Although I learned much from this experience and enjoyed working with the other astronomers, I believe that my abilities would be more usefully applied in some other way.

Medicine first attracted me because it requires a knowledge of several sciences, whereas most fields require (or encourage) knowledge of only one. In my senior research essay I will publish the results of an epidemiological investigation into correlations between high population density and certain pathologies among bacteria, laboratory rats, and humans. The data has been collected from experiments at Yale's Osborn Biology facility and from the Social Science Archives at Yale Computer Center. I hope to have this paper published in both biology and sociology journals.

My major involves sixteen courses, eight from sociology and eight from biology. Of course, in addition to these I have taken the required chemistry, physics, mathematics, and English. I have become especially interested in molecular biology, and now have a small library of books on this subject.

One of the most interesting experiences of the past three years was working in the emergency room of _____ Hospital in _____. I was part of the College Aide Program, which provided Yale students with an opportunity to observe hospital practices in return for volunteer work. I spent about half of my time in the emergency room in the medical and surgical trauma areas helping with suturing procedures, EKGs, IVs, and blood gases. The rest of my time was spent in the labs, helping with routine blood analysis. The shifts were four hours at a time, which was one-third of what many of the physicians worked, yet were still plenty tiring! However, I was so interested in what was happening that the time seemed to pass quickly. I gained a lot of respect and admiration for the doctors who had to deal with the great responsibility and pressure inherent to their profession, and decided that someday I would like to become one of them.

I have always been interested in issues of medical significance and was one of three student speakers (along with a number of academic figures) to make a presentation at the 1990 Bioethics Conference at _____. My talk was on the ethics of genetic engineering, a topic that is still a matter of controversy. At the time I was a freshman at Yale, and our biology department had just announced the results of some startling experiments with mouse embryos that had been genetically engineered.

All of these experiences have convinced me that medicine is an exciting field in which I believe I could make a worthwhile contribution while simultaneously gaining the personal satisfaction that accompanies such an important profession.

Essay 6

My decision to apply to medical school is a result of considerable preparation and thought, an evaluation of my own abilities, and some experience in the health field.

Among the attributes I believe a physician should possess are dedication, sincerity, and integrity. I believe that my peers consider me to have such qualities and I trust that these qualities should contribute to my professional success.

I've progressed through high school and college, both of which had demanding programs of study, and achieved superior grades. I always found science courses to be of special interest.

My decision to pursue a medical career stems from several motivating factors. Foremost, I have come to appreciate the inherent intellectual and emotional challenges involved in medicine during my research at _____ Hospital. While there I was involved in a research project dealing with the role of Ketoconazole in the treatment of fungal infections. This experience enabled me to directly view the clinical application of research. I have also been exposed to the emotional side of practicing medicine by participating in daily rounds and observing the patients' progress with physicians and other members of the research team. This activity was instrumental in allowing me to appreciate the vital role played by the physician in helping the patient emotionally as well as physically. As a member of this team, I used this opportunity to establish relationships by offering daily encouragement and explanations whenever possible. This unique medical exposure afforded me the opportunity of obtaining both intellectual and emotional satisfaction in a medical context.

The satisfactions derived from challenging intellectual and emotional pursuits have always motivated me to excel. This is underscored by my success as a youth leader in my church and as a coordinator of a blood drive for my school. My duties in the church involve weekly preparation of a portion of the Bible for presentation to the congregation. This entails approximately ten hours per week of preparation and requires a thorough understanding as well as memorization of the lengthy passages. Although extremely demanding of my time and concentration, the rewards of leadership and performing a job well make this task worth undertaking. I anticipate that this congregational leadership role will help me assume responsibilities as an active layman in my community later in my life.

As a coordinator of my school's blood drive, my major responsibility was donor recruitment. This entailed my allaying the fears of prospective donors and arranging all logistical aspects of the drive. My determination and hard work were rewarded by the outstanding achievement of the drive, as noted by the Red Cross for being the most successful drive in New York City.

I am well aware of the physical and emotional difficulties as well as the dedication required in a medical career. This realization has become evident to me through my close relationship with my brother-in-law who is currently a physician in postgraduate training. The demands and responsibilities of his work have often been communicated to me. The challenges and rewards however, are the factors that stand out as providing adequate compensation. I am confident that my personal attributes, coupled with my motivation refined through my various exposure to medicine, will lead me to a satisfying and fruitful career. I feel that I have already proved to myself that, when motivated, I can succeed at a challenging task. It is with this positive attitude that I seek to embark upon a medical career.

Essay 7

To the members of the Admission Committee:

I am applying for admission to your school with the aim of securing my M.D. degree as a basis for an eventual career in academic medicine. It is my goal to devote my professional activities to clinical practice, teaching, and research. This career goal evolved naturally during my adolescence, as well as during my college and graduate school studies.

I received my elementary school education at a small private school, where my initial interest in science developed. This interest was enhanced due to my close relationship with a cousin who was a medical technologist. By the time I was in my early teens, I had spent part of each summer in her hospital's laboratory observing the routine and being briefed in terms that were understandable. I became increasingly enthusiastic with my medical science exposure. Gradually, my horizons were expanded when I was fortunate to have the opportunity to observe the activities of the chief pathologist. I not only viewed specimen preparation procedures, but was given explanations of the clinical findings on both gross and microscopic levels. By the end of my freshman year of college, I had observed my first autopsy. Once I had this meaningful exposure, the stimulus to seek a medical career took on a self-propelling dimension. I realized how interesting and challenging the profession was and that it offered the satisfying opportunity to improve the quality of life of those I would have the opportunity to treat.

To attain my goal, I enrolled in a program of science and non-science studies at _____ College, and later, _____ University, where I elected to major in biology. As an upperclassman, I enrolled in some graduate level courses, took part in research, and wrote an honors thesis. I was the second person in the history of the Biology Department to graduate with departmental honors as well as summa cum laude.

My successful research activities, although exciting by themselves, stimulated my interest in a career in academic medicine. Because of the intimate student-graduate student-faculty relationships existing at my school, teaching came into the picture as part of my potential career activities. To further my ambition, I enrolled in our Masters Program and was offered a teaching assistantship. My graduate research so far has resulted in one paper (to be published shortly), another paper in preparation, and hopefully one commercial product. My successful teaching activities have covered a wide variety of undergraduate laboratory courses.

My academic achievements both as an undergraduate and graduate student have been consistently superior except for my sophomore year in college. At that time I was extremely preoccupied with my father's health, which was deteriorating because of emphysema. However, I gained a great deal of career inspiration from the dedicated team of medical personnel who pulled him through. Omitting this unrepresentative year, therefore, my cumulative average would be 3.76 (instead of 3.61), which is consistent with my 3.85 graduate school record.

In conclusion, I am convinced that I have the maturity, interest, and ability to undertake medical studies with a sense of enthusiasm and dedication. I hope you will afford me the opportunity to do so.

Essay 8

One might assume that since my father and grandfather are both physicians, the decision that I too must be a doctor would have been unquestioned. This may be true in many cases but the situation was quite the opposite for me. My decision to enter the medical profession is solely my own, made after a very prolonged period of introspection and soul-searching. My family did not seek to pressure me, but rather helped me to have a well-balanced view of this challenging profession. What I saw was the selfless dedication of my father to his family practice in a low-income area in central New Jersey. His major reward is, for the most part, the satisfaction of providing quality health care to the community he serves, which has always involved a great deal of physical and emotional commitment and self-sacrifice. Therefore, my decision is based not on an idealistic view but a very realistic one of the rewards that a medical career has to offer.

I have always had a great interest in farming. The idea of producing something with my own hands, managing my own affairs, and being my own boss has always meant a great deal to me. As a result, for the past six years I have been operating my own vegetable farm and produce stand. All the vegetables I sell I have grown myself. I have been careful to avoid treating my crops with pesticides and harmful chemicals. I found it especially enjoyable to deal directly with people and I related well to them to the point of building a sizable, steady clientele. In my work I have grown very found of the countryside and I enjoy working in a rural setting.

My love for plants and the soil contributed to my decision to major in biology at my college. After three years of undergraduate work I have found that the more I study biology, the more enthusiastic I become about the subject. This is reflected in my consistent A average in all my biology courses. My less than impressive overall performance during the first two years of college stems from my delay in firmly fixing my career goal until the end of sophomore year. As a result, I did not mobilize all of my intellectual resources toward achieving a strong academic record; however, once I made up my mind about my future, I began to demonstrate that I possess the necessary potential to meet the demands of medical school. I trust that my willingness to undertake the uphill journey to a medical career—although belatedly—will reflect favorably upon the genuineness of my commitment and the sincerity of my motivation. I am convinced that I can succeed in making a significant contribution to the well-being of the people I hope to serve.

After much though, I find that my fundamental reason for wanting to become a physician is simple: I want to establish a family practice in a rural area where dedicated physicians are sorely needed. I realize that the goal I have set may not, in the light of my initial college record, be easily attained. Nevertheless, I firmly believe that when my full record of achievement is reviewed, and the special circumstances discussed above are taken into consideration, I will merit the confidence of being offered a place in your freshman class.

Essay 9

"Mad Scientist" is the name my mother has affectionately called me since childhood. Even as a youngster, my favorite place was my father's laboratory in his medical office. On Sunday afternoons my father would take my four younger brothers and me to his office where we would spend hours viewing slides and "experimenting." It was in this lab that I developed my sense of curiosity, my love of science, and a spirit of adventure.

When I was 17 I left home and spent two years studying and traveling abroad. The experience of living 6,000 miles away from home in a milieu so different from my own provided me with a much broader view of the wide variety of existing culture. The most intriguing aspect of those years was the diversity of personalities I encountered. Among my classmates were natives of Yemen, Iran, England, and France. Every meal we shared resembled a model United Nations with students from many countries expressing varying opinions. I learned to relate to and understand people with whom I seemingly had little in common, and developed close and lasting friendships with them. This unique exposure will undoubtedly prove valuable to me in the years ahead in dealing with people as their physician.

I returned from overseas to pursue my educational and premedical career goals. I selected _____ University because of its academic excellence.

I worked with youth programs organized by the university and was recently appointed to head an educational program for high school students. I was also elected Senior Editor of the student newspaper. This position required an ability to express myself creatively in writing. It also required learning to work with a team while assuming a leadership role.

My summer experiences were an outgrowth of my scientific interests. I worked for a radiologist where I learned about human anatomy, about the fascinating methods now available through modern technology, and how to secure invaluable clinical information. I worked during the same summer with Dr. H., Director of the Rheumatic Diseases laboratory at _____ College of Medicine, studying the immunopathological process involved in cartilage erosion. The following summer I worked with Dr. S. of the Cardiology Department of the Medical School studying the microcirculation of the rat's coronary artery system. This laboratory work introduced me to such divergent procedures as gel electrophoresis and animal surgery and gave me a great respect for scientific inquiry. I am continuing my work with Dr. S. this summer, studying the effects of calcium channel blockers on the inotropy of the rat's myocardium.

All of my experiences mentioned above affected my career choice, and medicine offers a vast array of intellectual challenges. The coming decades will witness a continuation of the exciting technological revolution. I hope to be a part of this creative adventure. At the same time, medicine offers the ultimate in one's service to humanity. There is no greater pleasure than the ability to use one's intellect and abilities to alleviate human pain and suffering.

If accepted, I believe I will be an asset to your freshman class.

Essay 10

The gratification that I receive from working with and caring for others has been the major motivation behind my desire to become a doctor. My experience growing up as an only child has had much to do with my reaching out toward others, as I often felt isolated as a result of my parents' difficulty understanding English. When I show concern for another person it is because I know how important it can be to have someone show sincere interest and caring.

I have always been interested in serving the needs of others. At my school I was vice-president of a community service organization. I enjoyed working with those who shared the same interest. Some of my best experiences were working with concerned students on blood drives and fund-raisings. A particularly memorable experience was acting as co-chairman of the school's annual Muscular Dystrophy Marathon.

It is difficult to adequately describe the feelings I experience when my caring is rewarded with something as simple as being depended on and being considered a source of comfort. At the local hospital I formed a special relationship with a young patient suffering from multiple sclerosis. I spent many hours in her company, helping to feed her, and talking to her. More recently, I worked with a dedicated staff at another hospital, gift-wrapping hundreds of holiday presents for patients.

My earlier experiences influenced my decision to work this past year as an assistant in oral surgery, where I found great satisfaction comforting and relaxing patients before an operative procedure.

My interest in science has made becoming a doctor an ideal choice. I can remember very vividly the experience of seeing my mother admitted to a hospital because of a problem with her lungs. Before a diagnosis was reached, I wanted to know what was at stake and read all that I could about tuberculosis and cancer. (It turned out to be emphysema and she was successfully treated.) Several years later, this desire to learn about medicine was strongly reinforced as I sat totally absorbed watching open heart surgery. Another situation that has left a very strong impression occurred while I was a volunteer at the hospital's emergency room. I watched doctors and nurses working together under intense time pressure as they attempted to save an elderly man who had been hit by a truck. As I observed them, I could visualize myself being a part of their efforts to sustain life.

My firm commitment to my career goal has strengthened my determination during difficult periods. There were times when my ability to study effectively was disrupted by financial problems, illness, and a less than ideal living situation. In order to avoid a long commute, I often resorted to sleeping nights on dormitory floors and library couches.

Becoming a doctor is an extension of my interest in science and of my desire to lead a life that I consider all-absorbing. I strongly desire a career that involves a total commitment to learning and a responsibility for the welfare of others. The more lives I touch as a doctor, the more meaningful I feel my life becomes. Therefore, I would value the opportunity to pursue my studies at your institution.

APPENDIX D

MAJOR PROFESSIONAL ORGANIZATIONS

Aerospace Medical Association
P.O. Box 26128
Alexandria, Virginia 22313

American Academy of Allergy and Immunology
611 East Wells Street
Milwaukee, Wisconsin 53202

American Academy of Child and Adolescent Psychiatry
3615 Wisconsin, NW
Washington, DC 20016

American Academy of Dermatology
1567 Maple Avenue
Evanston, Illinois 60201

American Academy of Family Physicians
8880 Ward Parkway
Kansas City, Missouri 64114

American Academy of Neurology
3331 University Avenue SE
Suite 335
Minneapolis, Minnesota 55414

American Academy of Ophthalmology
655 Beach Street
P.O. Box 7424
San Francisco, California 94120

American Academy of Ophthalmology and Otalaryngology
15 Second Street SW
Rochester, Minnesota 55901

American Academy of Orthopedic Surgeons
222 South Prospect Avenue
Park Ridge, Illinois 60068

American Academy of Pediatrics
141 Northwest Point Boulevard
Elk Grove, Illinois 60009

American Academy of Physical Medicine and Rehabilitation
122 South Michigan Avenue
Suite 1300
Chicago, Illinois 60603

American Association of Colleges of Osteopathic Medicine
6110 Executive Boulevard
Rockville, Maryland 20852

American Association of Dental Schools
1625 Massachusetts Avenue NW
Washington, DC 20036

American Association of Neurological Surgeons
22 South Washington Street
Suite 100
Park Ridge, Illinois 60068

American Association of Opthalmology
1100 17th Street NW
Suite 304
Washington, DC 20036

American Association of Orthodontists
7477 Delmar Boulevard
St. Louis, Missouri 63130

American Association of Public Health Physicians
1703 Ridgemont
Austin, Texas 78723

American Board of Medical Specialties
One American Plaza
Suite 505
Evanston, Illinois 60201

American College of Allergy and Immunology
800 East Northwest Highway
Suite 1080
Palatine, Illinois 60067

American College of Cardiology
9111 Old Georgetown Road
Bethesda, Maryland 20014

American College of Chest Physicians
911 Busse Highway
Park Ridge, Illinois 60068

American College of Colon and Rectal Surgery
615 Griswold
Suite 1717
Detroit, Michigan 48226

American College of Emergency Physicians
P.O. Box 61991
Dallas, Texas 75261

American College of Gastroenterologists
13 Elm Street
Manchester, Massachusetts 01944

American College of Obstetricians and Gynecologists
600 Maryland Avenue SW
Suite 300
Washington, DC 20024

American College of Physicians
4200 Pine Street
Philadelphia, Pennsylvania 19104

American College of Preventive Medicine
1015 15th Street NW
Suite 403
Washington, DC 20005

American College of Radiology
1891 Preston White Drive
Reston, Virginia 22091

American College of Surgeons
55 East Erie Street
Chicago, Illinois 60611

American Council for Graduate Medical Education
535 North Dearborn Street
Chicago, Illinois 60610

American Dental Association
211 East Chicago Avenue
Chicago, Illinois 60611

American Federation for Clinical Research
6900 Grove Road
Thorofare, New Jersey 08086

American Geriatrics Society
770 Lexington Avenue
Suite 400
New York, New York 10021

American Hospital Association
840 North Lake Shore Drive
Chicago, Illinois 60611

American Medical Association
515 North Street
Chicago, Illinois 60610

American Medical Student Association
1890 Preston White Drive
Reston, Virginia 22091

American Medical Women's Association
801 North Fairfax Street
Alexandria, Virginia 22314

American Ophthalmological Society
Mayo Clinic
200 First Street SW
Rochester, Minnesota 55901

American Osteopathic Association
142 East Ontario Street
Chicago, Illinois 60611

American Osteopathic Healthcare Association
5301 Wisconsin Avenue NW
Washington, DC 20013

American Osteopathic Hospital Association
930 Busse Highway
Park Ridge, Illinois 60068

American Psychiatric Association
1400 K Street NW
Washington, DC 20005

American Rheumatism Association
1314 Spring Street NW
Atlanta, Georgia 36309

American Society of Anesthesiologists
515 Busse Highway
Park Ridge, Illinois 60068

American Society of Clinical Pathologists
2100 West Harrison Street
Chicago, Illinois 60612

American Society for Hematology
1101 Connecticut Avenue NW
Washington, DC 20036

American Society of Clinical Oncology
435 No. Michigan Avenue
Suite 1717
Chicago, Illinois 60611

American Society for Colon and Rectal Surgery
615 Griswold
Suite 1717
Detroit, Michigan 48226

American Society for Internal Medicine
1101 Vermont Avenue NW
Suite 500
Washington, DC 20005

American Society of Nephrology
1101 Connecticut Avenue NW
Washington, DC 20036

American Society of Plastic and Reconstructive Surgeons
444 East Algonquin Road
Arlington Heights, Illinois 60005

American Thoracic Society
1740 Broadway
New York, New York 10019

American Urological Association
6750 Loop South
Suite 900
Dallas, Texas 77401

Association of American Medical Colleges
2450 N Street NW
Washington, DC 20037

Association of Canadian Medical Colleges
151 Slater Avenue
Suite 1120
Ottawa, Ontario KIP 5NI
Canada

College of American Pathologists
5202 Old Orchard Road
Skokie, Illinois 60077

Educational Council for Foreign Medical Graduates
3624 Market Street
Philadelphia, Pennsylvania 19104

Endocrine Society
9650 Rorckville Park
Bethesda, Maryland 20014

Infectious Diseases Society of America
Office of the Secretary
Yale University School of Medicine
333 Cedar Street 201-LCI
New Haven, Connecticut 06510

National Dental Association
735 Fifteenth Street NW
Washington, DC 20005

National Medical Association
1720 Massachusetts Avenue NW
Washington, DC 20036

National Resident Matching Program
2450 N Street NW
Suite 201
Washington, DC 20037

Rehabilitation Physicians Association
1101 Vermont Avenue NW
Suite 500
Washington, DC 20005

Society of Critical Care Medicine
251 East Imperial Highway
Fullerton, California 92635

Society of Thoracic Surgeons
111 East Waker Drive
Chicago, Illinois 60604

APPENDIX E

ALTERNATIVE MEDICAL TERMINOLOGY _____

Allopathy

term coined by Dr. Samuel Hahnemann (1755–1843), the German founder of homeopathy. The name represents a combination of the Greek words *allos* (other) and *pathos* (suffering). It is a type of therapy aimed at healing a disease by producing a second condition that is different from the effects of that disease. The name now applies to all but osteopathic medical schools.

Acupuncture

Chinese technique for treating pain or disease in which needles are inserted in points along meridians that correspond to organs.

Alexander

Technique technique developed by an Australian actor as a method for improving posture so as to improve health.

Byur Veda

Indian healing approach that uses diet, herbs, exercise, massage, and scent, prescribed according to body type.

Bachs Flour Remedy

medicine made from flour and alcohol, based on the formulas of an English physician Edward Bachs (1886–1933).

Biofee

back a careful monitoring of body changes by which patients can learn to lower their blood pressure and alter other internal physiological functions.

Chelation Therapy

infusion of intravenous doses of an aminoxide. It is used to treat AIDS and other diseases and illnesses.

Shi

Chinese name for the invisible life force.

Chi Gong

a form of meditation or, as used by some, a type of hand healing.

Chiropractic

approach developed by D.D. Palmer (1845–1913), combining the Greek names *kheir* (hand) and *practios* (effective). He believed that 95% of illnesses could be cured by manipulating the spine. Most modern chiropractors primarily treat back problems.

Homeopathy

approach developed by Dr. Samuel Hahnemann. Combining the Greek word *homoest* (similar) and *pathos* (suffering), he treated symptoms on the principle that "like cures like." He prescribed substances that, in healthy patients, caused symptoms similar to those of the diseases he was treating.

Hydrotherapy

ancient remedy of bathing to promote health. Various combinations of minerals and temperatures are used.

Imagery

behavior therapy technique in which the patient is conditioned to replace feelings of anxiety with pleasant fantasies.

Iridology

examining the iris of the eye to diagnose illness.

Moxibustion

Asian treatment of burning herbs near the skin. The body should benefit from their penetration.

Naturapathy

system of therapy in which practitioners use natural means, such as herbal remedies, hydrotherapy, homeopathy, nutrition, manipulative modalities, acupuncture, and counseling for treatment.

Osteopathy

developed by Andrew Taylor Still (1828–1917), an American physician, who believed in applying musculoskeletal manipulation as a therapeutic approach. The profession has changed considerably since it was founded and has moved closer to allopathy.

Rolfing

deep massage technique developed by an American chemist, Dr. Ida Rolf.

Shiatsu

Japanese massage technique based on acupuncture concepts.

Traditional Chinese Medicine

system of healing using acupuncture, herbal medicine, moxibustion, massage, cupping, nutrition, and meditation. Its goal is to balance opposite and complementary aspects of being to enhance the flow of the life force (chi).

APPENDIX F

TRACKING TABLES _____

Applying to medical school requires the processing of all application material in a systematic manner. You must be conscious of deadlines and be aware that all required material must be submitted, or processing of your application will be delayed. Any prolonged delay can negatively impact on your chances for admission.

While medical schools have to handle hundreds of thousands of documents generated by more than 40,000 applicants, your contribution is to see that all material related to your own applications is submitted in a timely fashion. To facilitate that process, this appendix was developed and consists of a series of tracking tables that apply to the application process as a whole, MCAT registration, AMCAS and non-AMCAS school applications, and interviews. Using these tables will facilitate the orderly management of a challenging and critical part of your plan to secure a place in medical school. These tables will also serve to provide you with a record of what you have done and indicate the tasks ahead. It is also important to make copies of all important documents you send out.

The Appendix consists of:

Tracking Table 1: Application Process Sequence

Tracking Table 2: Medical College Admission Test (MCAT) Record

Tracking Table 3: Preliminary List of Medical Schools

Tracking Table 4: Final List of Medical Schools

Tracking Table 5: Application Schedule—AMCAS Schools

Tracking Table 6: Interview Record Form for AMCAS Schools

Tracking Table 7: Application Schedule—Non-AMCAS Schools

Tracking Table 1: *Application Process Sequence*
(*Check when complete*)

FRESHMAN YEAR

_____ Joined your school's premedical society and attended its meetings.
_____ Became personally acquainted with your premedical adviser.
_____ Discussed your career plans with your family physician.

SOPHOMORE YEAR

_____ Became familiar with the admission process.
_____ Got some hospital and/or research experience.

JUNIOR YEAR

_____ November–January: Preliminary MCAT Preparation
_____ February. Registered to take the MCAT.
_____ February–April. Intensive MCAT Preparation
_____ April. Took the MCAT.
_____ Solicited faculty recommendation from your advisory committee.
_____ May. Secured AMCAS and non-AMCAS Applications.
_____ Prepared first and revised drafts of your application essay.
_____ June. Completed AMCAS and non-AMCAS applications, including essays.
_____ Completed preliminary MCAT preparation for August examination.
_____ Advised premedical committee where to send recommendations.
_____ July–August. Completed intensive preparation if taking the fall MCAT.

SENIOR YEAR

_____ September. Checked with premedical advisory office to see if all supporting material is complete.
_____ Took or (retook) fall MCAT.
_____ October. Contacted medical schools to confirm that they received applications.
_____ Completed and submitted supplementary applications.
_____ November. Prepared for interviews.
_____ December–January. Attended interviews.
_____ February. Sent lower senior year transcript (if it helps you).
_____ March. Advised waiting-list schools of interest.
_____ Contacted schools you haven't heard from (by phone and/or letter) expressing interest.
_____ Asked advisor to contact schools on your behalf.
_____ April–August. You can still get an affirmative reply.
_____ Made sure that medical schools know your summer address.
_____ August. If you have still not been accepted, consider the options discussed earlier in the chapter for rejected applicants (see page 75). Don't give up hope; it may be worth trying again.

Tracking Table 2: *Medical College Admission Test (MCAT) Record*
(*Check when complete*)

1. _____ Secured MCAT Registration Packet (This can be obtained from your Premedical Advisory Office or MCAT Program, PO Box 4056, Iowa City, IA 52243. (319) 337–1357.

2. _____ Mailed MCAT Registration Form on ___/___/___/.

3. _____ Received MCAT Registration Permit on ___/___/___.

4. _____ Score reporting (if applicable). AMCAS, when forwarding a copy of your record (transmittal notification) to the medical schools you designate, includes your MCAT exam scores. Thus, you need only designate the non-AMCAS schools to which you want your scores sent. (The first six reports are included in the enrollment fee for the exam.) Sent to:

   _____   _____   _____

   _____   _____   _____

5. Sample test scores (see end of Chapter 4).
   Verbal reasoning _____
   Physical sciences _____
   Biological sciences _____
   Writing sample _____

6. MCAT Exam taken ___/___/___ (spring/fall).
   MCAT Scores
   Verbal reasoning _____
   Physical sciences _____
   Biological sciences _____
   Writing sample _____

7. Discussed MCAT scores with advisor ___/___/___.
   Recommendation: Don't retake _____ Retake _____
   Comments: _____

8. Repeat MCAT scores (spring/fall exam), Date taken ___/___/___
   Verbal reasoning _____
   Physical sciences _____
   Biological sciences _____
   Writing sample _____

9. Comparison of MCAT scores (if taken a second time).
   Verbal reasoning + _____ or – _____
   Physical sciences + _____ or – _____
   Biological sciences + _____ or – _____
   Writing sample + _____ or – _____

10. Comparison of performance: Achieved versus desirable scores for the medical schools to which I am applying (see Table 5.1)

SCHOOL	DESIRABLE SCORES VERBAL / PHYSICAL / BIOLOGICAL	MY SCORES VERBAL / PHYSICAL / BIOLOGICAL
_____	____ / ____ / ____	____ / ____ / ____
_____	____ / ____ / ____	____ / ____ / ____
_____	____ / ____ / ____	____ / ____ / ____
_____	____ / ____ / ____	____ / ____ / ____
_____	____ / ____ / ____	____ / ____ / ____
_____	____ / ____ / ____	____ / ____ / ____
_____	____ / ____ / ____	____ / ____ / ____
_____	____ / ____ / ____	____ / ____ / ____
_____	____ / ____ / ____	____ / ____ / ____
_____	____ / ____ / ____	____ / ____ / ____
_____	____ / ____ / ____	____ / ____ / ____
_____	____ / ____ / ____	____ / ____ / ____
_____	____ / ____ / ____	____ / ____ / ____
_____	____ / ____ / ____	____ / ____ / ____
_____	____ / ____ / ____	____ / ____ / ____
_____	____ / ____ / ____	____ / ____ / ____
_____	____ / ____ / ____	____ / ____ / ____
_____	____ / ____ / ____	____ / ____ / ____
_____	____ / ____ / ____	____ / ____ / ____
_____	____ / ____ / ____	____ / ____ / ____

Tracking Table 3: *Preliminary List of Medical Schools*

Based on your state of residency, school location, and tuition, as well as your academic credentials and MCAT scores, formulate a preliminary list of where you would conceivably apply. Use data taken from Table 5.1 (Chapter 5) and the profiles (Chapter 6) as well as Table 7.1, which gives the percentage of women (from which the percentage of men can be extrapolated) to see if your choices are realistic.

SCHOOL	AMCAS YES—NO	TUITION	PERCENTAGE MEN—WOMEN		CATALOG DATE REQD.—RECVD.	
1.						
2.						
3.						
4.						
5.						
6.						
7.						
8.						
9.						
10.						
11.						
12.						
13.						
14.						
15.						
16.						
17.						
18.						
19.						
20.						

Tracking Table 4: *Final List of Medical Schools*

After receiving your MCAT scores, you are in a more favorable position to prepare the definitive list of medical schools to which to apply. Doing so can be viewed as a four-step process.

1. Formulate, with the aid of Table 3.1, the approximate number of schools you think you should apply to in order to secure a place in the incoming freshman medical school class.

2. Determine if this number exceeds the number of schools recommended in Table 3.1. If it does, then using the criteria of affordability of tuition and the percentages of women and minorities accepted (if the last two are relevant), eliminate some schools from list. If further reduction is needed, note your academic credentials and the *mean* data for accepted students for schools you are considering (from Table 5.1), on the table below. You can eliminate schools where there is a wide divergence between the two sets of data.

   Another criterion that can be used for lowering the number of schools, aside from tuition, is the cost associated with an interview. This should be estimated and noted below. If your budget cannot tolerate such an expense and if there are no other mitigating circumstances in favor of the school (see below), it can be dropped from list.

3. If you have some uncertainty about eliminating a specific school, find out how many students from your school have been admitted to it over the last few years. If significant and you can afford it, keep the school on your list. (This information is also useful if you want or need to add schools to your list.)

4. Now check your list with your premedical adviser before acting on it, and make any needed adjustments.

Tracking Table 4: *Final List of Medical Schools*

SCHOOL	GPA	SCIENCE CUM	MCAT SCORES V	P	B	TOTAL TRAVEL COSTS	APPLYING YES	NO	DATE APPLIED
1.									
2.									
3.									
4.									
5.									
6.									
7.									
8.									
9.									
10.									
11.									
12.									
13.									
14.									
15.									
16.									
17.									
18.									
19.									
20.									

Tracking Table 5: *Application Schedule—AMCAS Schools*
(*check when complete*)

1. _____ Secured AMCAS Registration Packet. (This can be secured from your Premedical Advisory Office or from AMCAS, Association of American Medical Colleges, Section for Student Services, 2450 N Street NW, Suite 201, Washington, DC 20037, (202) 828-0600. Allow two weeks for delivery.)

2. _____ Received AMCAS Packet ___/___/___.

3. _____ Requested student copies of my college and/or university records (to accurately prepare application) from:
   Name _____   Date requested ___/___/___
   Name _____   Date requested ___/___/___
   Name _____   Date requested ___/___/___

4. _____ Completed and mailed application (certified, return receipt request recommended) on ___/___/___. (Made a copy for files before sending.)
   Note: earliest date for mailing is June 1.

5. _____ Arranged that my official transcripts be sent by the following colleges and/or universities:
   Name _____ Date requested ___/___/___ Rec'd by AMCAS ____
   Name _____ Date requested ___/___/___ Rec'd by AMCAS ____
   Name _____ Date requested ___/___/___ Rec'd by AMCAS ____

6. ___ Received Transmittal Notification on ___/___/___ Cycle form # _____

7. Phone log:
   Name _____ Phone # _____ Date _____
   Subject _____
   Name _____ Phone # _____ Date _____
   Subject _____
   Name _____ Phone # _____ Date _____
   Subject _____
   Name _____ Phone # _____ Date _____
   Subject _____
   Name _____ Phone # _____ Date _____
   Subject _____
   Name _____ Phone # _____ Date _____
   Subject _____
   Name _____ Phone # _____ Date _____
   Subject _____
   Name _____ Phone # _____ Date _____
   Subject _____
   Name _____ Phone # _____ Date _____
   Subject _____
   Name _____ Phone # _____ Date _____
   Subject _____

Tracking Table 6: *Interview Record Form for AMCAS Schools*
(*Duplicate for each school.*)

Medical School _____

Address _____
        (Street)   (City)   (State)   (Zip)

Phone # _____ FAX # _____

(*Check when completed*)

1. _____ Received interview invitation ___/___/___
2. _____ Interview accepted and scheduled for ___/___/___ at _____ AM _____ PM
3. _____ Travel instructions _____
   _____

4. _____ Information sources on school:
       Catalogue _____ available _____ requested ___/___/___
   Classmates (if already interviewed)
   Name _____ Phone _____
   Name _____ Phone _____
   Name _____ Phone _____
   Alumnus _____ Phone _____
   Alumnus _____ Phone _____

5. _____ Interviewers
   Name _____ Department _____
   Name _____ Department _____
   Name _____ Department _____

6. _____ Thank you note(s) sent ___/___/___
   Phone log:
   Name _____ Phone # _____ Date ___/___/___
   Subject _____
   Name _____ Phone # _____ Date ___/___/___
   Subject _____
   Name _____ Phone # _____ Date ___/___/___
   Subject _____
   Name _____ Phone # _____ Date ___/___/___
   Subject _____
   Name _____ Phone # _____ Date ___/___/___
   Subject _____

7. Comments _____
   _____
   _____
   _____
   _____
   _____
   _____
   _____
   _____
   _____
   _____
   _____
   _____

Tracking Table 7: *Application Schedule—Non-AMCAS Schools*

Medical School _____

Address _____

          (Street)   (City)   (State)   (Zip)

Phone # _____   FAX # _____

(*Check when completed*)

1. _____ Application and catalogue: Date requested ___/___/___
         Date received ___/___/___

2. _____ Application deadline ___/___/___

3. _____ MCAT score Request sending: ___/___/___, (*see also* Tracking Table 2)

4. _____ Completed (and duplicated) application ___/___/___

5. _____ Mailed application (certified, return receipt requested recommended),
         ___/___/___

6. Requested (for fee) the official college or university transcripts be sent from:
    Name _____ Date _____
    Name _____ Date _____
    Name _____ Date _____

7. _____ Requested letters of recommendation
    Premedical Committee   Date ___/___/___ Date sent ___/___/___
    Dr. _____ Date ___/___/___ Date sent ___/___/___
    Dr. _____ Date ___/___/___ Date sent ___/___/___
    Dr. _____ Date ___/___/___ Date sent ___/___/___

8. _____ Received secondary application

9. _____ Returned secondary application ___/___/___

10. _____ Received confirmation that application is complete ___/___/___

11. _____ Interview Offered _____   Not Offered _____
    If yes, interview scheduled _____ at _____ (AM/PM)

12. _____ Interviewers:
    Name _____ Department _____
    Name _____ Department _____
    Name _____ Department _____

13. _____ Sent thank you note(s) to interviewers ___/___/___

14. _____ Comments concerning interview: _____
_____
_____
_____
_____
_____
_____
_____
_____
_____
_____
_____
_____
_____

15. _____   Final action taken
        Accepted   _____   __/__/__
        Rejected   _____   __/__/__
        Waiting list   _____   __/__/__

16. _____   Ultimate decision on application (if wait-listed)
        Acceptance   _____
        Rejection   _____

17. _____   Phone log:

Name _____ Phone # _____ Date _____
Subject _____

Name _____ Phone # _____ Date _____
Subject _____

Name _____ Phone # _____ Date _____
Subject _____

Name _____ Phone # _____ Date _____
Subject _____

Name _____ Phone # _____ Date _____
Subject _____

Name _____ Phone # _____ Date _____
Subject _____

Name _____ Phone # _____ Date _____
Subject _____

Name _____ Phone # _____ Date _____
Subject _____

Name _____ Phone # _____ Date _____
Subject _____

Name _____ Phone # _____ Date _____
Subject _____

Name _____ Phone # _____ Date _____
Subject _____

Name _____ Phone # _____ Date _____
Subject _____

Name _____ Phone # _____ Date _____
Subject _____

Name _____ Phone # _____ Date _____
Subject _____

Name _____ Phone # _____ Date _____
Subject _____

Name _____ Phone # _____ Date _____
Subject _____

Name _____ Phone # _____ Date _____
Subject _____

APPENDIX G

REGIONAL MAPS

boldface type	=	both medical and dental school
regular type	=	medical school only
italic type	=	dental school only

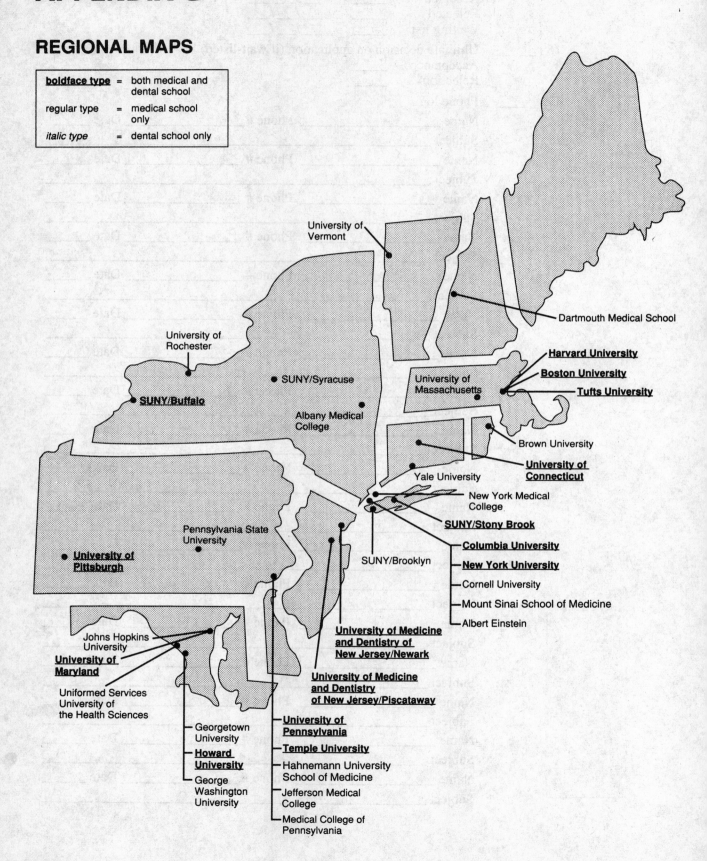

University of Vermont

Dartmouth Medical School

Harvard University

Boston University

Tufts University

Brown University

University of Rochester

University of Massachusetts

● SUNY/Syracuse

SUNY/Buffalo

Albany Medical College

University of Connecticut

Yale University

New York Medical College

SUNY/Stony Brook

Columbia University

New York University

Cornell University

Mount Sinai School of Medicine

Albert Einstein

Pennsylvania State University

University of Pittsburgh

SUNY/Brooklyn

University of Medicine and Dentistry of New Jersey/Newark

University of Medicine and Dentistry of New Jersey/Piscataway

Johns Hopkins University

University of Maryland

Uniformed Services University of the Health Sciences

Georgetown University

Howard University

George Washington University

University of Pennsylvania

Temple University

Hahnemann University School of Medicine

Jefferson Medical College

Medical College of Pennsylvania

Medical College
of Virginia

Eastern Virginia
Medical School

Duke University

**University of
North Carolina/
Chapel Hill**

East Carolina
University School
of Medicine

University of
South Carolina

**Medical University
of South Carolina**

Medical College of Georgia

Emory University

Morehouse School of Medicine

Mercer University

**University of
Florida**

**University of
Miami**

**West Virginia
University**

University of
Virginia

Bowman Gray
School of Medicine

Marshall University

University of
South Florida

**University of
Kentucky**

East Tennessee
State University

**University of
Tennessee**

**University
of Alabama**

University of
South Alabama

**Louisiana State
University/New Orleans**

Tulane University

**University of
Louisville**

**Meharry Medical
College**

Vanderbilt University

**University of
Mississippi**

University of
Arkansas

Louisiana
State
University/
Shreveport

University of
Texas/Galveston

**University of
Texas/Houston**

Baylor College
of Medicine

**University of
Oklahoma**

*Baylor College of
Dentistry*

University of
Texas/Dallas

Texas A & M
University

**University of
Texas/San Antonio**

Texas Tech
University

boldface type = both medical and
                    dental school

regular type = medical school
               only

italic type = dental school only

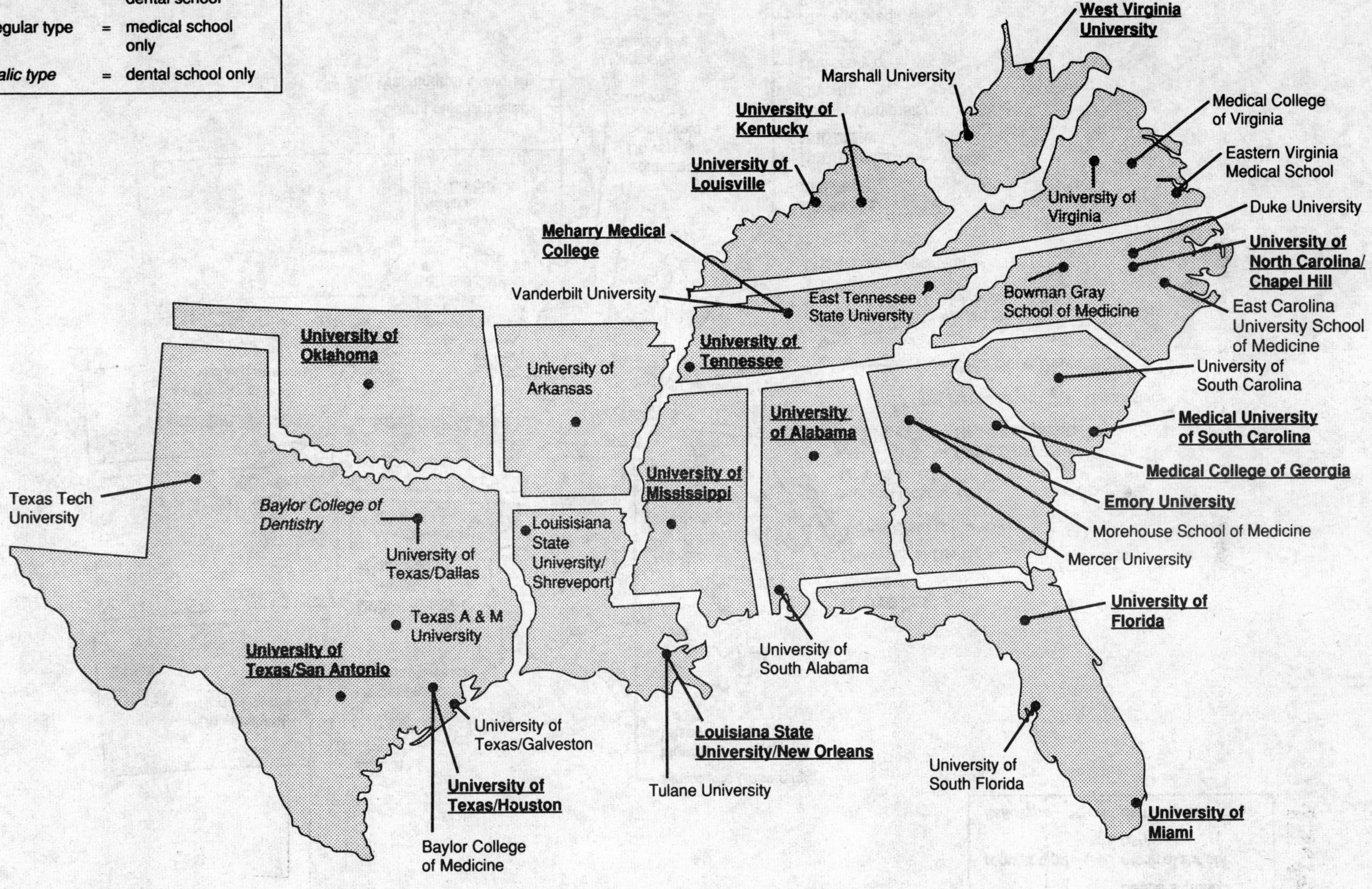

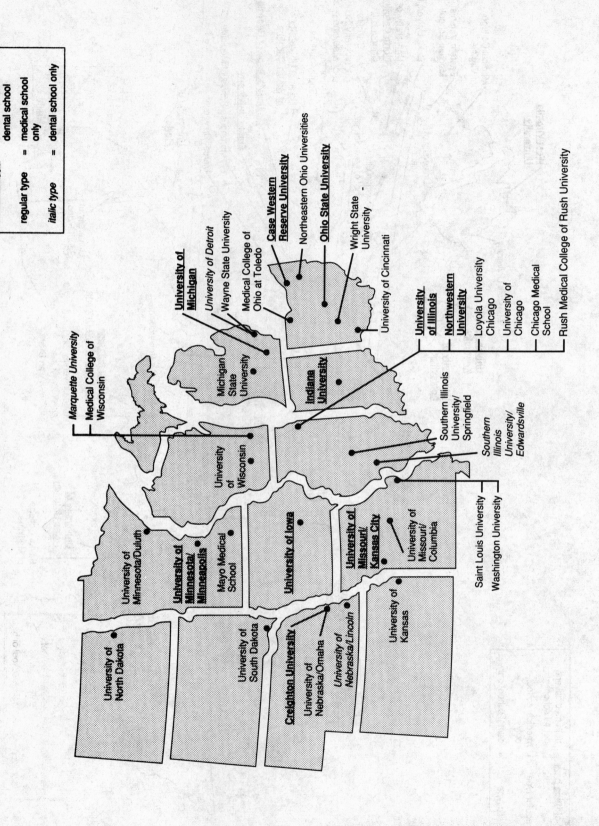

boldface type = both medical and dental school

regular type = medical school only

italic type = dental school only

Marquette University
Medical College of Wisconsin

University of Michigan

University of Detroit

Wayne State University

Medical College of Ohio at Toledo

Case Western Reserve University

Northeastern Ohio Universities

Ohio State University

Wright State University

University of Cincinnati

University of Illinois

Northwestern University

Loyola University Chicago

University of Chicago

Chicago Medical School

Rush Medical College of Rush University

Michigan State University

Indiana University

University of Wisconsin

Southern Illinois University/Springfield

Southern Illinois University/Edwardsville

University of Minnesota/Duluth

University of Minnesota/Minneapolis

Mayo Medical School

University of Iowa

University of Missouri/Kansas City

University of Missouri/Columbia

Saint Louis University

Washington University

University of North Dakota

University of South Dakota

Creighton University

University of Nebraska/Omaha

University of Nebraska/Lincoln

University of Kansas

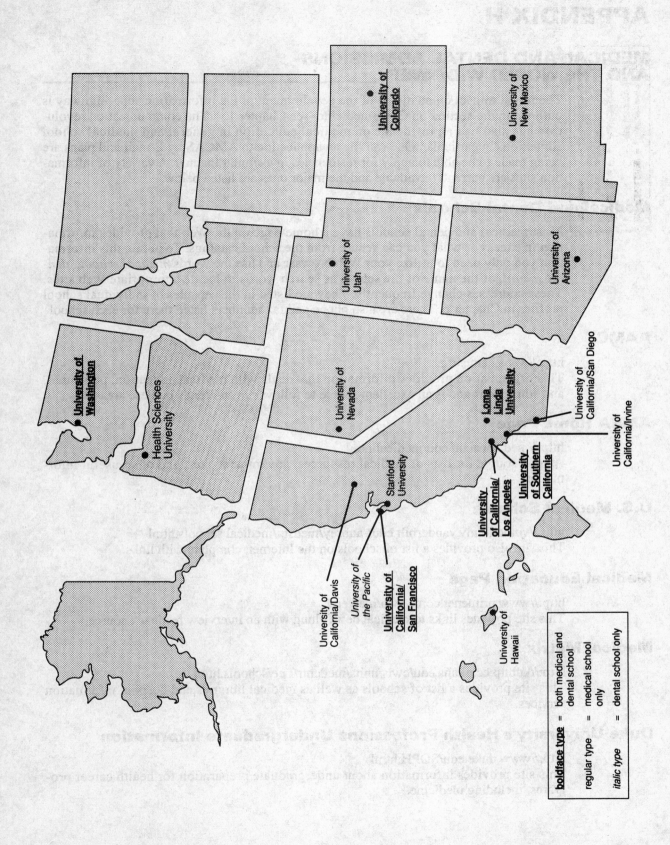

University of Colorado

University of New Mexico

University of Utah

University of Arizona

University of Washington

Health Sciences University

University of Nevada

Loma Linda University

University of California/San Diego

University of California/Irvine

Stanford University

University of California/Los Angeles

University of Southern California

University of California/Davis

University of the Pacific

University of California/San Francisco

University of Hawaii

boldface type = both medical and dental school

regular type = medical school only

italic type = dental school only

APPENDIX H

MEDICAL AND DENTAL ADMISSIONS AND THE WORLD WIDE WEB

The initial impact on medicine of the development of the information superhighway is outlined in the section on Cybermedicine (see Chapter 15). The communication revolution has also had an influence on medical education in general and medical school admissions in particular. One can file an application to AMCAS by E-mail and plans are being made to be able to apply for residencies in a similar manner. A variety of information sites are currently available and the major ones are listed below.

Medical and Dental Schools

Most medical and dental schools have a home page on the Web that provides information in excess of what you can secure from the school catalogs. To obtain this information you only need to utilize your Web browser and use the words *medical school*, *dental school*, or the name of the school as search words to locate appropriate Web sites. These addresses change frequently. They are listed in the capsules of individual school profiles in Chapter 6. There are also phone and fax numbers listed there for each school.

AAMC

http://www.aamc.org.
This organization provides information that deals with medical education, personnel, and admissions and is an excellent source to follow current trends in these areas.

AMSA Home Page

http://med.amsa.bu.edu/medical.html
A good source for lists of medical resources, government sites, and other useful information.

U.S. Medical Schools

http://vumclib.mv.vanderbilt.edu/-aubrey/medstu/medical schools.html
This site also provides a list of schools on the Internet, complete with links.

Medical Education Page

http://www.primenet.com/-gwa/med.ed./
This site provides links to medical news along with an interview feedback source.

Medical Matrix

http://kuhttp.cc.ukans.edu/cwis/units/medcntr/Lee/schools.html
This site provides a list of schools as well as medical libraries and hospital information services.

Duke University's Health Professions Undergraduate Information

http://www.duke.edu/SOPH.html
This site provides information about undergraduate preparation for health career programs, including medicine.

The Source

http://www.primenet.com/pulse/thesource.html
This site provides information concerning osteopathic medicine.

Achoo

http://www.achoo.com
This site is an information resource for the medical community.

BIBLIOGRAPHY

Abernethy, V. *Frontiers in Medical Ethics: Applications in a Medical Setting.* Cambridge, Massachusetts: Ballinger, 1982.

Belkin, L. *First Do No Harm.* New York: Simon and Schuster, 1993.

Bluestone, N. *So You Want to Be a Doctor?* New York: Lothrop, Lee and Shepard, 1981.

Bordley, J. and McGehee, H. *Two Centuries of American Medicine: 1776–1976.* Philadelphia: Saunders, 1976.

Brown, J. *Elizabeth Blackwell.* New York: Chelsea, 1989.

Brown, S. J., *Getting Into Medical School: The Complete Medical Student's Guidebook 7th ed.,* Hauppauge, N.Y.: Barron's Educational Series, Inc., 1989.

Callahan, D. *What Kind of Life: The Limit of Medical Progress.* New York: Simon and Schuster, 1990.

Coles, R. *The Call of Service.* New York: Houghton Mifflin, 1995.

Coombs, R. H. and St. John, J. *Making It in Medical School.* New York: SP Medical and Scientific Books, 1978.

Duffy, J. *The Healers: The Rise of the Medical Establishment.* New York: McGraw-Hill, 1976.

Eisenberg, H. *Night Calls.* New York: Arbor House, 1986.

Flexner, J. T. *Doctors on Horseback: Pioneers of American Medicine.* New York: Dover, 1979.

Hendrie, H. *Educating Competent and Human Physicians.* Indianapolis: Indiana University Press, 1990.

Heymann, J. *Equal Partners: A Physician's Call for a New Spirit of Medicine.* Boston: Little Brown, 1995.

Hilfiker, D. *Not all of Us Are Saints.* New York: Hill and Wang, 1995.

Hoffmeir, P. and Bonner, J. *From Residency to Reality.* New York: McGraw-Hill, 1990.

Hozed, J. L. *Pathways to a Career in Dentistry: A Source Book for Students Underrepresented in Dentistry.* Cambridge: Technical Education Research Center, 1976.

Jamieson, K. *Beyond the Double Bind: Women and Leadership.* New York: Oxford University Press, 1995.

Jonas, S. *Medical Mystery: The Training of Doctors in the United States.* New York: Norton, 1978.

Jeruchim, J. and Shapiro, P. *Women, Mentors, and Success.* New York: Baltantine Books, 1992.

Kaufman, M. *American Medical Education: The Formative Years, 1765–1910.* Westport, Conn.: Greenwood Press, 1976.

Kean, B. H. *One Doctor's Adventures among the Famous and Infamous from the Jungles of Panama to a Park Avenue Practice.* New York: Ballantine Books, 1990.

Klass, P. *A Not Entirely Benign Procedure.* New York: Putnam, 1987.

————— *Baby Docotor.* New York: Random House, 1992.

Klein, K. *Getting Better: A Medical Student's Story.* Boston: Little, Brown, and Co., 1980.

Klitzman, R. *A Year-long Night.* New York: Viking Penguin, 1989.

Knight, J. A. *Medical Student: Doctor in the Making.* New York: Appleton-Century-Crofts, 1973.

Knowles, J. H., ed. *Hospitals, Doctors, and the Public Interest.* Cambridge, Mass.: Harvard University Press, 1965.

Konner, M. *Becoming a Doctor.* New York: Viking, 1987.

Kronhaus, H. *Choosing a Practice.* New York: Springer, 1991.

Lander, L. *Defective Medicine: Risk, Anger, and the Malpractice Crisis.* New York: Farrar, Straus and Giroux, 1978.

Lasagna, L. *Life, Death and the Doctor.* New York: Knopf, 1968.

Lasser, M. H. *The Art of Learning Medicine.* New York: Appleton-Century-Crofts, 1974.

Laster, Leonard. *Choices after Medical School.* New York: Norton, 1995.

Lerner, M. R. *Medical School: The Interview and the Applicant.* Hauppauge, N.Y.: Barron's Educational Series, Inc., 1981.

Lippard, V. W. *A Half Century of American Medical Education, 1920–1970.* New York: Independent Publishers Group, 1974.

Loomis, F.A. *As Long as Life: The Memoirs of a Frontier Woman Doctor, Mary Canaga Rowland, 1873–1966.* Seattle, Wash.: Storm Peak Press, 1994.

Lygre, D. G. *Life Manipulation: From Test-Tube Babies to Aging.* New York: Walker, 1979.

Marion, Robert. *Learning to Play God.* New York: Fawcett, 1993.

_____ *The Intern Blues: The Private Ordeals of Three Young Doctors.* New York: Fawcett, 1990.

Mullen, F. *Vital Signs: A Young Doctor's Struggle with Cancer.* New York: Farrar, Straus, and Giroux, 1983.

Mumford, E. *Interns: From Students to Physicians.* Boston: Harvard University Press, 1970.

Noland, S. B. *Doctors: The Biography of Medicine.* New York: Knopf, 1988.

Nolen, W. A. *The Making of a Surgeon.* New York: Pocket Books, 1976.

_____ *A Surgeon's World.* New York: Fawcett, 1977.

Parati, C. *Breakthroughs: Astonishing Advances in Your Lifetime in Medicine, Science, and Technology.* Boston: Houghton Mifflin, 1980.

Pekkamen, J., M.D. *Doctors Talk about Themselves.* New York: Dell, 1988.

Raiber, J. K. *First Do No Harm.* New York: Villard, 1987.

Ramshell, M. (Ed.) *First Year as a Doctor: Real World Stories from America's M.D.s.* New York: Walker and Co., 1995.

Rabinowitz, P. M. *Talking Medicine: America's Doctors Tell Their Stories.* New York: Norton, 1981.

Reilly, P. *To Do No Harm: A Journey through Medical School.* New York: Auburn House, 1987.

Rogers, D. E. *American Medicine Challenges for the 1980s.* Cambridge, Mass.: Ballinger, 1978.

Rubin, T. I. *Emergency Room Diary.* New York: Grosset & Dunlap, 1972.

Seager, S. *Psych Ward.* New York: Putnam, 1991.

Seibel, H. R. and Guyer, K. E., *Barron's How to Prepare for the Medical College Admission Test, 7th edition.* Hauppauge, N.Y.: Barron's Educational Series, Inc., 1991.

Seltzer, R. *Down from Troy: A Doctor Comes of Age.* New York: Morrow, 1993.

Shapiro, E. C. and Lowenstein, L. M., eds. *Becoming a Physician: Development of Values and Attitudes in Medicine.* Cambridge, Mass.: Ballinger, 1979.

Silverstein, A. *Conquest of Death.* New York: Macmillan, 1979.

Starzl, T. *The Puzzle People: Memoirs, a Transplant Surgeon.* Pittsburgh, Pa.: University of Pittsburgh Press, 1993.

Stone, J. *The Country of Hearts: Journeys, in the Art of Medicine.* New York: Delacorte Press, 1991.

Swartz, Harold M. and Gottheil, Diane L., Eds. *The Education of Physical Scholars: Preparing for Leadership in the Health Care System.* Rockville, Maryland: Betz Pub. Co., Inc., 1993.

Verghese, A. *My Own Country.* New York: Simon and Schuster, 1995.

Virshup, B. *Coping in Medical School.* New York: Norton, 1985.

Waldenstein, J. G. *Reflections and Recollections From a Long Life with Medicine.* Rome: Ferrata Storti Foundation Publication, 1994.

Walters, B. et al. *Annotated Bibliography of Women in Medicine.* Toronto: Ontario Medical Association, 1993.

Warner, H. R. *Computer-Assisted Medical Decision Making.* New York: Academic Press, 1979.

Weatherall, D. *Science and the Quiet Art: The Role of Medical Research in Health Care.* New York: Norton, 1995.

Wischnitzer, S. *Futures in Health: A Guide to Podiatry, Optometry, Pharmacy and 56 Other Professions.* Hauppauge, N.Y.: Barron's Educational Series, Inc., 1985.

Zabarenko, R. *The Doctor Tree: Developmental Stages in the Growth of Physicians.* Pittsburgh: University of Pittsburgh Press, 1978.

Ziegler, E. *Emergency Doctor.* New York: Ballantine Books, 1987.

INDEXES

Index of Osteopathic School Profiles

Index of Dental School Profiles

SUBJECT INDEX